# EYE PATHOLOGY
## AN ATLAS AND BASIC TEXT

# EYE PATHOLOGY

## AN ATLAS AND BASIC TEXT

**RALPH C. EAGLE, JR., M.D.**

The Noel T. and Sara L. Simmonds Professor of Ophthalmic Pathology,
    Wills Eye Hospital
Professor of Ophthalmology and Pathology
Jefferson Medical College of Thomas Jefferson University
Director, Department of Pathology, Wills Eye Hospital
Coordinator, Section on Pathology, Lancaster Course in Ophthalmology
Director, Department of Continuing Medical Education, Wills Eye Hospital
Philadelphia, Pennsylvania

**W.B. SAUNDERS COMPANY**
*A Division of Harcourt Brace & Company*
Philadelphia • London • Toronto • Montreal • Sydney • Tokyo

**W.B. SAUNDERS COMPANY**

*A Division of Harcourt Brace & Company*

The Curtis Center
Independence Square West
Philadelphia, Pennsylvania 19106

**Library of Congress Cataloging-in-Publication Data**

Eagle, Ralph C.
    Eye pathology : an atlas and basic text / Ralph C. Eagle, Jr.
       p.    cm.
    ISBN 0–7216–7809–2
    1. Eye—Diseases.  2. Eye—Diseases Atlases.    I. Title.
    [DNLM: 1. Eye Diseases—pathology Atlases.    WW  17 E109a 1999]
  RE46.E316  1999
  617.7´1—dc21
  DNLM/DLC                    99–11310

EYE PATHOLOGY: AN ATLAS AND BASIC TEXT                    ISBN 0–7216–7809–2

Printed in the United States of America.

Last digit is the print number:    9   8   7   6   5   4   3   2   1

This book is dedicated . . .

to my teachers Myron Yanoff and Ramon L. Font . . .

to Ophthalmologist-In-Chief William S. Tasman for his

strong and unwavering support of Ophthalmic

Pathology at the Wills Eye Hospital . . .

and most of all . . .

to my dear wife Ewa for her strength, loyalty and love.

# PREFACE

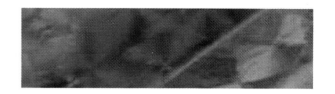

During the past two decades, the author has taught ophthalmic pathology to literally thousands of ophthalmologists-in-training at the Wills Eye Hospital Ophthalmology Review Course, the Harvard Intensive Review of Ophthalmology, and the Pathology Section of the Lancaster Course in Ophthalmology. Young physicians attending these review sessions repeatedly have voiced the need for a basic ophthalmic pathology review text that is fairly comprehensive, yet concise enough to be read and mastered in a relatively short time. High quality color illustrations are another request. This atlas and basic text is designed to fulfill this need. Although it is not encyclopedic, this textbook emphasizes eye diseases that comprise part of the traditional knowledge base of the well-trained ophthalmologist because they are important clinically or are frequently encountered by the practitioner.

This book is also designed to serve as an introductory text for medical students or residents who are beginning their ophthalmic studies. In addition, the text and atlas may benefit the surgical pathologist who wishes to learn more about eye pathology, and needs a short, well-illustrated reference by the grossing bench or microscope.

Why should one study ophthalmic pathology, anyway? Most would agree that an understanding of ocular disease and the pathogenic mechanisms that lead to blindness are prerequisites for quality ophthalmic practice. A physician cannot diagnose a disease that he has never heard of.

Nearly 14 years ago Dr. Frederick A. Jakobiec eloquently addressed this topic in his introduction to a special issue of the journal *Ophthalmology* dedicated to Basic Science and Ophthalmology. His words are equally true today . . .

"Unless one knows the natural course of a disease, it is not possible to decide whether an intervention has been efficacious or not. At a time when we are witnessing the progressive commercialization of ophthalmology and the slackening of traditional standards of professional behavior, one of the few remaining constraints that might prevent us from becoming high-tech mountebanks, peddling star wars' nostrums that are expensive and potentially meretricious, is our well-founded and ethically enhancing knowledge of ocular disease."

RALPH C. EAGLE, JR., M.D.

# ACKNOWLEDGMENTS

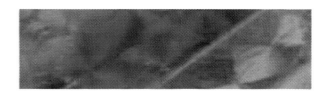

I would like to thank the following friends and colleagues who contribute specimens to the Ophthalmic Pathology Laboratory at the Wills Eye Hospital and have kindly shared clinical photographs that are included in this atlas. They include James J. Augsburger MD, Merrill Benson MD, Jurij Bilyk MD, Joseph Calhoun MD, Elizabeth Cohen MD, Edward Jaeger MD, Peter Laibson MD, Dr. med. Wolfgand Lieb, Irving Raber MD, Christopher Rapuano MD and Dario Savino-Zari MD. My special thanks go to my friends Jerry and Carol Shields who love ophthalmic pathology, and strongly support my laboratory with a wealth of exquisitely documented specimens.

I also thank the following physicians who permitted me to reprint figures from their papers: Jorge Alvarado MD, Edward Jaeger MD and Lorenz E. Zimmerman MD. Dr. Myron Yanoff allowed me to use several figures that originally were published in his textbooks. Dr. Ramon L. Font kindly provided a photomicrograph of retinal involvement in Whipple's disease. Specific citations are included in the figure legends.

The atlas contains some photomicrographs of microscopic sections that were distributed to the members of the Verhoeff-Zimmerman, Theobald and Eastern Ophthalmic Pathology Societies. I thank the following colleagues for sharing these rare and important cases and allowing me to photograph them: Harry Brown, MD, J. Douglas Cameron MD, Nongnart Chan MD, David G. Cogan MD, William C. Frayer MD, W. Richard Green MD, Frederick A. Jakobiec MD, Gordon K. Klintworth MD, PhD, Curtis Margo MD, Myron Yanoff MD, and Lorenz E. Zimmerman MD.

Excellent histological preparations are a requisite for high quality photomicrographs. I have always been fortunate to work with some of the best ocular histotechnologists in the United States. These histotechnical "artists" include Violetta Arbizo, Neena Panackal, Lili Grinshteyn and Faina Beloboradova at the Wills Eye Hospital, Dolores Ventura and the late Nestor Menocal at the Scheie Eye Institute, and Edna Prophet and Efrain Perez-Rosario at the Armed Forces Institute of Pathology.

I also must acknowledge the outstanding ophthalmic photographers who took most of the clinical photographs in this atlas. They include Bob Curtin, Jack Scully, Roger Barone, Jamie Nicholl and Terry Tomer at the Wills Eye Hospital and Bill Nyberg, Laurel Weeney and Tim Bennett at the Scheie Eye Institute.

Finally, I must thank the Women's Committee of the Wills Eye Hospital and the Noel T. and Sara L. Simmonds Endowment for their support of the Ophthalmic Pathology Laboratory at the Wills Eye Hospital.

# C O N T E N T S

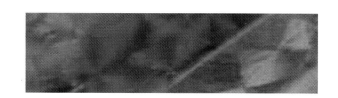

# ABOUT THE FIGURES

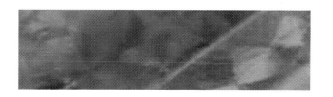

**A**ll of the photographs and photomicrographs that comprise the atlas were submitted to the publisher in the digital format as Adobe Photoshop™ 4.0 files. All but two of the photomicrographs were taken by the author. When possible, the transparencies were taken with Kodachrome™ 25 Professional film with a NCB10 daylight filter and a dydynium filter. The transparencies were scanned into Kodak PhotoCD™ format with a Kodak 2000 scanner at the Camera Shop, Inc.'s Visual Sound imaging facility in Lawrence Park, Pennsylvania. The digitized images were manipulated by the author using an Apple Macintosh Power PC™ 6100/60AV personal computer and the image editing program Adobe Photoshop™ 4.0 for the Macintosh. In most instances the 4.5 MB 1536 × 1024 pixel image on the PhotoCD was employed. The images were cropped to 11.5 × 7 cm at a resolution of 300 dpi and converted from the RBG to the CMYK color mode. The final figures averaged about 2.5 MB in size (range 1.1–4.3 MB). Images comprising a total 1.55 Gigabytes were submitted on 24 100 MB Iomega™ ZIP drives. In contrast, the text, references and figure legends comprised only 1.57 MB.

# CHAPTER 1

congenital anomalies are developmental disorders that are present at birth. Congenital malformations may be caused by mutant genes, chromosomal abnormalities, and major environmental factors such as infections, drugs and toxins, or radiation. In many instances the cause is unknown. Heritable disorders are genetically determined and may or may not affect the phenotype. Heritable traits may be manifest at birth, or they may become obvious later in life.

Etiologic factors that act early during embryogenesis (conception to 2 weeks) or the initial stages of ocular organogenesis (2 weeks to 3 months) tend to have profound effects on ocular development. The development of the eye commences about 24 days after fertilization when the optic pits form in the anterior part of the embryo's neuroectodermal plate. The pits subsequently evaginate to form the optic vesicles, which invaginate to form the optic cups 4 days later. The neuroectoderm comprising the inner layer of the optic cup is destined to form the neurosensory retina, the non-pigmented ciliary epithelium, and the posterior layer of iris epithelium. The outer layer of the optic cup gives rise to the retinal pigment epithelium, the pigmented ciliary epithelium, and the anterior layer of iris pigment epithelium, which includes the dilator muscle. The optic vesicles induce the formation of the lens placodes in the overlying surface ectoderm. The lens placodes invaginate to form the lens vesicles as the optic cups form. Transitory fissures in the outer wall of the optic cups form on day 29. These embryonic fissures give the hyaloid arteries access to the interior of the developing eye. The fissures subsequently are obliterated by fusion, which usually is complete by the sixth week of gestation. Abnormalities affecting each of these events may become manifest as severe developmental anomalies.

Primary anophthalmos is a rare anomaly caused by failure of optic vesicle evagination. Primary anophthalmos usually is bilateral and occurs sporadically in otherwise healthy individuals. Secondary anophthalmos is caused by suppression of the entire anterior part of the neural tube, which is lethal. The optic vesicle evaginates and then undergoes degeneration in consecutive anophthalmos. Histologic examination of the orbit usually discloses rudimentary neuroectodermal structures, which are absent in primary anophthalmos.

Synophthalmia/cyclopia is a striking anomaly caused by a failure of formation or induction of the anterior neural tube including the eye fields (Figs. 1–1, 1–2). Although it is often called a fusion anomaly, synophthalmia/cyclopia actually reflects a failure of complete bicentricity to emerge. The disorder is a continuum of anomalies that involves the brain, nose, orbits, and bones in addition to the eyes. Bicentricity fails to emerge at an early stage; cells that are induced as eye tissue complete all stages of development with a high degree of fidelity. The greatest degree of ocular differentiation occurs anteriorly and laterally; there is duplication of anterior ocular structures and fusion posteriorly with a single optic nerve. A rudimentary nose or nasal proboscis is present above the single midline orbit (Fig. 1–1). The proboscis is caused by faulty migration of the frontonasal processes. Failure of bicentricity also involves the forebrain, invariably producing a malformation called holoprosencephaly, which is marked by failure of the brain to divide into right and left hemispheres. Most patients with this clinical spectrum have synophthalmia; true cyclopia is rare. The lethal malformation usually is sporadic, but it may be a manifestation of trisomy 13. Autosomal dominant familial holoprosencephaly has been linked to mutations in the human sonic hedgehog gene on chromosome 7q36.

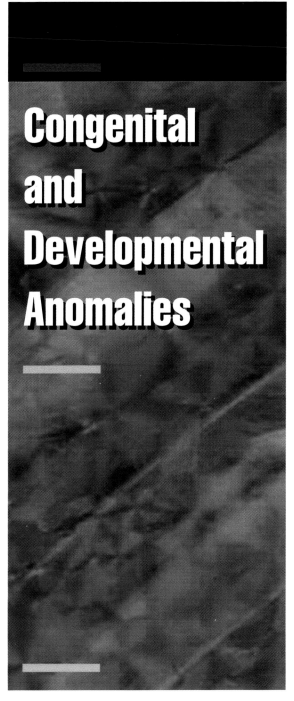

# Congenital and Developmental Anomalies

Congenital cystic eye is a rare anomaly caused by complete failure of optic vesicle invagination. Partial arrest of vesicle invagination probably causes extreme microphthalmos, which may simulate anophthalmos clinically. Congenital nonattachment of the retina is caused by faulty invagination and failure of the inner and outer layers of the optic cup to meet posteriorly.

Uveal colobomas are developmental anomalies caused by faulty closure of the embryonic fissure. Derived from the Greek word for "mutilation," coloboma is defined as "a condition where a portion of the structure of the eye is lacking." Colobomas typically are located inferonasally in the territory of the fissure. They can involve the iris, ciliary body, choroid, or any combination of the three and also may affect the optic nerve. Because the primary defect of a typical coloboma is in the neuroectoderm, absence of the mesectodermal uveal stroma is a secondary phenomenon. Occasionally the uveal tissue undergoes dysplasia or metaplasia, forming cartilage, muscle, or fat. An absolute scotoma is present in the region of the coloboma because the overlying retina is absent or dysplastic.

Although most colobomas are sporadic, they occasionally are inherited as isolated ocular defects, usually in an autosomal dominant fashion with incomplete penetrance. Colobomas are characteristic findings in several syndromes caused by the duplication or deletion of chromosomes or chromosomal fragments, such as trisomy 13. Colobomas in severely microphthalmic (less than 10 mm) eyes from infants with trisomy 13 often contain foci of hyaline cartilage and dysplastic retina (Figs. 1–3, 1–4).

Coloboma with cyst is a severe form of embryonic fissure anomaly characterized by a cystic outpouching of ectatic sclera that communicates with the interior of the eye through a posterior coloboma (Fig. 1–5). The intraocular contents protrude outward through the fissure, and the cyst is lined by a layer of atrophic or dysplastic neuroectodermal tissue. The cyst may become much larger than the eye (microphthalmos with cyst).

Atypical colobomas are not related to closure of the embryonic fissure and can occur anywhere. Macular colobomas probably result from intrauterine infections such as congenital toxoplasmosis.

Optic nerve aplasia usually is unilateral and occurs sporadically in individuals who have no systemic abnormalities. The optic nerve is absent, and the retina is avascular and lacks ganglion cells and axons.

Malformations that are localized to a single ocular structure usually are related to damage that occurs during the fetal period of ocular development (third to ninth months). Most are discussed in the chapters on individual ocular structures that follow.

## CHROMOSOMAL ANOMALIES

Ocular malformations occur in a number of chromosomal duplication or deletion syndromes. Down syndrome (trisomy 21) is the most common chromosomal syndrome and the most common cause of mental retardation. The "mongoloid" appearance of patients with Down syndrome is caused by upward and outward slanting of their palpebral fissures, which are almond shaped. Other ocular findings include epicanthal folds, significant refractive errors, especially high myopia, cataract, and strabismus, usually esotropia, which occurs in approximately 40%. Congenital ectropion, iris hypoplasia, keratoconus with acute hydrops, and an increased number of retinal vessels crossing the optic disk margin also occur.

Brushfield spots appear as a concentric ring of white or yellowish spots on the anterior surface of the iris in 85% of blue- or hazel-eyed patients with Down syndrome (Fig. 1–6). Brushfield spots are focal condensations of stromal collagen that are visible through the transparent anterior border layer of the blue iris and tend to be accentuated by concurrent iris atrophy. Discrete stromal condensations that resemble Brushfield spots, called Kruckmann-Wolfflin bodies, occur in some normal persons with blue or hazel eyes.

Severe ocular malformations, including anophthalmos, synophthalmia/cyclopia, microphthalmia, persistent hyperplastic primary vitreous (PHPV), retinal dysplasia, colobomas, and intraocular cartilage, occur in infants with trisomy 13 (Patau syndrome) (Figs. 1–3, 1–4). Affected infants have cleft lips and palates, cardiac and pulmonary defects, arrhinencephaly, and holoprosencephaly. Few survive the first year of life.

Epicanthal folds, ptosis, blepharophimosis, microphthalmos, corneal opacities, and congenital glaucoma are found in trisomy 18 (Edwards syndrome). It is the second most common autosomal trisomy.

Retinoblastoma occurs in the 13q- syndrome if the deletion includes the q1–4 band. The 22q+ syndrome includes microphthalmia, the posterior ulcer of von Hippel, and severe retinal dysplasia. Ocular abnormalities have been reported in the 18p-, 18q-, 18 ring chromosome, 5 p- (cri-du-chat), and 4 p- (Wolf-Hirschorn) syndromes.

## HERITABLE DISORDERS WITH OCULAR MANIFESTATIONS

A variety of heritable disorders caused by genetic mutations have ocular manifestations. Most cases of aniridia are caused by mutations in the *PAX6* gene on the short arm of chromosome 11. The term aniridia is a misnomer; most cases have severely hypoplastic irides that are hidden clinically by opaque limbal tissues (Figs. 1–7, 1–8). Aniridia is a spectrum of ocular disease that also includes foveal and optic nerve hypoplasia, cataract, secondary glaucoma, and corneal opacification. Eighty-five per cent of aniridic patients have autosomal dominant familial aniridia, which is an isolated ocular defect. The association of sporadic aniridia and Wilms' tumor or nephroblastoma, is called Miller syndrome and accounts for about 13% of cases. Miller syndrome is caused by deletions in the short arm of chromosome 11 that include both the *PAX6* gene and another closely linked tumor suppressor gene (*WT1*) involved in the pathogenesis of Wilms' tumor. The *PAX 6* gene plays a central role in ocular development throughout the animal kingdom. *PAX 6* mutations have been identified in patients with other anterior segment malformations, including Peters' anomaly and autosomal dominant keratitis.

A number of heritable ocular diseases are caused by mutant genes on the X chromosome and show X-linked recessive inheritance. They include color blindness (daltonism), juvenile X-linked retinoschisis, some cases of retinitis pigmentosa, the Nettleship-Falls type of ocular albinism, Fabry's disease, Hunter's disease, Norrie's disease, and Lowe syndrome. Incontinentia pigmenti (Bloch-Sulzberger) shows X-linked dominant inheritance. It occurs only in females and males with Klinefelter syndrome; it is lethal in normal males.

Other ocular disorders occur predominantly in males because they are caused by mutations in maternally transmitted mitochondrial DNA. They include Leber's hereditary optic neuropathy and the Kearns-Sayre, MERRF, and MELAS syndromes.

Autosomal recessively inherited disorders with prominent ocular manifestations include several types of albinism (foveal hypoplasia), systemic mucopolysaccharidoses including Hurler, Scheie, and Maroteaux-Lamy syndromes (corneal clouding), the lysosomal storage diseases Tay-Sachs disease and Niemann-Pick disease (macular cherry red spot), Wilson's disease (Kayser-Fleischer ring), the sickle hemoglobinopathies (neovascular sea fans), myotonic dystrophy (presenile cataract), alkaptonuria (sclera pigmentation), osteogenesis imperfecta (blue sclera), homocystinuria (ectopia lentis), and ocular-scoliotic Ehlers-Danlos syndrome (corneal and scleral rupture).

## PHAKOMATOSES

The term phakomatosis is applied to several heritable disorders that have important systemic and ocular findings. The primary phakomatoses include von Recklinghausen's neurofibromatosis, tuberous sclerosis, and von Hippel-Lindau disease, which are autosomal dominant disorders, and Sturge-Weber syndrome, which is sporadic. Advances in molecular genetics have made the basic concept of phakomatosis somewhat outdated. Mutations in recessive tumor suppressor genes have been identified in all three of the classic dominantly inherited phakomatoses.

Von Recklinghausen's neurofibromatosis (NF-1) is one of the most common hereditary diseases, because the NF-1 gene is quite large and is subject to mutation. The protein product of the NF-1 gene, which is located on chromosome 17, normally interacts with the protein product of the *ras* oncogene to dampen growth stimulatory signals. NF-1 is characterized by tumors composed of Schwann cells, which typically occur on the skin as multiple fibroma molluscum. Deforming elephantiasis neuromatosa is caused by diffuse neurofibromatous infiltration (Fig. 1–9). The presence of more than six cutaneous café au lait spots larger than 1.5 cm in diameter is a diagnostic criterion.

Ocular findings in NF-1 are numerous and include plexiform neurofibromas of the eyelid and orbit; an S-shaped lid fissure; congenital glaucoma, particularly if the upper lid is involved by neurofibromatous tissue; Lisch nodules on the iris; hamartomatous infiltration of the uvea with tactile corpuscle-like ovoid bodies (Figs. 1–10, 1–11); retinal and optic nerve gliomas; dysplasia of the sphenoid bone (Orphan Annie sign); pulsating exophthalmos; and a slightly increased risk for uveal melanoma. Lisch nodules (Figs. 1–12, 1–13) are the most common ocular manifestation of NF-1. These melanocytic hamartomas are a useful diagnostic criterion for NF-1 because they are found on the ante-

rior surface of the iris in nearly all affected adults and develop before cutaneous neurofibromas. Plexiform neurofibromas are composed of a plexus comprised of markedly enlarged nerves, which are swollen by a disorderly proliferation of Schwann cells and endoneural fibroblasts in a mucinous matrix (Fig. 1–14).

Neurofibromatosis type 2 (NF-2) is a totally separate disease caused by a gene located on chromosome 22. Bilateral schwannomas of the eighth cranial nerve are the disorder's classic manifestation. Ocular findings include presenile posterior subcapsular cataracts, epiretinal membranes, combined hamartoma of the retinal pigment epithelium (RPE) and retina, and optic nerve sheath meningiomas.

Tuberous sclerosis has been linked to two genes: one on chromosome 9 and one on chromosome 16. Tuberin, the protein product of the *TSC2* gene on chromosome 16, normally interacts with a *ras*-related protein called Rap1. The classic triad of tuberous sclerosis includes epilepsy, mental retardation, and facial lesions called adenoma sebaceum, which are angiofibromas. Astrocytic hamartomas and astrocytomas occur in the retina in about half of patients with tuberous sclerosis (Figs. 1–15, 1–16, 1–17). Astrocytomas overlying the optic disk have been called giant drusen of the optic nerve. Retinal astrocytomas may be confused clinically with retinoblastoma. More mature lesions typically contain calcospherites and have been called mulberry nodules. Large astrocytomas in the brain typically have a tuber-like appearance and may calcify, forming "brain stones." Subependymal giant cell astrocytomas are a characteristic finding. Visceral tumors include renal angiomyolipomas and cardiac rhabdomyomas. Pleural cysts predispose to spontaneous pneumothorax. Other skin lesions include subungual fibromas, shagreen patches, and ash leaf lesions.

Von Hippel-Lindau disease (angiomatosis retinae) is a hereditary cancer syndrome caused by germline mutations in the von Hippel-Lindau tumor suppressor gene located on chromosome 3p25. Cherry-like retinal angiomas with large feeding and draining vessels are the characteristic ocular manifestation of the syndrome (Fig. 1–18). These retinal lesions probably should be called retinal hemangioblastomas because they are identical histologically to the hemangioblastomas that may occur in the cerebellum in affected patients (Fig. 1–19). The retinal hemangioblastomas are bilateral in 50% of cases, can arise from the retina in an exophytic or endophytic fashion, may involve the optic disk or nerve, and often produce a Coats'-like exudative maculopathy. Patients are also at risk for pheochromocytoma and renal cell carcinoma.

Sturge-Weber syndrome (encephalotrigeminal angiomatosis) is a nonheritable congenital syndrome characterized by a facial port wine stain, or nevus flammeus, an ipsilateral hemangioma of the meninges and brain and "train track" intracranial calcification. Ocular findings include ipsilateral glaucoma and a diffuse cavernous hemangioma of the ipsilateral choroid (Fig. 1–20).

Other disorders that have been included with the phakomatoses are cavernous hemangioma of the retina, Wyburn Mason syndrome, organoid nevus (sebaceous nevus) syndrome, and ataxia telangiectasia. Large retinal arteriovenous malformations occur in the nonhereditary syndrome of Wyburn and Mason. About 20–30% of patients have associated midbrain arteriovenous malformations. The organoid nevus (sebaceous nevus) syndrome is characterized by cutaneous sebaceous nevi, seizures, epibulbar choristomas, and yellow fundus lesions that may represent intrascleral cartilage or bone. Ataxia-telangiectasia is a pleiotropic recessive disorder characterized by cerebellar ataxia, immunodeficiency, specific developmental defects, profound predisposition to cancer, and acute radiosensitivity. Ocular findings comprise telangiectatic conjunctival vessels and oculomotor disturbances. The *atm* gene normally is involved in DNA and cellular repair mechanisms.

Infections that occur during pregnancy and other harmful factors in the maternal environment, such as drugs, toxins, and radiation, may have devastating effects on the fetus. The most severe complications are associated with events that occur early in the first trimester. Maternal infections with ocular complications include rubella, toxoplasmosis, syphilis, cytomegalic inclusion disease, herpes simplex virus, and acquired immunodeficiency syndrome (AIDS). Drugs that cause congenital ocular anomalies include thalidomide, retinoic acid, lysergic acid diethylamide (LSD), cocaine, and ethanol (fetal alcohol syndrome).

# References

## General References

Duke-Elder S: The Iris. Congenital Deformities. Vol 3. Part 2. London: Henry Kimpton, 1964:565.
Mann I: The Development of the Human Eye. Orlando: Grune & Stratton, 1950.
Mann I: Developmental Abnormalities of the Eye. Philadelphia: Lippincott, 1957.
Pagon R: Ocular coloboma. Surv Ophthalmol 25:223, 1981.
Schubert HD: Schisis-like rhegmatogenous retinal detachment associated with choroidal colobomas. Graefes Arch Clin Exp Ophthalmol 233:74–79, 1995
Torczynski E, Jacobiec FA, Johnston MC, Font RL, Madewell JA: Synophthalmia and cyclopia: a histopathologic, radiographic, and organogenetic analysis. Doc Ophthalmol 44:311–378, 1977.
Waardenburg P, Franceschetti A, Klein D: Genetics and Ophthalmology. Springfield, IL: Charles C Thomas, 1961.

## Chromosomal Anomalies

Brushfield T: Mongolism. Br J Child Dis 21:241, 1924.
Donaldson D: The significance of spotting of the iris in mongols. Brushfield's spots. Arch Ophthalmol 65:26, 1961.
Hoepner J, Yanoff M: Ocular abnormalities in trisomy 13-15. Am J Ophthalmol 74:729, 1972.
Jaeger E: Ocular findings in Down's syndrome. Trans Am Ophthalmol Soc 78:808, 1980.
Wilcox LJ, Bercovitch L, Howard R: Ophthalmic features of chromosome deletion 4p- (Wolf-Hirschhorn syndrome). Am J Ophthalmol 86:834, 1978.

## Aniridia and Other Iris Anomalies

Davis A, Cowell JK: Mutations in the PAX6 gene in patients with hereditary aniridia. Hum Mol Genet 2:2093, 1993.
Duke-Elder S: Persistent pupillary membrane. In Congenital Deformities. Vol 3. Part 2. London: Henry Kimpton, 1964:775.
Eagle RJ: Iris pigmentation and pigmented lesions: an ultrastructural study. Trans Am Ophthalmol Soc 86:581, 1988.
Elsas F, Maumenee I, Kenyon K, et al: Familial aniridia with preserved ocular function. Am J Ophthalmol 83:718, 1977.
Gomes J, Eagle RJ, Gomes A, et al: Recurrent keratopathy after penetrating keratoplasty for aniridia. Cornea 15:457, 1996.
Graw J: Genetic aspects of embryonic eye development in vertebrates. Dev Genet 18:181, 1996.
Hanson IM, Fletcher JM, Jordan T, et al: Mutations at the PAX6 locus are found in heterogeneous anterior segment malformations including Peters' anomaly. Nat Genet 6:168, 1994.
Hittner H: Aniridia. In Ritch R, Shields M, Krupin T (eds) The Glaucomas. St. Louis: Mosby, 1989.
Mackman G, Brightbell F, Opitz J: Corneal changes in aniridia. Am J Ophthalmol 87:497, 1979.
Margo CE: Congenital aniridia: a histopathologic study of the anterior segment in children. J Pediatr Ophthalmol Strabismus 20:192, 1983.
Meisels H, Goldberg M: Vascular anastomoses between the iris and persistent primary vitreous. Am J Ophthalmol 88:179, 1979.
Miller R, Fraumeni JJ, Manning M: Association of Wilms' tumor with aniridia, hemihypertrophy, and other congenital malformations. N Engl J Med 270:922, 1964.
Mirzayans F, Pearce WG, MacDonald IM, et al: Mutation of the PAX6 gene in patients with autosomal dominant keratitis. Am J Hum Genet 57:539, 1995.
Nelson LB, Spaeth GL, Nowinski T, et al: Aniridia: a review. Surv Ophthalmol 28:621, 1984.

## Phakomatoses

Anonymous: Neurofibromatosis: conference statement, National Institutes of Health Consensus Development Conference. Arch Neurol 45:575, 1988.
Brownstein S: Neurofibromatosis. In Gold D, Weingeist T (eds) The Eye in Systemic Disease. Philadelphia, Lippincott, 1990:447.

Goldberg RE, Pheasant TR, Shields JA: Cavernous hemangioma of the retina: a four-generation pedigree with neurocutaneous manifestations and an example of bilateral retinal involvement. Arch Ophthalmol 97:2321–2324, 1979.

Grossniklaus HE, Thomas JW, Vigneswaran N, et al: Retinal hemangioblastoma: a histologic, immunohistochemical, and ultrastructural evaluation. Ophthalmology 99: 140–145, 1992.

Huson SM, Compston DA, Harper PS: A genetic study of von Recklinghausen neurofibromatosis in south east Wales. II. Guidelines for genetic counselling. J Med Genet 26:712, 1989.

Jakobiec FA, Font RL, Johnson FB: Angiomatosis retinae: an ultrastructural study and lipid analysis. Cancer 38: 2042–2056, 1976.

Lewis RA, Riccardi VM: Von Recklinghausen neurofibromatosis: incidence of iris hamartomata. Ophthalmology 88:348, 1981.

Lisch K: Ueber Beteiligung der Augen, insbesondere das Vorkommen von Irisknotchen bei der Neurofibromatose (Recklinghausen). Augenheilkunde 93:137, 1937.

Mindel JS, Rubenstein AE, Wallace S, et al: Congenital Horner's syndrome does not alter Lisch nodule formation. Ann Neurol 35:123, 1994.

Perry H, Font R: Iris nodules in von Recklinghausen neurofibromatosis: electron microscopic confirmation of their melanocytic origin. Arch Ophthalmol 100:1635, 1982.

Ragge NK, Falk RE, Cohen WE, Murphree AL: Images of Lisch nodules across the spectrum. Eye 7:95, 1993.

Robertson DM: Ophthalmic manifestations of tuberous sclerosis. Ann NY Acad Sci 615:17–25, 1991.

Sakurai T: Multiple neurofibroma patient showing multiple flecks on the anterior surface of the iris. Acta Soc Ophthalmol Jpn 39:87, 1935.

Ulbright TM, Fulling KH, Helveston EM: Astrocytic tumors of the retina: differentiation of sporadic tumors from phakomatosis-associated tumors. Arch Pathol Lab Med 108:160–163, 1984.

Williamson TH, Garner A, Moore AT: Structure of Lisch nodules in neurofibromatosis type 1. Ophthalmic Paediatr Genet 12:11, 1991.

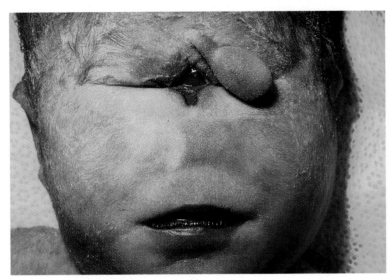

FIGURE 1–1 • **Synophthalmia, trisomy 13.** A pedunculated nasal proboscis is located above the single midline orbit.

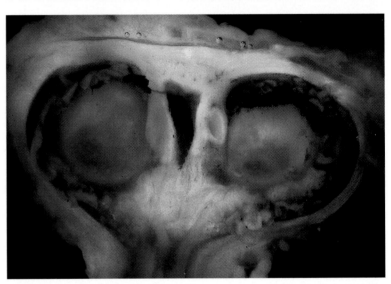

FIGURE 1–2 • **Synophthalmia, trisomy 13.** Small, synophthalmic eye from the infant shown in Figure 1–1 has two lenses and a single optic nerve. Septum between lenses contains two foci of hyaline cartilage. Mass of dysplastic retina fills vitreous cavity.

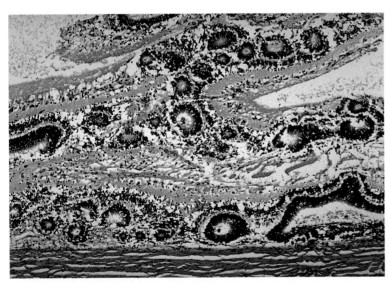

FIGURE 1–3 • **Coloboma and retinal dysplasia, trisomy 13.** Mass of disorderly dysplastic retina containing large multilayered rosettes adheres directly to the sclera within the coloboma. The choroid is absent. Hematoxylin-eosin, ×25.

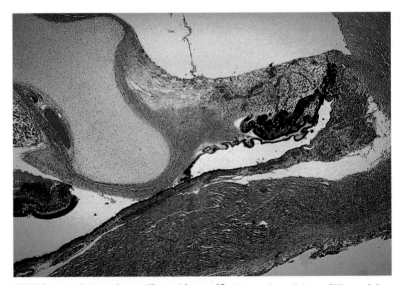

FIGURE 1–4 • **Intraocular cartilage, trisomy 13.** Mesenchymal tissue filling coloboma surrounds a focus of hyaline cartilage (at left) in a severely microphthalmic eye. Hematoxylin-eosin, ×10.

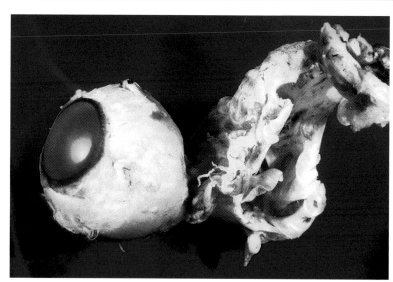

FIGURE 1–5 • **Microphthalmos with cyst.** Cystic outpouching of ectatic sclera is larger than microphthalmic eye. The lumen of the cyst was lined by atrophic neuroectodermal tissue, and it communicated with the interior of the eye through an optic nerve coloboma. The cyst ruptured intraoperatively.

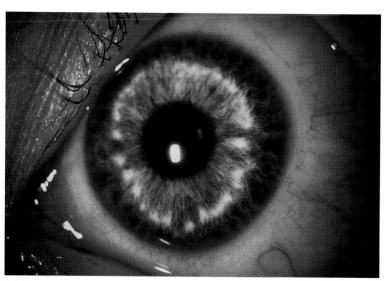

FIGURE 1–6 • **Brushfield spots, trisomy 21.** Focal stromal condensations form a ring of white spots in the middle third of the iris in a blue-eyed patient with Down syndrome. (Courtesy of Dr. Edward A. Jaeger. From Eagle RC Jr: Congenital, developmental and degenerative disorders of the iris and ciliary body . In: Albert DM, Jakobiec FA, eds. *Principles and Practice of Ophthalmology. Clinical Practice.* Vol 1. Philadelphia: Saunders, 1993:367–389)

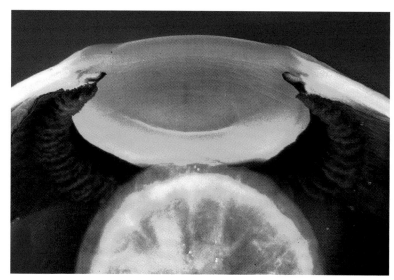

FIGURE 1–7 • **Aniridia.** Overhang of opaque limbal tissue hides skirt of hypoplastic iris in the peripheral anterior chamber. The lens dislocated during sectioning of eye obtained postmortem from an adult with familial aniridia.

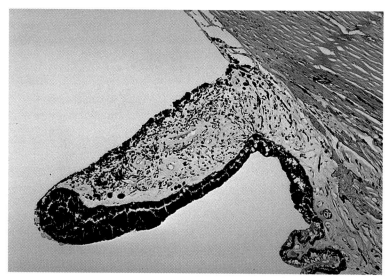

FIGURE 1–8 • **Aniridia.** Stubby hypoplastic iris leaflet from eye seen grossly in Figure 1–7 has thickened pigment epithelium and lacks sphincter and dilator muscles. Hematoxylin-eosin, ×25.

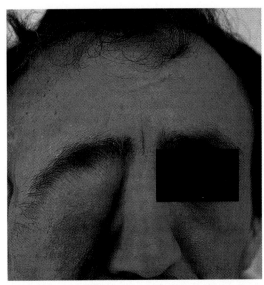

FIGURE 1–9 • **Elephantiasis neuromatosa, Von Recklinghausen's neurofibromatosis (NF-1).** Pendulous mass of hamartomatous tissue involves right upper lid and forehead. (Courtesy of Dr. Dario Savino-Zari, Caracas, Venezuela)

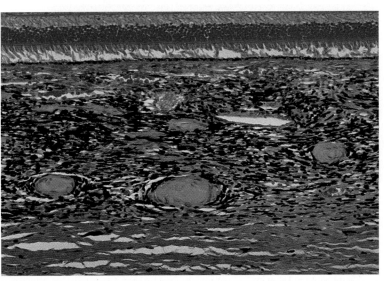

FIGURE 1–10 • **Choroidal infiltrate, NF-1.** The choroid is massively thickened by a hamartomatous infiltrate that contains an increased number of melanocytes and nonpigmented ovoid bodies that resemble tactile corpuscles. Hematoxylin-eosin, ×50.

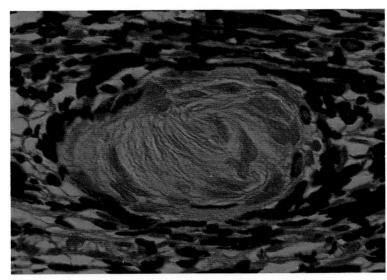

FIGURE 1–11 • **Ovoid body in choroidal infiltrate, NF-1.** Delicately laminated appearance of ovoid body reflects the presence of concentric Schwann cell processes. Hematoxylin-eosin, ×250.

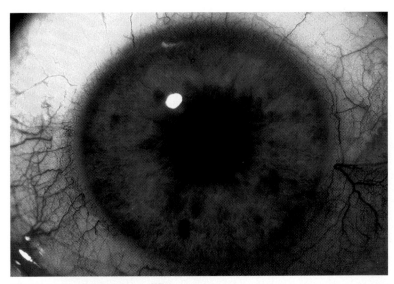

FIGURE 1–12 • **Lisch nodules, NF-1.** Multiple tan or pale brown dome-shaped nodules on the surface of the iris in a patient with NF-1. Lisch nodules occur in nearly all affected adults with NF-1 and are a useful diagnostic criterion.

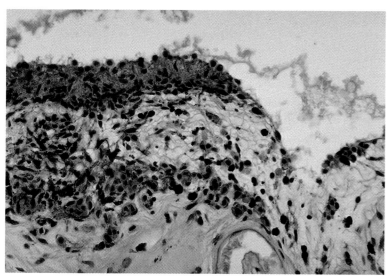

FIGURE 1–13 • **Lisch nodule, NF-1.** Focus of partially pigmented cells is seen on the anterior iridic surface and underlying stroma. Lisch nodules are melanocytic hamartomas. Hematoxylin-eosin, ×100.

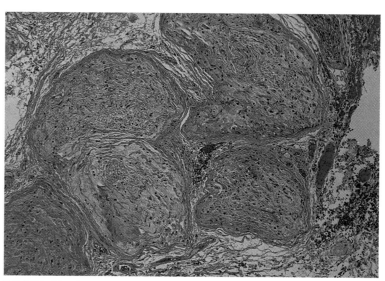

FIGURE 1–14 • **Plexiform neurofibroma, NF-1.** Markedly enlarged nerves forming a plexiform neurofibroma are swollen by a disorderly proliferation of Schwann cells and endoneural fibroblasts in a mucinous matrix. Hematoxylin-eosin, ×25.

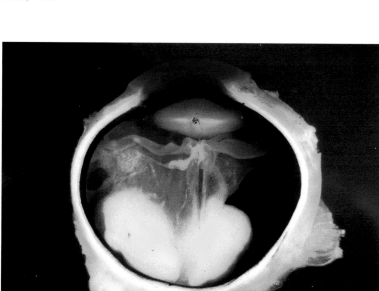

FIGURE 1–15 • **Retinal astrocytoma, tuberous sclerosis.** Large bilobed astrocytoma caused retinal detachment in a young girl with well documented tuberous sclerosis. The macroscopic appearance of the tumor resembles retinoblastoma.

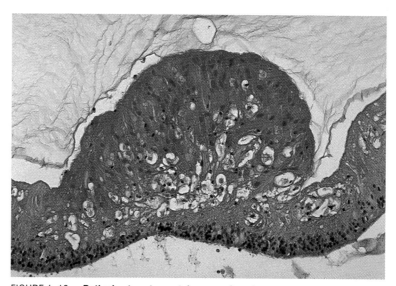

FIGURE 1–16 • **Retinal astrocytoma, tuberous sclerosis.** Small nodular astrocytoma arises from nerve fiber layer of the peripheral retina. The astrocytoma is comprised of large astrocytic cells with copious eosinophilic cytoplasm. Hematoxylin-eosin, ×100.

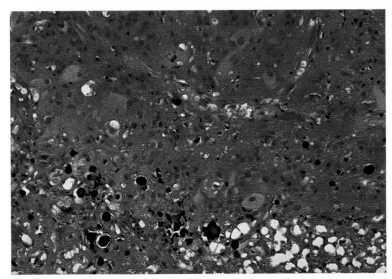

FIGURE 1–17 • **Giant cell retinal astrocytoma with calcospherites, tuberous sclerosis.** Photomicrograph of the tumor in Figure 1–15 shows large astrocytes with copious amounts of eosinophilic cytoplasm. A few basophilic spherules of calcium (calcospherites) are seen below. Other parts of the tumor were extensively necrotic. Hematoxylin-eosin, ×50.

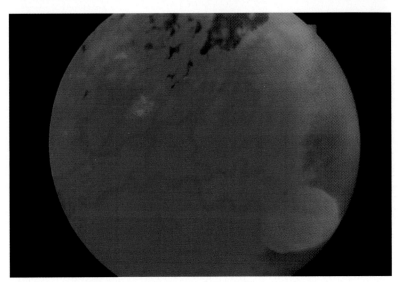

FIGURE 1–18 • **Retinal hemangioblastoma, von Hippel-Lindau disease.** A classic endophytic retinal angioma has large feeding and draining vessels.

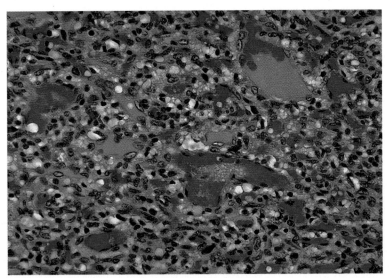

FIGURE 1–19 • **Retinal hemangioblastoma, von Hippel-Lindau disease.** This retinal tumor is comprised of capillaries and lipidized stromal cells. Histology of the retinal tumor is identical to that of a central nervous system hemangioblastoma. Hematoxylin-eosin, ×100.

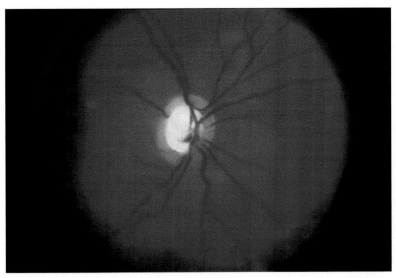

FIGURE 1–20 • **Sturge Weber syndrome.** Diffuse hemangioma obscures normal details of the choroid and imparts a "tomato ketchup" appearance to the fundus. Severe glaucomatous cupping is present.

# CHAPTER 2

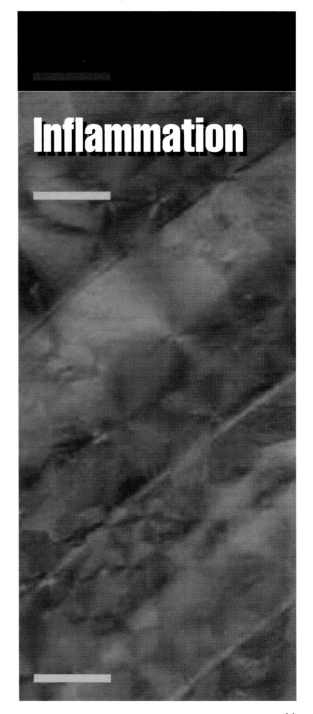

# Inflammation

During the evolutionary struggle for survival, a complex series of defense mechanisms has evolved (that in its totality we call inflammation). The inflammatory response involves a variety of specialized effector cells and a bewilderingly complex interplay of cells, mediators, and biochemical reactions that serve to protect the body against microorganisms and cancer. In addition, the inflammatory process includes mechanisms to repair and restore tissues damaged by foreign invaders, trauma, or chemical and physical agents. The wide spectrum of opportunistic infections and tumors that afflict patients who have the acquired immunodeficiency syndrome (AIDS) underscores generally how effective the intact immune system, the cornerstone of the inflammatory process, is in protecting us from potential invaders.

Fantone and Ward defined inflammation as "a reaction of the microcirculation characterized by movement of fluid and white blood cells from the blood into the extravascular tissues. This is frequently an expression of the host's attempt to localize and eliminate metabolically altered cells, foreign particles, microorganisms, or antigens." The inflammatory cells and the biochemical mediators of inflammation largely reside within the lumina of blood vessels. In contrast, most of the body's cells are located in the extravascular compartment, where invasion by microorganisms also generally begins. Hence inflammatory cells and macromolecules such as antibodies and components of the complement system must leave the vessels and enter the tissues if they are to combat microbial invaders or dispose of dead or damaged cells or other materials. Vasoactive inflammatory mediators such as histamine, serotonin, kinins, prostaglandins, and platelet-activating factor increase vascular permeability, allowing cells and antibodies access to the tissues. A second heterogeneous group of nonimmunoglobulin protein mediators called cytokines recruit and stimulate inflammatory cells. Cytokines are synthesized and secreted by inflammatory cells and include the interleukins, interferons, and colony stimulating factors. Other cell adhesion molecules, including integrins and cadherins, are involved in cellular homing, adhesion, and cell-to-cell interactions.

Increased vascular permeability is responsible for several of the cardinal manifestations of inflammation including *tumor* (swelling), *calor* (heat), and *rubor* (redness) (Fig. 2–1). Heat and redness reflect increased blood flow, and swelling reflects the collection of serum and other blood components in the extracellular space. Some inflammatory mediators (e.g., some of the prostaglandins) cause pain and stimulate the contraction of smooth muscle. Spasm of the ciliary muscle and sphincter muscles of the iris contributes to the pain of anterior uveitis, which usually is ameliorated by strong cycloplegic drugs such as atropine. Pain, pupillary miosis, and photophobia are helpful clinical markers that serve to differentiate iridocyclitis from conjunctivitis.

The increased vascular permeability that occurs with inflammation is readily evident to the ophthalmologist during slit lamp biomicroscopy. Aqueous humor normally is almost totally devoid of protein. The protein content rises when inflammation disrupts the blood–ocular barrier. A focused beam of light illuminating the anterior chamber becomes visible, just as a projector beam is visible in a smoky room. This phenomenon, termed aqueous "flare," or "ray," is caused by the Tyndall effect. The intensity of the aqueous flare correlates fairly well with the severity of the inflammation and may be roughly quantified and noted in the clinical record. Individual inflammatory cells also are evident on slit lamp examination as motes of light, and the quantity of cells can be roughly estimated and recorded. The cells normally move with the convection currents in the aqueous. (They sink anteriorly where the aqueous is cooled by the cornea and rise posteriorly where the aqueous is heated by the iris.) An absence of cellular convection currents may indicate clotting of fibrin-rich aqueous in a patient with severe vascular permeability. Adhesions readily form in the fibrin-rich milieu of ocular inflammation. Adhesions between the iris and the lens, called posterior synechias, can block the flow of aqueous humor through the pupil from the posterior chamber. The pupil is said to be secluded if its entire circumference is bound down by posterior synechias (seclusio pupillae). Secondary closed-angle glaucoma can develop if the synechias are not broken. Cycloplegic/mydriatic drugs help prevent these adhesions by dilating the pupil. Aggregates of inflammatory cells called keratic precipitates (KPs) form on the posterior surface of the cornea. The KPs may be small or large and lardaceous. The latter, which are often called "mutton fat" keratin precipitates, typically occur in eyes that have chronic granulomatous inflammation.

*Functio laesa,* or loss of function, is the final cardinal manifestation of inflammation. Although many common ocular inflammations such as conjunctivitis or chalazion are short-lived incapacitations or annoyances, severe inflammations or infections, particularly those that affect the interior of the eye, can cause blindness. Stereotyped inflammatory responses designed to protect the body against external invaders can totally destroy its delicate tissues. A small bacterial infection may be inconsequential in the skin, but it can totally destroy an eye. Even if an intraocular bacterial infection is expediently sterilized, the normal processes of regeneration and repair often cause blindness. A delicate membrane of connective tissue less than 1 mm long can profoundly affect visual acuity if it forms in an inopportune location. Likewise, minor

alterations in the structure of the transparent ocular media (cornea, lens, or vitreous) can markedly degrade their optical properties. One must also remember that the eye's neurosensory components are incapable of regeneration or repair, similar to central nervous system (CNS) tissue. Blindness caused by retinal damage or destruction is irrevocable and untreatable.

## CLASSIFICATION OF INFLAMMATION

Histopathologically, inflammation is categorized as acute or chronic based on the type of inflammatory cells found in the tissue or exudate. Acute inflammation usually is characterized by the presence of polymorphonuclear leukocytes, or "polys." Lymphocytes and plasma cells are found in chronic nongranulomatous inflammation, and their presence generally denotes involvement of the immune system. Activated macrophages or epithelioid histiocytes and inflammatory giant cells characterize chronic granulomatous inflammation.

### Polymorphonuclear Leukocytes

The polymorphonuclear leukocyte, neutrophil, or poly is the primary cell found in acute inflammation (Fig. 2–2). The poly is the body's first line of cellular defense. These cells phagocytize bacteria and other foreign material, and their cytoplasm contains many primary and secondary granules that harbor a wide variety of digestive enzymes they use to kill and digest microorganisms. Polys have pink cytoplasm and a multilobed (typically trilobed) nucleus in routine sections stained with hematoxylin and eosin (H&E). Degenerated polys with round karyorrhectic nuclei are frequently observed in focal collections of polys called abscesses. The term suppurative inflammation refers to the presence of an exudate called pus, which is composed of numerous polys and tissue destruction. Polys

do not proliferate at the site of inflammation. They are produced in the bone marrow and delivered via the bloodstream to the site of inflammation where they die. They are attracted to the site of injury by chemotactic gradients, adhere to receptors or adhesion molecules on the vascular endothelial cells (margination), and pass through the capillary wall into the tissue (diapedesis). The cell walls of polys have receptors for the Fc component of immunoglobulin. These Fc receptors aid in the phagocytosis of bacteria that have been combined with antibodies in a process called opsonization.

Clinically, acute inflammation is characterized by the presence of pus. Copious quantities of purulent exudate occur in patients who have hyperacute conjunctivitis, such as that caused by the gonococcus. A collection of polys called a hypopyon accumulates in the inferior part of the anterior chamber in eyes with acute keratitis or endophthalmitis. Vitreous abscesses form in the presence of acute purulent endophthalmitis. The polys in the vitreous abscess occasionally are arranged in a linear fashion, reflecting the orientation of the type II collagen fibrils that constitute the framework of the vitreous humor.

### Eosinophils

Eosinophilic leukocytes, or eosinophils, are recognized by their intensely eosinophilic orange granular cytoplasm and their bilobed nuclei (Fig. 2–3). Eosinophils are about the same size as polys. Their cytoplasmic granules have a characteristic rhomboid crystalloid configuration seen by electron microscopy. The eosinophil granules are rich in acid phosphatase and other lysosomal enzymes and also contain a unique eosinophilic major basic protein that is toxic to certain parasites and normal host cells. Eosinophils are involved in the phagocytosis of antigen–antibody complexes and are known to modulate inflammatory reactions mediated by mast cells. The presence of numerous eosinophils in tissue sections is highly suggestive of an allergic reaction or a parasitic infestation.

## Lymphocytes

Lymphocytes are mononuclear cells 7–8 $\mu$m in diameter. Lymphocytes appear as blue spheres in smears and tissue sections; their nuclei are round and intensely basophilic, and the cytoplasm is so scanty it is often inapparent (Fig. 2–4). Lymphocytes play a dominant role in chronic inflammation and in both humoral and cell-mediated immunity. Multiple subtypes of lymphocytes have been characterized. B lymphocytes are formed in the bone marrow and are involved in humoral immunity; they differentiate into plasma cells, the chief antibody-producing cells of the body. T lymphocytes, which originate in the thymus, include effector and regulatory subtypes. Effector T cells participate in delayed hypersensitivity and mixed lymphocyte reactions and are a prominent constituent of benign reactive lymphoid infiltrates. Regulator T cells [T-helper/amplifier (T4) and suppressor/cytotoxic (T8) cells] modulate the immune response. T4 cells, which are responsible for initiating the immune response, are preferentially infected and killed by human immunodeficiency virus (HIV), which binds to the CD4 receptor. Other lymphocyte subtypes include killer, natural killer, and null cells.

## Plasma Cells

Plasma cells are activated B lymphocytes and are the body's primary source of circulating antibodies. These antibody factories have a characteristic appearance (Fig. 2–5). Round and eccentrically located, the nucleus has dense clumps of chromatin that adhere to the inner surface of its membrane in a pattern that has been likened to a cart wheel or clock face. Unlike lymphocytes, plasma cells have an abundant amount of cytoplasm, which is largely occupied by rough endoplasmic reticulum (RER) used to synthesize immunoglobulin.

In routine sections stained with H&E the cytoplasm of plasma cells has a distinctly basophilic or purple hue caused by the affinity of the basic dye hematoxylin for ribosomal RNA in the RER. The Golgi apparatus of plasma cell is apparent with light microscopy as a lighter-staining crescent next to the nucleus called the perinuclear *hof* (German: courtyard). The cytoplasm of plasma cells may become eosinophilic as the cells produce large quantities of immunoglobulin. Eosinophilic crystals of immunoglobulin called Russell bodies occasionally form in the cytoplasm of plasma cells (Fig. 2–6). Usually round but occasionally square or even hexagonal, Russell bodies reflect the "terminal constipation" of plasma cells by immunoglobulin. They generally denote an inflammatory process of some chronicity and may be found intracellularly or free in the tissue. Dutcher bodies are similar, smaller crystalline inclusions of antibody molecules that appear to be intranuclear but actually reside in an intranuclear cytoplasmic inclusion. Positive staining with the periodic acid-Schiff (PAS) stain indicates that Russell or Dutcher bodies are composed of immunoglobulin A (IgA) or IgM molecules. A cell that contains multiple small intracytoplasmic Russell bodies is called a morula cell.

An inflammatory infiltrate composed of lymphocytes and varying numbers of plasma cells characterizes chronic nongranulomatous inflammation. Although lymphocytes and plasma cells occasionally constitute an acute inflammatory response to certain viral infections, the presence of these cells usually indicates that the immune system has been activated (Fig. 2–7). Special stains for microorganisms generally are nonrevealing in the presence of chronic nongranulomatous inflammation.

## Mast Cells

Mast cells are often called tissue basophils, although there is evidence that they are derived from neural crest rather than bone marrow. Mast cells play an important role in acute anaphylaxis (type I hypersensitivity reaction). IgE antibody molecules produced by allergic individuals bind to Fc receptors on the plasma membrane of mast cells. Subsequent interaction between the appropriate antigen and two IgE molecules causes mast cell degranulation and the release of potent vasoactive substances, including histamine, serotonin, and heparin, which have an immediate effect on vascular permeability. Severe itching and the acute onset of conjunctival edema or chemosis are clinical symptoms and signs of acute allergic conjunctivitis of the anaphylactic type.

Mast cells vaguely resemble plasma cells in tissue sections but have a centrally placed nucleus (Fig. 2–8). In routine H&E sections they lack the prominent array of basophilic granules disclosed by Wright's stain. The cytoplasm of mast cells is PAS-positive, and its constituent granules are stained intensely blue by the acid-fast stain. Mast cells are found in the conjunctival substantia propria in conjunction with allergic disorders such as vernal conjunctivitis and giant papillary conjunctivitis. They are also common in patients with some neoplasms, such as neurofibromas.

## Macrophages

The macrophage, or histiocyte, is the body's second line of cellular defense and its chief phagocytic cell. Macrophages are thought to be derived from circulating monocytes. They are relatively large mononuclear cells (larger than polys) that have an eccentric reniform or kidney shaped nucleus. Macrophages have a great capacity to phagocytize material, but unlike polys they cause little tissue damage. Prior to phagocytosis, newly formed macrophages have a modest amount of eosinophilic cytoplasm. In ophthalmic pathology, macrophages generally are characterized by the substances they have phagocytized, that is, those that have ingested blood-breakdown products such as hemosiderin and erythrocyte ghost cells, lipid material seen as foamy vacuoles, and other materials such as degenerated lens protein or melanin (Figs. 2–9, 2–10).

Macrophages play an important role as antigen-presenting cells during the initial stages of the immune response. They phagocytize and process antigenic material and present appropriate epitopes to helper T cells in conjunction with class II major histocompatibility molecules (called HLA-DR in humans) located in their cell membranes. During activation, macrophages produce a lymphokine called interleukin-1 (IL-1), which produces fever and is thought to induce the production of a second cellular messenger, IL-2, by the T cells. They also secrete a wide variety of powerful biologic molecules called monokines, which are important, even pivotal, participants in the inflammatory response.

## Epithelioid Histiocytes and Giant Cells

Under certain circumstances macrophages, or histiocytes, transform into more metabolically active forms called epithelioid cells or epithelioid histiocytes (Fig. 2–11). Activation typically occurs when the histiocytes encounter large quantities of antigenic material that is relatively insoluble or indigestible. Some microorganisms, particularly those that proliferate intracellularly, stimulate the formation of epithelioid histiocytes. Classic examples include the mycobacteria that cause tuberculosis and leprosy, fungi, and parasites such as schistosomes.

Epithelioid histiocytes are termed "epithelioid" (-oid = resembling; epithelioid = like epithelium) because these cells have abundant eosinophilic cytoplasm and superficially resemble simple epithelial cells (Fig. 2–12). If epithelioid histiocytes are observed histopathologically in a chronic inflammatory infiltrate, the inflammation is termed granulomatous. Epithelioid histiocytes are required for the diagnosis of

chronic granulomatous inflammation. Inflammatory giant cells are another characteristic feature of chronic granulomatous inflammation (Figs. 2–13, 2–14, 2–15). Inflammatory giant cells are a multinucleated syncytium formed by the fusion of epithelioid histiocytes.

Several kinds of inflammatory giant cells are recognized histopathologically. The Langhan's giant cell, which is typically seen in tuberculosis, has a peripheral rim of nuclei and homogeneous cytoplasm (Fig. 2–13). Foreign body giant cells have nuclei that are randomly dispersed or centrally located, and their cytoplasm contains particulates of foreign material in large vacuoles (Fig. 2–14). When an extremely large foreign body is encountered, numerous foreign body giant cells adhere to its outer surface, forming an encompassing cytoplasmic barrier that "insulates" the foreign material from the rest of the body. The Touton giant cell occurs with chronic lipogranulomatous inflammation (Fig. 2–15). The classic Touton giant cell is shaped like a target. The "bulls-eye" is a central zone of eosinophilic cytoplasm encircled by a ring of nuclei, which in turn is surrounded by an peripheral wreath of foamy lipidized cytoplasm. Although Touton giant cells classically are associated with juvenile xanthogranuloma (JXG), they also are found with other xanthogranulomatous disorders, such as Erdheim-Chester disease and necrobiotic xanthogranuloma.

## GRANULOMATOUS INFLAMMATION

### Background

By definition, to be classified as chronic granulomatous an inflammatory infiltrate must contain epithelioid histiocytes, inflammatory giant cells, or both. Clinically, the term granulomatous is applied to ocular inflammation when large lardaceous "mutton-fat" KPs

are observed. Mutton-fat KPs are miniature granulomas composed of aggregated epithelioid histiocytes. If granulomatous inflammation is noted clinically or histopathologically, a causative organism or specific etiologic agent should be sought. If granulomatous inflammation is encountered in tissue sections, it is imperative that stains for acid fast organisms, fungi, and bacteria (and occasionally silver stains for spirochetes) be performed. The specimen should also be examined with polarization microscopy to rule out the presence of foreign material, which may be inconspicuous. Sarcoidosis is a relatively common cause of granulomatous ocular inflammation (Figs. 2–12, 2–16). A diagnosis of exclusion, sarcoidosis should be suspected when a characteristic pattern of discrete noncaseating granulomas is found and special stains for microorganisms are negative. Granulomatous inflammation occasionally is a response to endogenous material. Examples include the response to lipid in chalazia and the thick layer of giant cells bordering keratin in the lumen of dermoid cysts with discontinuous epithelial linings.

### Patterns of Chronic Granulomatous Inflammation

The arrangement of the epithelioid histiocytes and other inflammatory cells differs for various chronic granulomatous disorders. These histologic patterns are often helpful in the diagnostic assessment of ocular specimens. Diffuse, discrete, and zonal patterns of granulomatous inflammation are recognized.

The diffuse pattern of chronic granulomatous inflammation characteristically occurs in sympathetic uveitis (ophthalmia) (see Fig. 3–8) and other diseases such as lepromatous leprosy. The epithelioid histiocytes and inflammatory giant cells are diffusely scattered among a background infiltrate composed of lymphocytes and plasma cells. The arrangement of the cellular elements has been likened to salt and pepper: The eosinophilic epithelioid histiocytes with their abundant cytoplasm, comprising the "salt," are diffusely dispersed within a "peppery" background of basophilic lymphocytes.

Discrete, well circumscribed aggregates of epithelioid histiocytes characteristically occur in sarcoidosis (Fig. 2–16). Hence the discrete pattern of chronic granulomatous inflammation is often called the sarcoidal pattern. The tubercles of epithelioid histiocytes and giant cells in sarcoidosis are sharply delimited from the surrounding infiltrate of round cells, comprised largely of helper T lymphocytes. The discrete granulomas in sarcoidosis are noncaseating, and they typically lack the cheesy, or caseous, central necrosis that is a characteristic feature of tuberculosis. Sarcoidosis is a diagnosis of exclusion, however, and special stains for microorganisms should always be performed. Discrete granulomas do occur in other diseases such as miliary tuberculosis and tuberculoid leprosy. In addition, polarization microscopy should be done to exclude particles of foreign material. Silica and beryllium can incite granulomatous inflammation, which can mimic sarcoidosis.

Concentric zones of inflammatory cells surround a central nidus of antigenic material in the zonal pattern of chronic granulomatous inflammation. The classic example in general pathology is the palisading granuloma that surrounds a nidus of devitalized collagen in rheumatoid arthritis. The classic examples of zonal granulomatous inflammation in the eye are rheumatoid scleritis (see Fig. 5–71) and the rare autoimmune disorder phacoanaphylactic endophthalmitis (phacoantigenic uveitis).

Phacoanaphylactic endophthalmitis (phacoanaphylaxis), or phacoantigenic uveitis, is a severe zonal granulomatous inflammatory reaction that is centered around the lens and follows trauma (Fig. 2–17). In the past, the avascular encapsulated lens was thought to be an immune-sequestered structure; and phacoanaphylaxis, in turn, was considered the body's attempt to reject this "foreign tissue" after its antigens were exposed by injury. These classic concepts are now known to be erroneous. The lens is *not* an immune sequestered structure; lens proteins or crystallins are expressed elsewhere in the body, and anti-lens antibodies have been found in the sera of normal individuals using modern sensitive assay techniques. Furthermore, if the immune sequestration theory were valid, phacoantigenic uveitis would be an extremely common disease in the current era of early extracapsular surgery. Residual undenatured lens material almost always remains in the capsular bag after planned extracapsular surgery. Despite this fact, phacoanaphylactic endophthalmitis remains a rare disease, and few cases have been documented after extracapsular surgery and intraocular lens implantation.

Phacoanaphylaxis is currently thought to be an immune complex disease (type III hypersensitivity reaction) involving loss of immune tolerance. Histopathologically, the zonal inflammatory reaction is centered around a lens whose capsule is ruptured, or fragments of lens substance (Fig. 2–17). The central zone of inflammatory cells that infiltrates the substance of the lens is comprised of polymorphonuclear leukocytes (first line of cellular defense). The polys are attracted by chemotactic molecules such as C5a that are generated when complement is activated by the formation of immune complexes of anti-lens antibodies and lens antigens. A second zone of granulomatous inflammation composed of epithelioid histiocytes (activated macrophages, the second line of cellular defense), and giant cells surrounds the inner collection of polys. A third zone of nongranulomatous inflammation containing granulation tissue, lymphocytes, and plasma cells occurs peripherally.

Granulation tissue forms during the reparative phase of inflammation and plays an important role in wound healing. Granulation tissue is composed of proliferating capillaries, activated fibroblasts with contractile properties called myofibroblasts, and a mixture of inflammatory cells including polys, lymphocytes, plasma cells, macrophages, and eosinophils (Fig. 2–18). The myofibroblasts are involved in scar contraction. A "pyogenic granuloma" is an inappropriate, exuberant proliferation of granulation tissue that typically arises after minor trauma (see Fig. 4–19).

## ENDOPHTHALMITIS AND PANOPHTHALMITIS

Endophthalmitis is defined as inflammation, usually acute and infectious in cause, that involves one or more of the ocular coats and adjacent intraocular cavities. Clinically, the term usually denotes an infection that involves the vitreous. As the name implies, panophthalmitis is a more extensive ocular infection that has spread to involve all of the ocular coats including the sclera and occasionally the orbit.

Endophthalmitis and panophthalmitis usually are caused by bacteria and less often by yeast and filamentous fungi. The ocular contents, especially the vitreous humor, comprise an excellent culture medium that supports the growth of relatively avirulent organisms including saprophytes. These intraocular infections usually are suppurative; that is, they are acute and characterized by the presence of myriad polys that accumulate in the vitreous cavity as a vitreous abscess. Tissue destruction, a hallmark of suppurative inflammation, is caused by the release of digestive enzymes by degenerating polys. The visual prognosis in endophthalmitis is often poor because the retina and other structures bordering the abscess may be destroyed.

Bacterial endophthalmitis usually presents 1–2 days postoperatively with severe pain, a turbid media, and a hypopyon. Eyes with acute purulent bacterial endophthalmitis typically contain a large solitary vitreous abscess (Fig. 2–19). Histopathology shows extensive necrosis and dissolution of uveal and retinal tissues and occasionally intraocular hemorrhage (Fig. 2–20). In contrast to the infiltrate of polys in the vitreous, the choroid often contains lymphocytes and plasma cells because Bruch's membrane acts as a natural barrier that confines the acute inflammation. In chronic cases, an ingrowth of granulation tissue from the uvea breaches the neuroepithelium and invades and organizes the vitreous abscess. Bacterial colonies are conspicuous in some cases, but extensive dispersion of ocular pigment can make identification of bacteria difficult. The clinical course of fungal endophthalmitis usually is more indolent than bacterial endophthalmitis. Multiple vitreous microabscesses are a characteristic finding in fungal endophthalmitis (Figs. 2–21, 2–22).

Endophthalmitis is said to be exogenous when the eye is invaded by organisms from the external environment. Exogenous endophthalmitis usually is caused by bacteria or fungi introduced during ocular surgery or penetrating trauma (Fig. 2–19). Other avenues of exogenous infection are infected corneal ulcers that perforate or infected filtering blebs in patients who have undergone fistulization surgery for glaucoma. Staphylococci, streptococci, gram-negative rods, and fungi are common causes of exogenous endophthalmitis. The term localized endophthalmitis refers to infection by relatively avirulent organisms, such as *Propionibacterium acnes* or *Candida parapsilosis*, which are sequestered within the lens capsular bag after extracapsular cataract extraction with intraocular lens implantation (Figs. 2–23, 2–24). Such infections tend to be chronic and smoldering and often incite a granulomatous response.

Endogenous endophthalmitis usually is caused by the hematogenous dissemination of organisms to the eye. Endogenous endophthalmitis can complicate septicemia, subacute bacterial endocarditis, meningococcemia, and systemic fungal infections such as candidiasis, aspergillosis, or nocardiosis in immunocompromised patients (Figs. 2–25, 2–26). The posterior segment usually harbors the bulk of the inflammatory process in an endogenous infection. Other important endogenous infections are the necrotizing retinitides caused by the herpesviruses cytomegalovirus (CMV), varicella zoster virus (VZV), and herpes simplex virus (HSV) and the protozoan parasite *Toxoplasma gondii*.

## VIRAL RETINITIS

Cytomegalovirus retinitis (Figs. 2–27, 2–28) is the most common opportunistic intraocular infection in patients who have AIDS, and it can also affect patients who are immunosuppressed following transplant surgery or cancer chemotherapy. Nearly one-third of AIDS patients develop CMV retinitis. CMV retinitis is a devastating ocular complication because it causes total retinal destruction and blindness if untreated.

Ophthalmoscopically, acute CMV infection causes coagulative necrosis and opacification of the retina, which appears yellowish white. Posterior retinal infections usually begin along vessels and often are marked by heavy infiltration and hemorrhage, which are responsible for an ophthalmoscopic appearance that has been likened to "crumbled cheese and ketchup." Peripheral lesions have a granular appearance and little or no hemorrhage.

The term cytomegalovirus is derived from the cellular enlargement that is a characteristic cytopathic effect of the virus (Fig. 2–28). In this regard CMV differs from the other herpesviruses that cause necrotizing retinitis. All retinal herpesvirus infections are characterized histopathologically by the presence of Cowdry type A intranuclear inclusions comprised of virions. The intranuclear inclusions found in cells infected by CMV are often called "owl's eye" inclusions because they typically are large and surrounded by a clear halo. Multiple intracytoplasmic inclusions also occur in cells infected with CMV.

Light microscopy discloses markedly enlarged abnormal retinal cells containing "owl's eye" inclusions in the necrotic retina (Fig. 2–28). Areas that are opaque clinically typically show full-thickness retinal destruction. The transition between healthy and totally necrotic retina is often abrupt. The underlying choroid contains acute and chronic inflammatory cells. CMV can also infect the retinal pigment epithelium (RPE). The vitreous in CMV retinitis is often relatively clear in contrast to the intense vitritis seen in ocular toxoplasmosis.

Necrotizing retinitis caused by herpes simplex or VZV occurs in acute retinal necrosis (ARN) or bilateral acute retinal necrosis (BARN) syndromes. Classic ARN syndrome occurs in presumably healthy patients who are not immunosuppressed, although a similar ocular infection is seen in immunosuppressed patients. The Cowdry type A intranuclear inclusions are smaller than the "owl's eye" inclusions of CMV, and cytomegaly is not observed. The visual prognosis in patients who have ARN is often poor because severe postinfectious retinal atrophy predisposes to retinal holes and detachment. VZV infection of the retina in AIDS patients causes the progressive outer retinal necrosis (PORN) syndrome, which begins with deep multifocal retinal opacification and rapidly progresses to total retinal necrosis (Fig. 2–29).

Eosinophilic viral inclusions are found postmortem in retinal neurons and glial cells in children who have subacute sclerosing panencephalitis (SSPE), which is thought to be a slow virus infection of the CNS due to the measles virus. SSPE can present with visual loss from a macular neuroretinitis (measles maculopathy). The average age at onset is age 7 years, and males are predominantly affected (3:1). As mental deterioration progresses toward decerebration, patients develop seizures and myoclonic jerks with distinctive electroencephalographic changes.

## TOXOPLASMA RETINOCHOROIDITIS

Ocular toxoplasmosis is an infestation by the obligatory intracellular protozoan parasite *Toxoplasma gondii,* whose definitive host is the cat. Toxoplasmosis is a retinochoroiditis; the neurotropic parasite infests the retina and CNS primarily. The multiplicative activity of the organisms themselves causes coagulative necrosis of retinal tissue; *Toxoplasma* proliferates in the cytoplasm of the parasitized retinal cells until the cells rupture. Infected portions of the retina are totally destroyed, and the area of primary retinal infection is usually sharply demarcated (Fig. 2–30). The primary retinitis is associated with a secondary chronic choroiditis, which may spread to involve the sclera, producing a focal or segmental panophthalmitis. An example of a zonal granulomatous inflammatory reaction modified by anatomy, the inflammatory infiltrate is confined to the choroid by the structural barrier of Bruch's membrane and usually contains epithelioid histiocytes.

The name *Toxoplasma* (toxon = bow) derives from the crescentic shape of the tachyzoites, which are the rapidly multiplying free form of the parasite. Tachyzoites occasionally are identified in the infected retina, but the diagnosis usually is confirmed by the identification of *Toxoplasma* cysts in sections stained with PAS (Fig. 2–31). *Toxoplasma* cysts are filled with hundreds of slowly proliferating bradyzoites, which are released when the cyst walls rupture. Reactivation of infection in adults is caused by the release of organisms that have remained encysted and dormant in the margins of old congenital chorioretinal scars.

In the United States most cases of ocular toxoplasmosis are acquired *in utero* by transplacental transmission of the parasite from a newly infected mother to her fetus. Congenital retinochoroiditis produces atrophic and pigmented crater-like chorioretinal scars, which typically are located in the macula and were once called atypical colobomas. The macular region is affected primarily because it is profusely vascularized, and the parasite is disseminated hematogenously. The old scars of ocular toxoplasmosis appear white because the sclera has been bared by full-thickness choroidal destruction. Intensely pigmented clumps of hyperplastic RPE are also typically found.

Active infection causes focal retinal opacification and necrosis and an intense inflammatory infiltrate in the vitreous comprised of histiocytes and lymphocytes. The intense vitritis markedly reduces visual acuity and may partially obscure the underlying focus of white, infected retina. The latter appearance has been likened to a "headlight in fog." Toxoplasmosis is one of the opportunistic infections that can occur in patients with AIDS.

## UVEITIS

Uveitis refers to inflammation of the uveal tract, the middle pigmented and heavily vascularized coat of the eye that includes the iris, ciliary body, and choroid. Endogenous chronic nongranulomatous iridocyclitis, a poorly understood immunologic disorder, is encountered most frequently in clinical practice. Uveitis is often idiopathic, but it may be associated with systemic disorders including juvenile rheumatoid arthritis, ankylosing spondylitis, Reiter syndrome, ulcerative colitis, regional enteritis, or Behçet's disease. Microscopy discloses an infiltrate of lymphocytes and plasma cells in the uveal stroma in eyes with nongranulomatous uveitis (Fig. 2–7). Russell bodies and morula cells may be common in chronic cases.

Clinical or pathologic evaluation may disclose a specific cause in patients who have chronic granulomatous uveitis. Sarcoidosis is the most common cause of granulomatous uveitis. Approximately 38% of patients with systemic sarcoidosis have ocular involvement at some point in their disease. Granulomatous intraocular inflammation can also be caused by tuberculosis, leprosy, syphilis, parasites, and fungal infections including candidiasis, coccidioidomycosis, histoplasmosis, blastomycosis, and sporotrichosis. Granulomatous inflammation is also found in sympathetic uveitis and Vogt-Koyanagi-Harada disease.

Behçet's disease is a systemic immune complex disease that causes occlusive vasculitis. Genital and oral aphthous ulcers and recurrent nongranulomatous iridocyclitis with hypopyon are characteristic manifestations and diagnostic criteria. Ocular involvement also is marked by retinal vasculitis, which leads to hemorrhagic retinal infarction and retinal detachment. Especially common in the Middle and Far East, Behçet's disease is associated with HLA phenotype HLA-B5 and its subtype HLA-Bw51. Patients who have ocular Behçet's disease usually become blind if they are not treated with immunosuppressive drugs.

## SEQUELAE OF OCULAR INFLAMMATION

The sequelae of ocular inflammation include corneal scarring and vascularization, band keratopathy, cataract, and secondary glaucoma. The latter is often closed angle in type and is caused by inflammatory posterior synechias between the iris and lens. Intraocular fibrosis and membranes are caused by the organization of inflammatory debris. A cyclitic membrane is a fibrous membrane that bridges the anterior part of the vitreous cavity behind the lens from ciliary body to ciliary body (Fig. 2–32). Cyclitic membranes are caused by fibrous organization of the anterior vitreous. Contraction of inflammatory membranes causes tractional detachment of the ciliary body or retina. Ocular hypotony and shrinkage frequently result from the disorganization and destruction of intraocular structures. Clinically, the term "phthisical" is applied to blind hypotonous eyes that are soft, are partially collapsed, and have a vaguely cuboidal shape caused by rectus muscle traction. The pathologic diagnosis phthisis bulbi (atrophia bulbi with shrinkage and disorganization) is reserved for eyes that are markedly atrophic and disorganized and have thickened folded sclera. The interior of such phthisical eyes usually is filled with scar tissue, and intraocular structures are unrecognizable. The term "atrophia bulbi with shrinkage" is used if intraocular structures can be identified (Fig. 2–33). Intraocular ossification (osseous metaplasia of the retinal pigment epithelium) is commonly observed in phthisical and atrophic eyes that have chronic retinal detachments (Fig. 2–34).

# References

### General References

Chensue SW, Ward PA: Inflammation. In Damjanov I, Linder J (eds) Anderson's Pathology. 10th ed. St. Louis: Mosby, 1996:387–415.

Cotran RS, Kumar V, Robbins SL: Inflammation and repair. In Cotran RS, Kumar V, Robbins SL (eds) Pathologic Basis of Disease. 5th ed. Philadelphia: Saunders, 1994: 51–92.

Fantone JC, Ward PA: Inflammation. In Rubin E, Farber JL (eds) Pathology. Philadelphia: Lippincott, 1994:32–67.

Gallin JI, Goldstein IM, Snyderman R (eds): Inflammation: Basic Principles and Clinical Correlates. New York: Raven, 1992.

Green WR: Inflammatory diseases and conditions of the eye. In Spencer W (ed) Ophthalmic Pathology: An Atlas and Textbook. Vol 3. Philadelphia: Saunders, 1996:1864–2110.

Howes EL, Rao NA: Basic mechanisms in pathology. In Spencer W (ed) Ophthalmic Pathology: An Atlas and Textbook. Vol 4. Philadelphia: Saunders, 1996: 2935–3044.

Naumann GOH, Naumann LR: Intraocular inflammations. In Naumann GOH, Apple DJ (eds) Pathology of the Eye. Springer: New York, 1986:99–184.

Ormerod LD, Margo CE: Changing patterns of ocular infectious disease. Ophthalmol Clin North Am 8:109–124, 1995.

Pepose JS, Holland GN, Wilhelmus KR (eds): Ocular Infection & Immunity. St. Louis: Mosby, 1996.

Proia AD: Inflammation. In Garner A, Klintworth GK (eds) Pathobiology of Ocular Disease. A Dynamic Approach. New York: Marcel Dekker, 1994:63–100.

Roitt I (ed): Essential Immunology. Oxford: Blackwell, 1988.

### Inflammatory Mediators

Albelda SM, Buck CA: Integrins and other cell adhesion molecules. Faseb J 4:2868–2880, 1990.

Albelda SM, Smith CW, Ward PA: Adhesion molecules and inflammatory injury. FASEB J 8:504–512, 1994.

Arai KI, Lee F, Miyajima A, Miyatake S, Arai N, Yokota T: Cytokines: coordinators of immune and inflammatory responses. Annu Rev Biochem 59:783–836, 1990.

Cochrane CG, Gimbrone MA Jr (eds) Cellular and Molecular Mechanisms of Inflammation. Signal Transduction in Inflammatory Cells. Part A. San Diego: Academic, 1992:1–195.

Cochrane CG, Gimbrone MA Jr (eds) Cellular and Molecular Mechanisms of Inflammation. Vascular Adhesion Molecules. San Diego: Academic, 1991:1–181.

Dinarello CA: Biology of interleukin 1. FASEB J 2: 108–115, 1988.

Harlan JM, Liu DY (eds): Adhesion. Its Role in Inflammatory Disease. New York: WH Freeman, 1992:1–202.

Kunkel SL, Remick DG (eds) Cytokines in Health and Disease. New York: Marcel Dekker, 1992:1–568.

Le J, Vilcek J: Tumor necrosis factor and interleukin 1: cytokines with multiple overlapping biological activities. Lab Invest 56:234–248, 1987.

Movat HZ: Tumor necrosis factor and interleukin-1: role in acute inflammation and microvascular injury. J Lab Clin Med 110:668–681, 1987.

### Inflammatory Cells

Adams DO, Hamilton TA: The activated macrophage and granulomatous inflammation. Curr Top Pathol 79: 151–167, 1989.

Becker EL: Leukocyte stimulation: receptor, membrane, and metabolic events: introduction and summary. Fed Proc 45:2148–2150, 1986.

Cochrane CG: Mechanisms coupling stimulation and function in leukocytes: introduction. Fed Proc 43:2729–2731, 1984.

Elsbach P, Weiss J: Oxygen-dependent and oxygen-independent mechanisms of microbicidal activity of neutrophils. Immunol Lett 11:159–163, 1985.

Fantone JC, Ward PA: Role of oxygen-derived free radicals and metabolites in leukocyte-dependent inflammatory reactions. Am J Pathol 107:395–418, 1982.

Johnston RB Jr: Current concepts: immunology: monocytes and macrophages. N Engl J Med 318:747–752, 1988.

Kay AB: The eosinophilic leukocyte. In Dale MM, Foreman JC (eds) Textbook of Immunopharmacology. Oxford: Blackwell, 1989:68–76.

Lewis CE, McGee GOD (eds): The Natural Immune System. The Macrophage. Oxford: IRL Press at Oxford University Press, 1992.

Thomas R, Lipsky PE: Monocytes and macrophages. In Kelley WN, Harris ED Jr, Ruddy S, Sledge CB (eds) Textbook of Rheumatology. 4th ed. Philadelphia: Saunders, 1993:286–303.

Van Furth R: Development and distribution of mononuclear phagocytes. In Gallin JI, Goldstein IM, Snyderman R (eds) Inflammation. Basic Principles and Clinical Correlates. New York: Raven, 1992:325–340.

Weiss SJ, LoBuglio AF: Phagocyte-generated oxygen metabolites and cellular injury. Lab Invest 47:5–18, 1982.

Weller PF: The immunobiology of eosinophils. N Engl J Med 374:1110–1118, 1991.

### Granulomatous Inflammation

Boros DL: Granulomatous inflammation. In Zembala M, Asherson GL (eds) Human Monocytes. San Diego: Academic, 1989:313–381.

Ferry AP: The histopathology of rheumatoid episcleral nodules: an extra-articular manifestation of rheumatoid arthritis. Arch Ophthalmol 82:77–88, 1969.

Font RL, Fine BS, Messmer E, et al: Light and electron microscopic study of Dalen-Fuchs nodules in sympathetic ophthalmia. Ophthalmology 90:66–75, 1982.

Jakobiec FA, Marboe CC, Knowles DM II, et al: Human sympathetic ophthalmia: an analysis of the inflammatory infiltrate by hybridoma-monoclonal antibodies, immunochemistry, and correlative electron microscopy. Ophthalmology 90:76–95, 1983.

Lubin JR, Albert DM, Weinstein M: Sixty-five years of sympathetic ophthalmia: a clinicopathologic review of 105 cases (1913–1978). Ophthalmology 87:109–121, 1980.

Marak GE: Phacoanaphylactic endophthalmitis. Surv Ophthalmol 36:325–329, 1992.

Obenauf CD, Shaw HE, Wyndor CF, et al: Sarcoidosis and its ocular manifestations. Am J Ophthalmol 86:648–655, 1978.

Rao NA, Marak GE, Hidayat AA: Necrotizing scleritis: a clinicopathologic study of 41 cases. Ophthalmology 92: 1542–1549, 1985.

To KW, Jakobiec FA, Zimmerman LE: Sympathetic uveitis. In Albert DM, Jakobiec FA (eds) Principles and Practice of Ophthalmology: Clinical Practice, Vol 1. Philadelphia: Saunders, 1994:496–503.

### Bacterial Endophthalmitis

Allen HF, Mangiaracine AB: Bacterial endophthalmitis after cataract surgery. Arch Ophthalmol 91:3–7, 1974.

Jensen AD, Naidoff MA: Bilateral meningococcal endophthalmitis. Arch Ophthalmol 90:396–398, 1973.

Meisler DM, Mandelbaum S: Propionibacterium-associated endophthalmitis after extracapsular cataract extraction: review of reported cases. Ophthalmology 96:54–61, 1989.

Meisler DM, Palestine AG, Vastein DW, et al: Chronic Propionibacterium endophthalmitis after extracapsular cataract extraction and intraocular lens implantation. Am J Ophthalmol 102:733–739, 1986.

O'Brien TP, Green WR: Endophthalmitis. In Mandell GL, Douglas RG Jr, Bennett JE (eds) Principles and Practice of Infectious Diseases. 4th ed. New York: Churchill Livingstone, 1993.

Piest KL, Kincaid MC, Tetz MR, et al: Localized endophthalmitis: a newly described cause of the so-called toxic lens syndrome. J Cataract Refract Surg 13:498–510, 1987.

Shammas HF: Endogenous E. coli endophthalmitis. Surv Ophthalmol 21:428–435, 1977.

**Fungal Endophthalmitis**

Abbott RL, Forster RK, Rebell G: Listeria monocytogenes endophthalmitis with a black hypopyon. Am J Ophthalmol 86:715–719, 1978.

Brod RD, Clarkson JG, Flynn HM Jr, et al: Endogenous fungal endophthalmitis. In Tasman W, Jaeger EA (eds) Duane's Clinical Ophthalmology. New York: Harper & Row, 1990:1–39.

Caya JG, Farmer SG, Williams GA, et al: Bilateral Pseudallescheria boydii endophthalmitis in an immunocompromised patient. Wis Med J 87:11–14, 1988.

Chen CJ: Nocardia asteroides endophthalmitis. Ophthalmic Surg 14:502–505, 1983.

Demicco DD, Reichman RC, Violette EJ, et al: Disseminated aspergillosis presenting with endophthalmitis: a case report and a review of the literature. Cancer 53:1995–2001, 1984.

Edwards JE Jr, Foos RY, Montgomerie JA, Gutz LB: Ocular manifestations of Candida septicemia: review of 76 cases of hematogenous Candida endophthalmitis. Medicine 53:47–75, 1974.

Ferry AP, Font RL, Weinberg RS, et al: Nocardial endophthalmitis: report of two cases studied histopathologically. Br J Ophthalmol 72:55–61, 1988.

Fine BS, Zimmerman LE: Exogenous intraocular fungus infections with particular reference to complications of intraocular surgery. Am J Ophthalmol 48:151–165, 1959.

Gregor RJ, Chong CA, Augsburger JJ, et al: Endogenous Nocardia asteroides subretinal abcess diagnosed by transvitreal fine-needle aspiration biopsy. Retina 9:118–121, 1989.

Ho PC, Tolentino FI, Baker AS: Successful treatment of exogenous Aspergillus endophthalmitis: a case report. Br J Ophthalmol 68:412–415, 1984.

McGuire TW, Bullock JD, Bullock JD Jr, et al: Fungal endophthalmitis: an experimental study with a review of 17 human ocular cases. Arch Ophthalmol 109:1289–1296, 1991.

Michelson PE, Stark WJ, Reeser F, Green WR: Endogenous Candida endophthalmitis: report of 13 cases and 16 from the literature. Int Ophthalmol Clin 11:125–147, 1971.

O'Brien TP, Green WR: Fungus infections of the eye and periocular tissues. In Garner A, Klintworth GK (eds) Pathology of Ocular Disease. A Dynamic Approach. 2nd ed. New York: Marcel Dekker, 1993.

Weishaar PD, Flynn HW Jr, Murray TG, et al. Endogenous aspergillus endophthalmitis: clinical features and treatment outcomes. Ophthalmology 105:57–65, 1998.

Wong KW, Tasman W, Eagle RC Jr, Rodriguez A: Bilateral Candida parapsilosis endophthalmitis. Arch Ophthalmol 115:670–672, 1997.

**AIDS**

Pepose JS, Holland GN, Nestor MS, et al: Acquired immune deficiency syndrome: pathogenic mechanisms of ocular disease. Ophthalmology 92:472–484, 1985.

Rajeev B, Rao NA: Advances in ocular pathology in AIDS. Ophthalmol Clin North Am 8:125–141, 1995.

Rao NA, Zimmerman PL, Boyer D, et al: A clinical, histopathologic, and electron microscopic study of Pneumocystis carinii choroiditis. Am J Ophthalmol 107:218–228, 1989.

**Viral Retinitis**

Culbertson WW, Blumenkranz MS, Haines H, et al: The acute retinal necrosis syndrome. 2. Histopathology and etiology. Ophthalmology 89:1317–1325, 1982.

Duker JS, Blumenkranz MS: Diagnosis and management of the acute retinal necrosis (ARN) syndrome. Surv Ophthalmol 35:327–343, 1991.

Fisher JP, Lewis ML, Blumenkranz M, et al: The acute retinal necrosis syndrome. 1. Clinical manifestations. Ophthalmology 89:1309–1316, 1982.

Font RL, Jenis EH, Tuck KO: Measles maculopathy associated with subacute sclerosing panencephalitis. Arch Pathol 96:168–174, 1973.

Holland GN: The progressive outer retinal necrosis syndrome. Int Ophthalmol 18:163–165, 1994.

Murray HW, Knox DL, Green WR, et al. Cytomegalovirus retinitis in adults: a manifestation of disseminated viral infection. Am J Med 63:574–584, 1977.

Pavesio CE, Mitchell SM, Barton K, Schwartz SD, Towler HM, Lightman S: Progressive outer retinal necrosis (PORN) in AIDS patients: a different appearance of varicella-zoster retinitis. Eye 9:271–276, 1995.

Pepose JS, Holland GN: Cytomegalovirus infections of the retina. In Ryan S (ed) Retina. 2nd ed. Vol 2. St Louis: Mosby, 1994:1559–1570.

**Uveitis**

Bell R, Font RL: Granulomatous anterior uveitis caused by Coccidioides immitis. Am J Ophthalmol 74:93–98, 1972.

Inomata H, Kohno T, Rao NA, et al: Vasculitis and intraocular neovascularization in Behçet's disease: histopathology of the early and advanced late stages. In Dernouchamps JP, Verougstraete C, Caspers-Velu L, et al (eds) Proceedings of the Third International Symposium on Uveitis. Brussels, Belgium, May 24–27, 1992. New York: Kugler, 1993:349–355.

Knox DL: Uveitis associated with systemic disease. In Albert DM, Jakobiec FA (eds) Principles and Practice of Ophthalmology: Clinical Practice. Vol 1. Philadelphia: Saunders, 1994:465–474.

Loewenfeld I, Thompson H: Fuchs' heterochromic cyclitis: a critical review of the literature. II. Etiology and mechanisms. Surv Ophthalmol 18:2, 1973.

Mullaney J, Collum LM: Ocular vasculitis in Behçet's disease: a pathological and immunohistochemical study. Int Ophthalmol 7:183–191, 1985.

O'Brien JM, Albert DM, Foster CS: Anterior uveitis. In Albert DM, Jakobiec FA (eds) Principles and Practice of Ophthalmology: Clinical Practice. Vol 3. Philadelphia: Saunders, 1994:1745–1770.

Park SS, To KW, Friedman AH, Jakobiec FA: Infectious causes of posterior uveitis. In Albert DM, Jakobiec FA (eds) Principles and Practice of Ophthalmology: Clinical Practice. Vol 1. Philadelphia: Saunders, 1994:450– 464.

**Parasitic Infection**

Anderson J, Font RL: Ocular onchocerciasis. In Binford CH, Connor DH (eds) Pathology of Tropical and Extraordinary Diseases. Vol II. Washington, DC: Atlas of Armed Forces Institute of Pathology, 1976:360.

Gagliuso DJ, Teich SA, Freidman AH, et al: Ocular toxoplasmosis in AIDS patients. Trans Am Ophthalmol Soc 88:63–86, 1990.

Naumann G, Gunders AE: Pathogenesis of the posterior segment lesion of ocular onchocerciasis. Am J Ophthalmol 75:82–89, 1973.

O'Connor GR: Manifestations and management of ocular toxoplasmosis. Bull NY Acad Sci 174:192–210, 1970.

Perkins ES: Ocular toxoplasmosis. Br J Ophthalmol 57:1–17, 1973.

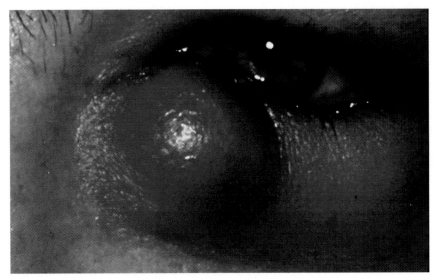

FIGURE 2–1 • **Acute dacryocystitis.** Signs of acute inflammation including swelling and erythema are evident in the region of the infected lacrimal sac and lower lid.

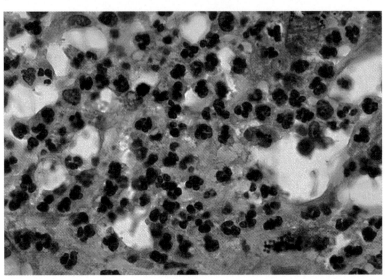

FIGURE 2–2 • **Polymorphonuclear leukocytes.** Polys have multilobed nuclei and eosinophilic cytoplasm. The polys in this field are well preserved. A few mononuclear histiocytes also are present in the acute inflammatory infiltrate. Hematoxylin-eosin, ×250.

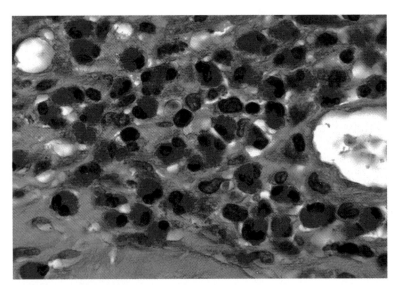

FIGURE 2–3 • **Eosinophils.** The cytoplasm of eosinophils contains intensely eosinophilic granules. The nuclei are bilobed. The presence of eosinophils usually suggests the presence of allergy or a parasite. Hematoxylin-eosin, ×250.

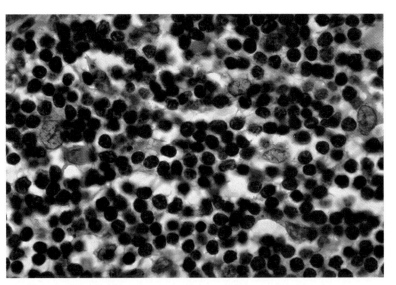

FIGURE 2–4 • **Lymphocytes.** Lymphocytes have round, intensely basophilic nuclei and scanty cytoplasm that usually is inapparent in routine light microscopic sections. Many subtypes of lymphocytes can be identified with special immunohistochemical stains. Hematoxylin-eosin, ×250.

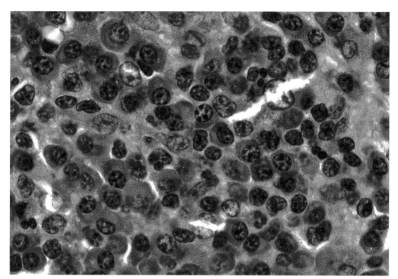

FIGURE 2–5 • **Plasma cells.** Plasma cells have round, eccentrically located nuclei with a cartwheel or clock face pattern of chromatin clumping. The cytoplasm is basophilic because it contains large quantities of ribosomal RNA used in antibody synthesis. The Golgi apparatus is evident light microscopically as a perinuclear "hof." Hematoxylin-eosin, ×250.

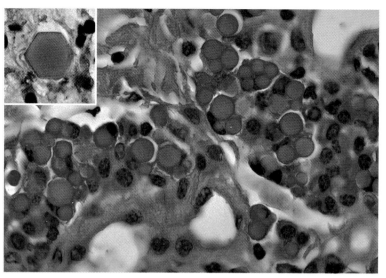

FIGURE 2–6 • **Russell bodies.** The uniformly eosinophilic spherules in this chronic inflammatory infiltrate are crystalloids of immunoglobulin called Russell bodies. A hexagonal Russell body is seen in the *inset*. Both figures: hematoxylin-eosin, ×250.

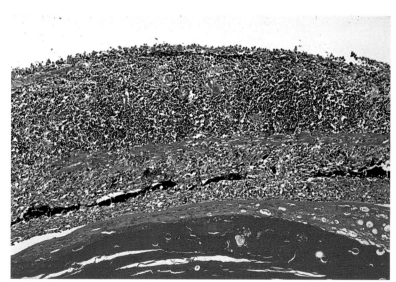

FIGURE 2–7 • **Iritis.** An infiltrate of lymphocytes and plasma cells massively thickens the stroma of the iris, which adheres to the anterior surface of the cataractous lens. The iris pigment epithelium is disrupted. No microorganisms were detected. Hematoxylin-eosin, ×50.

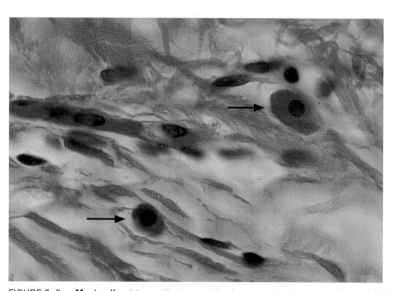

FIGURE 2–8 • **Mast cells.** Mast cells (arrows) in tissue sections have round, centrally located nuclei. The cytoplasm is mildly basophilic in routine sections stained with hematoxylin-eosin, and stains intensely with periodic acid-Schiff. Hematoxylin-eosin, ×250.

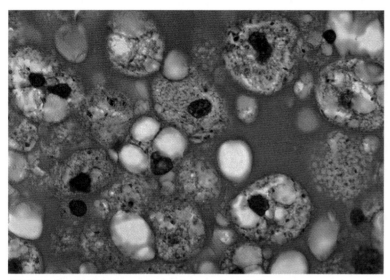

FIGURE 2–9 • **Lipid-laden macrophages, subretinal fluid.** The frothy vacuolated cytoplasm is filled with lipid vacuoles and scattered elliptical granules of RPE melanin. The surrounding subretinal fluid is protein-rich and intensely eosinophilic. The patient had radiation retinopathy. Hematoxylin-eosin, ×250.

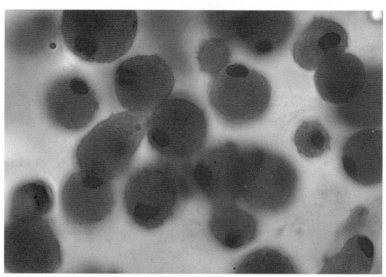

FIGURE 2–10 • **Lens-laden macrophages, phacolytic glaucoma.** These macrophages have copious quantities of eosinophilic cytoplasm that reflects the ingestion of degenerated lens protein released from an advanced cortical cataract. Hematoxylin-eosin, ×250.

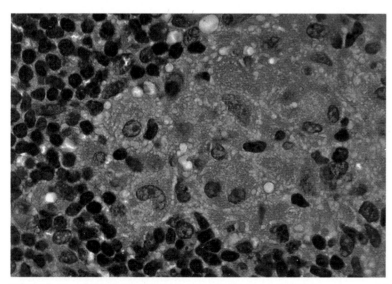

FIGURE 2–11 • **Epithelioid histiocytes, sarcoidosis.** Epithelioid histiocytes comprising the discrete granuloma have abundant quantities of eosinophilic cytoplasm and vesicular nuclei with nucleoli. Hematoxylin-eosin, ×250.

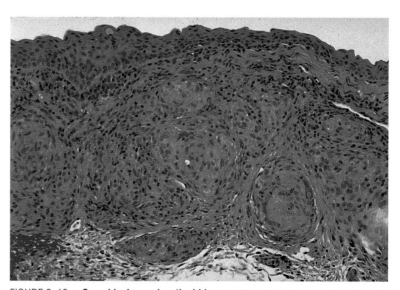

FIGURE 2–12 • **Sarcoidosis, conjunctival biopsy.** The substantia propria contains discrete granulomas composed of epithelioid histiocytes and giant cells. The epithelioid histiocytes resemble epithelial cells in the nonkeratinized conjunctival epithelium. Hematoxylin-eosin, ×50.

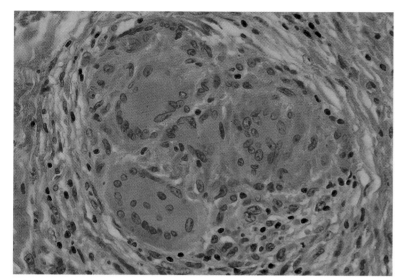

FIGURE 2–13 • **Inflammatory giant cells, Langhans' type.** The nuclei are located peripherally. The cytoplasm is uniformly eosinophilic. Langhans' giant cells are found in tuberculosis and other granulomatous diseases. Hematoxylin-eosin, ×100.

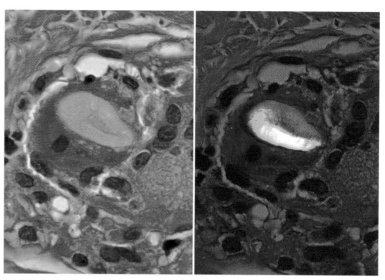

FIGURE 2–14 • **Foreign body giant cell.** The cytoplasm of the giant cell contains an oval cellulose fiber. The foreign body shows vivid birefringence during polarization microscopy (*right*). The nuclei of foreign body giant cells are arranged haphazardly. Hematoxylin-eosin with (right) and without (left) crossed polarizers, ×250.

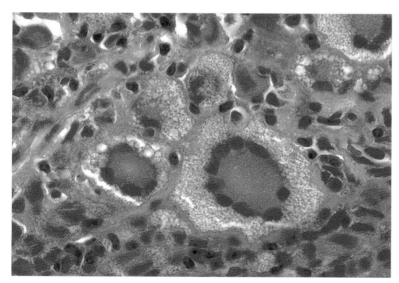

FIGURE 2–15 • **Touton giant cells, juvenile xanthogranuloma.** Fully developed Touton giant cells have a target configuration. A peripheral rim of frothy lipidized cytoplasm surrounds a ring of nuclei, which in turn encompasses a central bull's-eye of eosinophilic cytoplasm. Touton giant cells are found in juvenile xanthogranuloma and other xanthogranulomatous diseases. Hematoxylin-eosin, ×250.

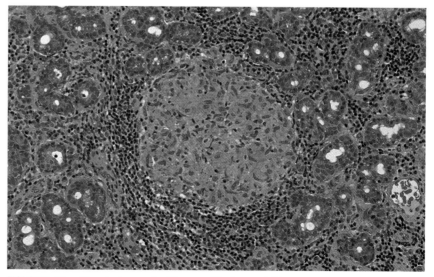

FIGURE 2–16 • **Chronic dacryoadenitis, sarcoidosis.** An infiltrate of lymphocytes, rich in helper T cells, surrounds a discrete noncaseating granuloma composed of epithelioid histiocytes and inflammatory giant cells. Scattered acini and ducts persist. Hematoxylin-eosin, ×50.

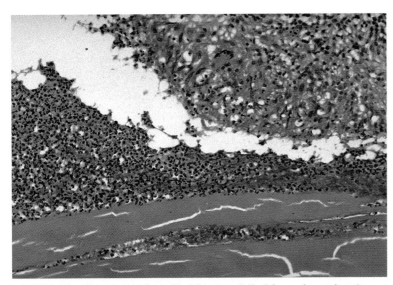

FIGURE 2–17 • **Phacoantigenic uveitis (phacoanaphylaxis), zonal granulomatous response.** Polymorphonuclear leukocytes infiltrating the substance of the ruptured lens (below) constitute the first zone of inflammatory cells. A second zone of epithelioid histiocytes surrounds the polys. The clear space separating the two zones of cells is a sectioning artifact. A third zone of nongranulomatous inflammation occurs peripherally. Hematoxylin-eosin, ×100.

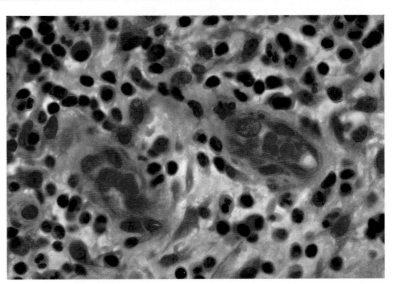

FIGURE 2–18 • **Granulation tissue.** Mixed inflammatory infiltrate comprised of lymphocytes, plasma cells, polys, and macrophages surrounds proliferating capillaries and spindle-shaped myofibroblasts. Hematoxylin-eosin, ×25.

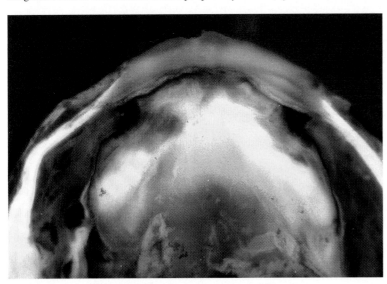

FIGURE 2–19 • **Acute endophthalmitis, secondary to *Bacillus cereus*.** A large abscess comprised of polymorphonuclear leukocytes fills the vitreous cavity. The exogenous infection developed rapidly after organisms were introduced through a corneal laceration. The anterior chamber is flat, and the choroid is detached. The retina was totally necrotic.

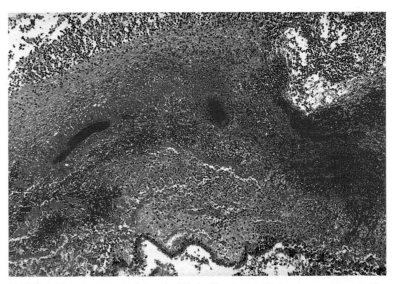

FIGURE 2–20 • **Acute bacterial endophthalmitis.** Polys fill the vitreous (above). The retina is almost totally necrotic and shows loss of its normal lamellar architecture. Focal hemorrhage is present. Hematoxylin-eosin, ×25.

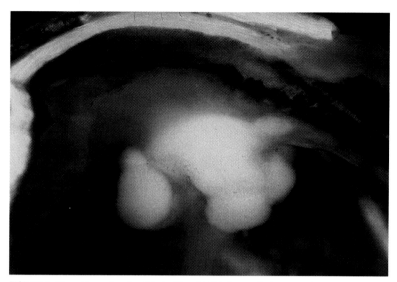

FIGURE 2–21 • **Fungal endophthalmitis.** Multiple small vitreous microabscesses are present. Vitreous microabscesses are a characteristic finding of fungal endophthalmitis.

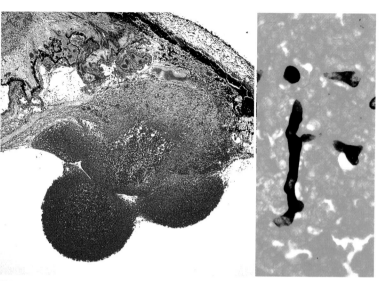

FIGURE 2–22 • **Fungal endophthalmitis.** Photomicrograph of the eye seen in Figure 2–21 shows characteristic microabscesses in the posterior chamber. Hematoxylin-eosin, ×10. *Inset:* Fungal hyphae in the center of a microabscess. Gomori methenamine silver, ×250.

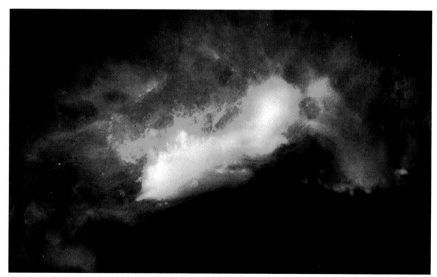

FIGURE 2–23 • *__Propionibacterium acnes-induced localized endophthalmitis.__* Large intracapsular colony of bacteria forms a whitish plaque within the excised lens capsular bag. Chronic granulomatous uveitis developed months after extracapsular cataract extraction.

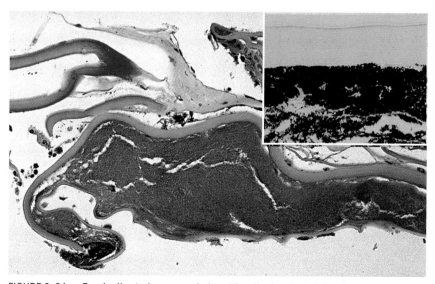

FIGURE 2–24 • *__Propionibacterium acnes-induced localized endophthalmitis.__* Large colony of sequestered diphtheroids forms a basophilic granular deposit within explanted lens capsular bag. Hematoxylin-eosin, ×50. *Inset:* Mass of pleomorphic gram-positive bacteria underneath the anterior lens capsule. Gram stain, ×250.

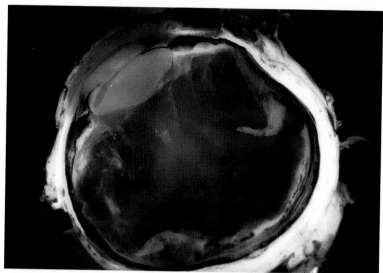

FIGURE 2–25 • **Endogenous fungal endophthalmitis, aspergillosis.** Posterior retina is thickened and necrotic, and posterior choroid is thickened. Inflammatory cells partially opacify the vitreous.

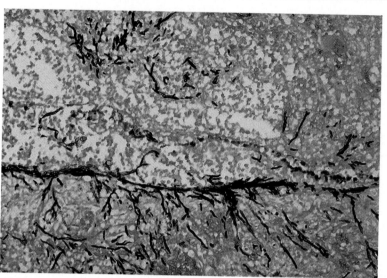

FIGURE 2–26 • **Endogenous fungal endophthalmitis, aspergillosis.** Characteristic linear array of fungal hyphae is seen on the inner surface of Bruch's membrane. Branching septate hyphae also infiltrate the retina and choroidal stroma. Gomori methenamine silver, ×50.

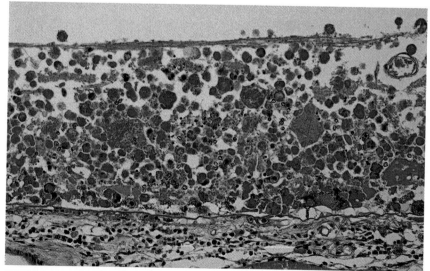

FIGURE 2–27 • **Cytomegalovirus retinitis.** Full-thickness destruction of the retina and RPE are present. Infected retina contains enlarged cells. The patient had received chemotherapy for lymphoma. Hematoxylin-eosin ×100. (Case presented by Dr. William C. Frayer at the 1998 meeting of the Verhoeff Society, Little Rock, AK)

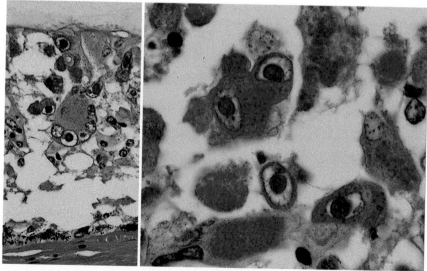

FIGURE 2–28 • **Cytomegalovirus retinitis, intranuclear inclusions.** Clear haloes surrounding large Cowdry type A intranuclear inclusions of cytomegalovirus impart "owl's eye" appearance to infected nuclei. Smaller cytoplasmic inclusions also are present. Multinucleated giant cell (at left) contains viral inclusion. Hematoxylin-eosin. Left ×100, right ×250. (Case presented by Dr. William C. Frayer at the 1998 meeting of the Verhoeff Society, Little Rock, AK)

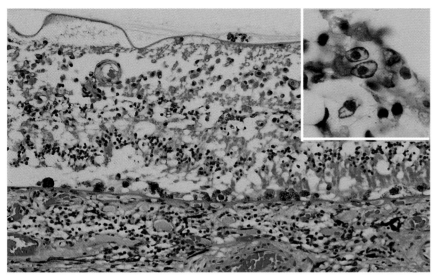

FIGURE 2–29 • **Progressive outer retinal necrosis (PORN) syndrome.** Necrosis involves all retinal layers including the RPE in a patient with AIDS. Hematoxylin-eosin, ×100. *Inset:* Cowdry type A intranuclear inclusions of varicella-zoster virus are seen. Hematoxylin-eosin, ×250. (Case presented by Dr. Curtis Margo at the 1994 meeting of the Verhoeff Society, Rochester, MN)

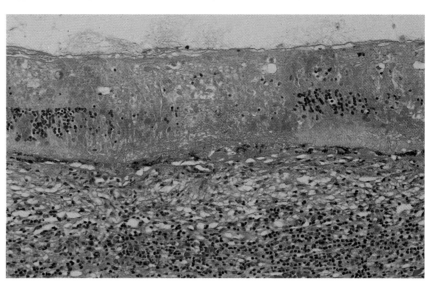

FIGURE 2–30 • *Toxoplasma retinochoroiditis.* The infected retina is almost totally necrotic. The choroid is thickened by chronic granulomatous inflammation. Hematoxylin-eosin, ×50.

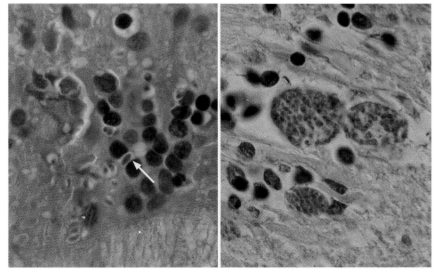

FIGURE 2–31 • *Toxoplasma retinochoroiditis.* Arrow denotes toxoplasma tachyzoite in largely necrotic retina (*left*). Intraretinal *Toxoplasma* cysts filled with bradyzoites are seen at right. Both figures: hematoxylin-eosin, ×250.

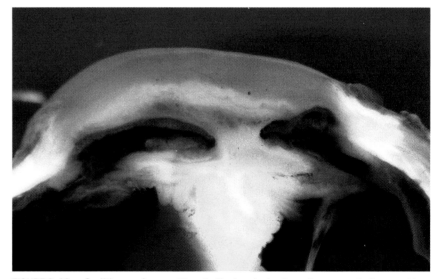

FIGURE 2–32 • **Cyclitic membrane.** Chronically detached retina adheres anteriorly to a white mass of fibrous connective tissue filling the posterior chamber. Cyclitic membranes are caused by fibrous organization of the vitreous.

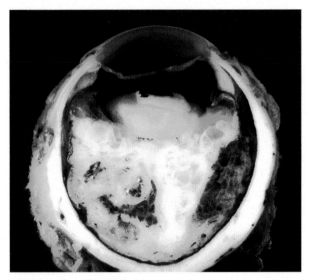

FIGURE 2–33 • **Atrophia bulbi.** Totally detached gliotic retina and metaplastic bone fills the disorganized interior of a chronically blind and painful eye. The angle is closed by peripheral anterior synechias. The pupil adheres to the lens at the site of a white anterior subcapsular cataract.

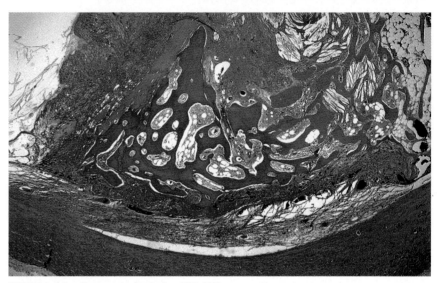

FIGURE 2–34 • **Osseous metaplasia of the RPE.** Large focus of metaplastic bone is present on the inner surface of choroid. Intraocular bone is often found in phthisical eyes with long-standing retinal detachments. Hematoxylin-eosin, ×10.

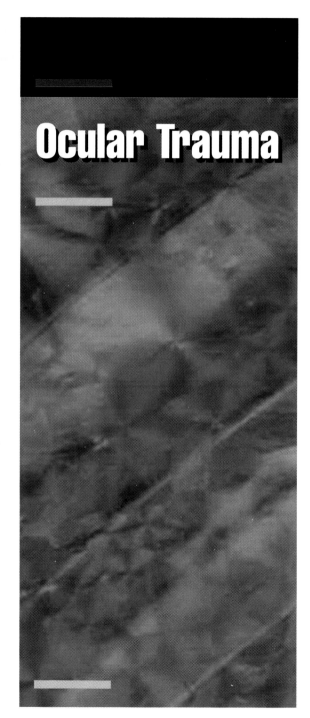

# CHAPTER 3

# Ocular Trauma

Many eyes that are enucleated have a past history of nonsurgical or surgical trauma. The eye can be totally destroyed by severe injuries that violate the integrity of its protective coats and scatter its contents. Less devastating injuries cause blindness by disrupting the normal anatomic and functional relations between the eye's highly specialized tissues. Retinal detachment, retinal avulsion anteriorly from the ora serrata or posteriorly from the optic nerve, avulsion of the optic nerve from the globe, irido- or cyclodialysis, lens dislocation, and choroidal rupture are examples.

By disrupting pristine anatomic relations, trauma exposes new surfaces on which cells can proliferate. These include the inner and outer surfaces of the retina after retinal detachment, the posterior face of the vitreous exposed by vitreous detachment, or the anterior chamber structures made accessible to surface epithelium by poorly apposed wounds in the cornea. Cellular proliferation on these newly exposed surfaces leads to permanent adhesions between structures, membrane formation, fibrosis, traction, retinal detachment, and glaucoma.

Hemorrhage commonly complicates trauma. The blood opacifies transparent ocular media such as the vitreous and may cause secondary glaucoma by occluding aqueous outflow pathways. In addition, intraocular hemorrhage causes expulsion and irrevocable loss of vital intraocular structures when it accumulates in the suprauveal space and fills the interior of the eye (expulsive choroidal hemorrhage). Blindness also can result when the body's normal mechanisms of regeneration and repair cause scarring that affects highly differentiated transparent tissues or when fibrous membranes exert traction on vital structures. For example, the fibrous organization of tracts of hemorrhage in the vitreous left by perforating missiles ultimately can cause tractional retinal detachment.

Trauma also predisposes to infection by destroying the eye's normal protective barriers. Infection is always a danger after ocular trauma, even such minor injuries as corneal abrasions. Organisms introduced by penetrating injuries or contaminated intraocular foreign bodies of metallic, vegetable, or even endogenous animal (e.g., hair, skin) composition can cause exogenous endophthalmitis.

The terms penetrating and perforating are commonly applied to ocular injuries that produce defects in the integrity of the ocular coats (Fig. 3–1). A penetrating injury partially cuts or tears a structure. A perforation is a through and through injury that completely cuts or tears through a structure. To use these terms properly one must specify the structure involved. For example, a corneal laceration is both a perforating injury of the cornea and a penetrating injury of the globe. Most corneal foreign bodies produce a small penetrating injury in the anterior stroma that is filled by the corneal epithelium, forming an epithelial facette (Fig. 3–2).

The ophthalmic pathology laboratory frequently processes eyes that have been ruptured by severe blunt trauma, have severe corneoscleral lacerations caused by sharp objects, or have been perforated by missiles such as BBs (Figs. 3–3, 3–4, 3–5). Pathologic examination of some severely traumatized eyes reveals a disrupted scleral shell filled with blood and scant remnants of intraocular tissue. Most cases show intraocular hemorrhage and loss or incarceration of intraocular structures. Massive intraocular hemorrhage typically involves the vitreous and the subretinal and suprauveal spaces. Loss of intraocular contents is caused by the space-occupying effect of expanding suprauveal hemorrhage and compression of the eye by the surrounding orbital tissue and forceful eyelid closure. Both mechanisms elevate the intraocular pressure and expel the intraocular tissues through the open wound. Tissues that are frequently lost or incarcerated in the wound include the iris, lens, ciliary body, vitreous, and occasionally the retina and choroid. Prolapsed intraocular tissue excised during the repair of corneoscleral lacerations should always be submitted for pathologic examination. If retina is found, the prognosis is poor.

Expulsive choroidal hemorrhage caused by an expanding suprauveal hematoma is a dreaded complication of ocular surgery. Intraoperative rupture of a sclerotic arteriole caused by the sudden hypotony of surgery causes an expanding hemorrhage in the suprachoroidal space. Spontaneous expulsive choroidal hemorrhage can also complicate corneal perforation in glaucomatous eyes (Figs. 3–6, 3–7).

## SYMPATHETIC UVEITIS

Expedient enucleation of eyes that are severely traumatized and hopelessly blind is strongly advised as prophylaxis against a rare autoimmune disorder called sympathetic uveitis, which affects and potentially can blind *both* eyes after unilateral trauma. Sympathetic uveitis (ophthalmia) is a severe bilateral granulomatous inflammation of the uveal tract that follows unilateral trauma or surgery, which usually is complicated by the incarceration of uveal tissue in the wound (Figs. 3–8, 3–9, 3–10). Blurred vision, photophobia, and signs of granulomatous inflammation develop in the uninjured (sympathizing) eye simultaneous with exacerbation of signs and symptoms in the injured (exciting) eye.

Sympathetic uveitis is thought to be an autoimmune response to antigenic material released by the injury.

Uveal pigment, retinal S-antigen, and interphotoreceptor retinoid-binding protein are possible antigens. Sympathetic uveitis occurs 2 weeks to 1 year after injury in about 90% of patients, most cases occurring during the 3 week to 3 month interval. Sympathetic uveitis generally does not develop if the injured eye is enucleated within 1 week of the injury. If enucleation of the injured eye is delayed, the noninjured eye remains at risk. There is some evidence that enucleation of the inciting eye decreases the severity of the inflammation in the sympathizing eye after bilateral uveitis develops.

Sympathetic uveitis is a clinicopathologic diagnosis. There must be a history of unilateral trauma followed by bilateral uveitis. Four characteristic features are found on histopathologic examination. The uvea is thickened by a diffuse granulomatous infiltrate composed of epithelioid histiocytes and inflammatory giant cells and lymphocytes of the T suppressor/cytotoxic subtype (Fig. 3–8). The choriocapillaris is not destroyed by the inflammation (sparing of the choriocapillaris). The epithelioid histiocytes and giant cells usually contain granules of phagocytized uveal pigment (Fig. 3–9). Nodular aggregates of epithelioid cells, which focally detach the retinal pigment epithelium, are found on the inner surface of Bruch's membrane (Fig. 3–10). These Dalen-Fuchs nodules are not pathognomonic for sympathetic uveitis because they also occur in sarcoidosis and Vogt-Koyanagi-Harada disease. The uveal infiltrate rarely contains plasma cells. Eosinophilia may be found in deeply pigmented patients, in whom the inflammation typically is more severe. Sympathetic uveitis usually spares the retina. One should consider another diagnosis if retinal involvement is found distant from the site of injury. Rare cases of sympathetic uveitis have been reported after ocular evisceration, probably related to antigenic material left behind in scleral emissarial canals, which typically are involved by granulomatous inflammation. Although their immunopathogenic mechanisms

differ, sympathetic ophthalmia and phacoantigenic uveitis may occur concurrently in a traumatized eye.

## CONTUSION INJURIES

Minor contusion injuries often cause abrasions of the corneal epithelium that rapidly heal by epithelial sliding (Fig. 3–11). Severe contusion injuries can rupture the cornea and sclera. A rupture caused by blunt trauma can occur directly at the site of impact. In other instances, the thinnest parts of the globe such as the limbus or the sclera behind the insertion of the rectus muscles or adjacent to the optic nerve are involved indirectly by force vectors transmitted by the essentially incompressible globe.

Contusion injuries need not disrupt the integrity of the cornea or sclera to wreak severe intraocular havoc. Ocular contusion injuries can rupture Descemet's membrane, the lens, or choroid, detach or avulse the retina from its attachments to the ora serrata (Fig. 3–12) or optic nerve, or fracture photoreceptor outer segments causing Berlin's edema or commotio retinae. Late cystoid macular degeneration or macular holes are common sequelae. Other anterior segment complications include lens dislocation, contusion rosette cataract (Fig. 3–13), postcontusion angle recession, iridodialysis, cyclodialysis, and hyphema.

Blood staining of the corneal stroma is a potential complication of chronic hyphema (Fig. 3–14). Whether corneal blood staining develops depends on the health of the corneal endothelium, the intraocular pressure, and the duration of the hyphema. Blood staining may occur within 48 hours if the intraocular pressure is high. The corneal stroma contains small particles of hemoglobin, not intact erythrocytes. Golden brown granules of hemosiderin are found in the cytoplasm of the keratocytes.

During a contusion injury of the anterior segment, the lens and iris act together as a ball valve that confines the aqueous humor to the anterior chamber. The incompressible aqueous humor conveys the force of the blow to the weakest parts of the anatomy, which are subject to damage. The iris may be ripped from the ciliary body at its root where it is thin (iridodialysis). In other cases the tenuous attachment of the ciliary muscle to the scleral spur is disrupted, causing detachment of the ciliary body or cyclodialysis (Fig. 3–15).

Tears into the anterior face of the ciliary body cause postcontusion angle recession (Figs. 3–16, 3–17). The tear usually extends between the external longitudinal fibers of the ciliary muscle and its radial and circumferential fibers, which are located centrally (Fig. 3–16). The injury usually detaches in the inner uveal part of the trabecular meshwork and disrupts the greater arterial circle of the iris, causing anterior chamber hemorrhage (hyphema). The root of the iris is displaced posteriorly by the tear. Afterwards gonioscopy discloses widening of the ciliary body band. Microscopic examination of acutely traumatized eyes often reveals ischemic necrosis of the iris and ciliary body. In chronic cases the residual ciliary muscle typically has a fusiform configuration, reflecting ischemic atrophy of its inner parts.

Postcontusion angle recession can cause late-onset unilateral open angle glaucoma. When they are stable, patients who have had hyphemas always should be gonioscoped to exclude traumatic angle recession. Fewer than 10% of patients who have postcontusion angle recession develop glaucoma. Microscopic examination of blind glaucomatous eyes with recessed angles that are enucleated typically reveals a new layer of Descemet's membrane on the inner surface of the damaged trabecular meshwork.

## INTRAOCULAR FOREIGN BODIES

Fragments of foreign material often are left inside the eye during perforating injuries (Fig. 3–18). How well the eye tolerates an intraocular foreign body depends on the chemical composition of the intruder and whether it is sterile or contaminated with microorganisms. Foreign bodies composed of vegetable matter are often contaminated with fungi and typically cause a violent inflammatory response. In contrast, foreign bodies of glass and plastic usually are inert and are well tolerated. Iron foreign bodies, which are relatively common, have a toxic effect on the retina, lens epithelium, and aqueous outflow pathways if they are chronically retained. Ferrous iron is more toxic than ferric iron. Ocular siderosis is marked by the deposition of iron in epithelial or neuroectodermal derivatives (epithelia of cornea, lens, and ciliary body; iris musculature; retina; and retinal pigment epithelium, or RPE) (Figs. 3–19, 3–20). An identical deposition of hematogenous iron (hemosiderosis) can complicate repeated chronic intraocular hemorrhage (Fig. 3–21). Foreign bodies comprised of more than 90% copper incite a severe sterile purulent reaction, and retained fragments of brass or bronze that contain 70–90% copper cause deposition in Descemet's membrane and the lens capsule (chalcosis) (Fig. 3–22). An analogous deposition of copper occurs in these thick basement membranes in Wilson's hepatolenticular degeneration and are responsible for the characteristic Kayser-Fleischer ring and sunflower cataract.

## CHEMICAL INJURIES

Chemical injuries by strong acids and alkalis usually involve the anterior part of the eye. The severity of the injury generally depends on the nature and strength of the agent and the duration of contact. Acid burns are nonprogressive and generally are less severe than alkali burns because penetration is limited by a buffering action of the tissues. Histology usually shows superficial coagulative necrosis of the conjunctival or corneal epithelium (or both). In contrast, alkali penetrates deeply, causing denaturation of protein, saponification of fat, and necrosis of intraocular structures (Figs. 3–23, 3–24). Alkali injuries usually are progressive because the alkali is difficult to neutralize and the necrosis of stromal fibroblasts precludes replacement or repair of denatured corneal collagen. In addition, vascular occlusion caused by necrosis of the vascular endothelium produces tissue ischemia. Collagenase produced by polymorphonuclear leukocytes infiltrating the necrotic stroma contributes to corneal dissolution and ulceration.

## WOUND HEALING

Many complications that occur after ocular surgery are related to poor wound healing. Ocular wounds heal by the formation of scar tissue. The mechanisms involved in wound healing differ depending on what ocular tissue is involved.

The healing of limbal wounds (most cataract incisions) involves a proliferation of granulation tissue derived from the episclera and the substantia propria of the conjunctiva. Epithelial migration and an early proliferation of granulation tissue rapidly seal the superficial aspect of well apposed wounds; and a plug of fibrin, which polymerizes on the exposed collagen in the wound, prevents leakage of aqueous humor. The posterior wound gapes slightly, and elastic Descemet's membrane curves inwardly. Granulation tissue enters the external part of the wound at about 8 days and has extended the full length of the wound by 2 weeks. By this time migrating endothelial cells have covered the posterior wound. These cells eventually synthesize a new layer of Descemet's membrane. The fibroblastic component of the granulation tissue produces collagen, which is initially randomly arranged. As the scar matures and becomes less vascularized, collagen is progressively produced, and the fibers mature and undergo reorientation.

Unlike the limbus, the central corneal is an avascular site. Hence granulation tissue is not involved in the healing of central corneal wounds (Fig. 3–25). Initially, the lips of the wound swell, functionally sealing the wound, which gapes anteriorly and posteriorly. A fibrin plug forms, and Descemet's membrane retracts and curves inwardly. Neighboring corneal endothelial cells are lost. The anterior surface of the wound is reepithelialized by surface epithelial sliding, which enters the gaping anterior part of the wound and fills it with an epithelial plug. The anterior surface of the wound usually is reepithelialized by 12 hours. At 3–4 days after an injury, stromal fibroblasts enter the wound and begin to elaborate collagen. The plug of surface epithelium regresses as stromal wound healing proceeds, and regression generally is complete by 2 weeks. At that time the sliding endothelium has extended across the posterior defect and has begun to lay down a new layer of Descemet's membrane. During the next 6 months the cellularity of the scarred area gradually decreases, and the character and orientation of the collagen becomes more regular.

Unsutured wounds of the iris do not heal. Iridectomies remain patent unless they are closed by pigment epithelial migration. Most wounds in the lens lead to cataract formation. Small rents in the capsule may be closed by posterior synechias and repaired by fibrous metaplasia of lens epithelium and capsular reformation. The sclera itself does not participate in the healing of defects. Full-thickness scleral wounds heal by an ingrowth of granulation tissue from the episclera and the superficial choroid.

## SURGICAL COMPLICATIONS

Poorly apposed or poorly healed limbal surgical wounds cause a variety of postoperative complications. Leaky wounds cause serous choroidal detachments and loss and flattening of the anterior chamber, which can lead to secondary angle closure or corneal endothelial damage due to lens corneal touch. Poorly healed wounds also allow microorganisms to enter the interior of the eye and can provide an avenue for surface epithelial invasion of the anterior chamber. Incarceration of uvea or vitreous in wounds can contribute to permanent fistula formation (vitreous wick) and increase the chance of postoperative infection or epithelial downgrowth.

Epithelial downgrowth is a complication of surgical or nonsurgical trauma in which corneal or conjunctival epithelium gains access to the anterior chamber and proliferates on the back of the cornea, the trabecular meshwork, the anterior surface of the iris, and on even more posteriorly located structures (Fig. 3–26; see also Fig. 7–17). Most cases occur after cataract surgery or penetrating keratoplasty. Patients typically present with a translucent sheet of epithelial cells that slowly grows down the back surface of the cornea. In occasional instances where posterior corneal epithelialization is not obvious, epithelial downgrowth may present several months postoperatively with pain, glaucoma, and intensifying inflammatory signs. Several mechanisms can obstruct aqueous outflow in eyes with epithelial downgrowth, including sheets of epithelium covering the trabecular meshwork, peripheral anterior synechia formation, and blockage of the trabecular meshwork by desquamated epithelial cells.

Histopathologically, the intraocular epithelium may approximate the normal surface epithelium in thickness, or it may be markedly attenuated. The advancing edge of the epithelial sheet on the posterior corneal surface typically is prominent. Epithelium growing on vascularized structures such as the iris often is thicker than that on the cornea. The anterior surface of the iris usually is flattened by the epithelial sheet. Occasionally, the epithelium extends through the pupil onto the iris pigment epithelium and ciliary body, and rarely it extends onto the inner surface of the peripheral retina, causing a tractional retinal detachment.

Clinically, the presence of epithelium on the iris can be confirmed by laser photocoagulation, which causes blanching. The prognosis of epithelial downgrowth usually is poor. Although some cases can be cured by extensive *en bloc* resection of ocular tissue, the intraocular epithelial proliferation is often diffuse, extensive, and impossible to eradicate. Experimental studies suggest that a healthy population of corneal endothelial cells tends to retard epithelial migration via cellular contact inhibition.

Fibrous ingrowth also complicates poor wound closure, particularly when there has been intraoperative vitreous loss (Fig. 3–27). Incarcerated vitreous serves as a growth scaffold for fibroblasts, which invade the interior of the eye, produce collagen, and transform the vitreous into a mass of fibrous scar tissue.

Fibrous metaplasia of the RPE is another major source of intraocular scarring. RPE hyperplasia and metaplasia typically occur after retinal detachment, which abolishes the outer retina's normal inhibitory effect on RPE proliferation. Papillary proliferation, the formation of large drusen-like structures, and pseudoadenomatous proliferation of the RPE ensue. The RPE synthesizes large quantities of extracellular matrix material, including granular drusenoid material, collagen, and ultimately bone. Massive fibrous and osseous metaplasia of the RPE are commonly found in chronically blind phthisical eyes, which often must be decalcified before they can be dissected. The bone always is found on the inner surface of Bruch's membrane. The bone is mature lamellar bone and may contain fatty marrow (see Fig. 2–32).

The term phthisis bulbi is applied clinically to blind hypotonous eyes that are soft, shrunken, partially collapsed, and have a vaguely cuboidal configuration caused by traction of the four rectus muscles. Pathologically, the diagnosis of phthisis bulbi (atrophia bulbi with shrinkage and disorganization) is reserved for profoundly atrophic globes that have markedly thickened, folded sclera and generally unrecognizable intraocular structures. If the intraocular structures can be identified, the term atrophia bulbi with shrinkage is used.

Superficial absorption of ultraviolet light causes punctate keratopathy (welder's flash, snow blindness). Relatively low doses of ionizing radiation can cause cataract. Radiation-induced occlusion of the retinal capillary bed is the cause of radiation retinopathy.

# References

**Surgical Trauma**

Apple DJ, Mamilis N, Loftfield K, et al: Complications of intraocular lenses: a historical and histochemical review. Surv Ophthalmol 29:1–54, 1984.

Apple DJ, Mamalis N, Olson RJ, Kincaid MC: Intraocular Lenses: Evolution, Designs, Complications and Pathology. Baltimore: Williams & Wilkins, 1989.

Bettman JW Jr: Pathology of complications of intraocular surgery. Am J Ophthalmol 68:1037–1050, 1969.

Cerasoli JR, Kasner D: A follow-up of vitreous loss during cataract surgery managed by anterior vitrectomy. Am J Ophthalmol 71:1040–1043, 1971.

Friedman AH, Henkind P: Corneal stromal overgrowth after cataract extraction. Br J Ophthalmol 54:528–534, 1970.

Gass JDM, Norton EWD: Cystoid macular edema and papilledema following cataract extraction. Arch Ophthalmol 76:646–661, 1966.

Kohnen T, Koch DD, Font RL: Lensification of the posterior corneal surface: an unusual proliferation of lens epithelial cells. Ophthalmology 104:1343–1347, 1997.

Kuchle M, Green WR: Epithelial ingrowth: a study of 207 histopathologically proven cases. Ger J Ophthalmol 5: 211–23, 1996.

Magnante DO, Bullock JD, Green WR: Ocular explosion after peribulbar anesthesia: case report and experimental study. Ophthalmology 104:608–615, 1997.

McDonnel PJ, Patel A, Green WR: Comparison of intracapsular and extracapsular cataract surgery: histopathologic study of eyes obtained postmortem. Ophthalmology 92: 1208–1225, 1985.

Sassani JW, John T, Cameron JD, Yanoff M, Eagle RC: Electron microscopic study of corneal epithelial endothelial interactions in organ culture. Ophthalmology 91: 553–557, 1984.

Swan KC: Fibroblastic ingrowth following cataract surgery. Arch Ophthalmol 89:445–449, 1973.

Von Domarius D, Naumann GOH: Accidental and surgical trauma and wound healing of the eye. In Naumann GOH, Apple DJ (eds) Pathology of the Eye. New York: Springer, 1986:185–248.

Wiener MJ, Trentacoste J, Pon DM, et al: Epithelial downgrowth: a 30-year clinicopathological review. Br J Ophthalmol 73:6–11, 1989.

Williams DK, Rentiers PK: Spontaneous expulsive choroidal hemorrhage: a clinicopathologic report of two cases. Arch Ophthalmol 83:191–194, 1970.

Winslow RL, Stevenson W III, Yanoff M: Spontaneous expulsive hemorrhage. Arch Ophthalmol 92:33–36, 1974.

Wolter JR: Expulsive hemorrhage: a study of histopathological details. Graefes Arch Clin Exp Ophthalmol 219: 155–158, 1982.

**Nonsurgical Trauma**

Barr CC, Mitchell D: Penetrating ocular injury caused by nylon cord fragment from electric lawn trimmer. Ophthalmic Surg 14:741–743, 1983.

Blanton FM: Anterior chamber angle recession and secondary glaucoma. Arch Ophthalmol 72:39–43, 1964.

Broderick JD: Corneal blood staining after hyphema. Br J Ophthalmol 56:589–593, 1972.

Cox MS, Schepens CL, Freeman HM: Retinal detachment due to ocular contusion. Arch Ophthalmol 76:678–685, 1966.

Dunn ES, Jaeger EA, Jeffers JB, Freitag SK: The epidemiology of ruptured globes. Ann Ophthalmol 24:405–410, 1992.

Esmaeli B, Elner SG, Schork MA, Elner VM: Visual outcome and ocular survival after penetrating trauma: a clinicopathologic study. Ophthalmology 102:393–400, 1995.

Gregor Z, Ryan SJ: Combined posterior contusion and penetrating injury in the pig eye. I. A natural history study. Br J Ophthalmol 66:793–798, 1982.

Gregor Z, Ryan SJ: Combined posterior contusion and penetrating injury in the pig eye. II. Histologic features. Br J Ophthalmol 66:799–804, 1982.

Hagler WS, North AW: Retinal dialysis and retinal detachment. Arch Ophthalmol 79:376–388, 1968.

Helveston EM: Eye trauma in childhood. Pediatr Clin North Am 22:501–511, 1975.

Honig MA, Barraquer J, Perry HD, Riquelme JL, Green WR: Forceps and vacuum injuries to the cornea: histopathologic features of twelve cases and review of the literature. Cornea 15:463–472, 1996.

Kempster RC, Green WR, Finkelstein D: Choroidal rupture: clinicopathologic correlation of an unusual case. Retina 16:57–63, 1996.

Manche EE, Goldberg RA, Mondino BJ: Air bag-related ocular injuries. Ophthalmic Surg Lasers 28:246–250, 1997.

Martin DF, Awh CC, McCuen BW, Jaffe GJ, Slott JH, Machemer R: Treatment and pathogenesis of traumatic chorioretinal rupture (sclopetaria). Am J Ophthalmol 117: 190–200, 1994.

Meredith TA, Gordon PA: Pars plana vitrectomy for severe penetrating injury with posterior segment involvement. Am J Ophthalmol 103:549–554, 1987.

Messmer EP, Gottsch J, Font RL: Blood staining of the cornea: a histopathologic analysis of 16 cases. Cornea 3: 205–212, 1984.

Pearlstein ES, Agapitos PJ, Cantrill HL, Holland EJ, Williams P, Lindstrom RL: Ruptured globe after radial keratotomy. Am J Ophthalmol 106:755–756, 1988.

Rudd JC, Jaeger EA, Freitag SK, Jeffers JB: Traumatically ruptured globes in children. J Pediatr Ophthalmol Strabismus 31:307–311, 1994.

Russell SR, Olsen KR, Folk JC: Predictors of scleral rupture and the role of vitrectomy in severe blunt ocular trauma. Am J Ophthalmol 105:253–257, 1988.

Ryan SJ: Penetrating ocular trauma and pars plana vitrectomy. Trans New Orleans Acad Ophthalmol 31:129–136, 1983.

Schein OD, Hibberd PL, Shingleton BJ, et al: The spectrum and burden of ocular injury. Ophthalmology 95:300–305, 1988.

Smiddy WE, Green WR: Retinal dialysis: pathology and pathogenesis. Retina 2:94–116, 1982.

Spalding SC, Sternberg P Jr: Controversies in the management of posterior segment ocular trauma. Retina 10:S76–82, 1990.

Sternberg P Jr, de Juan E Jr, Green WR, Hirst LW, Sommer A: Ocular BB injuries. Ophthalmology 91:1269–1277, 1984.

Winthrop SR, Cleary PE, Minckler DS, Ryan SJ: Penetrating eye injuries: a histopathological review. Br J Ophthalmol 64:809–817, 1980.

Wolff SM, Zimmerman LE: Chronic secondary glaucoma associated with retrodisplacement of the iris root and deepening of the anterior chamber secondary to contusion. Am J Ophthalmol 54:547–562, 1962.

**Sympathetic Uveitis**

Auw-Haedrich C, Loeffler KU, Witschel H: Sympathetic ophthalmia: an immunohistochemistry study of four cases. Ger J Ophthalmol 5:98–103, 1996.

Croxatto JO, Galentine P, Cupples HP, Harper D, Reader A, Zimmerman LE: Sympathetic ophthalmia after pars plana vitrectomy-lensectomy for endogenous bacterial endophthalmitis. Am J Ophthalmol 91:342–346, 1981.

Font RL, Fine BS, Messmer E, et al: Light and electron microscopic study of Dalen-Fuchs nodules in sympathetic ophthalmia. Ophthalmology 90:66–75, 1982.

Gass JD: Sympathetic ophthalmia following vitrectomy. Am J Ophthalmol 93:552–558, 1982.

Green WR, Maumenee AE, Sanders TE, et al: Sympathetic uveitis following evisceration. Trans Am Acad Ophthalmol Otolaryngol 76:625–644, 1972.

Jakobiec FA, Marboe CC, Knowles DM II, et al: Human sympathetic ophthalmia: an analysis of the inflammatory infiltrate by hybridoma-monoclonal antibodies, immunochemistry, and correlative electron microscopy. Ophthalmology 90:76–95, 1983.

Lubin JR, Albert DM, Weinstein M: Sixty-five years of sympathetic ophthalmia: a clinicopathologic review of 105 cases (1913–1978). Ophthalmology 87:109–121, 1980.

Marak GE. Phacoanaphylactic endophthalmitis. Surv Ophthalmol 36:325–329, 1992.

Morse PH, Duke JR: Sympathetic ophthalmitis: report of a case, proven pathologically, eight years after original injury. Am J Ophthalmol 68:508–512, 1969.

To KW, Jakobiec FA, Zimmerman LE: Sympathetic uveitis. In Albert DM, Jakobiec FA (eds) Principles and Practice of Ophthalmology: Clinical Practice. Vol 1. Philadelphia: Saunders, 1994:496–503.

Wilson MW, Grossniklaus HE, Heathcote JG: Focal post-traumatic choroidal granulomatous inflammation. Am J Ophthalmol 121:397–404, 1996.

**Intraocular Foreign Bodies**

Hanna C, Fraunfelder FT: Lens capsule change after intraocular copper. Ann Ophthalmol 5:9–12 , 1973.

Masciulli L, Andersen DR, Charles S: Experimental ocular siderosis in the squirrel monkey. Am J Ophthalmol 74:638–661, 1972.

Rosenthal AR, Appleton B, Hopkins JL: Intraocular copper foreign bodies. Am J Ophthalmol 78:671–678, 1974.

Seland JH: The nature of capsular inclusions in lenticular chalcosis: report of a case. Acta Ophthalmol (Copenh) 54:99–108, 1976.

Talamo JH, Topping TM, Maumenee AE, Green WR: Ultrastructural studies of cornea, iris and lens in a case of siderosis bulbi. Ophthalmology 92:1675–1680, 1985.

**Chemical Burns**

Brown SI, Weller CA, Akiya S: Pathogenesis of ulcers of the alkali-burned cornea. Arch Ophthalmol 83:205–208, 1970.

Hirst LW, Fogle JA, Kenyon KR, Stark WJ: Corneal epithelial regeneration and adhesions following acid burns in the rhesus monkey. Invest Ophthalmol Vis Sci 23:764–773, 1982.

**Radiation Injuries**

Bagan SM, Hollenhorst RW: Radiation retinopathy after irradiation of intracranial lesions. Am J Ophthalmol 88:694–697, 1979.

Brown GC, Shields JA, Sanborn G, Augsburger JJ, Savino PJ, Schatz NJ: Radiation retinopathy. Ophthalmology 89:1494–1501, 1982.

Brown GC, Shields JA, Sanborn G, Augsburger JJ, Savino PJ, Schatz NJ: Radiation optic neuropathy. Ophthalmology 89:1489–1493, 1982.

Buschke W, Friedenwald JS, Moses SG: Effect of ultraviolet irradiation on corneal epithelium: mitosis, nuclear fragmentation, post-traumatic cell movements, loss of tissue cohesion. J Cell Comp Physiol 26:147–164, 1945.

Cogan DG, Donaldson DD: Experimental radiation cataracts. I. Cataracts in the rabbit following single x-ray exposure. Arch Ophthalmol 45:508–522, 1951.

Noble KG, Kupersmith MJ: Retinal vascular remodelling in radiation retinopathy. Br J Ophthalmol 68:475–478, 1984.

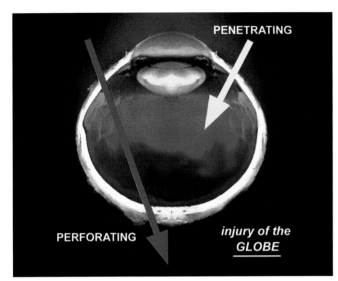

FIGURE 3–1 • **Penetrating and perforating ocular injuries.** A penetrating injury enters, but does not pass through, a structure. A perforation is a through-and-through injury that completely cuts or tears through a structure. The structure involved must be specified.

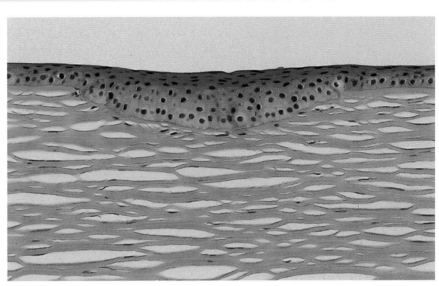

FIGURE 3–2 • **Epithelial facette, cornea.** Epithelium fills crater in Bowman's membrane and anterior stroma caused by corneal foreign body. Hematoxylin-eosin, ×100.

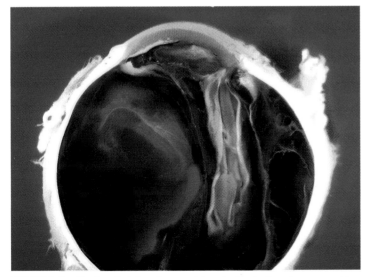

FIGURE 3–3 • **Ruptured globe.** Lens and detached retinal are incarcerated in a sutured limbal wound. The anterior chamber is flat, and part of the iris is absent. A massive suprauveal hemorrhage fills half of the posterior segment.

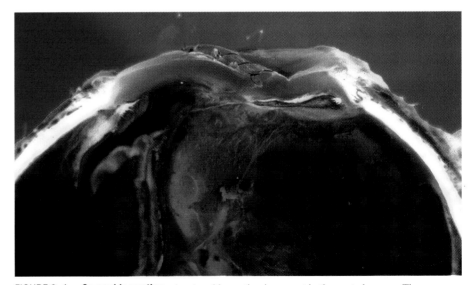

FIGURE 3–4 • **Corneal laceration.** A sutured laceration is present in the central cornea. The lens and half of the iris are absent, and the detached retina is drawn toward the wound. Most of the blood filling the interior of the eye is located in the suprauveal space.

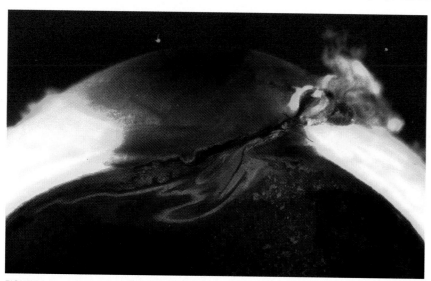

FIGURE 3–5 • **Uveal and retinal incarceration in a limbal wound.** Pigmented uveal tissue and an orange band of the detached retina extend extraocularly through the scleral wound. Degenerated blood fills the interior of the globe.

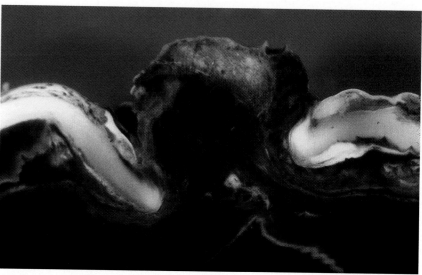

FIGURE 3–6 • **Spontaneous expulsive hemorrhage.** Knuckle of uveal tissue is expelled extraocularly through lips of gaping perforation in infected cornea by massive suprauveal hemorrhage. A hypopyon fills the residual anterior chamber.

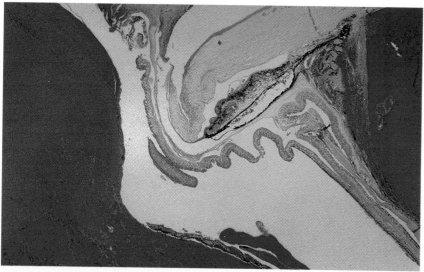

FIGURE 3–7 • **Spontaneous expulsive hemorrhage.** Detached retina and hemorrhagic detachment of choroid extend extraocularly through perforation in an infected cornea. Blood detaches the ciliary body at right. Neovascular glaucoma predisposed to acute keratitis and corneal perforation. Hematoxylin-eosin, ×5.

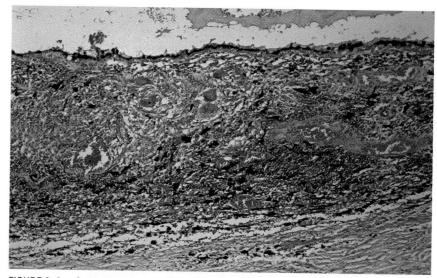

FIGURE 3–8 • **Sympathetic uveitis.** The choroid is massively thickened by a diffuse granulomatous infiltrate of epithelioid histiocytes, giant cells, and lymphocytes. The inflammation has spared the choriocapillaris. Hematoxylin-eosin, ×50.

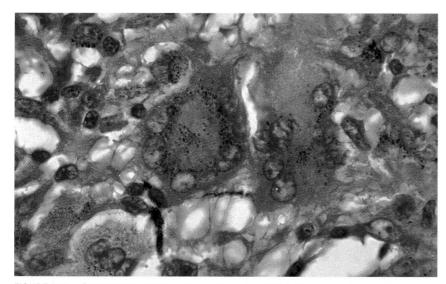

FIGURE 3–9 • **Sympathetic uveitis.** Giant cells in choroidal infiltrate contain granules of melanin pigment. Hematoxylin-eosin, ×5.

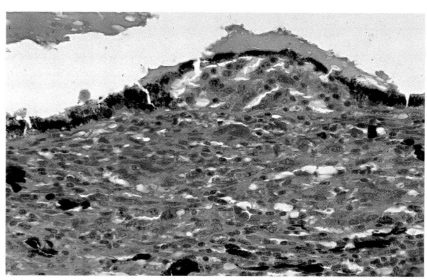

FIGURE 3–10 • **Dalen-Fuchs nodule, sympathetic uveitis.** Aggregate of epithelioid histiocytes on the inner surface of Bruch's membrane focally detaches the RPE. Underlying choroid contains diffuse granulomatous inflammatory infiltrate rich in epithelioid histiocytes. Hematoxylin-eosin, ×100.

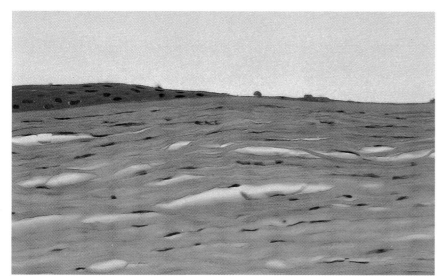

FIGURE 3–11 • **Corneal abrasion.** Sliding epithelium healing cornea abrasion has a tapering margin. Hematoxylin-eosin, ×100.

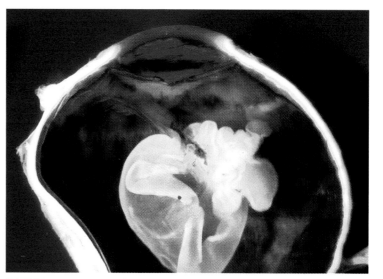

FIGURE 3–12 • **Anterior retinal avulsion, contusion injury.** The retina's attachments to the ora serrata have been disrupted. A hyphema fills the anterior chamber.

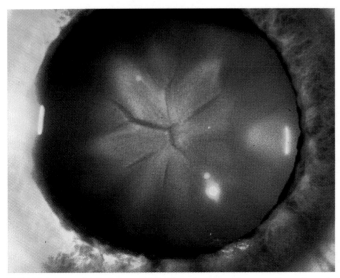

FIGURE 3–13 • **Contusion rosette cataract.** Petalliform configuration of traumatic cataract reflects damage to superficial lens fibers. This type of cataract serves as a clinical marker for an ocular contusion injury.

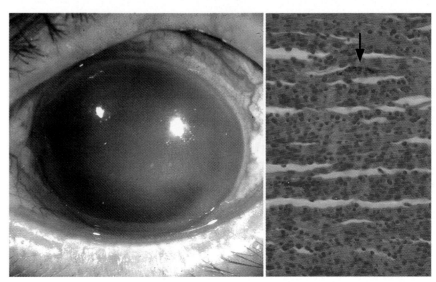

FIGURE 3–14 • **Corneal blood staining.** The corneal stroma contains small particles of hemoglobin that are much smaller than intact erythrocytes. One of the keratocytes contains granules of golden-brown hemosiderin pigment (arrow). Inset: hematoxylin-eosin, ×250.

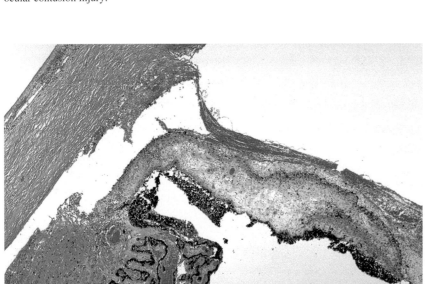

FIGURE 3–15 • **Cyclodialysis, contusion injury.** The ciliary body has been avulsed from its attachment to the scleral spur. The iris shows early necrosis. A hyphema is present. Hematoxylin-eosin, ×25.

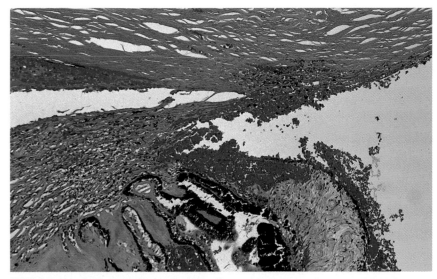

FIGURE 3–16 • **Acute contusion angle deformity.** Blood highlights a fresh tear in the face of the ciliary body caused by a contusion injury. Hematoxylin-eosin, ×50.

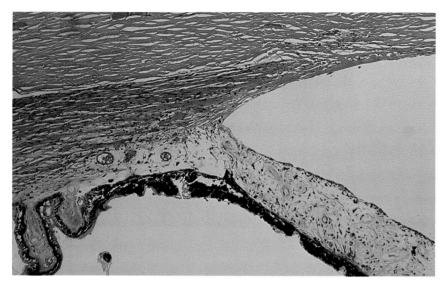

FIGURE 3–17 • **Postcontusion angle recession.** The iris root and ciliary processes are displaced posteriorly, and the residual ciliary muscle has a fusiform configuration. New Descemet's membrane covers the trabecular meshwork. Incidental pseudoexfoliation is present. Hematoxylin-eosin, ×50.

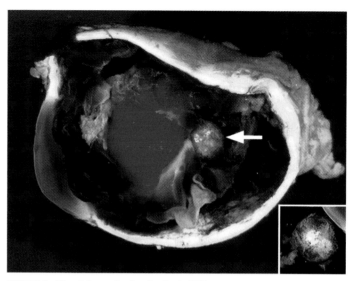

FIGURE 3–18 • **Intraocular foreign body (BB).** Arrow denotes a BB surrounded by blood and disrupted retina and choroid in the disorganized interior of a ruptured globe. A pars plana entrance wound is seen at top left. *Inset:* Foreign body.

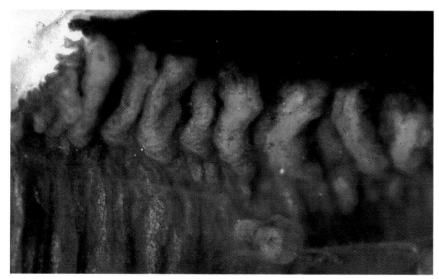

FIGURE 3–19 • **Siderosis.** Ciliary processes in eye with chronically retained intraocular iron foreign body show rusty discoloration.

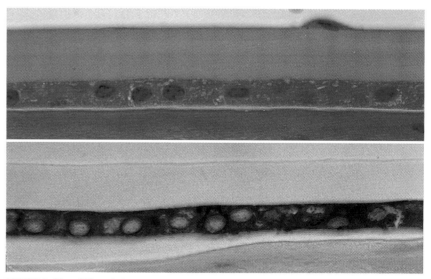

FIGURE 3–20 • **Siderosis lentis.** *Top:* Iron pigment in lens epithelium appears as brownish granules. Hematoxylin-eosin, ×250. *Bottom:* Prussian blue reaction for iron is intensely positive. Iron stain, ×250.

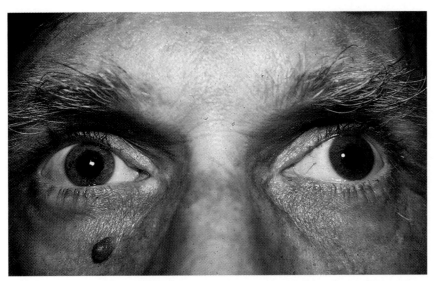

FIGURE 3–21 • **Heterochromia iridum, hemosiderosis.** Iris of a blind, exotropic left eye shows greenish discoloration caused by iron deposition. Chronic vitreous hemorrhage caused ocular hemosiderosis.

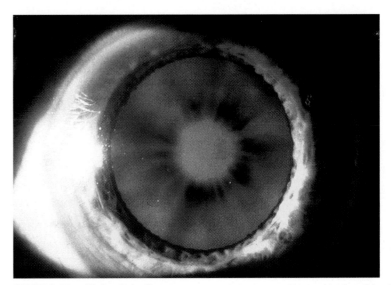

FIGURE 3–22 • **Chalcosis lentis.** A sunflower cataract caused by copper deposition in the lens capsule developed in this eye with an intraocular foreign body composed of copper alloy. The central disk of the "sunflower" corresponds to the diameter of the undilated pupil and the petals to radial ridges in the iris pigment epithelium. (Courtesy of Prof. Dr. med. Wolfgang Lieb, University of Würzburg, From Eagle RC Jr: Congenital, developmental and degenerative disorders of the iris and ciliary body. In Albert DM, Jakobiec FA, eds. *Principles and Practice of Ophthalmology. Clinical Practice.* Vol 1. Philadelphia: Saunders, 1993:367–389.)

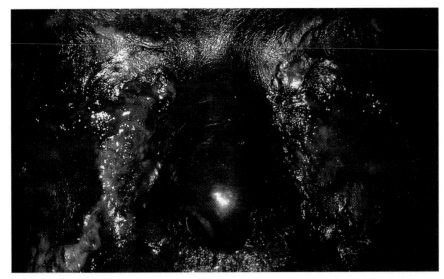

FIGURE 3–23 • **Alkali injury.** Patient was blinded by strong alkali drain cleaner poured on his eyes while asleep.

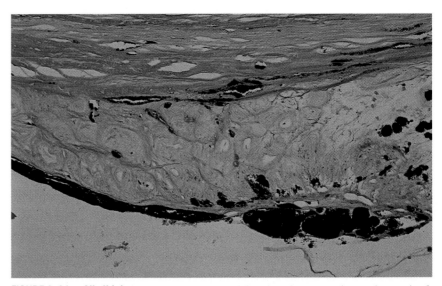

FIGURE 3–24 • **Alkali injury.** Alkali has penetrated deep into the eye causing total necrosis of the iris, which adheres to the posterior surface of the cornea. Necrotic iris and cornea appear acellular. Hematoxylin-eosin, ×50.

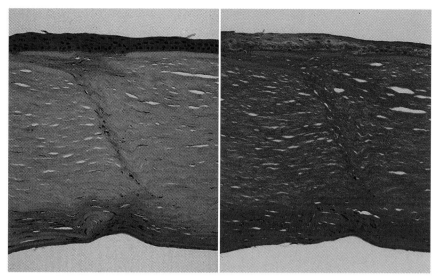

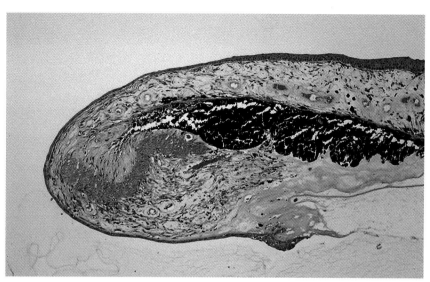

FIGURE 3–25 • **Scar of corneal laceration.** PAS stain (at right) highlights gap in Descemet's membrane in a scar of well healed and fairly well approximated corneal laceration. Right: Periodic acid-Schiff, ×50. Left: Hematoxylin-eosin, ×50.

FIGURE 3–26 • **Epithelial downgrowth.** A sheet of corneal epithelium introduced by trauma flattens the anterior iridic surface and extends through the pupil, which is bowed posteriorly by traction. Hematoxylin-eosin, ×50.

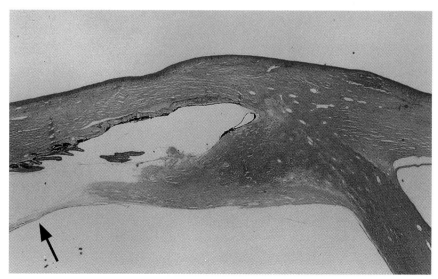

FIGURE 3–27 • **Fibrous ingrowth.** Thick membranes of dense collagenous connective tissue have formed on the scaffold of the vitreous incarcerated in a central corneal wound. An extensive anterior synechia is seen at top right. Arrow denotes anterior vitreous face. Hematoxylin-eosin, ×5.

# CHAPTER 4

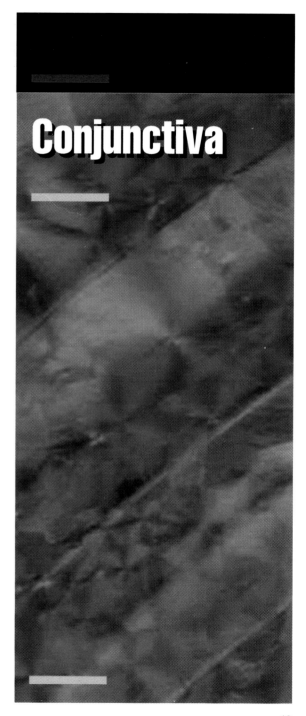

# Conjunctiva

The conjunctiva is a delicate mucous membrane that covers the anterior surface of the eyeball and the posterior surface of eyelids. The term conjunctiva is derived from Latin meaning "to bind together."

The nonkeratinized stratified columnar epithelium of the conjunctiva is two to five cells in thickness and contains mucous glands called goblet cells whose contents appear clear or bluish in routine hematoxylin-eosin (H&E) sections and are vividly periodic acid-Schiff (PAS)-positive (Fig. 4–1). Goblet cells are more numerous nasally, especially in the semilunar fold (plica semilunaris).

Topographically, the conjunctiva is divided into bulbar, forniceal, and tarsal (or palpebral) parts. The bulbar conjunctiva covers the surface of the eyeball and is freely movable. The stroma, or substantia propria, of the bulbar conjunctiva is composed of loose, areolar connective tissue and is easily ballooned-up by edema fluid (chemosis) or injected anesthetic. In contrast, the palpebral conjunctiva adheres firmly to the tarsal plate and does not move freely. Multiple gland-like epithelial invaginations or crypts called pseudoglands of Henle usually occur in the palpebral conjunctiva. The forniceal conjunctiva that arches around the superior and inferior cul-de-sacs is redundant and folded to facilitate eye movements. Several small accessory lacrimal glands of Krause are found underneath the forniceal conjunctiva, and accessory glands of Wolfring occur at the upper and lower margins of the tarsal plates. Lymphocytes and plasma cells normally are found in the conjunctival stroma and constitute part of the eye's normal defense mechanisms.

## DEVELOPMENTAL LESIONS

Congenital epibulbar dermoids are choristomatous masses that usually occur at the limbus temporally. They are comprised of coarse interweaving bundles of collagenous connective tissue and are covered by conjunctival or corneal epithelium or skin-like epithelium with epidermal appendages (Fig. 4–2). Epibulbar dermoids that contain cartilage or ectopic lacrimal gland tissue (or both) are called complex choristomas (Fig. 4–3). (A choristoma is a congenital tumor composed of tissue that is not normally found in an area.) Solid epibulbar dermoids should not be confused with dermoid cysts, which usually occur in the superotemporal orbit. Dermolipomas (lipodermoids) are solid dermoids comprised largely of adipose tissue (Fig. 4–4). These yellowish tan, soft fusiform tumors usually are located in the superotemporal quadrant. Bilateral epibulbar dermoids and dermolipomas occur in two thirds of patients with Goldenhar syndrome, which also includes vertebral anomalies, preauricular appendages, and aural fistulas. Epibulbar dermoids also occur in the organoid nevus (sebaceous nevus) syndrome. Other congenital lesions of the conjunctiva include ectopic lacrimal gland and episcleral osseous choristoma. Episcleral osseous choristomas are plaques of mature bone located in the superotemporal quadrant (Fig. 4–5).

## CONJUNCTIVITIS

Most inflammatory diseases of the conjunctiva are treated medically and are rarely seen in the ophthalmic pathologic laboratory, except as scrapings or smears. Conjunctivitis can be acute or chronic and can be caused by numerous infectious or noninfectious agents including bacteria, viruses, fungi, and protozoans. Allergy is another important cause of conjunctivitis.

The clinical manifestations of acute conjunctivitis include redness (conjunctival injection or hyperemia), chemosis, and exudation. The exudate in acute purulent bacterial conjunctivitis contains numerous polymorphonuclear leukocytes (polys) (Fig. 4–6). Histologic sections (obtained incidentally) show edema and infiltration of the conjunctival epithelium and substantia propria by polys and an exudate composed of a mixture of polys, fibrin, mucus, and necrotic cellular debris. Clinically, the presence of copious quantities of pus (hyperacute conjunctivitis) suggests the possibility of gonococcal infection.

Inflammatory membranes or pseudomembranes may develop in severely inflamed eyes. They adhere to the conjunctiva and are composed of fibrin and inflammatory cells. True membranes occur in Stevens-Johnson syndrome or bacterial infections by β-hemolytic *Streptococcus*, *Neisseria gonorrhoeae*, or *Corynebacterium diphtheriae*. True conjunctival membranes are firmly adherent to the epithelium, and bleeding occurs when removal is attempted.

Conjunctival pseudomembranes are less adherent and can be peeled without bleeding. Pseudomembranes may complicate infection by adenovirus 8 (epidemic keratoconjunctivitis, or EKC) and adenovirus 3 (pharyngoconjunctival fever, or PCF). They also form in patients with certain severe bacterial infections (*Staphylococcus*, *Streptococcus*, *Neisseria meningitidis*, *Pseudomonas*, coliforms) or complicate chemical burns, foreign bodies, benign mucous membrane pemphigoid, or ligneous conjunctivitis.

Ligneous conjunctivitis is a rare form of chronic pseudomembranous conjunctivitis marked by a massive accumulation of fibrin (Figs. 4–7, 4–8). The term ligneous refers to the firm, woody consistency of the large masses of fibrin that comprise the pseudomembranes. Ligneous conjunctivitis typically occurs in children and may recur in adults. Treatment is often challenging because the inflammation is persistent and the pseudomembranes frequently recur rapidly after excision. Histopathology shows two components: granulation tissue and sheets of intensely eosinophilic acellular amorphous material, which has been shown to be composed predominantly of fibrin by immunohistochemical stains (Fig. 4–8). The mass of fibrin also incorporates other serum components, such as immunoglobulin. The granulation tissue component (like all granulation tissue) is rich in acid mucopolysaccharide ground substance. Lesions that resemble those found in the conjunctiva can affect other mucous membranes including the larynx and vagina. Heritable defects in plasminogen have been identified in some patients with ligneous conjunctivitis who inherit the disorder as an autosomal recessive trait.

Acute anaphylactic conjunctivitis is marked by the abrupt onset of severe conjunctival edema (chemosis), mild injection, and itching. The latter is an important clinical symptom of ocular allergy. The release of inflammatory mediators such as histamine and serotonin by mast cells in the substantia propria causes the signs and symptoms in persons who are sensitized to antigens such as ragweed pollen or animal dander. Such atopic individuals produce immunoglobulin E (IgE), which is incorporated into the cell membranes of the mast cells. Mast cell degranulation occurs when the appropriate antigen is reencountered. The release of vasoactive substances markedly increases the permeability of conjunctival vessels, which leads to an outpouring of fluid that fills the areolar substantia propria of the bulbar conjunctiva, causing chemosis. Contact hypersensitivity to topical medications can cause severe ocular injection, itching, and eyelid erythema in postoperative patients.

## Chronic Conjunctivitis

Chronic follicular conjunctivitis and chronic papillary conjunctivitis are the conjunctiva's two basic patterns of response to chronic inflammatory stimuli. Chronic follicular conjunctivitis represents a reactive follicular hyperplasia of the population of lymphocytes that normally reside in the substantia propria. This lymphoid hyperplasia can be a reaction to a variety of stimuli. Conjunctival follicles are evident clinically as gray-white, round to oval elevations with an avascular center (Fig. 4–9). Microscopically, the substantia propria contains an intense basophilic infiltrate of benign lymphocytes and plasma cells that often has follicular centers (Fig. 4–10). The conjunctival epithelium overlying the lymphoid follicles is often thinned.

Conjunctival follicles occur in some types of acute viral conjunctivitis. They are typically observed in acute adenovirus infections such as EKC and PCF, herpes simplex virus (HSV) conjunctivitis, swimming pool conjunctivitis (Newcastle virus), and the acute hemorrhagic conjunctivitis caused by enterovirus 70.

Infectious causes of chronic follicular conjunctivitis include trachoma, psittacosis, *Moraxella,* and infectious mononucleosis. *Chlamydia,* small obligate intracellular parasites that are sensitive to antibiotics, cause trachoma, inclusion conjunctivitis, psittacosis, and lymphogranuloma venereum.

Trachoma is the most important infectious cause of blindness in the world. Trachoma is caused by serotypes A, B, and C of *Chlamydia trachomatis.* In endemic areas, trachoma is spread by direct contact with infected ocular secretions. Poor hygiene and insect vectors such as flies contribute to the spread of the disease.

Trachoma is marked by bilateral keratoconjunctivitis, which may be asymmetric. The initial infection involves the conjunctival epithelial cells and stimulates epithelial hyperplasia. Conjunctival smears stained with Giemsa stain show a mixed inflammatory exudate that contains lymphocytes and polys as well as large macrophages laden with phagocytized cellular debris called Leber cells. The conjunctival epithelial cells contain diagnostic basophilic intracytoplasmic inclusions of Halberstaedter and Prowaczek (Fig. 4–11). More specific direct immunofluorescence tests and enzyme immunoassays that facilitate the diagnosis are now available.

An intense infiltration of the substantia propria by chronic inflammatory cells follows the initial epithelial infection. Numerous lymphoid follicles occur on the upper tarsus. In florid cases, the follicles develop central areas of necrosis that can extend superficially, forming small ulcerations. Follicles also occur in the fornix and at the limbus. During the latter stages of the disease the remnants of follicles may be evident at the limbus as saucer-like depressions called Herbert's pits. As the disease progresses, papillary hypertrophy of the conjunctiva supplants the follicular response. Pannus formation is another characteristic feature of trachoma. The inflammatory pannus of trachoma is marked by a downgrowth of subepithelial vessels from the superior limbus that destroys Bowman's membrane. Scarring occurs during the late stages of trachoma. A linear scar called Arlt's line, which extends across the upper tarsus parallel to the lid margin, is one of the diagnostic criteria for trachoma listed by the World Health Organization. (Other diagnostic criteria include lymphoid follicles on the upper tarsus, a vascular pannus, and active limbal follicles or Herbert's pits. Two are diagnostic.)

Blindness in trachoma typically results from sequelae that develop during the cicatricial stage. Severe conjunctival drying and epidermalization result from the loss of epithelial goblet cells and obstruction of the ducts of the main and accessory lacrimal glands. Lid scarring also causes entropion and trichiasis, which predispose to severe corneal scarring, ulceration, and secondary bacterial infection.

Serotypes D through K of *C. trachomatis* cause inclusion conjunctivitis or paratrachoma in developed countries. Inclusion blenorrhea, an infantile form of inclusion conjunctivitis is an important cause of acute purulent conjunctivitis or ophthalmia neonatorum in the newborn. (Other causes include *N. gonorrhoeae* and a chemical conjunctivitis caused by Credé silver nitrate prophylaxis against gonococcal infection.) Infants acquire the disease from an infected mother during passage through the birth canal. Inclusion conjunctivitis is a venereal disease in adults. In contrast to the superior conjunctival involvement found in trachoma that has superior tarsal involvement, the follicles in inclusion conjunctivitis occur in the lower fornix.

Chronic follicular conjunctivitis can also be a response to cosmetics, topical medications such as atropine, eserine, or idoxuridine (IDU), viral particles shed by a molluscum contagiosum on the eyelid margin, or the feces of crab lice infesting the lashes (*Phthiriasis palpebrarum*). The lids and lashes should always be carefully (and expeditiously!) examined when unilateral follicles are encountered during the clinical examination.

Papillary hypertrophy is the second type of relatively nonspecific reaction that occurs in some patients with chronic conjunctivitis (Fig. 4–12). Papillary hypertrophy typically develops on the tarsal conjunctiva and is marked by proliferation of the conjunctival epithelium and hyperplasia of the substantia propria. Pale avascular valleys that contain deep infoldings of conjunctival epithelium separate individual papillae, which have a richly vascular stroma and a central tuft of blood vessels (Fig. 4–13). This contrasts with lymphoid follicles, which typically are avascular. Papillae contain a moderately intense infiltrate composed of a variety of inflammatory cells. Eosinophils and mast cells usually are present. The sheets of lymphocytes and follicular centers found in chronic follicular conjunctivitis are absent.

Giant papillae, which have been likened to cobblestones, occur on the superior tarsus in vernal conjunctivitis, a bilateral chronic recurrent disease that typically afflicts adolescents who have a history of atopy (Fig. 4–14). The term *vernal* reflects the characteristic exacerbation of signs and symptoms that occurs in the spring. Itching is a characteristic symptom, and patients have a thick, ropy discharge rich in eosinophils. Conjunctival smears contain eosinophils and eosinophilic granules. The large "cobblestone" papillae may abrade the cornea, producing painful shield-like abrasions of the superior corneal epithelium. A limbal variant of vernal conjunctivitis that has papillae at the superior limbus also occurs. The "limbal vernal" form is said to be more common in black patients. Horner-Trantas dots, which are intra- and subepithelial collections of eosinophils and cellular debris, occasionally occur near the limbus. Histopathologically, vernal conjunctivitis is characterized by papillary hypertrophy of the conjunctiva. The edematous fibrovascular core of the papillae contains an infiltrate of lymphocytes and plasma cells and numerous eosinophils.

Giant papillary conjunctivitis occurs in patients who chronically wear hard and soft contact lenses and even ocular prostheses. It is probably a cell-mediated hypersensitivity reaction stimulated by the accumulation of immunogenic material on the surface of foreign material. Giant papillary conjunctivitis shares similarities with vernal conjunctivitis but usually has fewer eosinophils.

Phlyctenular keratoconjunctivitis is thought to be a hypersensitivity reaction to bacterial proteins. It classically was associated with tuberculosis, but now most cases probably are related to staphylococcal blepharitis. Phlyctenular conjunctivitis is marked clinically by the presence of 2 to 3-mm whitish inflammatory nodules on the bulbar conjunctiva. A zone of dilated vessels surrounds the nodules, and the overlying epithelium is ulcerated. Microscopically the nodules are composed of acute and chronic inflammatory cells.

## Chronic Granulomatous Conjunctivitis

A chronic inflammatory infiltrate that includes epithelioid histiocytes and inflammatory giant cells occurs in several conjunctival diseases. Discrete noncaseating granulomas are found in biopsies from patients with sarcoidosis (see Fig. 2–12). The granulomas may be evident clinically as small yellowish tan nodules in the inferior fornix. Extensive subepithelial infiltration by sarcoidosis can stimulate symblepharon formation. The conjunctiva can be biopsied when sarcoidosis is suspected clinically, and a tissue diagnosis is required. A bilateral blind conjunctival biopsy is positive in about 50% of patients with sarcoidosis, despite the absence of obvious nodules or ocular inflammation clinically.

Granulomatous conjunctivitis with associated regional lymphadenopathy, usually a preauricular node, constitutes Parinaud's oculoglandular syndrome. The differential diagnosis of Parinaud's oculoglandular syndrome is rather extensive and includes a number of relatively rare infectious disorders caused by a variety of microorganisms including bacteria, spirochetes, *Chlamydia*, *Rickettsia*, fungi, and viruses.

Cat scratch fever is a relatively common cause of Parinaud's oculoglandular syndrome (Fig. 4–15). The disease is caused by *Bartonella henselae*, a bacterium that usually is inconspicuous in routine Gram stains because it is only faintly gram-negative. The infected conjunctiva contains an intense lymphoplasmocytic infiltrate with foci of necrosis. The Warthin-Starry silver stain often reveals masses of bacteria in the necrotic areas. There usually is a history of a cat scratch that typically does not involve the eye or face. Conjunctival involvement results from a bacteremia.

Granulomatous conjunctivitis in response to the irritating hairs or setae of certain species of caterpillars is called ophthalmia nodosa. The setae occasionally migrate into the anterior chamber causing severe intraocular inflammation.

Synthetic fiber granuloma is a foreign body giant cell reaction to a "fuzz ball" of synthetic fabric fibers lodged in the inferior conjunctival fornix (Fig. 4–16). Most cases have occurred in infants and young children. Synthetic fiber granuloma has been confused with ophthalmia nodosa histopathologically. Particulates of inorganic delustering agent incorporated into the fibers and knife chatter-marks on the ends of sectioned fibers serve to differentiate the synthetic fabric fibers from caterpillar setae.

Allergic conjunctival granuloma is a bilateral condition marked by the presence of yellowish nodules on the ocular surface, which is thought to be a response to parasitic infestation, probably by nematodes. Histopathology discloses granulomatous inflammation and eosinophilia centered around intensely eosinophilic deposits of antigen–antibody complexes called the Splendore-Hoeppli phenomenon. Nematode fragments are identified histologically in fewer than one fifth of cases.

Parasitic and mycotic infections of the conjunctiva are rare in the United States. Adult *Loa loa* worms that have migrated to the subconjunctival space occasionally are found in visitors from West and Central Africa. These worms causes itching, pain, and the disconcerting sensation of a mobile foreign body. Systemic infestation with *Trichinella spiralis* (trichinosis) causes fever, eosinophilia, periorbital swelling, edema of the eyelids and conjunctiva, and subconjunctival hemorrhages and petechiae. *Rhinosporidium seeberi,* an unusual fungus with a pathognomonic histologic appearance, causes strawberry-like papillary conjunctival granulomas studded with white microabscesses. Although rhinosporidiosis has been reported in the United States, most cases occur in India and Southeast Asia. Microsporidia and *Pneumocystis carinii* can cause conjunctivitis in patients with acquired immunodeficiency syndrome (AIDS) (Fig. 4–17).

Ocular cicatricial pemphigoid (OCP) is a systemic autoimmune disease with ocular and systemic manifestations. Thought to be a type II hypersensitivity reaction, OCP is believed to occur when environmental factors, probably viruses, stimulate genetically susceptible individuals to make autoantibodies against components of the conjunctival basement membrane (Fig. 4–18). A similar disease occurs in some patients receiving topical medication. Antibody deposition and complement activation cause chronic inflammation and stimulate fibroblasts to produce collagen causing abnormal conjunctival scarring. Conjunctival bullae rarely form in OCP. Progressive cicatrization causes foreshortening of the conjunctival fornices, symblepharon formation, and drying due to compromise of the lacrimal gland and meibomian gland ductules. The endstage of the disease is marked by epidermalization of the cornea and conjunctival epithelium and adherence of the lids to the globe. Routine conjunctival biopsies are nondiagnostic; specialized immunohistochemical procedures are required to show immunoglobulin or complement deposition in the epithelial basement membrane. These tests must be performed on fresh frozen-sectioned tissue.

Severe subepithelial fibrosis, symblepharon formation, severe ocular drying, and trichiasis complicate Stevens-Johnson syndrome (erythema multiforme), which is thought to be a type III hypersensitivity reaction to microbes or drugs characterized by circulating IgA containing immune complexes and lymphocytic vasculitis. Conjunctival involvement by pemphigus vulgaris is marked by bulla formation, but subepithelial scarring and symblepharon formation do not occur.

The normal reparative phase of the inflammatory response is marked by the production of granulation tissue, which plays an important role in wound healing. An inappropriate, exuberant proliferation of granulation tissue may develop on the surface of the globe or conjunctiva after surgery or trauma. The thoroughly ingrained term pyogenic granuloma is applied by ophthalmologists to these relatively common inflammatory tumors. The lesions are diagnosed as "exuberant granulation tissue (pyogenic granuloma)" to distinguish them from an acquired type of capillary hemangioma that dermatopathologists call pyogenic granuloma. (The latter lesions usually are relatively devoid of inflammatory cells and rarely occur on the conjunctiva or eyelid.) The richly vascular mass of exuberant granulation tissue usually has a smooth, rounded surface and generally is red or pink (Fig. 4–19). A paler hue may reflect superficial necrosis or adherent exudate. These lesions can arise rapidly, which serves to differentiate them from true neoplasms.

The mass of granulation tissue is composed of proliferating capillaries, activated fibroblasts with contractile properties called myofibroblasts, and a spectrum of acute and chronic inflammatory cells including polys, lymphocytes, plasma cells, histiocytes, and occasional eosinophils and mast cells (Fig. 4–20). The inflammatory infiltrate usually lacks epithelioid histiocytes and inflammatory giant cells unless it contains residual lipogranulomatous inflammation from a previously drained chalazion. The vessels in pyogenic granuloma usually radiate from the base or stalk of the lesion. This radial vascular pattern and the prominent inflammatory cell component differentiate pyogenic granuloma from hemangioma on histopathologic examination.

## DEGENERATIONS

Chronic light exposure damages the stromal connective tissue of the bulbar conjunctiva exposed in the interpalpebral fissure. This actinic damage is evident clinically as a yellowish white or gray-white opacification of the subepithelial tissue. In advanced cases a raised yellowish mound called a pinguecula forms near the limbus (Fig. 4–21). Microscopy discloses an acellular grayish granular deposit of extracellular matrix material underneath the limbal epithelium, which

usually is elevated and thinned (Fig. 4–22). Some pinguecula contain thickened vermiform fibrils of degenerated collagen; others contain deposits of hyaline material, such as those found in chronic actinic keratopathy. The damaged matrix material stains positively (black) with the Verhoeff-van Gieson stain for elastic tissue. Pretreatment with the enzyme elastase does not abolish positive staining for elastic tissue. Hence the term elastoid is applied. The degenerative process may involve the production of abnormal elastic tissue components by light damaged fibroblasts. Similar foci of elastotic degeneration often are found in pterygia.

Conjunctival amyloidosis usually is a localized phenomenon that occurs in healthy adults who do not have systemic amyloidosis (Fig. 4–23). The degeneration can involve any part of the conjunctiva. The subepithelial amyloid can form circumscribed polypoid, yellowish, waxy nodules on the epibulbar surface, or it may diffusely infiltrate the substantia propria. Light microscopy discloses relatively acellular amorphous deposits of eosinophilic hyaline material (Fig. 4–24). Special stains, usually congo red, and polarization microscopy are used to confirm the diagnosis.

## CONJUNCTIVAL CYSTS

Conjunctival cysts occur congenitally or may develop secondarily when surface epithelium is implanted in the stroma during surgery or trauma. Conjunctival inclusion cysts are lined by conjunctival epithelium, which may be attenuated. The lumen appears empty, or it may be filled with mucinous material, proteinaceous fluid, or both. Cysts also form when conjunctival crypts or pseudoglands of Henle become occluded and dilate. The proteinaceous luminal contents of such cysts occasionally undergo inspissation and even calcification, forming irritating concretions that literally feel like "grains of sand" in the eye. Another type of

conjunctival cyst is caused by blockage of an accessory lacrimal gland duct. Such cysts are analogous to sweat ductal cysts of eyelid skin. They have a clear, empty lumen and are lined by a dual layer of ductal epithelium.

## CONJUNCTIVAL TUMORS

There are three basic categories of conjunctival tumor. Most benign and malignant neoplasms of the conjunctiva arise from the squamous epithelium, associated melanocytes, or the lymphoid cells that normally reside in the substantia propria.

### Squamous Epithelial Lesions

Squamous epithelial lesions of the conjunctiva include benign papillomas, actinic keratoses, and a spectrum of intraepithelial neoplasia that can progress to invasive squamous cell carcinoma. Rare keratoacanthomas of the conjunctiva have been reported. Bilateral benign leukoplakic lesions occur on the conjunctiva and other mucous membranes in hereditary benign intraepithelial dyskeratosis.

Most papillomas of the conjunctiva are composed of multiple fronds, or finger-like projections, of conjunctival epithelium that enclose cores of vascularized connective tissue (Figs. 4–25, 4–26). The vessels in the fronds of the papilloma are visible through the transparent epithelium as multiple "hairpin" vascular loops. Conjunctival papillomas in children may be multiple, and they tend to recur after excision. Many probably are caused by human papilloma virus (HPV) infection.

The term papilloma signifies a growth pattern. Although most conjunctival papillomas are benign, malignant tumors of the squamous epithelium occasionally grow in a papillomatous fashion. In malignant lesions, the epithelium comprising the papillomatous growth is thickened and replaced totally or in part by atypical cells. The former is termed papillary squamous cell carcinoma *in situ*.

Squamous cell lesions of the conjunctiva tend to occur in the sun-exposed part of the conjunctiva near the limbus, where there is a population of proliferating stem cells. Clinically it is often impossible to distinguish between actinic keratoses, which recur infrequently after excision, and the spectrum of conjunctival intraepithelial neoplasia (CIN) (see below), which tends to recur, and includes cases of *in situ* and invasive squamous cell carcinoma.

Most actinic keratoses are focal leukoplakic lesions that occur on the surface of pinguecula or pterygia (Fig. 4–27). Histopathology discloses irregular focal acanthosis of the epithelium by atypical epidermoid cells, a surface plaque of parakeratosis, and actinic elastosis in the substantia propria (Fig. 4–28). Excisional biopsy is usually curative.

Conjunctival intraepithelial neoplasia is a spectrum of squamous epithelial disease, in which part or all of the conjunctival epithelium is replaced by the proliferation of a new clone of neoplastic cells spawned by a mutation in the basal germinative layer. Intraepithelial neoplasia is often called conjunctival dysplasia. The newer term CIN is derived from terminology applied to an analogous spectrum of intraepithelial malignancy that involves the uterine cervix. The term Bowen's disease should never be applied to the conjunctiva.

Most cases of CIN arise near the limbus in the interpalpebral part of the conjunctiva (Figs. 4–29, 4–30). The palpebral conjunctiva is rarely affected. Patients usually have a history of extensive sun exposure. In many cases the abnormal epithelium appears diffusely thickened and has a gelatinous appearance clinically. Leukoplakia may be present. More advanced lesions form epibulbar tumors that may have a vascularized, papillary configuration. Corneal involvement may be evident as contiguous areas of grayish epithelial thickening.

Microscopic examination typically shows an abrupt transition between the normal conjunctival epithelium and the affected part (Fig. 4–31). Compared to normal epithelium, the dysplastic epithelium shows increased cellularity, poor maturation, and a disorderly arrangement of its cells (Fig. 4–32). Part or all of the epithelium is replaced by the new clone of neoplastic cells. The basal part of the epithelium is replaced first because the mutational event occurs there. The involved epithelium is often massively thickened or acanthotic, sometimes measuring 8–10 times normal thickness. The abnormal cells may have a spindled configuration with scant cytoplasm or may show epidermoid differentiation with copious quantities of eosinophilic cytoplasm. Varying degrees of atypia are possible. Mitoses are not confined to the basal cell layer where mitotic activity normally takes place; they may be found throughout the thickened epithelium. Lesions caused by HPV infection may show koilocytosis (Fig. 4–33).

Depending on the amount of surface differentiation that persists, the lesion is roughly graded as mild, moderate, or severe dysplasia. If the entire thickness of the epithelium is replaced and there is no evidence of maturation or surface differentiation, the process is termed carcinoma *in situ* (Fig. 4–31). The malignant cells are still confined by the epithelial basement membrane in carcinoma *in situ*. Carcinoma *in situ* has a good prognosis because the cells have not gained access to the blood vessels and lymphatics in the conjunctival stroma.

Intraepithelial carcinoma can progress to invasive squamous cell carcinoma (Fig. 4–34). This occurs when tumor cells break through the epithelial basement membrane and invade the conjunctival stroma. Invasive squamous cell carcinoma does have a potential for metastatic spread (usually to regional lymph nodes), but the frequency of metastasis fortunately is low. In many cases the squamous cell carcinoma tends to be papillary in configuration and forms an exophytic mass on the surface of the globe (Fig. 4–35).

Most conjunctival squamous cell carcinomas remain superficial and rarely invade the eye or orbit. Most are successfully eradicated by local excision. Invasion of the eye or orbit occurs infrequently, but enucleation or orbital exenteration (or both) occasionally are required (Fig. 4–36). Poorly differentiated spindle cell carcinomas or mucoepidermoid carcinomas of the conjunctiva can behave aggressively, as can tumors in immunosuppressed patients. Mucoepidermoid carcinomas contain pools of mucous and goblet cells (Fig. 4–37). Positive immunohistochemical stains for cytokeratin may be necessary to differentiate spindle cell carcinoma from other spindle cell tumors (Fig. 4–38).

Hereditary benign intraepithelial dyskeratosis is an autosomal dominantly inherited trait characterized by keratinized plaques of hyperplastic epithelium that occur bilaterally in the limbal conjunctiva and are associated with ocular injection (Fig. 4–39). The surface plaque of keratin is composed of round or oval dyskeratotic cells found throughout the thickened epithelium (Fig. 4–40). The condition is always benign. Although cases have been reported elsewhere, most affected patients belong to a triracial isolate called the Haliwa Indians from Halifax and Warren Counties in North Carolina.

## Pigmented Lesions of the Conjunctiva

Most pigmented lesions of the conjunctiva are composed of melanocytes. Melanocytic lesions of the conjunctiva include racial melanosis, benign freckles and lentigines, several types of nevi, malignant melanomas, and primary acquired melanosis, which is often an *in situ* form of malignant melanoma. Conjunctival pigmentation can develop in certain systemic diseases such as Addison's disease and ochronosis (Fig. 4–41), or it may be caused by systemic (phenothiazines, tetracycline) or topical (epinephrine) drugs or the deposition of metals such as silver (argyrosis) (Fig. 4–42).

Conjunctival freckles, or ephelides, are flat patches of pigmentation. Histopathology shows increased pigmentation of the epithelial basal cell layer. An identical picture may be found in the early stages of primary acquired melanosis.

Conjunctival nevi are benign hamartomatous tumors composed of modified melanocytes called nevus cells derived embryologically from the neural crest (Figs. 4–43, 4–44, 4–45). Although nevi are considered to be congenital lesions, they often are detected toward the end of the first decade of life. Apparent growth and increased pigmentation of conjunctival nevi is often caused by elevated levels of hormones during puberty or pregnancy (Fig. 4–44). Excisional biopsy is usually performed for cosmetic reasons or when apparent enlargement or the deepening of pigmentation raises concern about possible malignant transformation.

Conjunctival nevi are classified topographically based on the location of the nevus cells in relation to the epithelium. The nevus cells are located at the epithelial–subepithelial junction in junctional nevi. Nevus cells are confined to the conjunctival stroma in subepithelial nevi, which are the counterpart of intradermal nevi in the skin. Most conjunctival nevi are compound nevi that have both junctional and subepithelial components (Fig. 4–45). Junctional activity tends to decrease markedly with age. Junctional nevi are rare during childhood and almost never occur in adults. Hence any lesion in an adult that appears to be a junctional nevus should be considered to be primary acquired melanosis until proven otherwise. Strictly subepithelial nevi generally are found in older adults.

Microscopically, nevus cells often form aggregates called nests. Polarity may be present; that is, more superficial nevus cells tend to be large, whereas cells deeper in the stroma tend to be small and may have a lymphocytoid appearance, reflecting scanty cytoplasm. Bland multinucleated nevoid giant cells are seen in some cases.

Most compound conjunctival nevi are cystic; the nevus contains cystic invaginations and occasionally solid rests of conjunctival epithelium (Fig. 4–45). These intralesional microcysts can be seen with the slit lamp in some cases, an observation that suggests the diagnosis. The pigment content of conjunctival nevi varies markedly. Some nevi are dark brown, whereas others are totally amelanotic and may appear pink if inflamed.

Blue nevi are composed of melanocytes located deep to the epithelium in the stroma or epibulbar tissues. Blue nevi are composed of bland dendritiform melanocytes. A deep blue nevus that typically involves the deep stroma, epibulbar connective tissue, and adnexal skin occurs in congenital oculodermal melanocytosis, or the nevus of Ota (Fig. 4–46). Patients with Ota's nevus typically have congenital hyperchromic heterochromia iridum (involved eye is darker) caused by a diffuse nevus of the ipsilateral uveal tract (Fig. 4–47). Caucasian patients with oculodermal melanocytosis are at risk for uveal, orbital, and central nervous system (CNS) malignant melanoma, but not conjunctival melanoma. Blue nevi appear blue or slate-gray because the longer wavelengths of light are absorbed or scattered as the light passes through the epithelium and connective tissue of the overlying conjunctiva (Fig. 4–48). The conjunctiva moves freely over the deeply situated pigmented cells (Fig. 4–49). If the conjunctival pigmentation moves, the pigment or pigmented cells are associated with the epithelium.

## Primary Acquired Melanosis and Conjunctival Melanoma

Although conjunctival melanomas can arise *de novo* or from preexisting nevi, almost three fourths develop from a form of *in situ* atypical melanocytic proliferation called primary acquired melanosis (PAM). Clinically, PAM appears as patchy acquired unilateral pigmentation of the conjunctiva that usually affects middle-aged or elderly white individuals (Fig. 4–50). The onset is insidious, and the pigmentation may wax and wane. The acquired and unilateral nature of the pigmentation serves to distinguish PAM from racial melanosis, which occurs bilaterally in heavily pigmented races. PAM can affect black patients, but it is exceedingly rare. PAM is important because about 20% of patients go on to develop invasive malignant melanoma.

Primary acquired melanosis has been classified into benign and malignant variants histopathologically. Invasive malignant melanomas arise from PAM with atypia. Benign PAM includes cases with freckle-like pigmentation of the epithelial basal cell layer or basal hyperplasia of benign-appearing melanocytes (Fig. 4–51). PAM with atypia shows atypical melanocytic hyperplasia that infiltrates and replaces part or all of the epithelium (Fig. 4–52). In some cases the atypical melanocytes eventually break through the epithelial basement membrane and invade the substantia propria, forming invasive conjunctival malignant melanoma (Fig. 4–53). Only 20% of patients go on to develop invasive melanoma if the hyperplasia of atypical melanocytes is confined to the basal part of the epithelium. If the atypical melanocytes include epithelioid cells or if there is extensive pagetoid intraepithelial spread or replacement of the epithelium by atypical cells (*in situ* melanoma), the prognosis is more guarded; 75% and 90% of these patients, respectively, develop malignant melanoma.

Patients with primary acquired melanosis should be followed closely with photographic documentation. Areas of conjunctiva that become thickened and are presumed to be melanoma should be biopsied excisionally. Multiple mapping biopsies to determine the extent of the disease have been recommended. Therapy is often challenging. In addition to local excision of nodules, extensive cryotherapy and topical chemotherapy with agents such as mitomycin C have been advocated. Orbital exenteration may be required if nodules of recurrent malignant melanoma invade the orbit. Such radical surgical therapy probably does not improve the prognosis for life but may be necessary to debulk the tumor and relieve local symptoms. Rarely, PAM is totally amelanotic and inapparent clinically. A nodule of invasive melanoma usually is the presenting sign of PAM sine pigmento.

Conjunctival melanomas are relatively rare tumors (Figs. 4–54, 4–55). There are about 10 uveal melanomas for every conjunctival melanoma in the Registry of Ophthalmic Pathology at the Armed Forces Institute of Pathology. Although its behavior is unpredictable, conjunctival melanoma has a better prognosis than uveal melanoma of the ciliary body or choroid. The overall mortality is about 26%. Most (75%) conjunctival melanomas appear to arise from PAM with atypia. Some patients do have a history of an antecedent presumed or biopsy-confirmed conjunctival nevus. Remnants of a nevus are found histopathologically in about one fourth of cases. Some conjunctival melanomas arise *de novo*.

Conjunctival melanomas do not behave like uveal tumors. Although they do contain spindle and epithelioid cells, the Callender classification for uveal melanoma is not applicable to them. Initially, conjunctival melanomas spread to regional lymph nodes, usually the preauricular or intraparotid nodes. Prognosis generally is poorer in patients with nodal metastases because the tumor cells gain access to blood vessels via anastomoses between vessels and lymphatics in the nodes. Some patients have been cured by the excision of involved nodes, however.

## Lymphoid Tumors

A spectrum of lymphoid tumors that includes reactive follicular hyperplasias, atypical lymphoid hyperplasias, and malignant lymphomas occurs in the conjunctiva. Many of the lymphomas are low-grade non-Hodgkin's B cell tumors of the mucosa associated lymphoid tissue (MALT) type.

Clinically, lymphoid infiltrates of the conjunctiva cause few symptoms because the infiltrate lacks a connective tissue stroma, is soft and elastic, and molds to the surrounding tissues. Conjunctival lymphoid tumors usually are salmon pink, reflecting the lesion's fine vascularity (Fig. 4–56). Conjunctival lymphoid lesions are covered by an intact layer of conjunctival epithelium. The surface may be smooth or pebbly and multinodular. The latter usually is seen with follicular hyperplasia or follicular lymphoma. Infiltrates typically present as a "salmon patch" in the fornix or on the epibulbar surface of the globe. In some instances the anterior aspect of an orbital lymphoid tumor is present underneath the conjunctiva. Imaging studies to exclude orbital involvement should be undertaken if there is uncertainty whether a lesion is purely conjunctival.

Histopathologically, follicular lymphoid hyperplasia (often called benign reactive lymphoid hyperplasia) is comprised of an infiltrate of mature well-differentiated lymphocytes, often with plasma cells, that contains benign reactive lymphoid follicles or germinal centers (Fig. 4–57). The reactive follicles are comprised of large, pale, mitotically active immunoblasts, and they harbor tingible body macrophages that contain basophilic bodies of apoptotic nuclear debris. These macrophages process antigen and present it to helper T cells to initiate the immune response. Specialized immunohistochemical stains show that B lymphocytes are concentrated in the follicular centers and the surrounding mantle zone. T lymphocytes predominate in the interfollicular zone between the germinal centers (see Fig. 15–13).

Although high grade conjunctival lymphoid tumors occasionally are diagnosed with routine light microscopy, many conjunctival lymphoid lesions are composed of a diffuse infiltrate of B lymphocytes without obvious cellular atypia (Fig. 4–58). Many of these tumors fall into an indeterminate category light microscopically and are called atypical lymphoid hyperplasias. Special immunohistochemical stains or flow cytometric analysis for cell surface markers show that most of these atypical lymphoid hyperplasias are diffuse monoclonal proliferations of B cells consistent with well-differentiated lymphocytic lymphomas. Antibodies such as L-26 (for B cells) and UCHL (for T cells) can differentiate B and T cells in routine paraffin sections, but immunoglobulin light chains (which are necessary to demonstrate monoclonality) often are too fragile to be detected. If lymphoma is suspected clinically and sufficient quantities are available, it is prudent to forward fresh tissue to the laboratory for immunophenotypic analysis by flow cytometry or immunostaining of frozen sections.

Conjunctival lymphoma generally has an excellent prognosis. Systematized lymphoma rarely presents in the conjunctiva. Lymphoma confined to the conjunctiva is associated with systemic lymphoma (prior, concurrent, or subsequent) in about 20% of cases.

## CARUNCULAR LESIONS

The caruncle is a small nodular island of skin surrounded by conjunctiva near the medial canthus. It is covered by keratinized epithelium and has sweat glands and pilosebaceous units with delicate hairs. Caruncular masses include nevi, papillomas, senile sebaceous gland hyperplasia, inclusion cysts, and oncocytomas. The latter are comprised of modified glandular epithelial cells with copious amounts of eosinophilic cytoplasm that is replete with mitochondria (Fig. 4–59). Rare cases of sebaceous carcinoma arise in the caruncle.

## References

**Developmental Lesions**

Cunha RP, Cunha MC, Shields JA: Epibulbar tumors in children: a survey of 282 biopsies. J Pediatr Ophthalmol Strabismus 24:249–254, 1987.

Dreizen NG, Schachat AP, Shields JA, Augsburger JJ: Epibulbar osseous choristoma. J Pediatr Ophthalmol Strabismus 20:247–249, 1983.

Eijpe AA, Koornneef L, Bras J, Verbeeten B Jr, Peeters FL, Zonneveld FW: Dermolipoma: characteristic CT appearance. Doc Ophthalmol 74:321–328, 1990.

Elsas FJ, Green WR: Epibulbar tumors in childhood. Am J Ophthalmol 79:1001–1007, 1975.

Gonnering RS, Fuerste FH, Lemke BN, Sonneland PR: Epibulbar osseous choristomas with scleral involvement. Ophthal Plast Reconstr Surg 4:63–66, 1988.

Lucarelli MJ, Ceisler EJ, Talamo JH, Jakobiec FA: Complex choristoma. Arch Ophthalmol 114:498–499, 1996.

Melki TS, Zimmerman LE, Chavis RM, Ellsworth R, O'Neill JF: A unique epibulbar osseous choristoma. J Pediatr Ophthalmol Strabismus 27:252–254, 1990.

Oakman JH Jr, Lambert SR, Grossniklaus HE: Corneal dermoid: case report and review of classification. J Pediatr Ophthalmol Strabismus 30:388–391, 1993.

Pittke EC, Marquardt R, Mohr W: Cartilage choristoma of the eye. Arch Ophthalmol 101:1569–1571, 1983.

Pokorny KS, Hyman BM, Jakobiec FA, Perry HD, Caputo AR, Iwamoto T: Epibulbar choristomas containing lacrimal tissue: clinical distinction from dermoids and histologic evidence of an origin from the palpebral lobe. Ophthalmology 94:1249–1257, 1987.

Roth DB, Shields JA, Shields CL, Eagle RC Jr: Lacrimal gland choristoma of the conjunctiva simulating a squamous cell carcinoma. J Pediatr Ophthalmol Strabismus 31:62–64, 1994.

Shields JA, Eagle RC, Shields CL, et al. Epibulbar osseous choristoma: computed tomography and clinicopathologic correlation. Ophthalmic Pract 15:110–112, 1997.

Shields JA, Shields CL, Eagle RC Jr, Arevalo F, De Potter P: Ophthalmic features of the organoid nevus syndrome. Trans Am Ophthalmol Soc 94:65–86, 1996.

Sugar HS: The oculoauriculo-vertebral syndrome of Goldenhar. Am J Ophthalmol 62:678–682, 1966.

## Conjunctivitis

Allansmith MR, Baird RS, Greiner JV: Vernal conjunctivitis and contact lens-associated giant papillary conjunctivitis compared and contrasted. Am J Ophthalmol 87:544–555, 1979.

Dawson CR, Jones BR, Tarizzo ML: Guide to Trachoma Control. Geneva: World Health Organization, 1981:7.

Eagle RC Jr, Brooks SJS, Katowitz JA, et al: Fibrin as a major constituent of ligneous conjunctivitis [letter]. Am J Ophthalmol 101:493, 1986.

Foster CS: The pathophysiology of ocular allergy: current thinking. Allergy 50:6–9; discussion 34–38, 1995.

Hidayat AA, Riddle PJ. Ligneous conjunctivitis: a clinicopathologic study of 17 cases. Ophthalmology 94:949–959, 1987.

MacCallan AF: The epidemiology of trachoma. Br J Ophthalmol 15:369–411, 1931.

Schuster V, Mingers AM, Seidenspinner S, et al: Homozygous mutations in the plasminogen gene of two unrelated girls with ligneous conjunctivitis. Blood 90:958–966, 1997.

## Granulomatous Conjunctivitis

Bergmans AM, Groothedde JW, Schellekens JF, et al: Etiology of cat scratch disease: comparison of polymerase chain reaction detection of Bartonella (formerly Rochalimaea) and Afipia felis DNA with serology and skin tests. J Infect Dis 171:916–923, 1995.

Margo CE, Hamed LM. Ocular syphilis. Surv Ophthalmol 37:203–220, 1992.

Nichols CW, Eagle RC Jr, Yanoff M, Menocal NG: Conjunctival biopsy as an aid in the evaluation of the patient with suspected sarcoidosis. Ophthalmology 87:287–291, 1980.

Obenauf CD, Shaw HE, Wyndor CF, et al: Sarcoidosis and its ocular manifestations. Am J Ophthalmol 86:648–655, 1978.

Spektor FE, Eagle RC Jr, Nichols CW: Granulomatous conjunctivitis secondary to Treponema pallidum. Ophthalmology 88:863–865, 1981.

Wear DJ, Raga HM, Zimmerman LE, et al: Cat scratch disease bacilli in the conjunctiva of patients with Parinaud's oculoglandular syndrome. Ophthalmology 92:1282–1287, 1985.

Weinberg JC, Eagle RC Jr, Font RL, et al: Conjunctival synthetic fiber granuloma: a lesion that resembles conjunctivitis nodosa. Ophthalmology 91:867–872, 1984.

## Parasitic and Mycotic Infections

Ashton N, Cook C: Allergic granulomatous nodules of the eyelid and conjunctiva: the XXXV Edward Jackson memorial lecture. Am J Ophthalmol 87:1–28, 1978.

Connor DH, Neafie RC, Meyers WM: Loiasis. In Binford CH, Connor DH (eds) Pathology of Tropical and Extraordinary Diseases. Washington, DC: Armed Forces Institute of Pathology, 1976.

Diesenhouse MC, Wilson LA, Corrent GF, Visvesvara GS, Grossniklaus HE, Bryan RT: Treatment of microsporidial keratoconjunctivitis with topical fumagillin. Am J Ophthalmol 115:293–298, 1993.

Friedberg DN, Stenson SM, Orenstein JM, et al. Microsporidial keratoconjunctivitis is acquired immunodeficiency syndrome. Arch Ophthalmol 108:504–508, 1990.

Reidy JJ, Sudesh S, Klafter AB, Olivia C: Infection of the conjunctiva by Rhinosporidium seeberi. Surv Ophthalmol 41:409–413, 1997.

Ruggli GM, Weber R, Messmer EP, Font RL, Moll C, Bernauer W: Pneumocystis carinii infection of the conjunctiva in a patient with acquired immune deficiency syndrome. Ophthalmology 104:1853–1856, 1997.

## Ocular Cicatricial Pemphigoid

Mondino BJ, Ross AN, Rabin BS: Autoimmune phenomena in ocular cicatricial pemphigoid. Am J Ophthalmol 83:443–450, 1977.

Power WJ, Neves RA, Rodriguez A, Dutt JE, Foster CS: Increasing the diagnostic yield of conjunctival biopsy in patients with suspected ocular cicatricial pemphigoid. Ophthalmology 102:1158–1163, 1995.

Sacks EH, Jakobiec FA, Wieczorek R, et al: Immunophenotypic analysis of the inflammatory infiltrate in ocular cicatricial pemphigoid: further evidence for a T cell-mediated disease. Ophthalmology 96:236–243, 1989.

Tyagi S, Bhol K, Natarajan K, Livir-Rallatos C, Foster CS, Ahmed AR: Ocular cicatricial pemphigoid antigen: partial sequence and biochemical characterization. Proc Natl Acad Sci USA 93:14714–14719, 1996.

## Amyloidosis

Blodi FC, Apple DJ: Localized conjunctival amyloidosis. Am J Ophthalmol 88:346–350, 1979.

Knowles DM, Jakobiec FA, Rosen M, Howard G: Amyloidosis of the orbit and adnexae. Surv Ophthalmol 19:367–384, 1975.

O'Donnell B, Wuebbolt G, Collin R: Amyloidosis of the conjunctiva. Aust NZ J Ophthalmol 23:207–212, 1995.

## Conjunctival Tumors

Grossniklaus HE, Green WR, Luckenbach M, Chan CC: Conjunctival lesions in adults: a clinical and histopathologic review. Cornea 6:78–116, 1987.

McLean IW, Burnier MN, Zimmerman LE, Jakobiec FA. Tumors of the eye and ocular adnexa, In Atlas of Tumor Pathology. Third Series. Fascicle 12. Washington, DC: Armed Forces Institute of Pathology, 1994.

Seitz B, Fischer M, Holbach LM, Naumann GO: [Differential diagnosis and prognosis of 112 excised epibulbar epithelial tumors.] Klin Monatsbl Augenheilkd 207: 239–246, 1995.

Shields JA, Shields CL, De Potter P: Surgical management of conjunctival tumors: the 1994 Lynn B. McMahan lecture. Arch Ophthalmol 115:808–815, 1997.

**Squamous Epithelial Tumors**

Brown HH, Glasgow BJ, Holland GN, Foos RY: Keratinizing corneal intraepithelial neoplasia. Cornea 8:220–224, 1989.

Cohen B, Green WR, Iliff N, et al: Spindle cell carcinoma of the conjunctiva. Arch Ophthalmol 98:1809–1813, 1980.

Erie JC, Collyer SK, Campbell RJ: Dehydrated cucumber slice as a mount for conjunctival biopsy specimens. Am J Ophthalmol 99:539–541, 1985.

Erie JC, Liesegang TJ, Campbell RJ: Conjunctival and corneal intraepithelial neoplasia: experience at the Mayo Clinic 1920–1983. Ophthalmology 93:176–183, 1986.

Illif WF, Marbeck R, Green WR: Invasive squamous cell carcinoma of the conjunctiva. Arch Ophthalmol 93: 119–122, 1975.

Lass JH, Grove AS, Papale JJ, et al: Detection of human papillomavirus DNA sequences in conjunctival papillomas. Am J Ophthalmol 95:670–674, 1983.

Lee GA, Hirst LW: Ocular surface squamous neoplasia. Surv Ophthalmol 39:429–450, 1995.

Mauriello JA Jr, Napolitano J, McLean I: Actinic keratosis and dysplasia of the conjunctiva: a clinicopathological study of 45 cases. Can J Ophthalmol 30:312–316, 1995.

McDonnell JM, McDonnell PJ, Sun YY: Human papillomavirus DNA in tissues and ocular surface swabs of patients with conjunctival epithelial neoplasia. Invest Ophthalmol Vis Sci 33:184–189, 1992.

Odrich MG, Jakobiec FA, Lancaster WD, et al: A spectrum of bilateral squamous conjunctival tumors associated with human papillomavirus type 16. Ophthalmology 98: 628–635, 1991.

Pizzarello LD, Jakobiec FA: Bowen's disease of the conjunctiva: a misnomer. In Jakobiec FA (ed) Ocular and Adnexal Tumors. Birmingham, AL: Aesculapius, 1978: 553–571.

Rao NA, Font RL: Mucoepidermoid carcinoma of the conjunctiva: a clinicopathologic study of five cases. Cancer 38:1699–1709, 1976.

Schubert HD, Farris RL, Green WR: Spindle cell carcinoma of the conjunctiva. Graefes Arch Clin Exp Ophthalmol 233:52–53, 1995.

Waring GO, Roth AM, Ekins MB: Clinical and pathologic description of 17 cases of corneal intraepithelial neoplasia. Am J Ophthalmol 97:547–559, 1984.

**Melanocytic Lesions**

Brownstein S, Jakobiec FA, Wilkinson RD, Lombardo J, Jackson WB: Cryotherapy for precancerous melanosis (atypical melanocytic hyperplasia) of the conjunctiva. Arch Ophthalmol 99:1224–1231, 1981.

De Potter P, Shields CL, Shields JA, Menduke H: Clinical predictive factors for development of recurrence and metastasis in conjunctival melanoma: a review of 68 cases. Br J Ophthalmol 77:624–630, 1993.

Dutton JJ, Anderson RL, Schelper RL, et al: Orbital malignant melanoma and oculodermal melanocytosis: report of two cases and a review of the literature. Ophthalmology 91:497–507, 1984.

Eagle RC Jr: Iris pigmentation and pigmented lesion: an ultrastructural study. Trans Am Ophthalmol Soc 87: 581–687, 1989.

Folberg R, Jakobiec FA, Bernardino VB, et al: Benign conjunctival melanocytic lesions: clinicopathologic features. Ophthalmology 96:436–461, 1989.

Folberg R, Jakobiec FA, McLean IW, Zimmerman LE: Is primary acquired melanosis of the conjunctiva equivalent to melanoma in situ? Mod Pathol 5:2–5; discussion 5:6–8, 1992.

Folberg R, McLean IW, Zimmerman LE: Conjunctival melanosis and melanoma. Ophthalmology 91:673–678, 1984.

Folberg R, McLean IW, Zimmerman LE: Malignant melanoma of the conjunctiva. Hum Pathol 16:136–143, 1985.

Folberg R, McLean IW, Zimmerman LE: Primary acquired melanosis of the conjunctiva. Hum Pathol 16:129–135, 1985.

Jakobiec FA: The ultrastructure of conjunctival melanocytic tumors. Trans Am Ophthalmol Soc 82:599–752, 1984.

Jakobiec FA, Folberg R, Iwamoto T: Clinicopathologic characteristics of premalignant and malignant melanocytic lesions of the conjunctiva. Ophthalmology 96: 147–66, 1989.

Jakobiec FA, Rini FJ, Fraunfelder FT, et al: Cryotherapy for conjunctival primary acquired melanosis and malignant melanoma. Ophthalmology 95:1058–1070, 1988.

Liesegang TJ: Pigmented conjunctival and scleral lesions. Mayo Clin Proc 69:151–161, 1994.

Liesegang TJ, Campbell RJ: Mayo Clinic experience with conjunctival melanomas. Arch Ophthalmol 98:1385–1389, 1980.

Paridaens AD, McCartney AC, Hungerford JL: Multifocal amelanotic conjunctival melanoma and acquired melanosis sine pigmento. Br J Ophthalmol 76:163–165, 1992.

Paridaens AD, Minassian DC, McCartney AC, Hungerford JL: Prognostic factors in primary malignant melanoma of the conjunctiva: a clinicopathological study of 256 cases. Br J Ophthalmol 78:252–259, 1994.

**Lymphoid Lesions**

Knowles DM, Jakobiec FA, McNally L, Burke JS: Lymphoid hyperplasia and malignant lymphoma occurring in the ocular adnexa (orbit, conjunctiva, and eyelids): a prospective multiparametric analysis of 108 case during 1977 to 1987. Hum Pathol 21:959–973, 1990.

Margo CE: Orbital and ocular adnexal lymphoma: evolving concepts. Ophthalmol Clin North Am 8:167–177, 1995.

Medeiros LJ, Harris NL: Immunuhistologic analysis of small lymphocytic infiltrates of the orbit and conjunctiva. Hum Pathol 21:1126–1131, 1990.

**Miscellaneous Lesions**

Kiratli H, Shields CL, Shields JA, DePotter P: Metastatic tumours to the conjunctiva: report of 10 cases. Br J Ophthalmol 80:5–8, 1996.

Margo CE, Grossniklaus HE: Intraepithelial sebaceous neoplasia without underlying invasive carcinoma. Surv Ophthalmol 39:293–301, 1995.

**Tumors of the Caruncle**

Chang WJ, Nowinski TS, Eagle RC Jr: A large oncocytoma of the caruncle. Arch Ophthalmol 113:382, 1995.

Hirsch C, Holz FG, Tetz M, Volcker HE: Clinical aspects and histopathology of caruncular tumors. Klin Monatsbl Augenheilkd 210:153–157, 1997.

Massry GG, Holds JB, Kincaid MC, Patrinely JR: Sebaceous gland hyperplasia of the caruncle. Ophthal Plast Reconstr Surg 11:32–36, 1995.

Rodman RC, Frueh BR, Elner VM: Mucoepidermoid carcinoma of the caruncle. Am J Ophthalmol 123:564–565, 1997.

Shields CL, Shields JA, White D, Augsburger JJ: Survey of lesions of the caruncle. Trans Pa Acad Ophthalmol Otolaryngol 38:528–534, 1986.

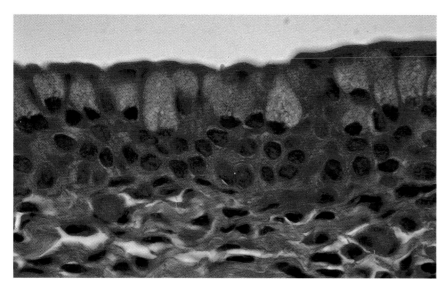

**FIGURE 4–1 • Conjunctival epithelium.** The stratified squamous epithelium of the conjunctiva is nonkeratinized and contains mucin producing goblet cells, which are most numerous in the nasal bulbar conjunctiva. Chronic inflammatory cells normally are present in the substantia propria. Hematoxylin-eosin, ×250.

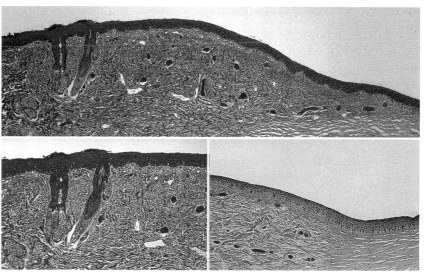

**FIGURE 4–2 • Solid epibulbar dermoid.** Epidermis-like epithelium with epidermal appendages covers apex of epibulbar choristoma and merges with nonkeratinized ocular surface epithelium on its sloping margin. The stroma is comprised of coarse interweaving bundles of collagen. Hematoxylin-eosin. Top ×25, bottom left ×50, bottom right ×50.

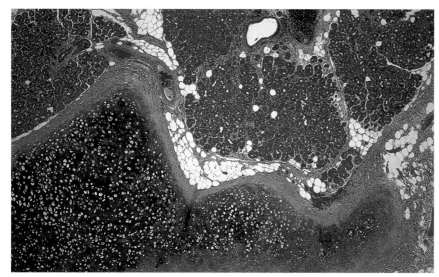

**FIGURE 4–3 • Complex choristoma, conjunctiva.** A choristoma is a congenital tumor composed of tissue that is not normally found in an area. This epibulbar complex choristoma contains hyaline cartilage, ectopic lacrimal gland, and fat. The surface of the choristoma was lined by skin-like epithelium with epidermal appendages. Hematoxylin-eosin, ×10.

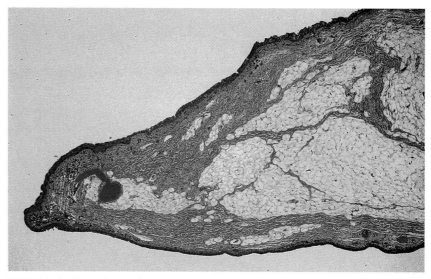

**FIGURE 4–4 • Dermolipoma (lipodermoid).** A dermolipoma is a solid epibulbar dermoid comprised largely of adipose tissue. Most dermolipomas occur on the superotemporal surface of the globe. Hematoxylin-eosin, ×10 .

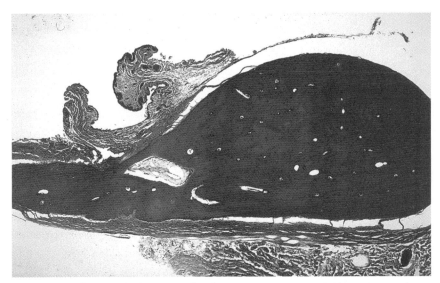

FIGURE 4–5 • **Osseous choristoma, conjunctiva.** This rare type of epibulbar choristoma is composed of a plaque of mature bone. Most occur in the superotemporal quadrant. Hematoxylin-eosin, ×10 .

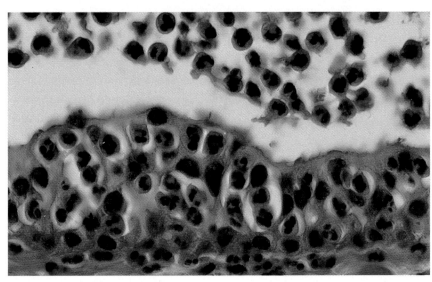

FIGURE 4–6 • **Acute purulent conjunctivitis.** Polys infiltrate the edematous conjunctival epithelium and are the major cellular constituent of the purulent exudate. The focus of acute conjunctivitis was found incidentally in a tumor resection specimen. Hematoxylin-eosin. ×250.

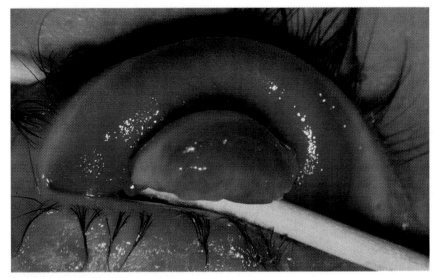

FIGURE 4–7 • **Ligneous conjunctivitis.** Inflammatory mass on upper palpebral conjunctiva had a firm, woody consistency. It recurred several times and was composed largely of fibrin. (Courtesy of Dr. Joseph Calhoun, Wills Eye Hospital)

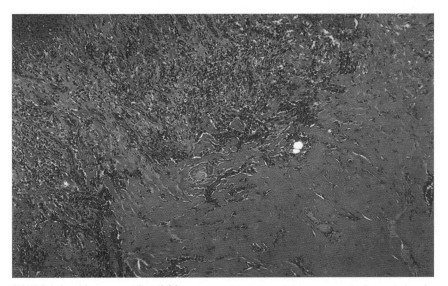

FIGURE 4–8 • **Ligneous conjunctivitis.** Ligneous conjunctivitis is composed of granulation tissue (*top*) and sheets of intensely eosinophilic acellular amorphous fibrin (bottom). Ligneous conjunctivitis has been linked to defects in the plasminogen gene. Hematoxylin-eosin, ×25.

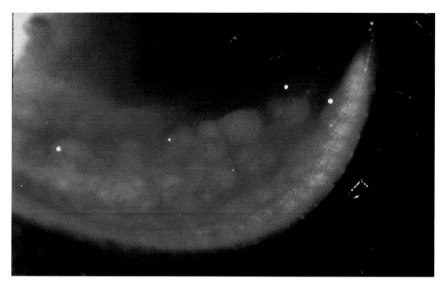

FIGURE 4–9 • **Chronic follicular conjunctivitis.** Conjunctival follicles are caused by reactive follicular hyperplasia of the tissue's normal resident population of lymphocytes. The round to oval, gray-white elevations are avascular centrally.

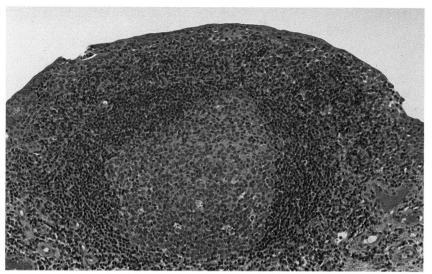

FIGURE 4–10 • **Conjunctival follicle.** The follicle is composed of an avascular sheet of basophilic lymphocytes. A germinal center is present. The overlying epithelium is thinned. Hematoxylin-eosin, ×25.

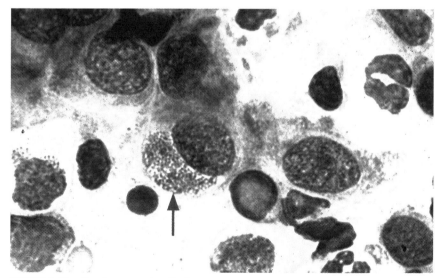

FIGURE 4–11 • **Trachoma, conjunctival smear.** Arrow denotes large basophilic intracytoplasmic inclusion of Halberstaedter and Prowaczek in an epithelial cell. The inflammatory exudate includes both polys and lymphocytes. Giemsa, ×250.

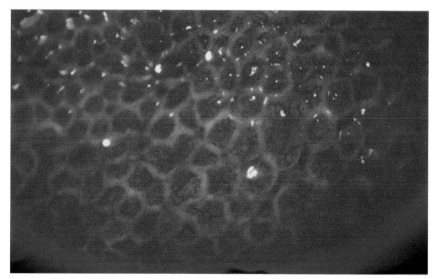

FIGURE 4–12 • **Conjunctival papillae.** Avascular valleys separate papillae on the superior tarsal conjunctiva. Fine vessels are seen in the center of the papillae. (Courtesy of Dr. Dario Savino-Zari, Caracas, Venezuela)

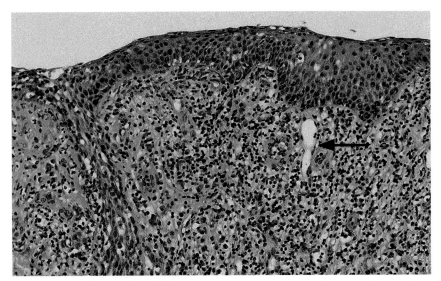

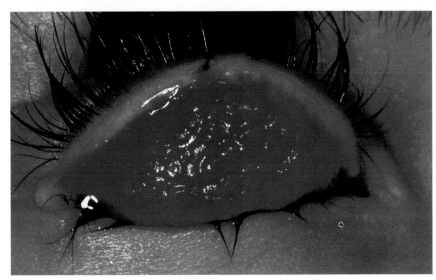

FIGURE 4–13 • **Vernal conjunctivitis.** Infolding of conjunctival epithelium (at left) extends into the valley separating two large "cobblestone" papillae. Arrow points to a central vessel in the papilla. Moderately intense inflammatory infiltrate includes chronic inflammatory cells and eosinophils. Hematoxylin-eosin, ×50.

FIGURE 4–14 • **Vernal conjunctivitis.** Large cobblestone papillae blanket superior tarsal conjunctiva.

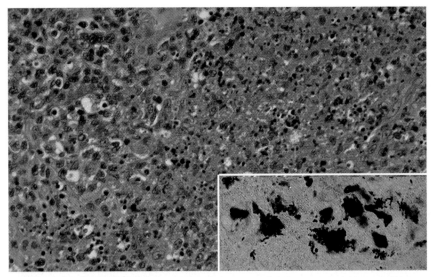

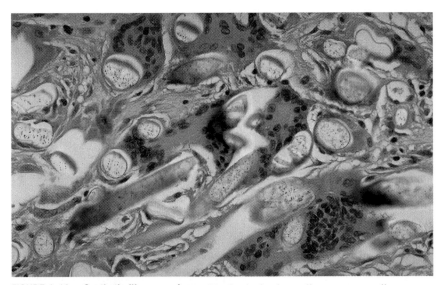

FIGURE 4–15 • **Cat scratch disease, conjunctiva.** The intense chronic inflammatory infiltrate contains a focus of necrotic karyorrhectic cells. Hematoxylin-eosin, ×100. *Inset:* Silver stain discloses masses of bacteria (*Bartonella henselae*). Warthin-Starry, ×250. The patient developed unilateral granulomatous conjunctivitis and a preauricular node after being scratched by a cat.

FIGURE 4–16 • **Synthetic fiber granuloma.** Foreign body giant cells encompass yellow synthetic fabric fibers that contain dark particulates of delustering agent added to opacify the plastic. Hematoxylin-eosin, ×100.

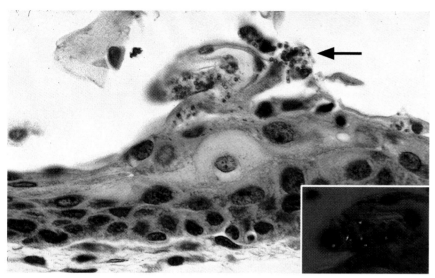

FIGURE 4–17 • **Microsporidial keratoconjunctivitis.** Arrow points to minute microsporidial parasites (*Encephalitozoon hellem*) in conjunctival epithelium from an AIDS patient with chronic keratoconjunctivitis. Hematoxylin-eosin, ×250. *Inset:* Polarization microscopy discloses birefringent polar bodies. Hematoxylin-eosin, ×250. (Case presented by Dr. Ramon L. Font at the 1992 meeting of Eastern Ophthalmic Pathology Society, Jekyll Island, GA)

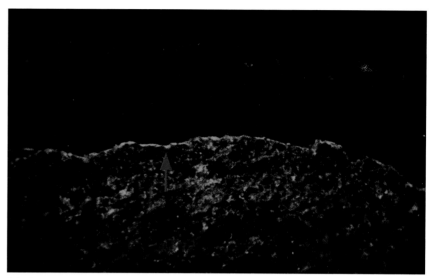

FIGURE 4–18 • **Ocular cicatricial pemphigoid.** Immunofluorescent microscopy discloses deposition of IgA in conjunctival basement membrane (arrow). Immunofluorescence, ×250. (Courtesy of Dr. C. Stephen Foster, Boston, MA)

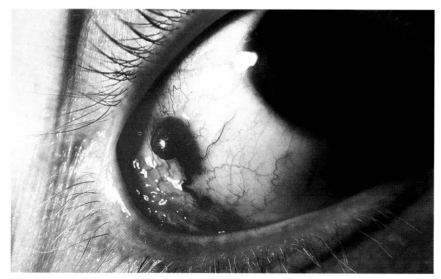

FIGURE 4–19 • **"Pyogenic granuloma."** Round, smooth, red mass of granulation tissue developed after strabismus surgery.

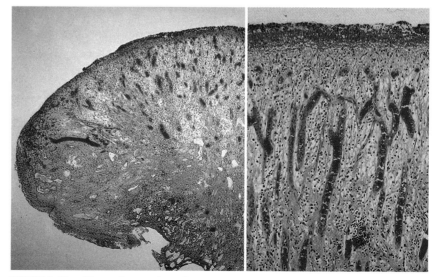

FIGURE 4–20 • **"Pyogenic granuloma."** Exuberant proliferation of granulation tissue forms smooth-surfaced pedunculated mass. Radially oriented vessels and inflammatory cells are seen at higher magnification (*right*). Hematoxylin-eosin. Left ×10, right ×25.

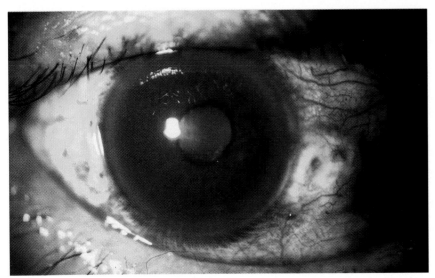

FIGURE 4–21 • **Pinguecula.** The yellowish mounds near the limbus are caused by actinic damage to conjunctival stromal connective tissue.

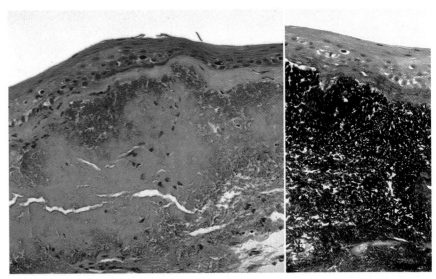

FIGURE 4–22 • **Pinguecula.** Grayish deposit of elastotic degeneration elevates the limbal epithelium. Deposit has granular and hyalinized areas. *Inset:* Intense positive staining for elastic tissue that is not quenched by pretreatment with elastase. Left: hematoxylin-eosin, ×100; right: Verhoeff-van Gieson, ×125.

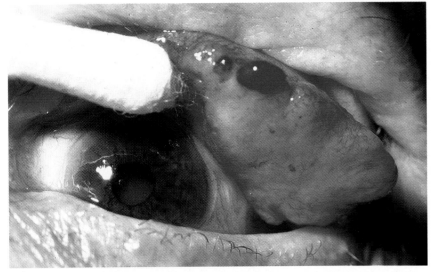

FIGURE 4–23 • **Conjunctival amyloidosis.** Large amyloid deposit forms a yellowish mass on the tarsal surface of the upper lid. Sebaceous carcinoma was suspected clinically.

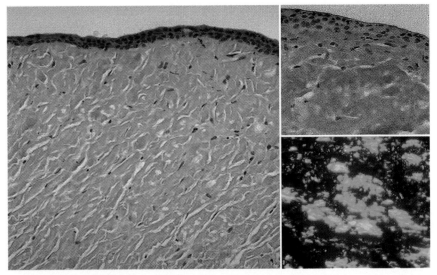

FIGURE 4–24 • **Conjunctival amyloidosis.** Substantia propria contains extensive eosinophilic deposit of acellular amorphous amyloid. Hematoxylin-eosin, ×25. Amyloid shows positive (orange) staining with congo red (*top inset*) and apple green birefringence with polarization microscopy (*bottom inset*). Top inset: congo red, ×50; bottom inset: congo red with crossed polarizers, ×50.

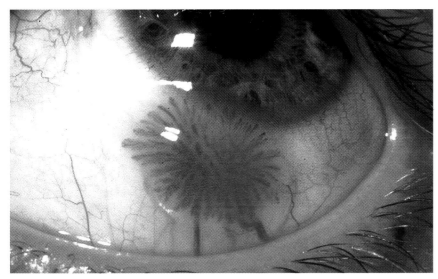

FIGURE 4–25 • **Conjunctival papilloma.** Vessels in fibrovascular cores of epithelial fronds are visible as hairpin vascular loops through transparent conjunctival epithelium. This benign epithelial tumor occurred in a child.

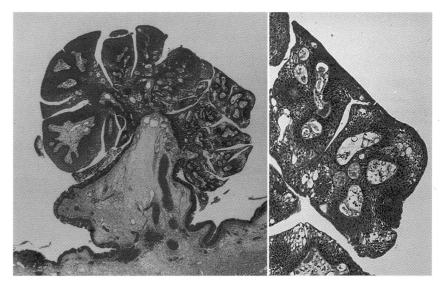

FIGURE 4–26 • **Conjunctival papilloma.** Benign pedunculated tumor is comprised of multiple fronds of conjunctival epithelium that surround cores of fibrovascular tissue. Hematoxylin-eosin, ×10. *Inset:* Fronds are seen at higher magnification. Hematoxylin-eosin, ×50.

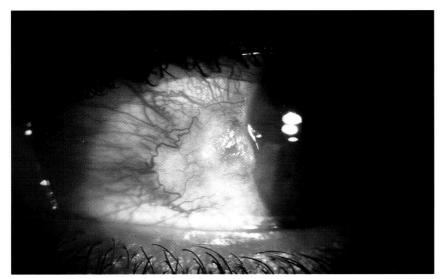

FIGURE 4–27 • **Actinic keratosis, conjunctiva.** Elevated leukoplakic lesion is located near the limbus in the exposed interpalpebral part of the conjunctiva. Leukoplakia indicates keratin-producing squamous cell lesion.

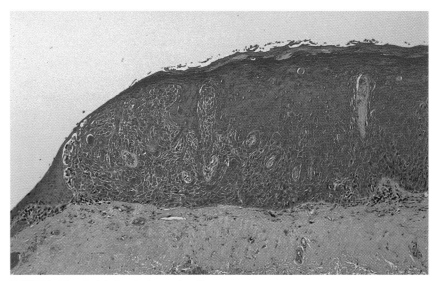

FIGURE 4–28 • **Actinic keratosis, conjunctiva.** Hyperkeratosis and parakeratosis are present on the surface of a thick plaque of epidermoid cells that arises abruptly from normal epithelium. The underlying stroma shows actinic elastosis. Hematoxylin-eosin, ×50.

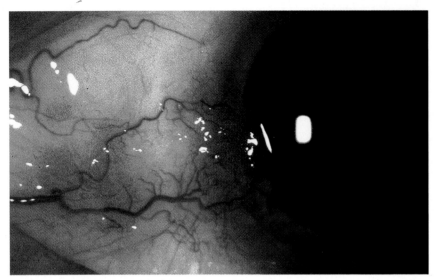

FIGURE 4–29 • **Conjunctival intraepithelial neoplasia.** A gelatinous lesion has arisen from exposed interpalpebral conjunctiva at the limbus. Excisional biopsy is required for definitive diagnosis of conjunctival squamous lesions.

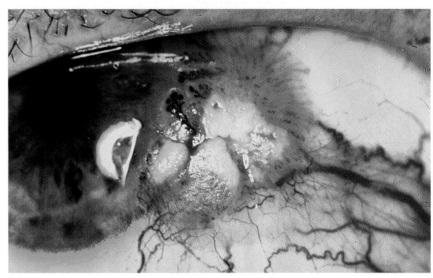

FIGURE 4–30 • **Squamous cell carcinoma, conjunctiva.** Limbal tumor is leukoplakic, indicating keratin production. Peripheral corneal invasion and prominent feeder vessels are evident.

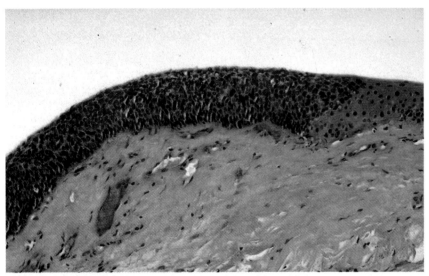

FIGURE 4–31 • **Conjunctival intraepithelial neoplasia (carcinoma *in situ*).** The epithelium at left has been totally replaced by atypical squamous cells and appears hypercellular and basophilic compared to the segment of normal limbal epithelium at right. The transition is characteristically abrupt. The carcinoma is *in situ* because the epithelial basement membrane is intact. Hematoxylin-eosin, ×100.

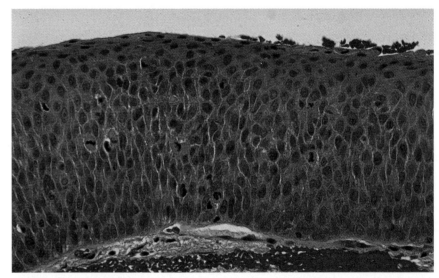

FIGURE 4–32 • **Conjunctival intraepithelial neoplasia (severe dysplasia).** The thickened epithelium is largely replaced by atypical cells, but surface differentiation persists. The epithelial basement membrane is intact. Mitotic figures are present within the acanthotic epithelium. Hematoxylin-eosin, ×200.

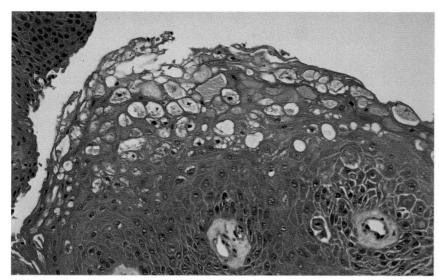

FIGURE 4–33 • **Koilocytosis, conjunctival papilloma.** Cells with pyknotic nuclei and vacuolated cytoplasm serve as light microscopic markers for human papillomavirus infection. *In situ* hybridization disclosed HPV 6/11. Hematoxylin-eosin, ×100.

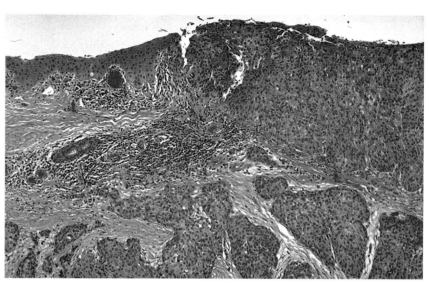

FIGURE 4–34 • **Invasive squamous cell carcinoma, conjunctiva.** Nests and islands of squamous cell carcinoma invade the substantia propria at right. The tumor cells have broken through the epithelial basement membrane. A characteristically abrupt junction separates the tumor from a segment of normal limbal conjunctiva at left. Hematoxylin-eosin, ×50.

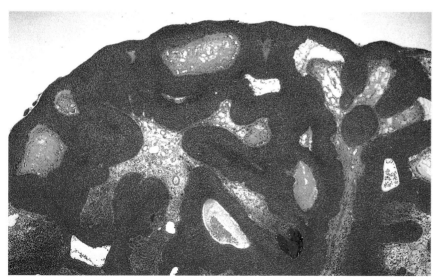

FIGURE 4–35 • **Papillary squamous cell carcinoma *in situ*.** The epithelial component of exophytic papillary lesion is totally comprised of highly atypical squamous epithelium consistent with carcinoma *in situ*. Hematoxylin-eosin, ×10.

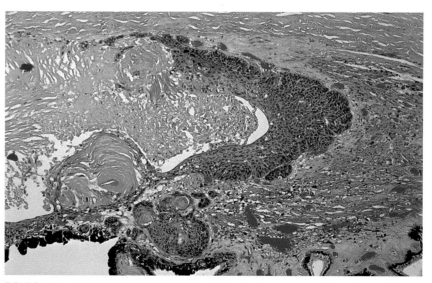

FIGURE 4–36 • **Anterior chamber invasion by conjunctival squamous cell carcinoma.** Tumor lines the angle and iris surface and infiltrates the iris stroma. Desquamated keratin fills the anterior chamber. Hematoxylin-eosin, ×50.

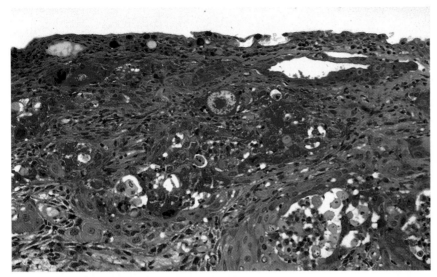

FIGURE 4–37 • **Mucoepidermoid carcinoma, conjunctiva.** PAS stain highlights focal mucin production by conjunctival carcinoma. Mucoepidermoid carcinoma of the conjunctiva can behave aggressively. Periodic acid-Schiff, ×100.

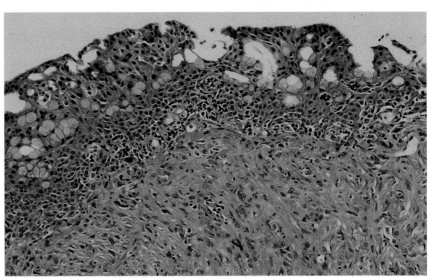

FIGURE 4–38 • **Spindle cell carcinoma, conjunctiva.** Spindle cell carcinomas are aggressive, poorly differentiated squamous cell carcinomas. Immunohistochemical stains may be necessary to differentiate spindle cell carcinoma from other spindle cell tumors. Hematoxylin-eosin, ×100. (Case presented by Dr. Gordon K. Klintworth at the 1997 meeting of the Eastern Ophthalmic Pathology Society, New York, NY)

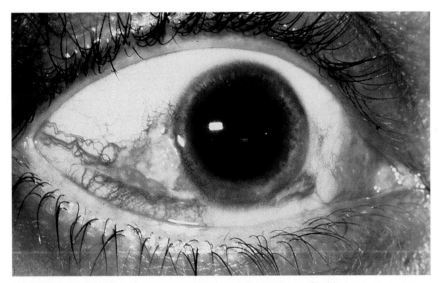

FIGURE 4–39 • **Hereditary benign intraepithelial dyskeratosis, conjunctiva.** Two leukoplakic lesions are present. The other eye and buccal mucosa also were involved. The patient traced her ancestry to Halifax County, North Carolina. (From Shields CL, Shields JS, Eagle RC: Hereditary benign intraepithelial dyskeratosis. Arch Ophthalmol 105:422–423, 1987. Copyright 1987, American Medical Association)

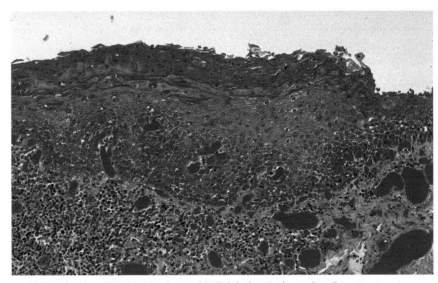

FIGURE 4–40 • **Hereditary benign intraepithelial dyskeratosis, conjunctiva.** Parakeratin plaque composed of plump dyskeratotic cells covers acanthotic epithelium. Single dyskeratotic cells are seen in the deeper part of the benign lesion. The underlying substantia propria contains a heavy infiltrate of lymphocytes. Hematoxylin-eosin, ×50.

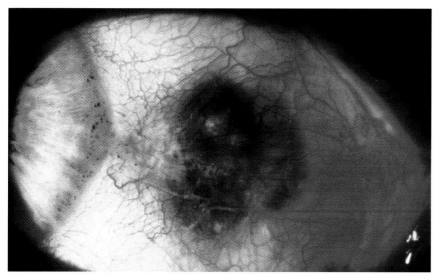

FIGURE 4–41 • **Ochronosis.** Brownish deposit of homogentisic acid discolors sclera near the insertion of the medial rectus tendon. A few globules of pigment are seen in the peripheral cornea.

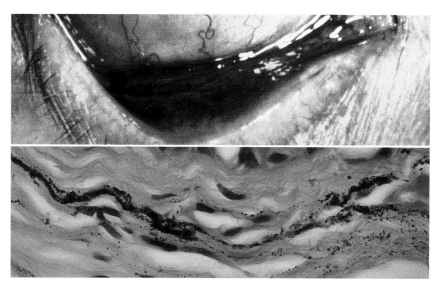

FIGURE 4–42 • **Argyrosis, conjunctiva.** Chronic administration of silver containing eye drops has caused grayish discoloration of the forniceal conjunctiva. Photomicrograph (*bottom*) shows deposition of silver granules in the substantia propria. Hematoxylin-eosin, ×250.

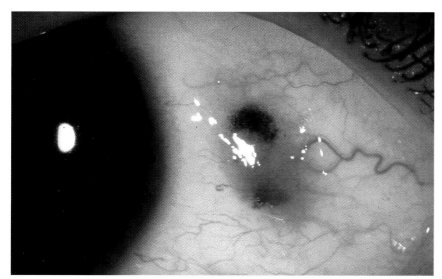

FIGURE 4–43 • **Conjunctival nevus.** Nevus is variably pigmented. (Photograph courtesy of Dr. Jerry A. Shields, Wills Eye Hospital)

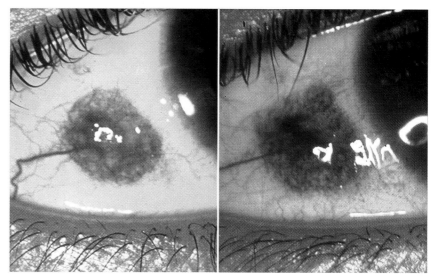

FIGURE 4–44 • **Hormone-induced changes in conjunctival nevus.** Compound cystic nevus was photographed at age 11 (*left*) and age 13 (*right*). Cytologically benign lesion appears larger and more intensely pigmented after menarche. The nevus contains multiple cysts.

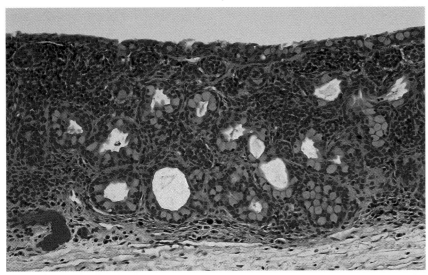

**FIGURE 4–45 • Amelanotic compound cystic nevus, conjunctiva.** Nevus contains characteristic cystic rests of conjunctival epithelium with goblet cells. Nevus cells are present at the junctional position and in the substantia propria. Hematoxylin-eosin, ×50.

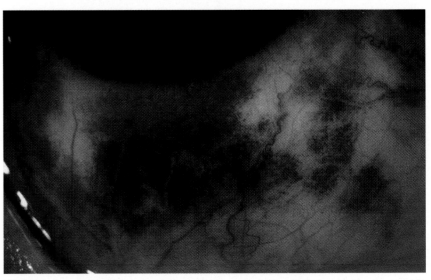

**FIGURE 4–46 • Congenital ocular melanocytosis.** Patchy, slate gray pigmentation is caused by dendritiform melanocytes deep in epibulbar tissues beneath conjunctiva. (Courtesy of Dr. Jerry A. Shields, Wills Eye Hospital)

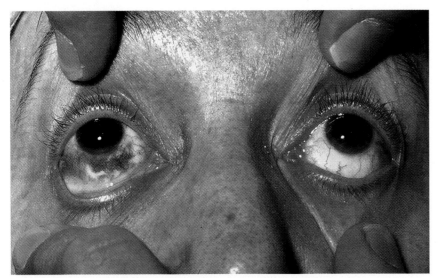

**FIGURE 4–47 • Congenital oculodermal melanocytosis (Nevus of Ota).** Affected right eye has slate gray epibulbar pigmentation, subtle pigmentation of adnexal tissues, and hyperchromic heterochromia iridum caused by a diffuse uveal nevus that predisposes Caucasians to uveal malignant melanoma. (From Eagle RC Jr: Iris pigmentation and pigmented lesion: an ultrastructural study. *Transact Am Ophthalmol Soc* 87:581–587, 1989)

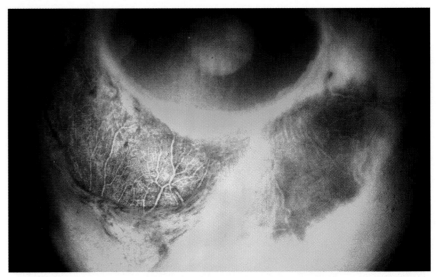

**FIGURE 4–48 • Congenital oculodermal melanocytosis (nevus of Ota).** Epibulbar pigment exposed by conjunctival rip appears brown. Tyndall effect makes pigment underneath the intact conjunctiva appear gray. Eye was obtained postmortem from patient illustrated in Figure 4–47. (From Eagle RC Jr. Congenital, developmental and degenerative disorders of the iris and ciliary body. In Albert DM, Jakobiec FA, eds. *Principles and Practice of Ophthalmology. Clinical Practice.* Vol 1. Philadelphia: Saunders, 1993:367–389)

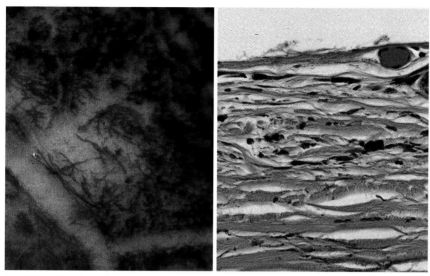

FIGURE 4–49 • **Epibulbar pigmentation, nevus of Ota.** Dendritiform shape of melanocytes is seen at high magnification in the photograph at left. Photomicrograph show melanocytes in episcleral tissues. Hematoxylin-eosin, ×100.

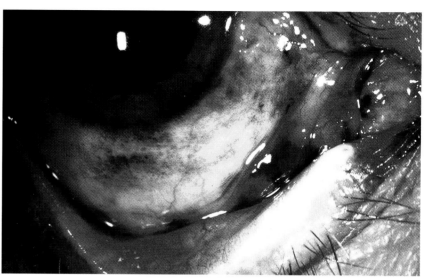

FIGURE 4–50 • **Primary acquired melanosis.** Patchy conjunctival pigmentation developed slowly in a middle-age Caucasian man. The pigment moved with the conjunctiva. Primary acquired melanosis is an important precursor of conjunctival melanoma. (Courtesy of Dr. Jerry A. Shields, Wills Eye Hospital)

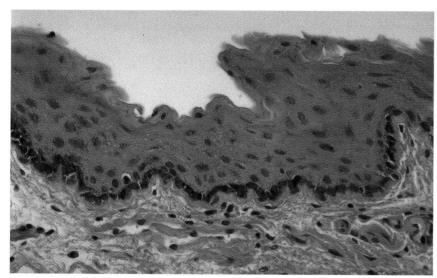

FIGURE 4–51 • **Primary acquired melanosis without atypia.** The basal cell layer of the conjunctiva is pigmented. Atypical melanocytic hyperplasia is not seen. Hematoxylin-eosin, ×250.

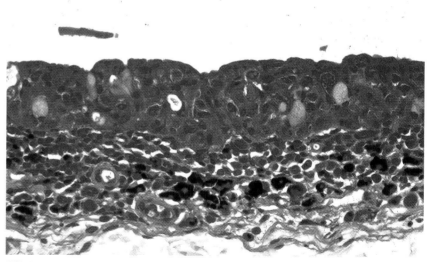

FIGURE 4–52 • **Primary acquired melanosis with atypia.** The epithelium is replaced by atypical melanocytes that include epithelioid cells. The basement membrane is intact. Hematoxylin-eosin, ×250.

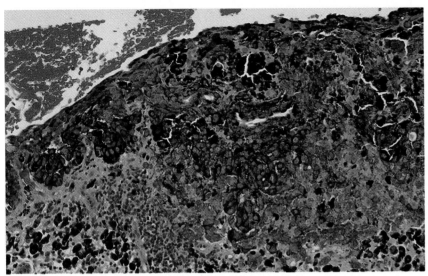

FIGURE 4–53 • **Malignant melanoma arising from PAM with atypia.** The atypical melanocytes have broken through the epithelial basement membrane, forming an invasive malignant melanoma. About 75% of conjunctival melanomas appear to arise from PAM with atypia. Hematoxylin-eosin, ×50.

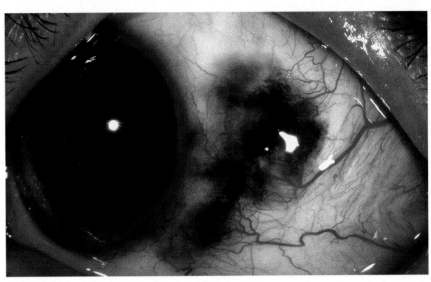

FIGURE 4–54 • **Conjunctival malignant melanoma.** (Courtesy of Dr. Jerry A. Shields, Wills Eye Hospital)

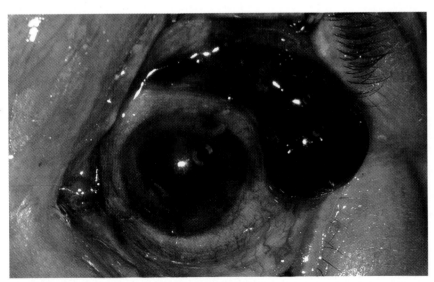

FIGURE 4–55 • **Conjunctival malignant melanoma.** Primary acquired melanosis is present. (Courtesy of Dr. Jerry A. Shields, Wills Eye Hospital)

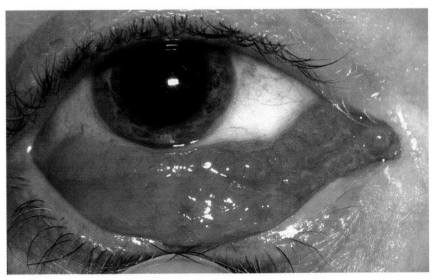

FIGURE 4–56 • **Follicular lymphoma, conjunctiva.** Conjunctival lymphomas are typically a salmon color.

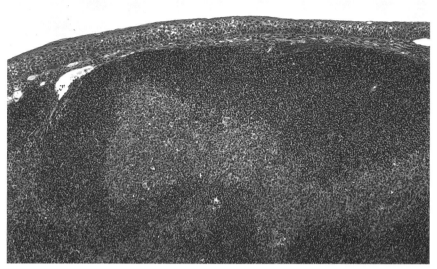

FIGURE 4–57 • **Follicular lymphoid hyperplasia, conjunctiva.** Heavy infiltrate of lymphoid cells filling the substantia propria contains germinal centers. Hematoxylin-eosin, ×25.

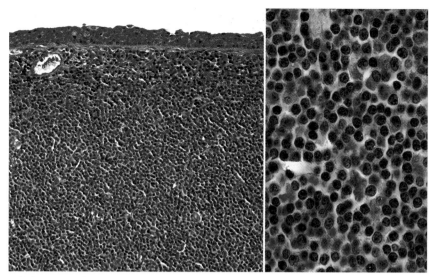

FIGURE 4–58 • **Conjunctival lymphoma, low grade.** Substantia propria contains diffuse infiltrate of well-differentiated lymphocytes, seen at high magnification in the *inset* (right). Flow cytometric analysis disclosed a monoclonal proliferation of B lymphocytes. Many conjunctival lymphomas are low-grade non-Hodgkin's B cell tumors of the mucosa associated lymphoid tissue (MALT) type. Hematoxylin-eosin. Main figure ×50, inset ×250.

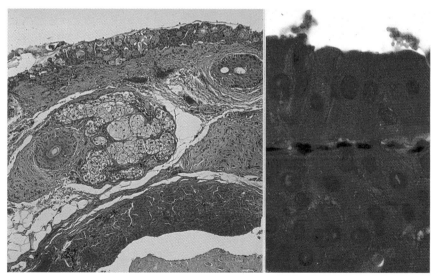

FIGURE 4–59 • **Oncocytoma, caruncle.** Benign cystadenomatous tumor deep in the caruncle is composed of tall bland epithelial cells with copious eosinophilic cytoplasm seen at higher magnification in the *inset*. The association of conjunctival epithelium with pilosebaceous units identifies the area as the caruncle. Hematoxylin-eosin. Main figure ×25, inset ×250.

# CHAPTER 5

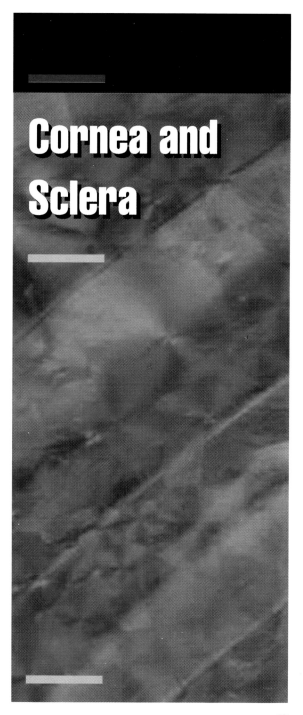

# Cornea and Sclera

T he cornea is the transparent anterior part of the eye's tough fibrous outer coat and is the eye's principal refractive element. The bulk of the cornea is comprised of interweaving lamellae of type I collagen fibers, which are spaced in an exquisitely regular fashion. Artifactitious clefts separate the stromal lamella in routine histologic sections. The stroma contains flattened dendritiform fibroblast-like cells called keratocytes (Fig. 5–1). A nonkeratinized epithelium five cells in thickness covers the anterior surface of the cornea (Fig. 5–2). It is composed of basal cells, wing cells, and flattened surface squamous cells. The epithelium normally has an inconspicuous basement membrane and rests on a hyaline band of modified stroma called Bowman's membrane. A delicate monolayer of flattened endothelial cells, derived embryologically from the neural crest, lines the posterior surface of the cornea (Fig. 5–3). The endothelium secretes a thick basement membrane called Descemet's membrane, which stains intensely with the periodic acid-Schiff (PAS) stain.

## DEVELOPMENTAL ANOMALIES

The corneal epithelium is a surface ectodermal derivative. The corneal endothelium and stroma are derived from successive waves of migrating mesectodermal cells of neural crest origin.

Developmental anomalies of the cornea include microcornea, defined as being less than 11 mm in greatest diameter; and megalocornea, which is more than 13 mm. Cornea plana is a bilateral familial trait (autosomal dominant or recessive) characterized by corneal flattening and peripheral opacification. The cornea in sclerocornea resembles sclera. The epithelium is thickened, Bowman's membrane is absent, and the anterior third of the stroma is scarred and vascularized. Solid dermoids and complex choristomas are discussed in Chapter 4.

The Axenfeld-Reiger syndrome is a spectrum of developmental anomalies that affects the peripheral cornea, the angle, and the iris. The terms angle cleavage syndrome and mesodermal dysgenesis were commonly applied to this disorder in the past. Axenfeld-Reiger syndrome is important because about half of affected patients develop glaucoma. Prominence and anterior displacement of Schwalbe's line into clear cornea, which is called posterior embryotoxon of Axenfeld, occurs in many patients (Fig. 5–4). Processes of iris stroma often bridge the angle and insert onto the posterior embryotoxon (Axenfeld's anomaly). Patients may have iris stromal abnormalities including hypoplasia and multiple, slit, and false pupils.

Axenfeld-Reiger syndrome is inherited as a autosomal dominant trait. Affected patients may have developmental defects of the face (maxillary hypoplasia) and teeth (anodontia, oligodontia, microdontia, and peg-like incisors). Shields postulated that the ocular abnormalities in Axenfeld-Reiger syndrome are consistent with a developmental arrest of certain anterior ocular structures derived from neural crest and occurring late in gestation.

A spectrum of developmental anomalies that includes the posterior ulcer of von Hippel and Peters' anomaly causes congenital opacities in the central cornea (Figs. 5–5, 5–6, 5–7). Histopathology shows a central concave defect in the posterior corneal stroma. The corneal endothelium and Descemet's membrane are absent in the posterior ulcer, and there is a corresponding area of central corneal edema and opacification. Bowman's layer may be thickened or absent. The

69

crystalline lens adheres to or is incarcerated within the posterior ulcer in some cases of Peters' anomaly (Fig. 5–7). Iridocorneal adhesions may insert into the periphery of the posterior corneal defect. Mutations in the *PAX 6* gene have been discovered in some patients with Peters' anomaly. The concave defect in the posterior cornea is lined by endothelium and Descemet's membrane in posterior keratoconus.

## CORNEAL INFLAMMATION

### Acute Keratitis and Corneal Ulceration

The anterior surface of the cornea is an interface between the eye and the external environment. Mechanisms that protect the cornea from infection include the five-cell thick layer of corneal epithelium, mucous strands made by the conjunctival goblet cells that can ensnare microorganisms, and tears that can wash them away. In addition, the tears contain natural antimicrobial substances such as lactoferrin, lysozyme, and antibodies. The latter are produced by lymphocytes and plasma cells, which are always found in the stroma of the conjunctiva and the parenchyma of the lacrimal gland.

Normally, these mechanisms are remarkably effective. Corneal infection usually develops when these normal protective mechanisms are compromised (e.g., when a contaminated foreign body perforates the epithelium and inoculates the corneal stroma or when the epithelium is abraded or damaged by chronic bullous keratopathy). Finally, a few organisms, most notably *Neisseria gonorrhoeae*, have the ability to invade through an intact epithelium.

Infiltration of the stroma by polymorphonuclear leukocytes (polys) occurs in acute bacterial keratitis (Figs. 5–8, 5–9). The polys collect in the clefts between adjacent stromal lamellae. Digestive enzymes released by the dying inflammatory cells cause stromal necrosis, which has a smudged basophilic appearance in routine hematoxylin-eosin (H&E) sections. Collagenase made by the corneal epithelium may contribute to dissolution of the stroma. Organisms such as *Pseudomonas* also produce potent enzymes that contribute to corneal destruction. *Pseudomonas* keratitis is characterized by marked stromal edema and dissolution with rapid corneal perforation. The infection can also spread posteriorly into the sclera as a sclerokeratitis (Fig. 5–10).

The epithelium, Bowman's membrane, and the anterior stroma are lost in a corneal ulcer. Corneal perforation results when the infection destroys the full-thickness stroma. Occasionally, a bulging dome of intact, elastic Descemet's membrane called a descemetocele persists in the floor of the incipient perforation (Fig. 5–11). Polys collect in the lower part of the anterior chamber as a hypopyon and typically adhere to the posterior cornea directly underneath the ulcer. The endothelium is often damaged. The tissue Gram stain may disclose myriad microorganisms in the infected corneal or none at all. Bacteria are often found in relatively noninflamed parts of the stroma bordering the inflammatory infiltrate. Perforation or impending perforation of the cornea is an indication for emergent penetrating keratoplasty (corneal transplantation). Cyanoacrylate tissue adhesive is used to seal corneal perforations. Although the "crazy glue" is lost during processing, its presence is marked by a telltale scalloped pattern on the anterior corneal surface.

Infectious pseudocrystalline keratopathy (Fig. 5–12) usually is caused by avirulent strains of streptococci, which proliferate in the relatively noninflamed stroma, forming large interlamellar bacterial colonies that have a vaguely crystalline configuration on biomicroscopy. This relatively rare disorder typically occurs in corneal grafts that have undergone chronic corticosteroid therapy. The bacteria are sequestered by a glycocalyx, whose formation is stimulated by steroid therapy.

Fungal keratitis (Figs. 5–13, 5–14, 5–15, 5–16) is rarer than bacterial keratitis, is more prevalent in the South, and often complicates corneal injuries by vegetable matter or steroid therapy in debilitated hosts. Eighty per cent of corneal ulcers in the United States are caused by *Aspergillus, Candida,* or *Fusarium* species. Clinically, fungal ulcers often have a deep crater with raised edges and may have smaller satellite lesions (Fig. 5–13). The fungal hyphae readily permeate the stroma and can perforate Descemet's membrane and invade the anterior chamber, placing the patient at risk for fungal endophthalmitis (Figs. 5–14, 5–15).

Fungal organisms may not be detected in superficial smears or scrapings because the hyphae are often found deep in the bed of the ulcer or in the relatively viable stroma of the ulcer wall (Fig. 5–16). Hence corneal biopsy may be required to establish the diagnosis. Fungi and yeast are best shown by the PAS stain or special stains for fungus such as the Gomori methenamine silver (GMS) silver impregnation stain. The nonspecific fluorescent calcofluor white stain demonstrates fungi well and is a helpful technique for screening corneal scrapings, but it must be used with a fluorescence microscope.

*Mycobacterium tuberculosis, Mycobacterium leprae,* and several strains of atypical mycobacteria such as *M. chelonei* rarely cause corneal infection. Special stains for acid-fast organisms and microbiologic cultures are used to diagnosis mycobacterial keratitis (see Fig. 15–10). The diagnosis is often unsuspected and is frequently delayed.

### Viral Keratitis

Herpes simplex (HSV) keratitis (Figs. 5–17, 5–18, 5–19, 5–20) is the most common corneal infection that causes visual loss in the United States and Europe. Most cases of herpetic keratitis are caused by HSV type I, which causes infection above the waist. The classic clinical manifestation of early ocular herpesvirus infection is dendritic keratitis, a superficial ulcerating infection of the corneal epithelium that has a characteristic branching configuration (Fig. 5–17). Viral cultures are positive in 75% of cases, and smears show Cowdry type A intranuclear viral inclusions in the infected epithelial cells. The primary epithelial infection tends to be self-limited, lasting 7–10 days with complete recovery and disappearance of virus from the primary site of infection. However, recurrences are common because the virus remains in a latent state in the trigeminal ganglion where its DNA has been incorporated into the genome of the neurons. Poorly understood trigger mechanisms reactivate the virus, which travels down the sensory nerve to cause overt recurrent disease. One in four cases of primary HSV keratitis recur. The recurrence rate rises to 50% after an initial recurrence.

A more serious, potentially blinding form of ocular herpesvirus infection affects the corneal stroma. Although the pathogenesis of herpes stromal keratitis is not entirely understood, an immunologic response to viral antigens shed from infected corneal epithelial or endothelial cells probably is the basis for nonulcerative HSV disciform keratitis. Experimental evidence in a murine model suggests that the disorder is an autoimmune response to antigens shared by the cornea and HSV type I. The necrotizing form of HSV stromal keratitis may involve viral invasion and low grade replication in the stroma.

Light microscopy of corneal buttons with chronic herpes stromal keratitis typically reveals scarring and vascularization of the stroma and infiltration by chronic inflammatory cells (Figs. 5–18, 5–19). The presence of lymphocytes, plasma cells, and histiocytes in the inflammatory infiltrate in many cases provides evidence for an immunologic response. The inflammatory infiltrate frequently includes epithelioid histiocytes, which may occur anywhere in the stroma although they characteristically coalesce to form giant cells near Descemet's membrane (Fig. 5–19). A giant cell reaction to Descemet's membrane is not pathognomonic for chronic HSV keratitis, but it is highly suggestive. In many cases there is thinning and scarring of the chronically inflamed cornea with loss of Bowman's membrane and anterior stroma. Progressive stromal loss can lead to corneal perforation in chronic herpetic keratitis. Compensatory hyperplasia of the corneal epithelium is often found in areas of extensive stromal loss (Fig. 5–20). Viral inclusions are not found by light microscopy in the stroma in herpes stromal keratitis. Virions and viral antigens have been detected electron microscopically and immunocytochemically, however.

Varicella zoster virus (VZV), another member of the herpesvirus family, also causes a dendritic keratitis. Zoster dendrites lack the rounded terminal bulbs that typically occur at the end of the branches of HSV dendrites and are not full-thickness epithelial ulcerations as are HSV dendrites (Fig. 5–17).

Focal subepithelial infiltrates occur in the corneas of patients who have epidemic keratoconjunctivitis (EKC), which generally is caused by adenovirus types 8 and 19. The subepithelial infiltrates develop in the later noninfectious stage of the disease and are thought to be comprised of lymphocytes attracted by viral antigens. EKC is often a severe, temporarily incapacitating infection that is highly contagious. Ophthalmologists should take care to avoid infecting themselves and other patients. Patients with EKC usually have preauricular adenopathy.

## Interstitial Keratitis

In a generic sense, the term interstitial keratitis refers to any nonulcerative inflammation of the corneal stroma. (HSV disciform keratitis is a form of interstitial keratitis.) Other causes of stromal or interstitial keratitis include tuberculosis and leprosy, protozoan parasites such as *Acanthamoeba*; onchocercal microfilaria; systemic disorders such as sarcoidosis, Hodgkin's disease, and mycosis fungoides; foreign bodies such as caterpillar setae and plant material; and drugs including gold and arsenic.

In common usage, however, the term interstitial keratitis almost always implies the severe stromal keratitis that affects patients with congenital syphilis during the first or second decade of life. Acute luetic interstitial keratitis is marked clinically by a "salmon patch" of intense stromal vascularization and severe photophobia. Lymphocytes infiltrate the edematous stroma. The late sequelae of old syphilitic interstitial keratitis can be relatively subtle: a faint diffuse nebulous opacification of the stroma and residual nonperfused ghost vessels that are located deep in the corneal stroma. They are best disclosed by the biomicroscopic technique of sclerotic scatter.

Histopathologically, Bowman's membrane usually is absent. The stroma is free of inflammation, and fine vessels that usually do not contain blood are seen in the posterior third of the stroma, often just anterior to Descemet's membrane (Fig. 5–21). Part of the stroma may have a rarefied vacuolated appearance and stains intensely for acid mucopolysaccharide. Descemet's membrane is often thickened, and it may be studded with irregular guttate excrescences. The thickening of Descemet's membrane may be massive. Relucent strands and networks of basement membrane material are found on the posterior corneal surface in exceptional cases (Fig. 5–22).

Luetic interstitial keratitis occasionally develops in acquired syphilis, in which corneal involvement is often unilateral and sectoral. The association of nonluetic interstitial keratitis and deafness is called Cogan syndrome. Cogan syndrome is thought to be an autoimmune disorder.

## Parasitic Keratitis

Protozoan parasites, including microsporidians and the freshwater amebas *Acanthamoeba castellani* and

*A. polyphaga*, cause unusual corneal infections. Microsporidial keratoconjunctivitis has been reported in patients with acquired immunodeficency syndrome (AIDS) who have cats as household pets. The parasite infects the epithelium of the cornea and conjunctiva (see Fig. 4–17).

*Acanthamoeba* keratitis, initially reported in 1974, is closely linked to the development and widespread use of soft contact lenses. *Acanthamoeba* keratitis classically afflicts soft contact lens wearers who use contaminated homemade saline solutions or wear their lenses while swimming or bathing in hot tubs. The keratitis is usually extremely painful. Although cases can respond to medical therapy, penetrating keratoplasty (corneal transplantation) may be necessary. The initial stages of *Acanthamoeba* keratitis may be confused with herpetic keratitis if clinical suspicion is low. A ring or annular infiltrate is a characteristic feature of *Acanthamoeba* keratitis but usually develops in the later stages of the disease.

Microscopically, *Acanthamoeba* keratitis is often marked by focal detachment or desquamation of the corneal epithelium. In contrast to bacterial or fungal keratitis, the anterior stroma contains only a relatively sparse infiltrate of inflammatory cells, mainly polys and macrophages (Fig. 5–23). Stromal necrosis is usually inconspicuous, and stromal vascularization generally is not observed despite a lengthy course that may last months prior to keratoplasty. Amebic cysts in the stroma and epithelium are readily found in routine H&E-stained sections (Fig. 5–24). The cyst walls stain with PAS, GMS, and Giemsa. The chitinous walls of the *Acanthamoeba* cysts are round or oval. The cytoplasm often retracts from the cyst wall in tissue sections. The cysts contain a round nucleus with a distinct nucleolus. Trophozoites are usually difficult to identify because they resemble macrophages.

*Acanthamoeba* keratitis can be diagnosed using corneal biopsies or smears. The nonspecific fluorescent calcofluor white stain is most helpful during the rapid screening of smears. *Acanthamoeba* is cultured on agar plates overlaid with a layer of *Escherichia coli*. The amebas produce diagnostic linear tracks on the surface of the plates as they graze on the bacteria.

Onchocerciasis is a major cause of blindness in parts of Africa and South and Central America. This infestation by the parasite *Onchocerca volvulus* is called river blindness because its vector, the black simulian fly, breeds in swift-running mountain streams. Pairs of adult *Onchocerca* breed in characteristic nodules in the skin of infested individuals. The female worm releases myriad microfilariae that migrate to all parts of the body. Necrotic microfilariae incite focal inflammation. Microfilariae are often found in the corneal stroma, where they produce keratitis with a characteristic nummular (coin-shaped) pattern. Secondary closed angle glaucoma caused by anterior uveitis is a major cause of blindness in endemic areas. Chorioretinal degeneration, also an allergic reaction to the parasite, is another important cause of blindness. Slit lamp examination may disclose microfilariae in the anterior chamber in heavily infested patients. The tiny nematodes are photophobic, and they quickly swim behind the iris when the lamp is turned on. Patients are treated by surgical removal of parasitic nodules and the anthelmintic drug ivermectin.

## PERIPHERAL CORNEAL ULCERS

Although bacterial and fungal ulcers usually involve the central cornea, a variety of ulcerations affect its periphery. Most important are the peripheral corneal ulcerations that may herald the presence of a systemic vasculitis such as Wegener's granulomatosis, periarteritis nodosa, systemic lupus erythematosus, or rheumatoid arthritis.

Mooren's ulcer begins peripherally and progressively extends across the cornea. This lesion has a characteristic overhanging margin (Fig. 5–25). Mooren's ulcer usually is a unilateral disease of elderly patients in the United States. A severe, bilateral form of the disease affects young individuals in Africa. Mechanisms that may be involved in the pathogenesis of Mooren's ulcer include ischemic necrosis, collagenase produced by limbal tissues, or an immunologic reaction. Some cases of Mooren's ulcer have been linked to chronic hepatitis C infection.

Terrien's ulcer is a slowly progressive, bilateral, trough-like thinning of the stroma that begins superiorly in male patients. The epithelium remains intact, but Bowman's membrane and the superficial stroma are lost. Vascularization and occasional lymphocytes and plasma cells are found in the ectatic stroma.

Toxins produced by staphylococci cause infiltrates and superficial ulcerations in the peripheral cornea.

## PTERYGIUM

Pterygium (Figs. 5–26, 5–27) is a degenerative disease of the cornea so named because of the lesion's fanciful resemblance to the membranous wing of an insect (*pter* is the Greek word for wing). Pterygia, which occur on the ocular surface exposed in the interpalpebral fissure, can be bilateral. Clinically, a wedge-shaped ingrowth of conjunctival tissue slowly invades the periphery of the nasal cornea. Pterygium initially is a cosmetic blemish, but it can cause visual loss if it invades the pupillary axis. Pterygium is not a neoplasm; the degenerative process may involve transdifferentiation of the cornea epithelium into conjunctiva-like tissue related to the death of corneal limbal stem cells. When a sector of corneal stem cells in the limbal palisades of Vogt is destroyed experimentally, conjunctival cells migrate centrally into the corresponding sector of the cornea and retain their conjunctival characteristics. Prolonged light exposure is thought to play an important role in stem cell damage. Pterygia are more common in southern latitudes and typically occur in individuals who work outdoors. Other environmental factors, such as wind or dust, also may play a pathogenetic role.

Microscopically, many pterygia resemble conjunctiva with a highly vascular stroma. Solar elastosis of collagen usually is present but is relatively inconspicuous in some cases. Bowman's membrane is absent. The epithelium may show focal corneal and conjunctival characteristics. In some cases it is thickened and even dysplastic. Pterygia should be examined histopathologically to exclude the possibility of an unsuspected neoplasm. In addition to squamous malignancies, amelanotic melanomas occasionally are misdiagnosed clinically as pterygia.

## OTHER CORNEAL DEGENERATIONS

Calcific band keratopathy is a superficial opacity that extends across the part of the cornea exposed in the interpalpebral fissure (Fig. 5–28). It is caused by calcification of Bowman's membrane and the anterior stroma. A clear interval separates the band of superficial calcification from the limbus, and the opacity usually contains small, circular holes. Calcific band keratopathy can complicate chronic uveitis or longstanding glaucoma; it also it complicates systemic disorders of calcium metabolism including hypercalcemia, vitamin D intoxication, milk-alkali syndrome, hypophosphatemia, and Fanconi syndrome. Histopathology discloses basophilic granules in Bowman's membrane and the superficial stroma. The alizarin red and von Kossa stains for calcium are positive. The chelating agent EDTA is often used to treat calcific band keratopathy. A noncalcific form of band keratopathy related to chronic actinic keratopathy also occurs. The granules are larger and stain positively with the elastic stain.

Chronic actinic keratopathy (Fig. 5–29) and climatic droplet keratopathy are two of many names applied to a degenerative disorder marked by the deposition of multiple spherules of yellow hyaline material in the anterior cornea. The disorder is also called spheroidal degeneration and Labrador keratopathy. The degeneration is particularly prevalent in areas where intense glare is reflected from ice (Labrador) or sand (the Dahlac Islands of the Indian Ocean). Other synonyms such as oleoguttate dystrophy stress the resemblance of the corneal deposits to droplets of oil. In H&E-stained sections the droplike deposits of amorphous hyaline material usually are light gray or amphophilic. The material stains intensely with the Verhoeff-van Gieson elastic stain, and the positive reaction is not quenched by pretreatment with elastase like the elastotic degeneration in pinguecula and pterygium. The hyaline deposits autofluoresce under ultraviolet light and are said to behave similarly when illuminated with the slit lamp's cobalt blue filter. In some cases tiny globules of hyaline material are concentrated in Bowman's membrane, mimicking calcific band keratopathy. In advanced cases, concurrent corneal scarring can severely decrease visual acuity.

Salzmann's nodular degeneration was once called Salzmann's nodular dystrophy. It is now recognized that this typically unilateral disorder is not heritable and is best classified as a secondary degenerative process of uncertain cause. Clinically the corneal epithelium is focally elevated by white mounds of dense collagenous connective tissue. Salzmann's nodular degeneration resembles a massive focal pannus histopathologically. Mounds of relatively acellular hyaline connective tissue elevate the corneal epithelium anterior to the plane of Bowman's membrane, which may be destroyed.

Lipid deposition occurs in the peripheral corneal stroma in arcus senilis or gerontoxon, a relatively common aging change. Fat stains performed on frozen sections disclose a concurrent deposit in the perilimbal sclera, which is inapparent clinically. Similar corneal deposition in male subjects less than age 40 may signify a hyperlipemic state that can predispose to cardiovascular disease. Lipid keratopathy is a secondary phenomenon caused by lipid deposition in a heavily vascularized stroma (Fig. 5–30).

A corneal keloid (Fig. 5–31) is a hypertrophic scar that massively thickens the corneal stroma. Elevated and exposed, the corneal epithelium on the surface of the keloid typically undergoes epidermalization and transforms into opaque skin-like tissue. Large corneal keloids often develop in patients who have corneal staphylomas. In such cases the posterior surface of the cornea is lined by atrophic remnants of iris, mainly iris pigment. A staphyloma is an ectasia (area of thinning) lined by uveal tissue. "Uveal" is derived from the Latin word *uva* meaning grape. *Staphyle* means a "bunch of grapes" in Greek. The latter prefix signifies the involvement of uveal tissue. Corneal staphylomas and keloids are a common sequelae of keratomalacia and measles keratitis in underdeveloped countries.

The tear film functions as the true anterior surface of the cornea, whose health depends on an adequate supply of properly constituted tears. Disorders of tear production and composition include deficiencies in the aqueous component, the mucinous wetting agent produced by the goblet cells, or abnormalities in the most superficial lipid layer. Minor degrees of ocular drying are encountered often in clinical practice. If an eye is totally dry, the cornea becomes opaque.

Keratoconjunctivitis sicca is marked by corneal drying, superficial punctate keratopathy (punctate staining), and filamentary keratitis composed of strands of detached of corneal epithelium and mucous. Keratoconjunctivitis sicca and xerostomia are characteristic features of the autoimmune disorder Sjögren syndrome. Drying of the mouth and eyes is caused by infiltration and destruction of the acini of the salivary glands and the main and accessory lacrimal glands by T lymphocytes. Myoepithelial islands persist in the lymphoid infiltrate (lymphoepithelial lesion of Godwin). About 10% of affected patients develop malignant lymphoma.

Corneal epithelial keratinization and epidermalization occur in severe vitamin A deficiency. Patients have xerophthalmia and night blindness caused by deficient rod photopigment. A process of bland corneal melting called keratomalacia frequently leads to corneal perforation (Fig. 5–32). Malnourished children in underdeveloped countries and vitamin A deficient alcoholics in the United States are at risk. Bitot's spot, a clinical marker for xerophthalmia, is an elevated dry area of epithelium with a foamy appearance.

A corneal delle (pl. dellen) is a focal area of corneal thinning with superficial surface ulceration located central to an elevated lesion at the limbus. Dellen probably are caused by focal dehydration of the corneal stroma related to deficient focal corneal wetting.

Neurotrophic or neuroparalytic keratopathy is a corneal epitheliopathy that may complicate fifth nerve lesions. The keratopathy develops rapidly after surgical sectioning of the trigeminal nerve interrupts poorly understood trophic factors.

The term pannus is applied to a flat superficial scar of the anterior cornea (Fig. 5–33). Two types of pannus are recognized histopathologically. The paradigmatic inflammatory pannus occurs in trachoma and is marked by a subepithelial ingrowth of inflamed fibrovascular tissue from the limbus, which destroys Bowman's membrane. Degenerative pannus is commonly found in corneas with chronic edema and bullous keratopathy. Microscopically, a layer of connective tissue is found interposed between the base of the epithelium and Bowman's membrane, which remains intact. In contrast to an inflammatory pannus, the subepithelial scar of degenerative pannus does not necessarily grow in from the limbus. Cells, which probably are stromal fibroblasts, migrate into the space between Bowman's membrane and the detached epithelium and synthesize collagen. This fibrous scar

forms the pannus and may alleviate the painful bullous keratopathy at the expense of visual acuity. In rare instances amyloid is deposited secondarily underneath the epithelium.

## KERATOCONUS

Keratoconus is an enigmatic bilateral degenerative disorder characterized by progressive thinning or ectasia of the central stroma that imparts a conical configuration to the cornea (Figs. 5–34, 5–35, 5–36). Keratoconus usually presents around puberty with visual loss caused by severe astigmatism. Most cases of keratoconus do not appear to be heritable, but the degeneration can complicate several systemic disorders including trisomy 21, Ehlers-Danlos syndrome, Leber's congenital amaurosis, and atopic dermatitis. Keratoconus occurs in approximately 5% of patients with Down syndrome and frequently is associated with the acute onset of severe corneal edema called corneal hydrops. Keratoconus in patients with atopic dermatitis, Down syndrome, and Leber's congenital amaurosis, a congenital photoreceptor degeneration, could be related to forceful eye rubbing or the oculodigital reflex. The latter is a behavioral pattern seen in visually and mentally handicapped children who repeatedly strike their eyes with their thumbs to induce flashes of light or phosphenes mechanically.

The consistency of the cornea in keratoconus is abnormal; the sectioned cornea almost invariably assumes an irregular wavy configuration on a microslide, which immediately suggests the diagnosis. Higher magnification discloses central or apical thinning of the stroma, which can be reduced to less than one-tenth normal thickness in exceptional cases. Characteristic dehiscences in Bowman's membrane, which often have a wavy configuration, are common (Fig. 5–35). Some cases exhibit apical scarring with increased fibroblastic activity and new collagen production. The

corneal epithelium usually is intact and irregular in caliber, with areas of thinning and compensatory hyperplasia. Descemet's membrane usually is thin, and the endothelium is well preserved. A rupture in Descemet's membrane is found if acute hydrops has occurred. If the hydrops had resolved prior to corneal transplantation, the gap in Descemet's membrane is lined by a thin layer of new Descemet's membrane synthesized by endothelial cells that have migrated into the defect. Special stains show iron deposition in the corneal epithelium encircling the cone. This deposit is evident clinically as a Fleischer ring, one of the several eponymic iron lines of the cornea (Fig. 5–36). Other iron lines include the Hudson-Stähli line (across the low third of the cornea), the Stocker line (in front of a pterygium), and the Ferry line (next to a filtering bleb). The basic defect in keratoconus is uncertain but may be related to abnormal degradation of the corneal extracellular matrix. Abnormal levels of tissue metalloproteinase inhibitors have been identified in some cases.

Pellucid degeneration of the cornea resembles keratoconus histopathologically but is located in the periphery of the cornea.

## CORNEAL DYSTROPHIES

In classic ophthalmic usage, the term dystrophy usually denotes an inherited, relatively symmetric bilateral disease that is unassociated with vascularization or inflammation in its early stages. The pathology is, or appears to be, localized to an ocular tissue. Dystrophies usually are not evident at birth but become clinically evident later in life. The etymologic derivation of the word dystrophy is outdated because it refers to poor nutrition. The term usually is applied to hereditary diseases of the cornea and macula.

Advances in molecular biology have markedly increased our understanding of these rare, interesting disorders. Several corneal dystrophies are now known to be caused by allelic mutations in a gene encoding a single corneal protein. Macular corneal dystrophy type I appears to be the ocular manifestation of an otherwise innocuous systemic enzyme deficiency. Meesman's epithelial dystrophy is caused by an abnormality in the gene for a protein that is expressed only in the corneal epithelium.

Corneal dystrophies have been classified topographically as epithelial, subepithelial, stromal, and endothelial based on the location of the clinical and pathologic findings. New classification schemes based on specific metabolic defects undoubtedly will be introduced in the future as our understanding of molecular genetics increases.

Meesmann's dystrophy (Fig. 5–37) is a relatively benign autosomal dominantly inherited disorder of the corneal epithelium. The eponym Stocker-Holt dystrophy is applied to a somewhat similar disorder. Clinically, Meesmann's dystrophy is characterized by the presence of myriad small punctate vacuoles in the corneal epithelium, which are best seen by retroillumination. Fluorescein dye typically pools in the vacuoles that have migrated to the corneal surface. Although recurrent epithelial erosions are possible, good vision is the rule. Histopathologically, both the epithelium and its basement membrane are thickened, and the epithelium has a disorderly appearance. In addition to small intraepithelial cystoid spaces, the epithelium contains cells that have a hyalinized appearance. Electron microscopy has disclosed intracellular aggregates of homogeneous "peculiar substance" thought to be condensed cytoskeletal material. Meesmann's corneal dystrophy is caused by mutations in the genes for cornea-specific keratins K3 and K12 which cause increased fragility of the corneal epithelium.

The terms anterior basement membrane dystrophy and map-dot-fingerprint dystrophy (Figs. 5–38, 5–39) have been applied to a corneal disorder marked by a spectrum of epithelial abnormalities including reduplication and intraepithelial segments of corneal epithelial basement membrane, intraepithelial cystoid spaces filled with devitalized cellular debris, and focal subepithelial scarring. The disorder is autosomal dominant and usually is seen in healthy middle-aged women who may have slightly reduced visual acuity. The clinical subtypes of the dystrophy often coexist. The microcystic form of the dystrophy (called Cogan's microcystic dystrophy) shows multiple intraepithelial cysts filled with white putty-like cellular debris (Fig. 5–38). The devitalized cells that fill the cystoid spaces are trapped by duplication of the epithelium, which prevents their desquamation. Parallel relucent lines that may represent basement membrane material separating sheets of duplicated epithelium are seen in the fingerprint subtype. Irregular, geographically shaped areas of subepithelial scarring characterize map-like changes. The corneal epithelial basement membrane is often thickened (Fig. 5–39).

Although cases undoubtedly occur in patients without corneal edema, epithelial abnormalities that are similar to those found in map-dot-fingerprint dystrophy are found histopathologically in many chronically edematous corneas. Histopathologic evidence suggests that bullous detachment of the epithelium is the primary event that leads subsequently to secondary abnormalities such as reduplication and intraepithelial cyst formation. It is possible that the primary dystrophy is caused by a defective molecule involved in corneal epithelial adhesion.

Granular, lattice, Avellino, and Reis-Bücklers dystrophies have been shown to be associated with different mutations of the beta ig-H3 gene (transforming growth factor-beta-inducible gene H3) on the long arm of chromosome 5. The corneal epithelium is rich in the gene's protein product keratoepithelin. The different clinical manifestations of these dystrophies presumably reflect variations in the aggregation or precipitation of the several mutant forms of keratoepithelin in the cornea.

Reis-Bücklers dystrophy and Thiel-Behnke's honeycomb dystrophy (Figs. 5–40, 5–41, 5–42, 5–43, 5–44) are two relatively similar disorders that primarily affect the epithelium, Bowman's layer, and the anterior stroma of the cornea. Both dystrophies present with recurrent erosions during the first decade and are characterized biomicroscopically by diffuse subepithelial scarring that markedly reduces visual acuity (Fig. 5–40). Histopathologically, the epithelium in both dystrophies is irregular in caliber and has a sawtoothed appearance. A thick multilaminar pannus, composed of alternating layers of collagen and an abnormal material that has the same tinctorial characteristics as the deposits in granular corneal dystrophy, elevates the epithelium anterior to the plane of Bowman's layer. Bowman's layer usually is destroyed. The material is more eosinophilic than normal stromal collagen and stains intensely red with Masson trichrome (Figs. 5–42, 5–43). The material initially collects underneath the epithelium and probably predisposes to recurrent erosions by interfering with epithelial adhesion. The multilaminated pannus likely results from repeated episodes of synthesis, epithelial detachment, and scarring. Reis-Bucklers dystrophy is caused by a mutation in the beta ig-H3 gene on chromosome 5.

Reis-Bücklers dystrophy and Thiel-Behnke's dystrophy are distinguished histologically and electron microscopically by the morphology of the abnormal deposits. Reis-Bücklers dystrophy resembles a superficial variant of granular corneal dystrophy; the mutant keratoepithelin forms small, sharply angulated crystalloids that are intensely Masson trichrome-positive and osmiophilic on transmission electron microscopy (Figs. 5–42, 5–44). The subepithelial deposits in Thiel-Behnke dystrophy are less pronounced, more amorphous, and less intensely acid-fuchsinophilic with Masson trichrome (Figs. 5–43). The deposits are composed of proteinaceous "curly filaments" seen by electron microscopy (Fig. 5–44). Patients with the latter findings have been erroneously reported in the American literature as having Reis-Bücklers dystrophy. The European literature indicates that the patients who were reported by Reis and Bückler had a form of superficial granular dystrophy.

Primary gelatinous drop-like dystrophy or familial subepithelial corneal amyloidosis is a rare type of heritable corneal amyloidosis in which the amyloid accumulates in focal mounds underneath the epithelium. The amyloid is composed of the antimicrobial protein lactoferrin produced by the lacrimal gland.

Granular, macular, and lattice dystrophies are the three classic dystrophies of the corneal stroma. As noted above, granular dystrophy, lattice dystrophy type I, a third stromal dystrophy called Avellino dystrophy (which combines features of both lattice and granular dystrophies), and Reis-Bücklers dystrophy are caused by disparate mutations in the beta ig-H3 gene on the long arm of chromosome 5. This gene codes for a protein called keratoepithelin.

Granular corneal dystrophy (also known as Groenow type I or Bückler type I) is the most benign of the corneal stromal dystrophies (Figs. 5–45, 5–46, 5–47). Visual loss develops relatively late in life. Granular dystrophy is inherited as an autosomal dominant trait. Slit lamp examination shows multiple white crumb or ring-shaped opacities in the central cornea of both eyes. Most are superficial. The opacities are separated by clear corneal stroma—hence the excellent visual acuity. Histologically, the deposits of mutant keratoepithelin resemble hyaline "rock candy." The material is more eosinophilic and less PAS-positive than the surrounding normal stroma and exhibits intense acid fuchsinophilia (red staining) with Masson trichrome (Figs. 5–46, 5–47). The granular deposits also stain intensely with the myelin stain luxol fast blue, are negative for mucopolysaccharide, and are less birefringent on polarization microscopy than normal stromal collagen. Electron microscopy discloses electron dense crystalloids, which may exhibit a regular periodicity. Granular corneal dystrophy can recur in the graft after corneal transplantation. When it does,

the granular material typically accumulates in the anterior cornea underneath the epithelium.

Lattice corneal dystrophy type I (also known as Bücklers type III or Biber-Haab-Dimmer) is an autosomal dominantly inherited form of amyloidosis that is confined to the cornea (Figs. 5–48, 5–49). The amyloid is comprised of a mutant form of keratoepithelin. Lattice corneal dystrophy typically begins during the first decade of life, and penetrating keratoplasty is indicated during the fourth or fifth decade. Surgery may be necessary earlier in cases with anterior amyloid deposition and scarring.

Clinically, the amyloid deposits form a characteristic latticework of branching relucent lines in the corneal stroma, which once were thought to be degenerating corneal nerves (Figs. 5–48). Histopathology reveals smudgy round or oval deposits of eosinophilic amyloid material in the stroma that stain positively with the amyloid stains congo red, crystal violet, and thioflavine T. The amyloid has a characteristic apple-green birefringence and dichroism when sections stained with congo red are examined with polarization microscopy (Figs. 5–49). The material is also PAS positive. Diffuse deposits of amyloid occur superficially and cause recurrent erosions in some cases, which may mimic Reis-Bücklers dystrophy. Lattice dystrophy can recur in the graft. In recurrences, the amyloid first accumulates superficially underneath the epithelium and in suture tracts.

Lattice dystrophy type II, or the Meretoja syndrome, is a type of autosomal dominantly inherited familial amyloidosis that is unrelated to the gene for keratoepithelin on chromosome 5. The amyloid deposits in the cornea and nerves are comprised of a protein called gelsolin, which is involved in actin metabolism. The corneal deposits in Meretoja syndrome typically are located in the midperipheral cornea and may represent amyloid degeneration of corneal nerves. Visual loss tends to be less severe than in lattice dystrophy type I. Patients also have amyloid neuropathy with cranial

nerve palsies, dry itchy skin, and mask-like "hound dog" facies with protruding lips.

Macular corneal dystrophy is the most severe of the classic corneal stromal dystrophies (Figs. 5–50, 5–51, 5–52). Although rare in the United States, macular dystrophy is common in Saudi Arabia and is the most common indication for corneal transplantation in Iceland. Unlike the other classic stromal dystrophies, which are dominant, macular corneal dystrophy is an autosomal recessive trait. Most patients require corneal transplantation in their twenties. The term macular refers to grayish opacities with indistinct borders that are found in the superficial stroma and begin axially (Fig. 5–50). The stroma is diffusely hazy between the macules. The haze involves the entire stroma and extends peripherally to the limbus.

Macular corneal dystrophy is a heterogeneous disorder that has been classified as a localized corneal mucopolysaccharidosis. Macular corneal dystrophy type I appears to be caused by defective sulfonization of keratan sulfate. Patients with macular dystrophy type I are deficient in corneal keratan sulfate, and they lack keratan sulfate in their serum and cartilage as well. The latter does not appear to have adverse consequences. Keratan sulfate is a major constituent of the cornea's ground substance. The lack of sulfated keratan causes abnormal hydration of the stroma, which degrades its optical properties. The hazy, poorly hydrated cornea in macular dystrophy is usually much thinner than normal (Fig. 5–51). This contrasts with the cloudy corneas in systemic mucopolysaccharidoses such as Hurler's disease, which are massively thickened. The abnormal nonsulfated keratan is insoluble and accumulates in the cytoplasm of keratocytes, in corneal endothelial cells, and as large extracellular deposits in the subepithelial stroma. The latter constitute the macules seen clinically.

The cytoplasm of the keratocytes and endothelial cells has a frothy vacuolated appearance in routine H&E sections, and the extracellular deposits are comprised of large vesicular granules that are mildly basophilic and PAS positive. The histochemical stains of choice for macular corneal dystrophy are the colloidal iron and alcian blue stains for acid mucopolysaccharide (glycosaminoglycans) (Figs. 5–52). Immunohistochemical stains for keratan sulfate have also been employed experimentally.

Schnyder's crystalline dystrophy is an autosomal dominantly inherited disorder characterized by the deposition of needle-shaped polychromatic crystals of cholesterol in the anterior corneal stroma (Fig. 5–53). A prominent arcus senilis is also present. Diffuse stromal clouding may necessitate penetrating keratoplasty during the fifth decade. Some patients have elevated serum lipids and xanthelasmas. A subtle pattern of stromal vacuolization is seen in routine sections because the lipid is dissolved during routine processing (Fig. 5–54). Stromal lipid deposition causes severe diffuse corneal clouding in rare heritable disorders of lipid metabolism, including lecithin acyl transferase (LCAT) deficiency, fish eye disease, and Tangier disease. The histopathologic findings are relatively subtle (Fig. 5–55).

François-Neetan's fleck dystrophy (dystrophie mouchetée) usually is an incidental finding clinically because visual acuity is unaffected. Ultrastructurally, the keratocytes are swollen and contain mucin and lipid. The inheritance pattern is autosomal dominant, and the dystrophy occasionally occurs unilaterally.

Congenital hereditary stromal dystrophy is a stationary, autosomal dominantly inherited disorder marked by bilateral corneal clouding. The cornea is normal in thickness, but its collagen fibers are one-half normal diameter (15 nm).

Pre-Descemet's dystrophy and deep filiform dystrophy may be the same disorder. The first is marked by fine flour-like opacities called cornea farinata, which are thought to be an age-related degenerative change. The keratocytes of deep filiform dystrophy are enlarged and contain fat and phospholipid inclusions.

## CORNEAL EDEMA, BULLOUS KERATOPATHY, AND ENDOTHELIAL DYSTROPHIES

Corneal edema caused by endothelial damage or disease (endothelial decompensation) is a major indication for corneal transplantation. In many cases the endothelial damage is related to prior intraocular surgery (aphakic or pseudophakic bullous keratopathy). The edema may also be caused by primary endothelial disease. The endothelial dystrophies of the cornea include Fuchs' dystrophy (which is relatively common) and congenital hereditary endothelial dystrophy and posterior polymorphous dystrophy of Schlichting (which are rare).

The corneal endothelium is a relatively fragile monolayer of approximately 400,000 cells; it synthesizes and rests on a thick layer of basement membrane material called Descemet's membrane (Fig. 5–3). The corneal endothelium is derived embryologically from neural crest, as are the corneal stroma and most other anterior segment tissues. Mature endothelial cells do not divide, and the endothelium generally is incapable of regeneration or repair.

The corneal endothelium plays an important role in the maintenance of corneal transparency. The transparency and optical properties of the cornea depend on an exquisitely regular spacing of the collagen fibrils in the stroma, which requires the stroma to be in a state of relative dehydration. The corneal endothelium maintains this state of relative stromal dehydration by acting as a barrier to aqueous humor and as an ion-fluid pump. If the endothelium is damaged or depleted, typically during surgery, aqueous humor enters the stroma; and the glycosaminoglycan-rich ground substance swells, separating the collagen fibrils. This action causes edema and degrades corneal transparency and optical function.

Histopathologically, an edematous cornea is thickened and may show partial obliteration of artifactitious interlamellar stromal clefts. The margins of the lamellae appear somewhat indistinct, and the edematous stroma is pale and has a frothy appearance, which has been likened to cotton candy (Fig. 5–56). As secondary epithelial edema develops, the basal cells often have a pale, edematous appearance (Fig. 5–57). Fluid accumulates in the spaces between cells and underneath the epithelium, forming focal bullous areas of epithelial detachment called bullous keratopathy (Fig. 5–58). Bullous keratopathy is a painful condition because the anterior cornea's rich supply or sensory nerve endings are exposed when the epithelial bullae rupture, which they often do. The cornea is also predisposed to infection because the normally protective epithelial layer has been compromised. A degenerative pannus (Fig. 5–33) is found in many corneas with chronic edema and bullous keratopathy. This opaque layer of connective tissue is interposed between the base of the epithelium and Bowman's layer, which is intact. Secondary epithelial changes similar to those found in anterior basement membrane dystrophy are also fairly common.

The stromal and epithelial changes of corneal edema described above are relatively nonspecific. They occur in corneas with damaged or dysfunctional endothelium (endothelial decompensation) from a variety of causes including aphakic and pseudophakic bullous keratopathy (PBK), most cases of corneal graft failure, and Fuchs' dystrophy. If bullous keratopathy and stromal edema are observed histopathologically, the pathologist should immediately direct his or her attention to Descemet's membrane and the endothelium where the diagnosis can be made.

Fuchs' dystrophy, the most common corneal dystrophy, presents during adult life with corneal edema and bullous keratopathy, which are caused by a primary defect in the corneal endothelium. This primary dystrophy of the corneal endothelium is readily diagnosed clinically and histopathologically by characteristic changes in Descemet's membrane (Figs. 5–59, 5–60, 5–61, 5–62).

Descemet's membrane in Fuchs' dystrophy typically is thickened and studded with anvil- or mushroom-shaped guttate excrescences of abnormal basement membrane material produced by the dystrophic endothelial cells (Figs. 5–59, 5–60). The term cornea guttata ("droplike cornea"; gutta = drop) is often applied to Fuchs' dystrophy and to cases of endothelial dystrophy prior to the onset of endothelial decompensation and bullous keratopathy. The guttae (guttata is an adjective!) are evident on slit lamp biomicroscopy as tiny drop-like relucences on the posterior corneal surface. Histopathologically, guttae that have been buried by a newly elaborated posterior layer of Descemet's membrane are often found, especially in the central cornea (Fig. 5–61). Thickening and multilamination of Descemet's membrane also is observed. In rare cases Descemet's membrane is diffusely thickened and lacks guttate excrescences (Fig. 5–62). The endothelium typically is atrophic, but a moderate number of corneal endothelial cells usually persist. The severe endothelial loss that characterizes most cases of PBK is unusual in Fuchs' dystrophy. The cytoplasm of the residual endothelial cells usually contain round granules of melanin pigment from the iris pigment epithelium. Such retrocorneal pigmentation in the fundus red reflex suggests the diagnosis during ophthalmoscopy or retinoscopy. The endothelial pigmentation in Fuchs' dystrophy is irregular in shape, unlike the vertically oriented Krukenberg spindle of pigmentary glaucoma, suggesting that the pattern of pigmentation is governed by an endothelial abnormality and not the circulation of aqueous humor.

Pseudophakic bullous keratopathy is an iatrogenic disease caused by direct or delayed endothelial damage associated with cataract surgery and intraocular lens implantation. In recent years PBK has been one of the most common indications for corneal transplantation.

In PBK, Descemet's membrane is not thickened and is regular in caliber without guttate excrescences (Fig.

5–63). The endothelium usually is severely atrophic and may appear totally absent (Fig. 5–64). Bullous keratopathy may be severe; total epithelial desquamation is found in some cases. Degenerative pannus formation is encountered less often than in Fuchs' dystrophy, probably because PBK has a more acute course.

An almost identical picture of corneal edema caused by endothelial decompensation occurs in most transplanted corneas that have failed, requiring repeat penetrating keratoplasty. An eosinophilic retrocorneal fibrous membrane is found on the posterior surface of Descemet's membrane in most failed grafts. If a retrocorneal fibrous membrane is observed microscopically, the periphery of the edematous cornea should be examined carefully for the wound of prior penetrating keratoplasty.

The cornea is also edematous in congenital hereditary endothelial dystrophy (CHED). The literature concerning CHED is somewhat confusing. Atrophic endothelium and massive thickening of Descemet's membrane have been reported in some cases. However, some reports have emphasized the association of massive corneal edema and normal appearing endothelium (Fig. 5–65). An inherited defect in endothelial function has been postulated in such cases.

Although the cornea is not edematous, characteristic endothelial abnormalities do occur in posterior polymorphous dystrophy. The corneal endothelial cells have many properties of corneal epithelial cells (Figs. 5–66, 5–67). They usually grow in a multilayered fashion, and electron microscopy discloses cytoplasmic tonofilaments and numerous surface microvilli. In addition, the abnormal endothelial cells express surface epithelial cytokeratins. Although some autosomal recessive cases have been reported, most cases of posterior polymorphous dystrophy are inherited as an autosomal dominant trait. Clinically, irregular blebs or vacuoles surrounded by a grayish area of mild opacification are observed at the level of Des-

cemet's membrane. The heterogeneous spectrum of disease seen in some kindreds also includes congenital corneal clouding, trough or gutter-shaped lesions of the posterior cornea, and peripheral anterior synechia formation resembling that seen in the iridocorneal endothelial (ICE) syndrome but is bilateral. The gutters can be confused with old Descemet's tears caused by obstetric forceps injuries, but they lack relucent margins.

Corneal edema occurs in some patients who have the ICE syndrome, which is characterized by unilateral glaucoma and secondary iris abnormalities caused by a proliferation of abnormal corneal endothelial cells. This disease spectrum includes the Cogan-Reese and Chandler syndromes and essential iris atrophy. The ICE syndrome is discussed further in Chapter 7.

## CORNEAL MANIFESTATIONS OF SYSTEMIC DISEASE

Copper deposition in the peripheral part of Descemet's membrane manifests clinically as a Kayser-Fleischer ring in patients with Wilson's hepatolenticular degeneration (Fig. 5–68). An analogous deposit of copper in the anterior lens capsule causes sunflower cataract (see Fig. 3–21). Corneal copper deposition has been reported in patients with primary biliary cirrhosis, familial cholestatic cirrhosis, and monoclonal gammopathies associated with multiple myeloma and pulmonary carcinoma.

Deposits of immunoglobulin in the cornea may herald the presence of protein dyscrasias such as multiple myeloma or Waldenström's macroglobulinemia (Fig. 5–69). The corneal deposition is protean in its manifestations. Deep polymorphic infiltrates occur in some patients; and others develop polychromatic crystals in the corneal epithelium.

Other causes of corneal crystals include cystinosis, gout, Bietti's crystalline dystrophy, and injury by the sap of plants such as the aroid *Dieffenbachia*, which contains crystalline raphides. Cystine crystals dissolve in water; preservation necessitates fixation of the cornea in absolute alcohol.

Cysts of the pars plana and pars plicata are common in multiple myeloma. The cysts in affected patients contain myeloma protein or Bence Jones protein, which is precipitated by fixation, causing the cysts to become milky white (see Fig. 8–52). Pars plana cysts found incidentally in elderly patients are filled with hyaluronic acid and are not opacified by fixation (see Figs. 8–50, 8–51).

## CORNEAL TRANSPLANTATION

Corneal transplantation, or penetrating keratoplasty, involves excising a central disk or button of full-thickness cornea and replacing it with a new transparent tissue obtained postmortem from a donor. Corneal transplantation is often successful without systemic immunosuppression because the cornea is an avascular structure. Surgery is less successful in eyes with corneal vascularization.

Corneal edema caused by endothelial damage or dystrophy is the most common indication for corneal transplantation in the United States. This category includes pseudophakic or aphakic bullous keratopathy and Fuchs' dystrophy. Most "failed grafts" also are edematous due to endothelial loss. Keratoconus is another common indication for transplantation. Other diseases treated by penetrating keratoplasty are interstitial keratitis, visually disabling scars, corneal dystrophies, and infectious keratopathies including chronic herpes simplex stromal keratitis and bacterial or fungal ulcers. Surgery is performed for acute keratitis when perforation has occurred or is imminent, or occasionally when the identity of the pathogenetic organism is uncertain.

## SCLERA

Scleral specimens are relatively uncommon and typically are inflammatory in nature. A superficial infiltrate of lymphocytes and plasma cells is seen with benign episcleritis. A necrotizing zonal pattern of granulomatous inflammation analogous to that seen in rheumatoid nodules characterizes the severe scleritis that complicates rheumatoid arthritis (Figs. 5–70, 5–71). In nodular episcleritis the granulomatous reaction is limited to the episcleral tissues. In severe cases of rheumatoid scleritis (scleromalacia perforans) areas of severe scleral thinning appear blue clinically because there is increased visibility of the underlying pigmented uvea. Patients who have rheumatoid scleritis are susceptible to the development of fatal cardiac and pulmonary manifestations of their rheumatoid disease. Posterior scleritis can mimic a primary uveal neoplasm. Scleritis and peripheral corneal ulceration can complicate systemic lupus erythematosus, polyarteritis nodosa, Wegener's granulomatosis, and relapsing polychondritis.

## References

### General References

Rodrigues MM, Hidayat AA, Choe HS: Advances in corneal pathology. Ophthalmol Clin North Am 8:83–107, 1995.
Spencer WH: Cornea. In Spencer WH (ed) Ophthalmic Pathology: An Atlas and Textbook. Philadelphia: Saunders, 1985:229–388.
Starck T, Hersh PS, Kenyon KR: Corneal dysgeneses, dystrophies and degenerations. In Albert DM, Jakobiec FA (eds) Principles and Practice of Ophthalmology: Clinical Practice. Vol 1. Philadelphia: Saunders, 1994:13–77.

### Developmental Lesions

Kanai A, Wood TC, Polack FM, et al: The fine structure of sclerocornea. Invest Ophthalmol Vis Sci 10:687–694, 1971.
Simpson WA, Parsons MA: The ultrastructural pathological features of congenital microcoria: a case report. Arch Ophthalmol 107:99, 1989.

### Axenfeld-Rieger Syndrome

Alkemade P: Dysgenesis Mesodermalis of the Iris and the Cornea. Assen, The Netherlands: Charles C Thomas, 1969.
Henkind P, Siegel IM, Carr RE: Mesodermal dysgenesis of the anterior segment: Rieger's anomaly. Arch Ophthalmol 73:810–817, 1965.
Reese A, Ellsworth R: The anterior chamber cleavage syndrome. Arch Ophthalmol 75:307, 1966.
Rieger H: Dysgenesis mesodermalis Corneae et Iridis. Z Augenheilkd 86:333, 1935.
Shields MB: Axenfeld-Rieger syndrome: a theory of mechanism and distinctions from the iridocorneal endothelial syndrome. Trans Am Ophthalmol Soc 81:736–784, 1983.
Shields M: Axenfeld-Rieger syndrome. In Ritch R, Shields M, Krupin T (eds) The Glaucomas. St Louis: Mosby, 1989.
Shields M, Buckley E, Klintworth G, et al: Axenfeld-Rieger syndrome: a spectrum of developmental disorders. Surv Ophthalmol 29:387, 1985.
Waring GI, Rodrigues M, Laibson P: Anterior chamber cleavage syndrome: a stepladder classification. Surv Ophthalmol 20:3, 1975.

### Peters' Anomaly

Hanson IM, Fletcher JM, Jordan T, et al: Mutations at the PAX6 locus are found in heterogeneous anterior segment malformations including Peters' anomaly. Nat Genet 6: 168, 1994.
Hennekam RC, Van Schooneveld MJ, Ardinger HH, et al: The Peters'-plus syndrome: description of 16 patients and review of the literature. Clin Dysmorphol 4:283–300, 1993.
Townsend W, Font R, Zimmerman L: Congenital corneal leukomas: 1. Central defects in Descemet's membrane. Am J Ophthalmol 77:80, 1974.
Townsend W, Font R, Zimmerman L: Congenital corneal leukomas. 2. Histopathological findings in 13 eyes with central defects in Descemet's membrane. Am J Ophthalmol 77:192, 1974.
Traboulsi EI, Maumenee IH: Peters' anomaly and associated congenital malformations. Arch Ophthalmol 110:1739–1744, 1992.

### Bacterial Keratitis

Dugel PU, Holland GN, Brown HH: Mycobacterium fortuitum keratitis. Am J Ophthalmol 105:661–669, 1988.

Elder MJ, Stapleton F, Evans E, Dart JK: Biofilm-related infections in ophthalmology. Eye 9:102–109, 1995.

Meisler DM, Langston RH, Naab TJ, Aaby AA, McMahon JT, Tubbs RR: Infectious crystalline keratopathy. Am J Ophthalmol 97:337–343, 1984.

Rhem MN, Wilhelmus KR, Font RL: Infectious crystalline keratopathy caused by Candida parapsilosis. Cornea 15: 543–545, 1996.

## Herpetic Keratitis

Cook SD, Hill JH: Herpes simplex virus: molecular biology and the possibility of corneal latency. Surv Ophthalmol 36:140–148, 1991.

Dawson CR, Togni B, Moore TE Jr: Structural changes in chronic herpetic keratitis studied by light and electron microscopy. Arch Ophthalmol 79:740–747, 1968.

Font RL: Chronic ulcerative keratitis caused by herpes simplex virus. Arch Ophthalmol 90:382–385, 1973.

Hendricks RL: An immunologist's view of herpes simplex keratitis: Thygeson lecture 1996. Cornea 16:503–506, 1997.

Liesgang TJ: Biology and molecular aspects of herpes simplex and varicella-zoster virus infections. Ophthalmology 99:781, 1992.

Pepose JS: Herpes simplex keratitis: role of viral infection versus immune response. Surv Ophthalmol 35:345–352, 1991.

Prenbenga LW, Laibson PR: Dendritic lesions in herpes zoster ophthalmicus. Arch Ophthalmol 90:268, 1973.

Zhao Z-S, Granucci F, Yeh L, et al: Molecular mimicry by herpes simplex virus-type I: autoimmune disease after viral infection. Science 279:1344–1347, 1998.

## Epidemic Keratoconjunctivitis

Dawson CR, Hanna L, Wood TR, et al: Adenovirus type 8 keratoconjunctivitis in the United States. III. Epidemiological, clinical and microbiologic features. Am J Ophthalmol 69:473–480, 1970.

Laibson PR, Dhiri S, Oconer J, Ortolan G: Corneal infiltrates in epidemic keratoconjunctivitis: response to double-blind corticosteroid therapy. Arch Ophthalmol 84:36–40, 1970.

## Interstitial Keratitis

Char DH, Cogan DG, Sullivan WR: Immunologic study of non-syphilitic interstitial keratitis with vestibulo-auditory symptoms. Am J Ophthalmol 80:491–494, 1975.

Waring GO, Font RL, Rodrigues MM, Mulberger RD: Alterations of Descemet's membrane in interstitial keratitis. Am J Ophthalmol 81:773–785, 1976.

## Acanthamoeba Keratitis

Auran JD, Starr MB, Jakobiec FA: Acanthamoeba keratitis: a review of the literature. Cornea 62:2–26, 1987.

Garner A. Pathogenesis of acanthamoebic keratitis: hypothesis based on a histological analysis of 30 cases. Br J Ophthalmol 77:366–370, 1993.

Marines HC, Osato MS, Font RL: The value of calcofluor white in the diagnosis of mycotic and Acanthamoeba infections of the eye and ocular adnexa. Ophthalmology 94: 23–26, 1987.

Paul EV, Zimmerman LE: Some observations on the ocular pathology of onchocerciasis. Hum Pathol 1:581–594, 1970.

## Peripheral Corneal Ulcerations

Austin P, Green WR, Sallyer DC, et al: Peripheral corneal degeneration and occlusive vasculitis in Wegener's granulomatosis. Am J Ophthalmol 85:311–317, 1978.

Brown SI: Mooren's ulcer: histopathology and proteolytic enzymes of adjacent conjunctiva. Br J Ophthalmol 59: 670–674, 1975.

Brown SI, Mondino BJ, Rabin BS: Autoimmune phenomenon in Mooren's ulcer. Am J Ophthalmol 82: 835–840, 1976.

Frayer WC: The histopathology of perilimbal ulceration in Wegener's granulomatosis. Arch Ophthalmol 64:88–94, 1960.

Guyer DR, Barraquer J, McDonnell PJ, Green WR: Terrien's marginal degeneration: clinicopathologic case reports. Graefes Arch Clin Exp Ophthalmol 225:19–27, 1987.

Moazami G, Auran JD, Florakis GJ, Wilson SE, Srinivasan DB: Interferon treatment of Mooren's ulcers associated with hepatitis C. Am J Ophthalmol 119:365–366, 1995.

## Corneal Degenerations

Austin P, Jakobiec FA, Iwamoto T: Elastodysplasia and elastodystrophy as the pathologic bases of ocular pterygia and pinguecula. Ophthalmology 90:96–109, 1983.

Barchiesi BJ, Eckel RH, Ellis PP: The cornea and disorders of lipid metabolism. Surv Ophthalmol 36:1–22, 1991.

Cogan DG, Albright F, Bartter FC: Hypercalcemia and band keratopathy: report of nineteen cases. Arch Ophthalmol 40:624–638, 1940.

Cursino JW, Fine BS: A histologic study of calcific and non-calcific band keratopathy. Am J Ophthalmol 82:395–404, 1976.

Freedman A: Climatic droplet keratopathy. I. Clinical aspects. Arch Ophthalmol 89:193–197, 1973.

Freedman A: Labrador keratopathy and related diseases. Can J Ophthalmol 8:286–290, 1973.

Gray RH, Johnson GJ, Freedman A: Climatic droplet keratopathy. Surv Ophthalmol 36:241–253, 1992.

Hogan MJ, Alvarado J: Pterygium and pinguecula: electron microscopic study. Arch Ophthalmol 78:174–186, 1967.

Klintworth GK: Chronic actinic keratopathy—a condition associated with conjunctival elastosis (pingueculae) and typified by characteristic extracellular concretions. Am J Pathol 67:327–342, 1972.

Rodrigues MM, Laibson PR, Weinreb S: Corneal elastosis: appearance of band-like keratopathy and spheroidal degeneration. Arch Ophthalmol 93:111–114, 1975.

Vannas A, Hogan MJ, Wood I: Salzmann's nodular degeneration of the cornea. Am J Ophthalmol 79:211–219, 1975.

## Vitamin A Deficiency

Sjögren H, Bloch K: Keratoconjunctivitis sicca and the Sjögren syndrome. Surv Ophthalmol 16:145–159, 1971.

Smith RS, Farrell T, Bailey T: Keratomalacia. Surv Ophthalmol 20:213–219, 1975.

Venkataswamy G: Ocular manifestations of vitamin A deficiency. Br J Ophthalmol 51:854–859, 1967.

## Keratoconus

Barraquer-Somers E, Chan CC, Green WR: Corneal epithelial iron deposition. Ophthalmology 90:729–734, 1983.

Kenney MC, Chwa M, Opbroek AJ, Brown DJ: Increased gelatinolytic activity in keratoconus keratocyte cultures: a correlation to an altered matrix metalloproteinase-2/tissue inhibitor of metalloproteinase ratio. Cornea 13:114–124, 1994.

Kenney MC, Nesburn AB, Burgeson RE, Butkowski RJ, Ljubimov AV: Abnormalities of the extracellular matrix in keratoconus corneas. Cornea 16:345–351, 1997.

Klintworth GK, Damms T: Corneal dystrophies and keratoconus. Curr Opin Ophthalmol 6:44–56, 1995.

Krachmer JH, Feder RS, Belin MW: Keratoconus and related noninflammatory corneal thinning disorders. Surv Ophthalmol 28:293–322, 1984.

Kremer I, Eagle RC, Rapuano CJ, Laibson PR: Histologic evidence of recurrent keratoconus seven years after keratoplasty. Am J Ophthalmol 119:511–512, 1995.

### Epithelial and Bowman's Membrane Dystrophies

Burns RP: Meesman's corneal dystrophy. Trans Am Ophthalmol Soc 66:530–635, 1968.

Irvine AD, Corden LD, Swensson O, et al: Mutations in cornea-specific keratin K3 or K12 genes cause Meesmann's corneal dystrophy. Nat Genet 16:184–187, 1997.

Klintworth GK: Proteins in ocular disease. In Garner A, Klintworth GK (eds) Pathobiology of Ocular Disease: A Dynamic Approach. 2nd ed. Part B. New York: Marcel Dekker, 1994:973–1032.

Klintworth GK, Valnickova Z, Kielar RA, et al: Familial subepithelial corneal amyloidosis: a lactoferrin-related amyloidosis. Invest Ophthalmol Vis Sci 38:2756–2763, 1997.

Kuchle M, Green WR, Volcker HE, Barraquer J: Reevaluation of corneal dystrophies of Bowman's layer and the anterior stroma (Reis-Bucklers and Thiel-Behnke types): a light and electron microscopic study of eight corneas and a review of the literature. Cornea 14:333–354, 1995.

Kuwabara T, Ciccarelli EC: Meesmann's corneal dystrophy: a pathological study. Arch Ophthalmol 71:676–682, 1964.

Li S, Edward DP, Ratnakar KS, Reddy M, Tso MO: Clinico-histopathological findings of gelatinous droplike corneal dystrophy among Asians. Cornea 15:355–362, 1996.

Perry HD, Fine BS, Caldwell DR: Reis-Bücklers dystrophy: a study of eight cases. Arch Ophthalmol 97:664–670, 1979.

Rodrigues MM, Fine BS, Laibson PR, et al: Disorders of the corneal epithelium—a clinicopathologic study of dot, geographic and fingerprint patterns. Arch Ophthalmol 92:475–482, 1974.

Small KW, Mullen L, Barletta J, et al: Mapping of Reis-Bucklers' corneal dystrophy to chromosome 5q. Am J Ophthalmol 121:384–390, 1996.

Waring GO, Rodrigues MM, Laibson PR: Corneal dystrophies. I. Dystrophies of the epithelium, Bowman's layer and stroma. Surv Ophthalmol 23:71–122, 1978.

Weber FL, Babel J: Gelatinous drop-like dystrophy: a form of primary corneal amyloidosis. Arch Ophthalmol 98:144–148, 1980.

Yee RW, Sullivan LS, Lai HT, et al: Linkage mapping of Thiel-Behnke corneal dystrophy (CDB2) to chromosome 10q23-q24. Genomics 46:152–154, 1997.

### Stromal Dystrophies

Edward DP, Thonar EJ, Srinivasan M, et al: Macular dystrophy of the cornea: a systemic disorder of keratan sulfate metabolism. Ophthalmology 97:1194–1200, 1990.

Garner A, Tripathi RC: Hereditary crystalline stromal dystrophy of Schnyder. II. Histopathology and ultrastructure. Br J Ophthalmol 56:400–408, 1972.

Gaynor PM, Zhang WY, Weiss JS, Skarlatos SI, Rodrigues MM, Kruth HS: Accumulation of HDL apolipoproteins accompanies abnormal cholesterol accumulation in Schnyder's corneal dystrophy. Arterioscler Thromb Vasc Biol 16:992–999, 1996.

Hassell JR, Klintworth GK: Serum sulfotransferase levels in patients with macular corneal dystrophy type I. Arch Ophthalmol 115:1419–1421, 1997.

Hirano K, Klintworth GK, Zhan Q, et al: Beta ig-H3 is synthesized by corneal epithelium and perhaps endothelium in Fuchs' dystrophic corneas. Curr Eye Res 15:965–972, 1996.

Hogan MJ, Albarado J: Ultrastructure of lattice dystrophy of the cornea: a case report. Am J Ophthalmol 64(Suppl):656–660, 1967.

Jonasson F, Oshima E, Thonar EJ, Smith CF, Johannsson JH, Klintworth GK: Macular corneal dystrophy in Iceland: a clinical, genealogic, and immunohistochemical study of 28 patients. Ophthalmology 103:1111–1117, 1996.

Jones ST, Zimmerman LE: Histopathologic differentiation of granular, macular, and lattice dystrophies of the cornea. Am J Ophthalmol 51:394–410, 1961.

Kivela T, Tarkkanen A, Frangione B, Ghiso J, Haltia M: Ocular amyloid deposition in familial amyloidosis, Finnish: an analysis of native and variant gelsolin in Meretoja's syndrome. Invest Ophthalmol Vis Sci 35:3759–3769, 1994.

Klintworth GK: Lattice corneal dystrophy: an inherited variety of amyloidosis restricted to the cornea. Am J Pathol 50:371–399, 1967.

Klintworth GK, Chang TS, Culbertson WW: Central cloudy corneal dystrophy of Francois: a clinicopathologic study. Arch Ophthalmol 115:1058–1062, 1997.

Klintworth GK, Oshima E, al-Rajhi A, al-Saif A, Thonar EJ, Karcioglu ZA: Macular corneal dystrophy in Saudi Arabia: a study of 56 cases and recognition of a new immunophenotype. Am J Ophthalmol 124:9–18, 1997.

Mannis MJ, Krachmer JH, Rodrigues MM, Pardos GJ: Polymorphic amyloid degeneration of the cornea: a clinical and histopathologic study. Arch Ophthalmol 99:1217–1223, 1981.

McCarthy M, Innis S, Dubord P, White V: Panstromal Schnyder corneal dystrophy: a clinical pathologic report with quantitative analysis of corneal lipid composition. Ophthalmology 101:895–901, 1994.

Meretoja J: Familial systemic paramyeloidosis with lattice dystrophy of the cornea, progressive cranial neuropathy, skin changes and various internal symptoms: a previously unrecognized heritable syndrome. Ann Clin Res 1:314–324, 1969.

Munier FL, Korvatska E, Djemai A, et al: Kerato-epithelin mutations in four 5q31-linked corneal dystrophies Nat Genet 15:247–251, 1997.

Nicholson DH, Green WR, Cross HE, et al: A clinical and histopathological study of François-Neetens speckled corneal dystrophy. Am J Ophthalmol 83:554–560, 1977.

Purcell JJ Jr, Rodrigues M, Chishti MI, Riner RN, Dooley JM: Lattice corneal dystrophy associated with familial systemic amyloidosis (Meretoja's syndrome). Ophthalmology 90:1512–1517, 1983.

Shearman AM, Hudson TJ, Andresen JM, et al: The gene for Schnyder's crystalline corneal dystrophy maps to human chromosome 1p34.1-p36. Hum Mol Genet 5:1667–1672, 1996.

Starck T, Kenyon KR, Hanninen LA, et al: Clinical and histopathologic studies of two families with lattice corneal dystrophy and familial systemic amyloidosis (Meretoja syndrome). Ophthalmology 98:1197–1206, 1991.

Stone EM, Mathers WD, Rossenwasser GOD, et al: Three autosomal dominant corneal dystrophies map to chromosome 5q. Nat Genet 6:47–51, 1994.

Vance JM, Jonasson F, Lennon F, et al: Linkage of a gene for macular corneal dystrophy to chromosome 16. Am J Hum Genet 58:757–762, 1996.

Varssano D, Cohen EJ, Nelson LB, Eagle RC Jr: Corneal transplantation in Maroteaux-Lamy syndrome. Arch Ophthalmol 115:428–429, 1997.

Weller RO, Rodger FC: Crystalline stromal dystrophy: histochemistry and ultrastructure of the cornea. Br J Ophthalmol 64:46–52, 1980.

### Endothelial Dystrophies

Adamis AP, Filatov V, Tripathi Bj, Tripathi RC: Fuchs' endothelial dystrophy of the cornea. Surv Ophthalmol 38:149–168, 1993.

Chan C, Green WR, Barraquer J: Similarities between posterior polymorphous and congenital hereditary endothelial dystrophies: a study of 14 buttons in 11 cases. Cornea 1:155–172, 1982.

Cibis G, Krachmer J, Phelps C, et al: Iridocorneal adhesions in posterior polymorphous dystrophy. Trans Am Acad Ophthalmol Otolaryngol 81:770, 1976.

Cibis G, Krachmer J, Phelps C, et al: The clinical spectrum of posterior polymorphous dystrophy. Arch Ophthalmol 95:1529, 1977.

Hanna C, Fraunfelder FT, McNair JR: An ultrastructure study of posterior polymorphous dystrophy of the cornea. Ann Ophthalmol 9:1371–1378, 1977.

Heon E, Mathers WD, Alward WL, et al: Linkage of posterior polymorphous corneal dystrophy to 20q11. Hum Mol Genet 4:485–488, 1995.

Levy SG, Moss J, Noble BA, McCartney AC: Early-onset posterior polymorphous dystrophy. Arch Ophthalmol 114:1265–1268, 1996.

Levy SG, Moss J, Sawada H, Dopping-Hepenstal PJ, McCartney AC: The composition of wide-spaced collagen in normal and diseased Descemet's membrane. Curr Eye Res 15:45–52, 1996.

McCartney AC, Kirkness CM: Comparison between posterior polymorphous dystrophy and congenital hereditary endothelial dystrophy of the cornea. Eye 2:63–70, 1988.

Sekundo W, Lee WR, Kirkness CM, Aitken DA, Fleck B: An ultrastructural investigation of an early manifestation of the posterior polymorphous dystrophy of the cornea. Ophthalmology 101:1422–1431, 1994.

Toma NM, Ebenezer ND, Inglehearn CF, Plant C, Ficker LA, Bhattacharya SS: Linkage of congenital hereditary endothelial dystrophy to chromosome 20. Hum Mol Genet 4:2395–2398, 1995.

Wilson DJ, Weleber RG, Klein ML, Welch RB, Green WR: Bietti's crystalline dystrophy: a clinicopathologic correlative study. Arch Ophthalmol 107:213–221, 1989.

**Cornea in Systemic Disease**

Auran JD, Donn A, Hyman GA: Multiple myeloma presenting as vortex crystalline keratopathy and complicated by endocapsular hematoma. Cornea 11:584–585, 1992.

Lois N, Kowal VO, Cohen EJ, et al: Indications for penetrating keratoplasty and associated procedures, 1989–1995. Cornea 16:623–629, 1997.

Ramsay AS, Lee WR, Mohammed A: Changing indications for penetrating keratoplasty in the west of Scotland from 1970 to 1995. Eye 11:357–360, 1997.

Stirling JW, Henderson DW, Rozenbilds MA, Skinner JM, Filipic M: Crystalloidal paraprotein deposits in the cornea: an ultrastructural study of two new cases with tubular crystalloids that contain IgG kappa light chains and IgG gamma heavy chains. Ultrastruct Pathol 21:337–344, 1997.

Tso MO, Fine BS, Thorpe HE: Kayser-Fleischer ring and associated cataract in Wilson's disease. Am J Ophthalmol 79:479–488, 1975.

**Sclera**

Benson WE, Shields JS, Tasman W, Crandall AS: Posterior scleritis, a cause of diagnostic confusion. Arch Ophthalmol 97:1482–1486, 1979.

Ferry AP: The histopathology of rheumatoid episcleral nodules: an extra-articular manifestation of rheumatoid arthritis. Arch Ophthalmol 82:77–88, 1969.

Foster CS, Forstot SL, Wilson LA: Mortality rate in rheumatoid arthritis patients developing necrotizing scleritis peripheral ulcerative keratitis: effects of systemic immunosuppression. Ophthalmology 91:1253–1263, 1984.

Norn MS: Scleral plaques. I. Incidence and morphology. Acta Ophthalmol (Copenh) 52:96–106, 1974.

Rao NA, Marak GE, Hidayat AA: Necrotizing scleritis: a clinicopathologic study of 41 cases. Ophthalmology 92:1542–1549, 1985.

Watson PG, Hayreh SS: Scleritis and episcleritis. Br J Ophthalmol 60:163–191, 1976.

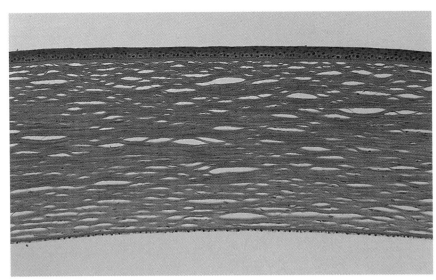

FIGURE 5–1 • **Normal cornea.** The corneal epithelium rests on Bowman's membrane. Most of the cornea is composed of collagenous stroma that contains keratocytes and artifactitious clefts. Posteriorly, a monolayer of endothelial cells rests on Descemet's membrane. Hematoxylin-eosin, ×50.

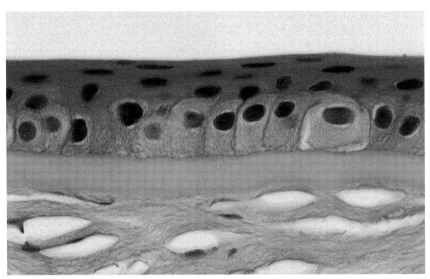

FIGURE 5–2 • **Corneal epithelium.** Five cells thick, the corneal epithelium is composed of basal cells, wing cells, and flattened superficial squamous cells. Bowman's membrane is the hyaline band of modified stroma underneath the epithelium. The clear spaces in the stroma are artifactitious clefts between lamellae. There is edema of the basal epithelium. The thin epithelial basement membrane is not evident in this section. Hematoxylin-eosin, ×250.

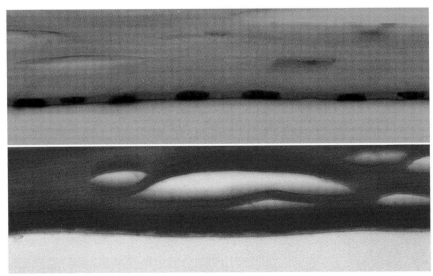

FIGURE 5–3 • **Corneal endothelium and Descemet's membrane.** The flattened monolayer of corneal endothelial cells lining the posterior cornea rests on Descemet's membrane, a thick basement membrane secreted by the endothelial cells. Descemet's membrane stains intensely with the PAS stain (bottom). Top: hematoxylin-eosin, ×250; bottom: periodic acid-Schiff, ×250.

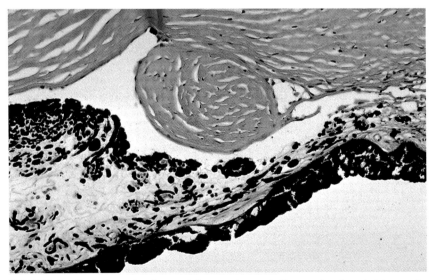

FIGURE 5–4 • **Posterior embryotoxon.** A large oval mound of connective tissue is interposed between the end of Descemet's membrane (Schwalbe's line) and the trabecular meshwork. This infant had multiple anterior segment anomalies. Hematoxylin-eosin, ×50.

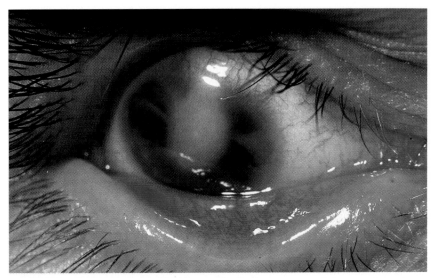

FIGURE 5–5 • **Peters' anomaly with iridocorneal adhesions.** Bands of iris stroma insert into the margin of the central corneal opacity. The lens was adherent to the posterior cornea centrally. Both eyes were affected. (Courtesy of Dr. Irving Raber, Wills Eye Hospital)

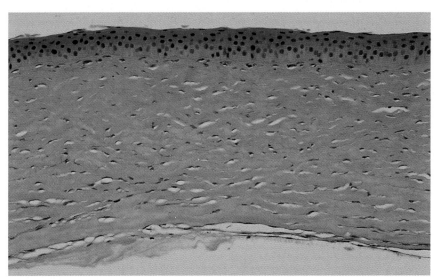

FIGURE 5–6 • **Posterior ulcer of von Hippel.** The endothelium and Descemet's membrane are absent in the region of a central posterior ulcer. The collagenous lamellae of the posterior stroma are thickened and irregular. Bowman's membrane is absent, and the epithelium is mildly thickened. A central corneal opacity was present clinically. Hematoxylin-eosin, ×50.

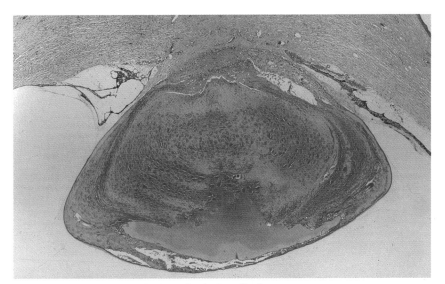

FIGURE 5–7 • **Peters' anomaly, keratolenticular adhesion.** The cataractous crystalline lens adheres to a posterior ulcer in the central cornea. The iris also attaches to the margin of the ulcer. The patient had fetal alcohol syndrome. (Case courtesy of Dr. Nongnart Chan, Philadelphia, PA)

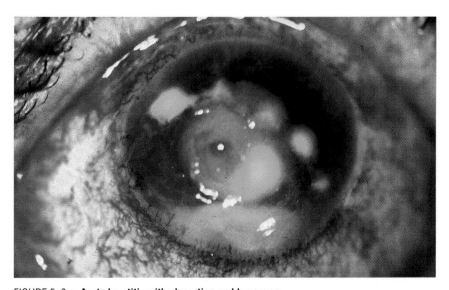

FIGURE 5–8 • **Acute keratitis with ulceration and hypopyon.**

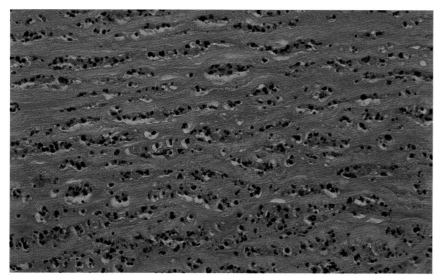

FIGURE 5–9 • **Acute keratitis.** Polymorphonuclear leukocytes accumulate in the clefts between the stromal lamellae. Most of the polys have pyknotic nuclei. Hematoxylin-eosin, ×100.

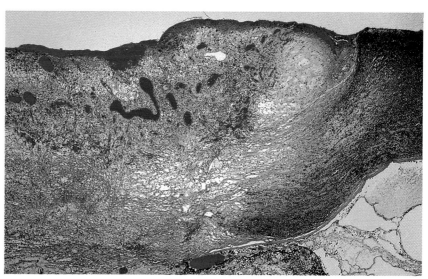

FIGURE 5–10 • ***Pseudomonas sclerokeratitis.*** *Pseudomonas* keratitis often extends posteriorly as an infectious scleritis. The acutely inflamed cornea (at right) appears blue reflecting heavy infiltration by polys. Proteolytic enzymes released by the gram negative rods have dissolved the limbal sclera. The angle is closed. Hematoxylin-eosin, ×10.

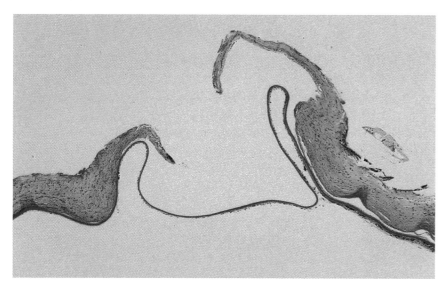

FIGURE 5–11 • **Descemetocele, acute keratitis.** An intact layer of Descemet's membrane persists in the bed of a deep corneal ulcer. The anterior layers of the cornea have been destroyed by inflammation. Hematoxylin-eosin, ×10.

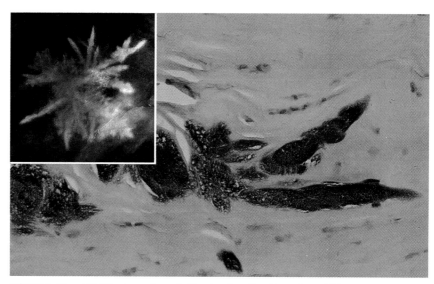

FIGURE 5–12 • **Infectious pseudocrystalline keratopathy.** Large basophilic colonies of relatively avirulent streptococci distend interlammellar clefts in a noninflamed part of the corneal stroma. Hematoxylin-eosin, ×100. *Inset:* Radiating crystalline appearance of a bacterial colony.

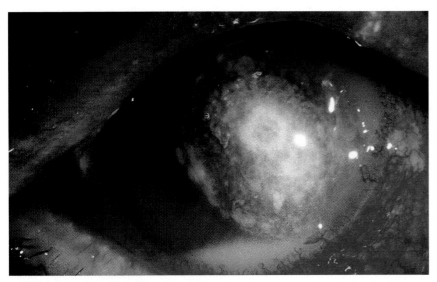

FIGURE 5–13 • **Fungal keratitis.** Aspergillus was cultured. Satellite lesions and a hypopyon are present. (Courtesy of Dr. Peter Laibson, Wills Eye Hospital)

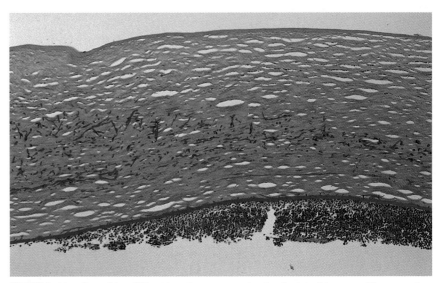

FIGURE 5–14 • **Fungal keratitis.** Note the numerous hyphae in the mid-stroma. The corneal epithelium is absent. A hypopyon adheres to the posterior cornea. Periodic acid-Schiff, ×25.

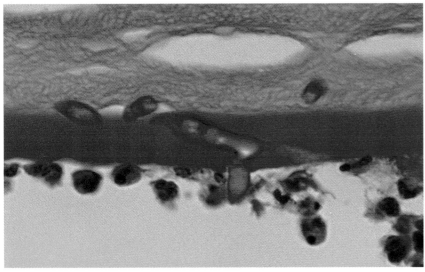

FIGURE 5–15 • **Fungal keratitis.** PAS-positive septate fungal hypha perforates Descemet's membrane and invades the anterior chamber, which contains polymorphonuclear leukocytes. Periodic acid-Schiff, ×250.

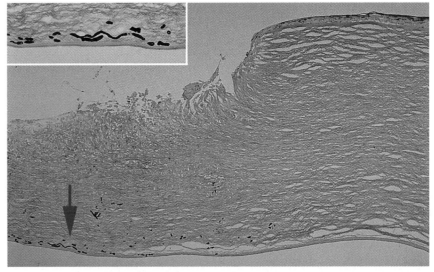

FIGURE 5–16 • **Deep hyphae, fungal keratitis.** The corneal epithelium and anterior stroma are absent in the ulcerated area at left. Arrow points to GMS-stained hyphae in the deep stroma near Descemet's membrane. *Inset:* Hyphae are seen at higher magnification. A superficial scraping of the ulcer bed was negative for fungus. Gomori methenamine silver. Main figure ×50, inset ×100.

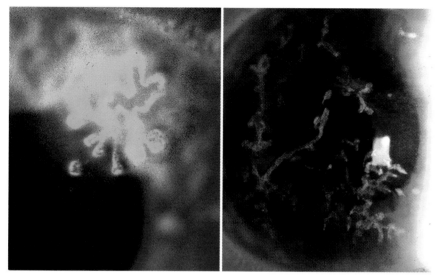

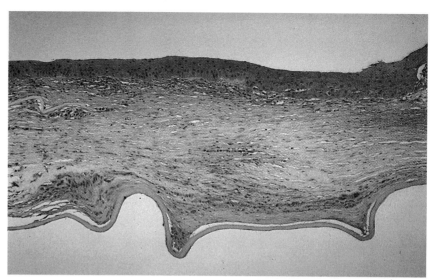

FIGURE 5–17 • **Viral dendritic keratitis, HSV and VZV.** Branching herpes simplex virus (HSV) dendrite (at left) is full-thickness ulceration with terminal bulbs. Dendritiform lesions of varicella-zoster virus (VZV) keratitis (at right) are comprised of heaped-up epithelium. HSV dendrite is stained with fluorescein dye. (Courtesy of Dr. Peter Laibson, Wills Eye Hospital)

FIGURE 5–18 • **Chronic herpetic stromal keratitis.** The stroma is thin, scarred, and chronically inflamed. The inflammatory infiltrate contains lymphocytes, plasma cells, and epithelioid histiocytes. Bowman's membrane is largely destroyed, and the epithelium is irregularly thickened. Descemet's membrane is folded. Hematoxylin-eosin, ×50.

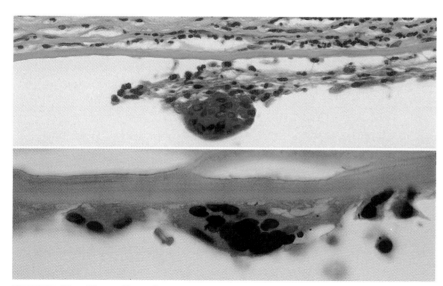

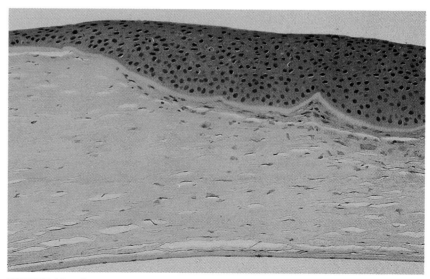

FIGURE 5–19 • **Giant cell reaction to Descemet's membrane, chronic HSV keratitis.** Although characteristic, this finding is not pathognomonic for HSV. Hematoxylin-eosin. Top: ×100, bottom ×250.

FIGURE 5–20 • **Compensatory epithelial hyperplasia, chronic HSV keratitis.** The epithelium is markedly thickened overlying an area of stroma loss. Bowman's membrane persists in the area of stromal thinning. Hematoxylin-eosin, ×50.

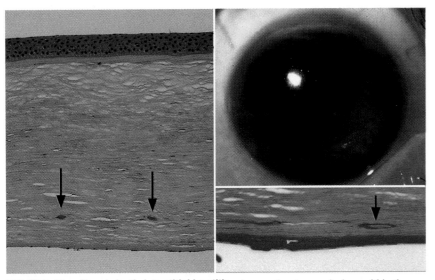

FIGURE 5–21 • **Chronic luetic interstitial keratitis.** Arrows denote vessels deep within the non-inflamed corneal stroma. Anterior stroma has lucent vacuolated appearance. Note the faint nebulous opacification of the cornea. *Inset:* Thickening of Descemet's membrane is seen. Hematoxylin-eosin. Main figure ×50, inset: Periodic acid-Schiff, ×100.

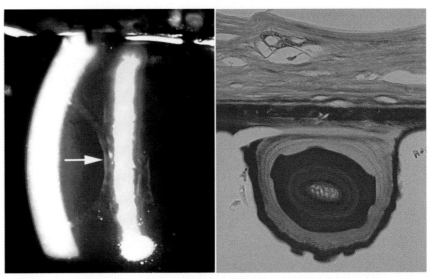

FIGURE 5–22 • **Descemet's membrane thickening, chronic luetic interstitial keratitis.** Arrow in clinical photograph denotes a relucent mass of hypertrophic Descemet's membrane on the posterior cornea. Photomicrograph shows a thick cylinder of PAS-positive basement membrane material studded with guttate excrescences on irregularly thickened Descemet's membrane. Periodic acid-Schiff, ×50. (Clinical photograph courtesy of Dr. Irving Raber, Wills Eye Hospital)

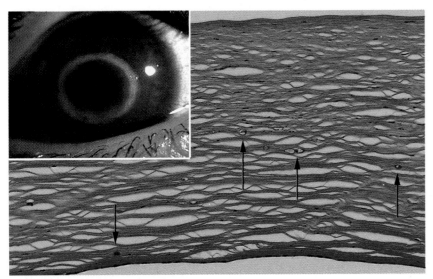

FIGURE 5–23 • **Acanthamoeba keratitis.** Arrows denote amebic cysts in minimally inflamed corneal stroma. The epithelium is absent. Clinical photograph shows characteristic late ring infiltrate. Hematoxylin-eosin, ×50. (Clinical photo courtesy of Dr. Elizabeth Cohen, Wills Eye Hospital)

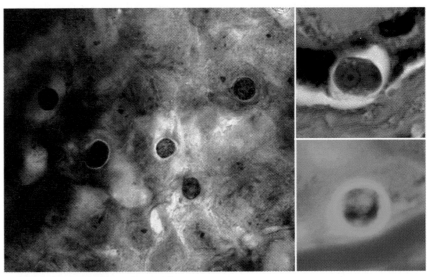

FIGURE 5–24 • **Acanthamoeba keratitis.** Acanthameba cysts are seen in epithelial smear stained with Giemsa. *Insets:* Sections stained with hematoxylin-eosin, (*top inset*) and calcofluor white (*bottom inset*). Cytoplasmic retraction from the cyst wall and a round nucleus with a distinct nucleolus are evident in routine section. Main figure: Giemsa, ×100; top inset: hematoxylin-eosin, ×250; bottom inset: calcofluor white, ×250.

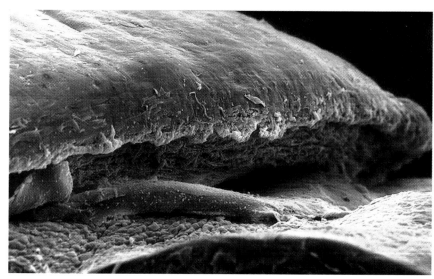

FIGURE 5–25 • **Mooren's ulcer.** Scanning electron micrograph shows characteristic overhanging margin of ulcer. ×125.

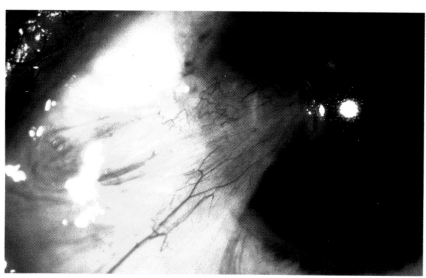

FIGURE 5–26 • **Pterygium.** Wedge-shaped ingrowth of conjunctival tissue invades the periphery of the nasal cornea. (Courtesy of Dr. Peter Laibson, Wills Eye Hospital)

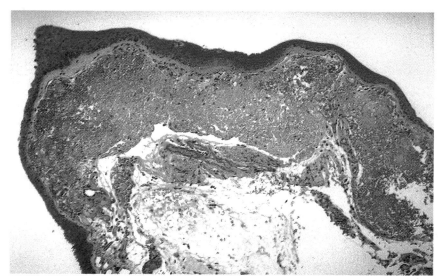

FIGURE 5–27 • **Pterygium.** There is extensive actinic elastosis of the substantia propria in this example. Hematoxylin-eosin, ×50.

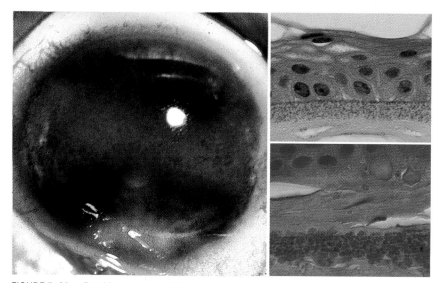

FIGURE 5–28 • **Band keratopathy.** Clinical photograph shows a band of superficial opacification involving the interpalpebral part of the cornea. *Top inset:* Fine basophilic granules of calcium stipple Bowman's layer. *Bottom inset:* Larger granules of actinic elastosis are found in noncalcific band keratopathy. Hematoxylin-eosin. Top inset ×250, bottom inset ×250.

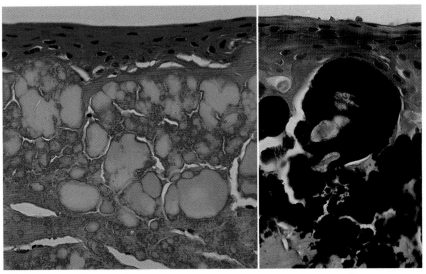

FIGURE 5–29 • **Chronic actinic keratopathy.** Anterior stroma contains amphophilic deposits of amorphous hyaline material. Hematoxylin-eosin, ×100. *Inset:* There is intense positive staining of deposits. Verhoeff-van Gieson elastic stain, ×125.

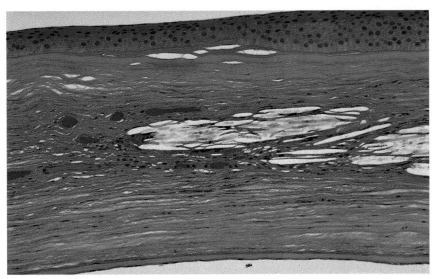

FIGURE 5–30 • **Lipid keratopathy.** The scarred and vascularized stroma contains cholesterol clefts, reflecting secondary lipid deposition. Hematoxylin-eosin, ×50.

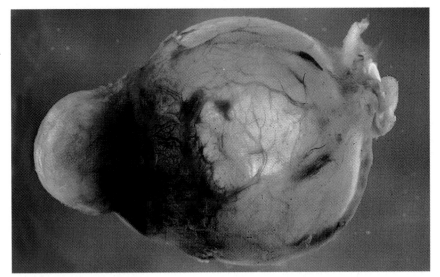

FIGURE 5–31 • **Corneal staphyloma.** The cornea is massively thickened by a hypertrophic scar (corneal keloid) that was lined internally by atrophic iris. The eye was enucleated from a child in an underdeveloped country.

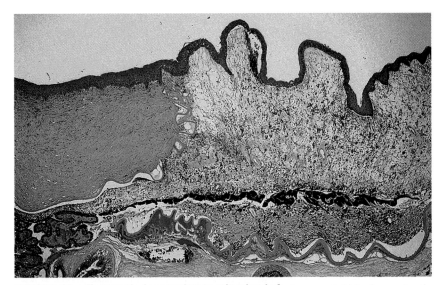

FIGURE 5–32 • **Keratomalacia secondary to avitaminosis A.** Incarcerated iris plugs a sharply margined perforation in the center of a noninflamed cornea. Avitaminosis A was caused by dietary deficiency in a chronic alcoholic. Hematoxylin-eosin, ×25.

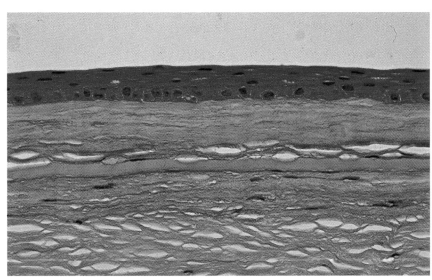

**FIGURE 5–33 • Degenerative pannus, chronic corneal edema.** A thick layer of relatively acellular connective tissue is interposed between the corneal epithelium and intact Bowman's membrane. Hematoxylin-eosin, ×100.

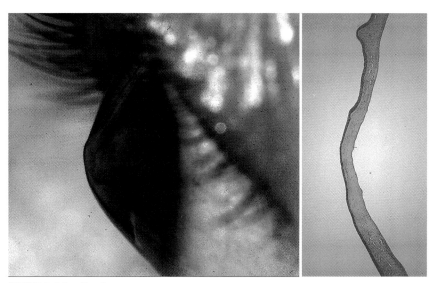

**FIGURE 5–34 • Keratoconus.** Clinical photograph shows the conical shape of the cornea. *Inset:* Sectioned ectatic cornea had a wavy configuration. Inset: hematoxylin-eosin, ×10.

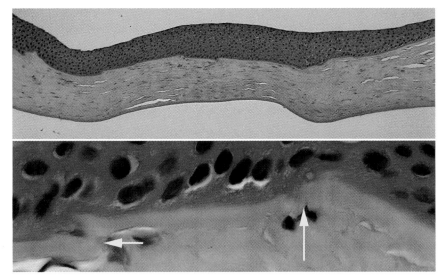

**FIGURE 5–35 • Keratoconus.** Photomicrograph (*top*) shows severe thinning of apical stroma and compensatory hyperplasia of the epithelium. Arrows point to dehiscences in Bowman's membrane (*bottom*). Hematoxylin-eosin. Top ×25, bottom ×250.

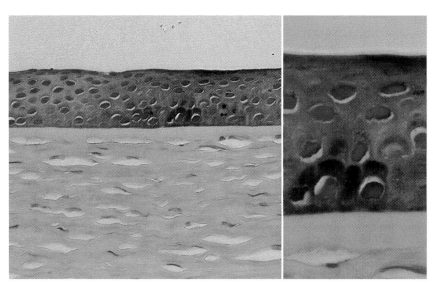

**FIGURE 5–36 • Keratoconus, Fleischer ring.** Iron stain shows focal deposition of iron in corneal epithelium surrounding the cone. Perls' stain for iron. Left ×100, right ×250.

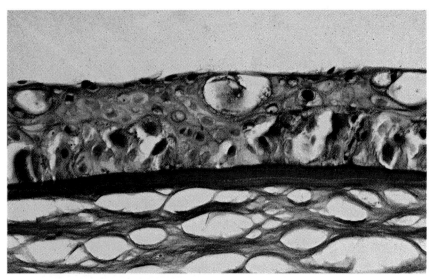

FIGURE 5–37 • **Meesmann's epithelial dystrophy.** The epithelium is thickened and contains small cystoid spaces. The epithelial basement membrane is markedly thickened. Periodic acid-Schiff, ×250.

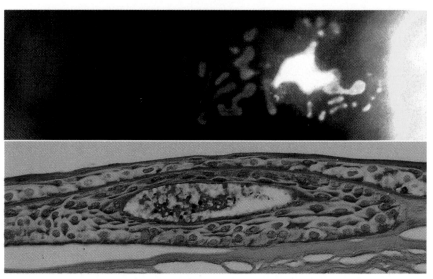

FIGURE 5–38 • **Cogan's microcystic dystrophy.** Slit lamp discloses intraepithelial deposits of putty-like cellular debris. Photomicrograph (*bottom*) shows devitalized cellular debris trapped by duplication of the epithelium. Periodic acid-Schiff, ×100.

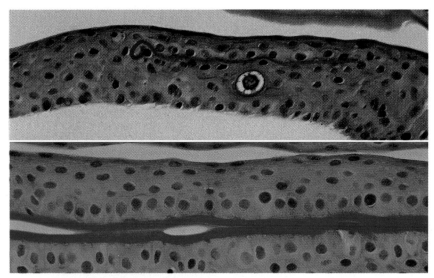

FIGURE 5–39 • **Map-dot-fingerprint dystrophy.** Photomicrographs of corneal scrapings show a small intraepithelial cyst with an intraepithelial segment of the basement membrane (above) and marked thickening of the epithelial basement membrane (below). Periodic acid-Schiff, ×100 .

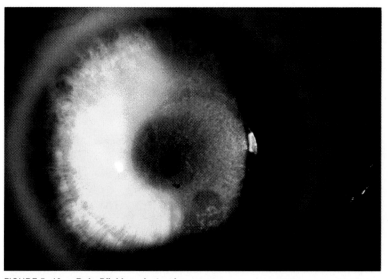

FIGURE 5–40 • **Reis-Bücklers dystrophy.** Slit lamp discloses diffuse subepithelial scarring. (Courtesy of Dr. Peter Laibson, Wills Eye Hospital)

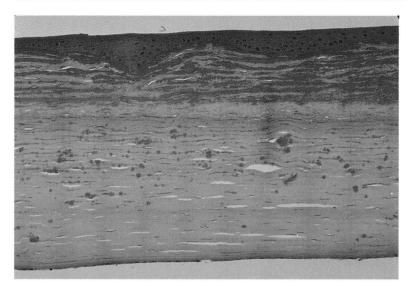

FIGURE 5–41 • **Reis-Bücklers dystrophy.** The "saw-toothed" epithelium rests on a thick multilaminar pannus composed of alternating layers of collagen and more eosinophilic material. Bowman's membrane has been destroyed. Smaller deposits of eosinophilic material are seen in the stroma. Hematoxylin-eosin, ×100.

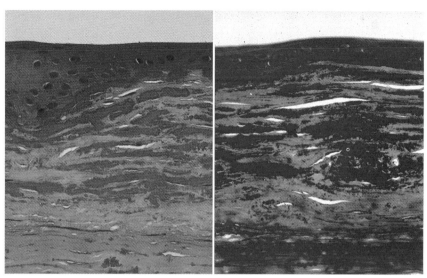

FIGURE 5–42 • **Reis-Bücklers dystrophy.** Abnormal material comprising part of multilaminar pannus is more eosinophilic than stromal collagen (*left*) and stains red with Masson trichrome (*right*), like deposits in granular corneal dystrophy. Left: hematoxylin-eosin, ×250; right: Masson trichrome, ×250.

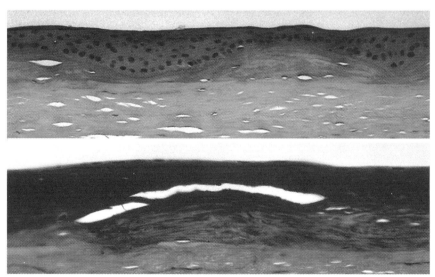

FIGURE 5–43 • **Thiel-Behnke dystrophy.** This Bowman's membrane dystrophy is characterized by epithelial "saw-toothing," destruction of Bowman's layer, and a multilaminar pannus containing intensely eosinophilic material that stains red with Masson trichrome. Top: hematoxylin-eosin, ×100; bottom: Masson trichrome, ×100.

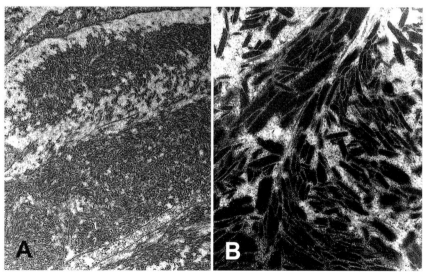

FIGURE 5–44 • **Electron microscopy, Bowman's membrane dystrophies.** TEM shows that abnormal material in Thiel-Behnke dystrophy (A) is comprised of "curly filaments." Osmiophilic crystalloids resembling deposits in granular corneal dystrophy are found in Reis-Bücklers dystrophy (B).

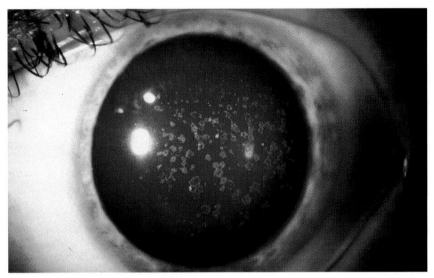

FIGURE 5–45 • **Granular corneal dystrophy.** Multiple white, crumb or ring-shaped opacities are present in the central cornea. The stroma is clear between the opacities.

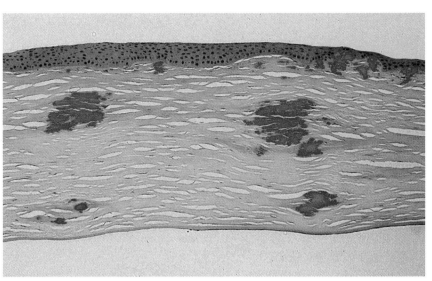

FIGURE 5–46 • **Granular corneal dystrophy.** Irregular "rock candy" deposits of mutant kera-toepithelin are more intensely eosinophilic than the surrounding normal stroma. Hematoxylin-eosin, ×50.

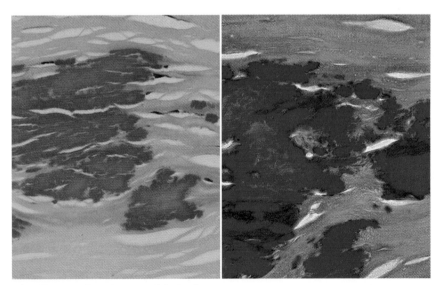

FIGURE 5–47 • **Granular corneal dystrophy.** Stromal deposits in granular corneal dystrophy are intensely eosinophilic (*left*) and show intense acid fuchsinophilia (red staining) with Masson trichrome (*right*). Left: hematoxylin-eosin, ×100; right: Masson trichrome, ×100.

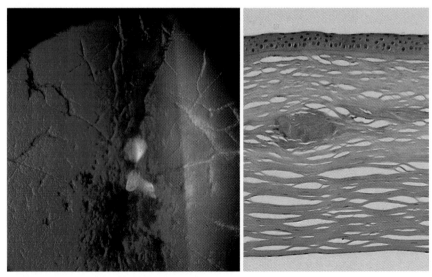

FIGURE 5–48 • **Lattice corneal dystrophy type I.** Slit lamp shows characteristic latticework of branching relucent lines in corneal stroma. Corresponding stromal deposits of amyloid are eosinophilic but have a more smudgy appearance that deposits in granular dystrophy. Hema-toxylin-eosin, ×100. (Clinical photograph courtesy of Dr. Peter Laibson, Wills Eye Hospital)

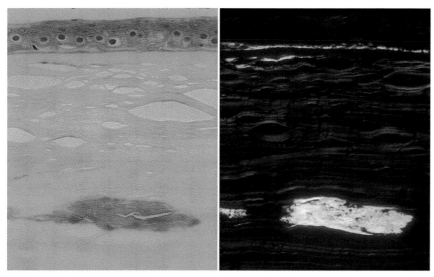

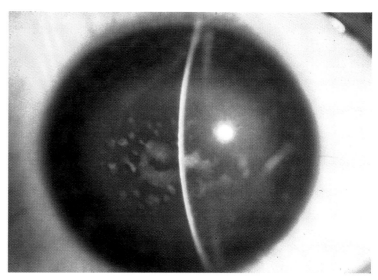

FIGURE 5–49 • **Lattice corneal dystrophy type I.** Amyloid deposits stain positively with congo red stain for amyloid (*left*) and show characteristic apple green birefringence with polarization microscopy. Left: congo red, ×80; right: congo red with crossed polarizers, ×80.

FIGURE 5–50 • **Macular corneal dystrophy.** The entire cornea is diffusely hazy. Grayish macules with indistinct borders are present axially. The cornea is not thickened. (Courtesy of Dr. Christropher Rapuano, Wills Eye Hospital)

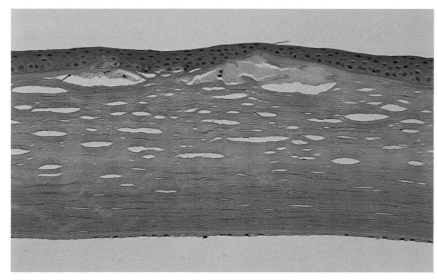

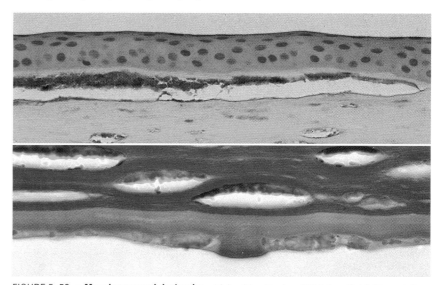

FIGURE 5–51 • **Macular corneal dystrophy.** Large subepithelial extracellular deposits of abnormal nonsulfated keratan correspond to macules seen clinically. The stroma is thin. A few guttae stud Descemet's membrane.

FIGURE 5–52 • **Macular corneal dystrophy.** Alcian blue (*top*) and Hale's colloidal iron stain for acid mucopolysaccharide (*bottom*) disclose material thought to be nonsulfated keratan in large subepithelial extracellular deposit and in cytoplasm of keratocytes and endothelial cells. Note guttate excrescence on Descemet's membrane. Top: alcian blue, ×100; bottom: Hale's colloidal iron, ×250.

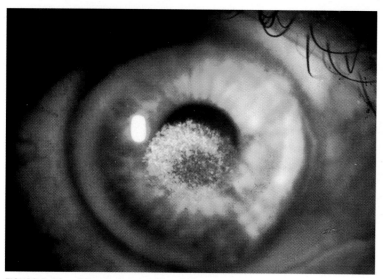

FIGURE 5–53 • **Schnyder's crystalline dystrophy.** A deposit of cholesterol crystals is present in the axial stroma. A prominent arcus senilis is also present.

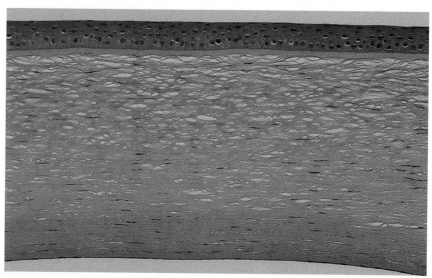

FIGURE 5–54 • **Schnyder's crystalline dystrophy.** Empty clefts and vacuoles that contained lipid in vivo are concentrated in the anterior stroma. No vessels or inflammation are present. Hematoxylin-eosin, ×50.

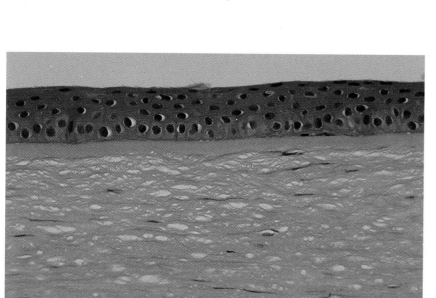

FIGURE 5–55 • **Primary lipid dystrophy.** The anterior stroma contains empty lipid vacuoles that are smaller and fewer in number than those in Schnyder's crystalline dystrophy (compare with Figure 5–54). Hematoxylin-eosin, ×100.

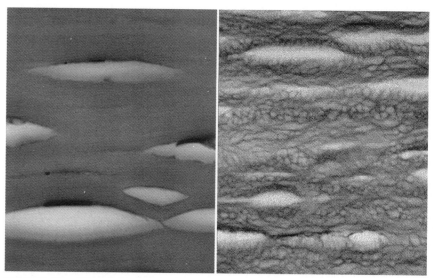

FIGURE 5–56 • **Corneal stromal edema.** Collagenous lamella of edematous cornea (*right*) have a frothy "cotton candy" appearance compared to compact lamellae of normal cornea (*left*). Hematoxylin-eosin, ×250.

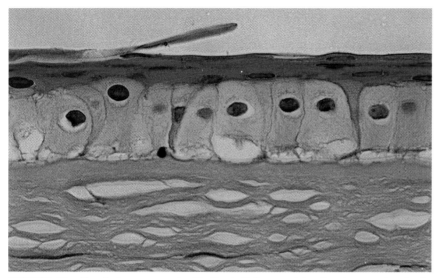

FIGURE 5–57 • **Basal edema, corneal epithelium.** Cells comprising the edematous basal cell layer of corneal epithelium have swollen lucent cytoplasm. Hematoxylin-eosin, ×250.

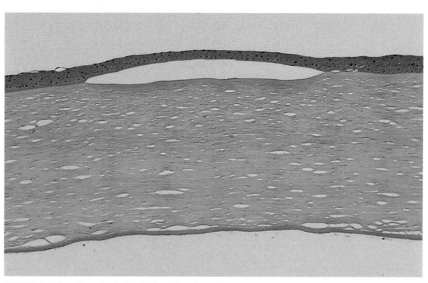

FIGURE 5–58 • **Pseudophakic bullous keratopathy.** The epithelium has detached from the edematous cornea, forming a bulla. Descemet's membrane is regular in caliber. The endothelium is markedly atrophic. Hematoxylin-eosin, ×25.

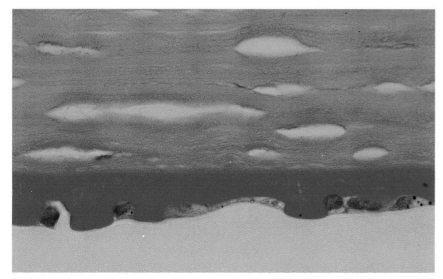

FIGURE 5–59 • **Fuchs' dystrophy.** Descemet's membrane is irregular in caliber and studded with guttate excrescences. Some of the residual endothelial cells contain melanin granules. Periodic acid-Schiff, ×250.

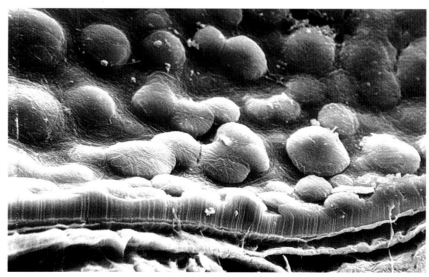

FIGURE 5–60 • **Fuchs' dystrophy.** Mushroom or anvil-shaped excrescences stud the posterior surface of Descemet's membrane. The specimen is oriented epithelial side down. Scanning electron micrograph, ×300.

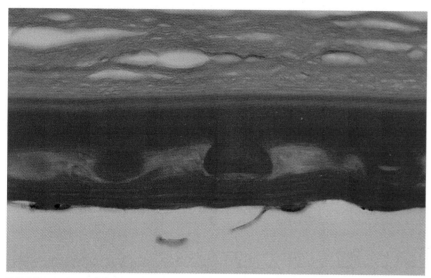

FIGURE 5–61 • **Fuchs' dystrophy, buried guttae.** Guttae have been "buried" by a newly synthesized layer of extracellular matrix material. The endothelium is markedly atrophic. Buried guttae typically occur in the center of the cornea. Periodic acid-Schiff, ×250.

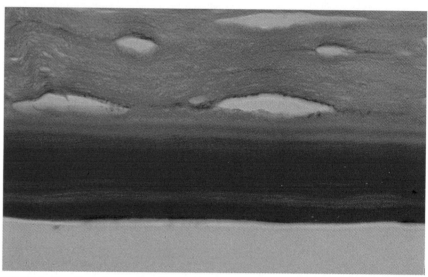

FIGURE 5–62 • **Nonguttate endothelial dystrophy.** Descemet's membrane is diffusely thickened and multilaminated. The endothelium is atrophic. Periodic acid-Schiff, ×250.

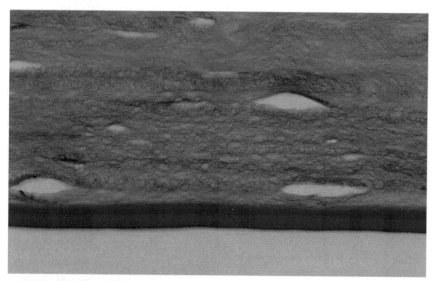

FIGURE 5–63 • **Pseudophakic bullous keratopathy.** Descemet's membrane is regular in caliber and lacks guttae. The stroma is edematous, and no endothelial cells are present. Periodic acid-Schiff, ×250.

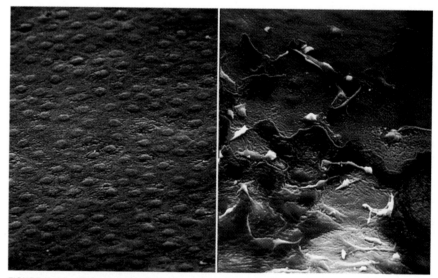

FIGURE 5–64 • **Pseudophakic bullous keratopathy.** Appearance of markedly atrophic endothelium from edematous corneal button shown by scanning electron microscopy (*right*) contrasts with a regular mosaic of normal control endothelium (*left*). Residual cells in this specimen are large and polymorphic, and Descemet's membrane is partially denuded. Scanning electron microscopy. Left ×640, right ×320.

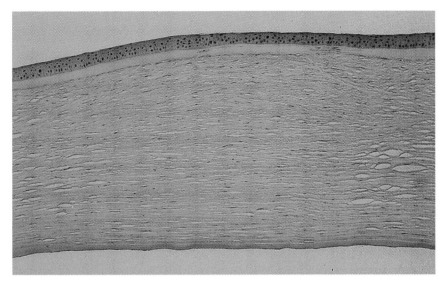

FIGURE 5–65 • **Congenital hereditary endothelial dystrophy.** The corneal stroma is massively edematous, but the endothelium appears well preserved. Bowman's layer is thickened. Hematoxylin-eosin, ×25.

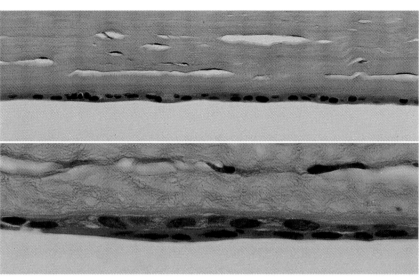

FIGURE 5–66 • **Posterior polymorphous dystrophy.** The corneal endothelium is hypercellular. Multilayered growth, a surface epithelial characteristic, is seen (*bottom*). Hematoxylin-eosin. Top ×100, bottom ×250.

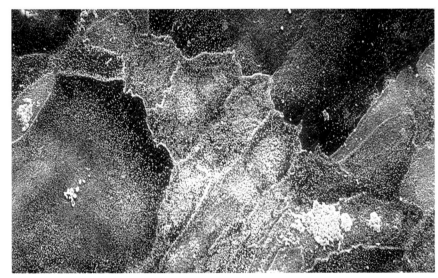

FIGURE 5–67 • **Posterior polymorphous dystrophy.** Endothelial cells disclosed by scanning electron microscopy vary markedly in size and shape. Numerous microvilli are present on the surface of the cells. ×1000.

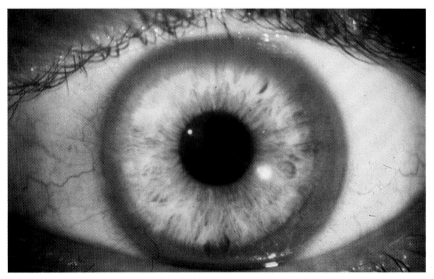

FIGURE 5–68 • **Kayser-Fleischer ring, Wilson's disease.** Brownish ring in peripheral cornea is caused by copper deposition in Descemet's membrane.

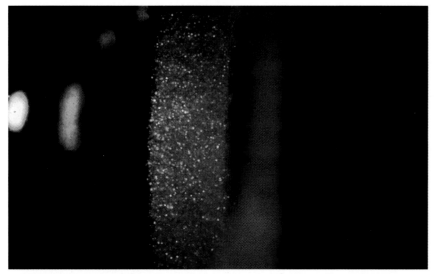

FIGURE 5–69 • **Corneal crystals, multiple myeloma.** Myriad polychromatic crystals in the corneal epithelium were the presenting manifestation of multiple myeloma. (Courtesy of Dr. Dario Savino-Zari, Caracas, Venezuela)

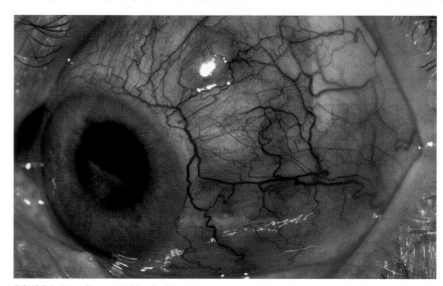

FIGURE 5–70 • **Rheumatoid scleritis.** Thinned areas of the sclera appear blue because there is increased visibility of the underlying uveal tract.

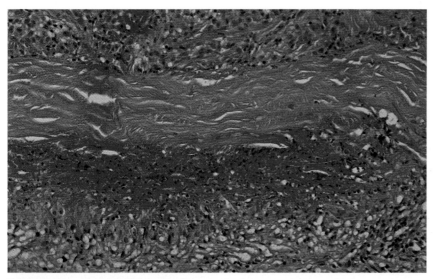

FIGURE 5–71 • **Rheumatoid scleritis.** Note the zonal pattern of granulomatous inflammation identical to that found in a rheumatoid nodule. A palisading granuloma of epithelioid histiocytes surrounds a sequestrum of residual devitalized scleral collagen. Necrosis is evident as smudgy basophilic foci along the lower border of the sequestrum. Hematoxylin-eosin, ×50.

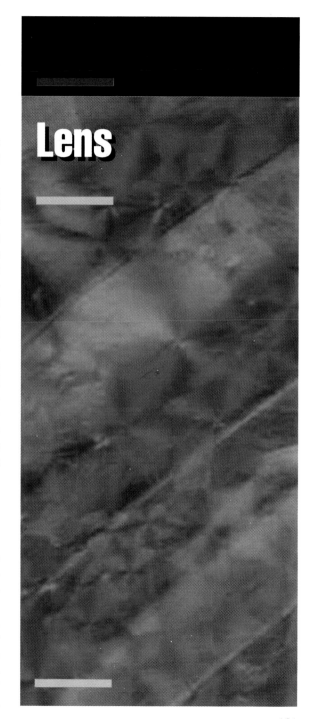

# CHAPTER 6

# Lens

The crystalline lens is situated in the posterior chamber behind the iris (Fig. 6–1). The lens is the only large, transparent cellular tissue in the body and the only intraocular structure derived embryologically from the surface ectoderm. Early during gestation the surface ectoderm overlying the optic vesicle thickens to form the lens placode, which subsequently invaginates to form the lens vesicle, as the neuroectodermal optic vesicle invaginates to form the optic cup. The epithelial cells of the posterior part of the vesicle elongate anteriorly, forming the primary lens fibers that fill the cavity of the optic vesicle. These fibers persist as the central embryonic nucleus in the adult lens. The anterior layer of cells remains as the anterior lens epithelium throughout life (Fig. 6–2). Secondary lens fibers are formed by division of lens epithelial cells near the equator of the lens. These long, strap-like cells (7–8 mm in length) extend from the anterior pole to the posterior pole of the lens, totally enveloping the nucleus. The formation of secondary lens fibers continues throughout life; new fibers are laid down in concentric lamellae peripherally in an onion-like fashion. The nuclei of the newly formed peripheral lens fibers form a curved bow near the equator (Fig. 6–3).

These highly specialized epithelial cells lose their nuclei shortly after formation. They are tightly packed in a nearly paracrystalline fashion and are joined together by ball and socket joints that minimize extracellular space. The lens has no vessels or nerves and is almost totally devoid of connective tissue, except for its thick enveloping capsule of basement membrane. The anterior capsule is much thicker than the posterior capsule, whose caliber is less than the diameter of an erythrocyte (Fig. 6–2). Like other basement membranes, the lens capsule stains intensely with periodic acid-Schiff (PAS) stain. The lens epithelial cells retain the ability to synthesize collagen and may do so under pathologic conditions.

The primary optical function of the lens is focusing or accommodation. The eye's major refractive element is the cornea, whose power is about 45 diopters. The power of the lens is only 10 diopters. Divergent light rays from near objects must be bent or refracted more to focus them sharply on the retina. When a near object (e.g., this page) is examined, the ciliary muscle contracts, relaxing the tension on the zonular fibers that form the suspensory ligament of the lens. The ciliary muscle is a circular, or sphincter, muscle. Its central aperture becomes smaller when it contracts. When distant objects are examined and the eye is at rest and not accommodating, the zonular fibers pull on the lens and flatten it. Relaxation of the zonular fibers during accommodation allows the lens to assume a more spherical configuration, which has a shorter radius of curvature and greater refractive power. Refractive power is inversely proportional to the radius of curvature of a lens.

## CONGENITAL ANOMALIES OF THE LENS

The posterior surface of the lens from an infant's eye often has a dimpled configuration called posterior umbilication (Fig. 6–4). Posterior umbilication is an artifact caused by fixation and is not present *in vivo*.

The surface of the lens has a conical configuration in lenticonus. Lenticonus can be anterior or posterior and probably is caused by focal thinning of the lens capsule. Anterior lenticonus usually is bilateral and may be associated with Alport syndrome (hereditary hemorrhagic nephritis and deafness), which is caused by an inherited abnormality in type IV, or basement membrane, collagen. The lens capsule in Alport syndrome is thin and has linear dehiscences. The renal disease presumably is caused by analogous abnormalities in the glomerular basement membrane.

Posterior lenticonus usually is a unilateral sporadic condition that is not associated with other ocular or systemic disease. When the lens is retroilluminated, the lenticonus often appears as an "oil droplet."

Lens colobomas (lens notching) are secondary phenomena caused by a focal absence of zonular fibers in a contiguous coloboma of the ciliary body. Rarely, lens colobomas herald the presence of a pediatric ciliary body neoplasm, usually a medulloepithelioma.

Congenital or developmental cataracts are often hereditary and may be inherited in an autosomal dominant fashion. Developmental cataracts can affect different parts of the lens. Anterior pyramidal cataract is a congenital form of anterior subcapsular cataract. The opacity underneath the anterior lens capsule is a white plaque of dense collagen.

Faulty resorption of the embryonic hyaloid vascular system that nourishes the developing lens *in utero* can give rise to a spectrum of posterior polar opacities, the most severe of which is persistent hyperplastic primary vitreous (PHPV). A congenital anomaly often found in microophthalmic eyes (see Figs. 11–31, 11–32, 11–33), PHPV is characterized by a retrolental plaque of vascularized connective tissue that is thought to represent part of the embryonic primary vitreous. The tips of the ciliary processes are attached to the margins of this retrolental plaque. As the eye enlarges, the ciliary processes are drawn centrally and stretched; they may be seen clinically when the pupil is dilated. PHPV produces leukocoria (a white pupil) and is an important lesion in the differential diagnosis of the childhood retinal malignancy retinoblastoma. Goldberg suggested that the term persistent fetal vasculature (PFV) be used for this syndrome.

An innocuous spot called Mittendorf's dot marks the site where the hyaloid artery was attached to the posterior lens capsule *in utero*. Mittendorf's dot, best seen on retroillumination, is found in about 25% of normal individuals. A patent hyaloid artery persists in some adults. Posterior remnants of the hyaloid artery and Bergmeister's papilla may be evident as vascular loops and glial veils on the optic disk.

Zonular cataracts are marked by the opacification of a single zone of lens fibers. Lamellar cataract is a form of zonular cataract that results when an opacified group of lens fibers is buried by the subsequent formation of clear healthy cortex (Fig. 6–5). Damage to developing lens fibers during an attack of neonatal tetany is a classic cause of lamellar cataract. Analogous to tree rings, the opacified fibers serve as a clinical marker that allows one to estimate roughly when an insult occurred during lens development.

The clinical triad that comprises Gregg syndrome of rubella-induced embryopathy includes cataract, deafness, and cardiac anomalies such as patent ductus arteriosus. Rubella cataracts are typically dense, pearly white, and nuclear. Lens epithelial nuclei may persist for decades in the embryonic nucleus of a rubella cataract. Virus has been cultured from rubella cataracts several years after birth. Congenital cataract and glaucoma occur together in patients who have Lowe syndrome, an X-linked oculocerebrorenal syndrome characterized by renal rickets and aminoaciduria. The lens in Lowe syndrome is small and discoid in shape and may have capsular incresences. Obligate female carriers of Lowe syndrome may have punctate opacities and plaque-like posterior subcapsular cataracts. Cataracts occur frequently in Down syndrome (trisomy 21).

## CATARACT

Cataract is opacification or optical dysfunction of the crystalline lens. Cataract is a common, economically important cause of visual loss. Derived from the Greek word for waterfall, the term cataract probably refers to the white appearance of some senile cataracts, likened to rapidly flowing "white water."

Cataract is the endstage, or final common pathway, of lens pathology. Although lens opacification often occurs as the result of aging, a host of other factors can cause cataracts, including trauma, drugs, toxins, radiation, inborn errors of metabolism, and concurrent ocular or systemic disease.

Cataract is essentially a clinical diagnosis denoting loss of optical function. It may be relatively difficult to diagnose cataract histopathologically, especially after modern surgical techniques such as phacoemulsification. Furthermore, it is nearly impossible to estimate the effect the pathology has on vision in most cases. Visual function is best determined by the ophthalmologist during a clinical examination. In institutions where cataracts are still submitted to the pathology laboratory, it is generally done to document that surgery was performed. Histopathologic examination usually is not performed.

Although a bewildering variety of lens opacities have been described clinically, only four basic types of cataract are recognized histopathologically: cortical, nuclear, anterior subcapsular, and posterior subcapsular. Each differs in its pathogenesis and histology.

Some degree of nuclear sclerosis (Figs. 6–6, 6–7) develops in all individuals as they age. The inevitability of nuclear sclerotic cataract is inherent in the lens's normal pattern of growth and development. The lens is derived from surface ectoderm, and it grows continuously, albeit slowly, throughout life, like skin. Growth of the lens results from the continuous addition of new secondary lens fibers around its circumference. The formation of the new lens fibers buries the older fibers, which are sequestered centrally in the lens nucleus. (Mature skin cells are desquamated.) With the passage of years, the older cells gradually degenerate. This is not surprising because mature lens cells are anucleate and lack the metabolic machinery for protein synthesis and repair. Eventually, the highly specialized lens proteins called crystallins become denatured, and the cytoplasm of the lens fibers becomes increasingly dehydrated. The degenerative process is also marked by the accumulation of a yellow-brown pigment called urochrome, which is probably related to photooxidation (Fig. 6–6).

Histopathologically, nuclear sclerosis is marked by increased eosinophilia, homogeneity of the lens nucleus, and an absence of the artifactitious cracks that normally occur between lens fibers during microtomy (Fig. 6–7). As the nucleus becomes denser, its index of refraction, and hence its refractive power, increases, causing lenticular myopia ("grandma's second sight"). Presbyopic patients often find that they are able to read without their reading glasses, as they develop nuclear sclerosis and become progressively myopic. Nuclear sclerosis also distorts color vision because the yellow-brown urochrome pigment accumulates in the lens and filters out blue wavelengths of light. After nuclear sclerotic cataracts are removed, patients may complain about "blue vision." In advanced nuclear sclerosis, cataracts may be amber-colored (brunescent) or even black (cataracta nigra). Calcium oxalate crystals occasionally are found in lenses with nuclear sclerosis. These oval crystals exhibit vivid rainbow-like birefringence during polarization microscopy (Fig. 6–8).

Cortical cataract (soft cataract) is marked by degeneration of the fiber cells comprising the lens cortex. The incipient stage of cortical cataract is marked clinically by the development of vacuoles or clefts containing clear, watery fluid (water clefts). As the disease progresses, the foci of degenerated cortical material appear white in direct illumination and as black shadows in retroillumination. The cortical opacities often begin near the equator and may involve a wedge-shaped sector of cortex. Birefringent crystals of cholesterol and insoluble amino acids develop in some cases. The term "Christmas tree cataract" is applied to cataracts that contain many crystals.

Histopathologically, cortical degeneration is marked by clefts and spaces in the cortex filled with liquefied cortex, which oozes from fractured lens fibers. Spherules of degenerated lens cytoplasm called morgagnian globules typically are seen (Fig. 6–9). Total cortical liquefaction characterizes advanced cases called morgagnian cataracts (Figs. 6–10, 6–11). Morgagnian cataracts are typically swollen and intumescent because the osmotic effect of the degenerated cortical material causes the lens to imbibe aqueous humor. In some patients the swollen lens may precipitate closed-angle glaucoma (phacomorphic glaucoma). The sclerotic nucleus typically resists liquefaction and sinks inferiorly in the capsular bag of liquefied cortex (Fig. 6–10). The milky, fluid cortex often contains crystals of cholesterol. The denatured lens protein can leak through the intact lens capsule in advanced cases and stimulate a bland macrophagic response. This may lead to a secondary open-angle glaucoma called phacolytic glaucoma, which is caused by obstruction of the trabecular meshwork by macrophages that have ingested lens material and free high-molecular-weight lens protein (see Figs. 2–10, 7–25). Dystrophic calcification is often found in the degenerated cortex of long-standing cataracts. Blind, painful eyes occasionally contain totally calcified lenses that are rock-hard and cannot be sectioned without prior decalcification.

The two other histologic subtypes of cataract—anterior subcapsular cataract and posterior subcapsular cataract—are caused by abnormalities in the anterior lens epithelium. Anterior subcapsular cataract is marked histopathologically by a white plaque of dense collagenous connective tissue that forms underneath the anterior lens capsule (Fig. 6–12). Characteristic sinuous folds in the anterior capsule are caused by contraction of the fibrous tissue (Fig. 6–13). The subcapsular collagen is synthesized by lens epithelial cells. The cells are found within the plaque surrounded by capsules of basement membrane material that evidence their lens epithelial lineage. In some instances, a sec-

ond, delicate, new layer of lens capsule is found underneath the anterior subcapsular fibrous plaque. This layer is synthesized by lens epithelial cells that have migrated underneath the plaque. Adhesions between the iris and lens (posterior synechias), anterior segment inflammation, or both often stimulate the proliferation and fibrous transformation of the lens epithelium. Although anterior subcapsular cataracts frequently are found in blind, painful eyes in the ophthalmic pathology laboratory, they are not often observed clinically because they typically are obscured by posterior synechias and pupillary membranes. Capsular fibrosis, which causes capsular opacification and wrinkling after planned extracapsular cataract extraction (ECCE) surgery, reflects an identical process of lens epithelial proliferation and fibrous transformation (Fig. 6–14).

With posterior subcapsular cataract, lens epithelial cells migrate posteriorly underneath the lens capsule behind the lens equator where the monolayer of anterior lens epithelium normally terminates. Noxae such as inflammation or ciliary body tumors stimulate the abnormal epithelial migration. Situated aberrantly at the posterior pole of the lens, the lens epithelial cells attempt to form new secondary lens fibers, but abortive lens fibers called Wedl or bladder cells result (Fig. 6–15). Filled with lens protein, the Wedl cells are large, are round or oval, and have a single nucleus. Posterior subcapsular cataracts tend to interfere with near vision early because the opacity is located near the nodal point of the eye's visual system. Patients with posterior subcapsular cataract also are prone to develop severe glare symptoms, especially during night driving. The nuclei of bladder or Wedl cells serve to distinguish them from morgagnian globules, which are round, anucleate spherules of lens protein.

Cells analogous to Wedl cells called Elschnig's pearls can form on or within the lens capsular bag after planned extracapsular surgery. This postoperative proliferation of lens cells may resemble a mass of fish eggs clinically (Fig. 6–16).

## Complicated Cataracts

Complicated cataracts (cataracta complicata) are caused by concurrent ocular disease. Cataract formation can complicate chronic uveitis in patients who have sarcoidosis or the type of juvenile rheumatoid arthritis that is pauciarticular, rheumatoid factor (RF)-seronegative, and anti-nuclear antibody (ANA)-positive. Unilateral cataract, mild asymptomatic uveitis, and depigmentation of the iris stroma are the classic clinical manifestations of Fuchs' heterochromic cyclitis (Fig. 6–17).

Posterior subcapsular cataracts form in some patients who have retinitis pigmentosa. It is unclear how cataract formation is related to heritable defects in photopigments such as rhodopsin.

Intraocular tumors, particularly ciliary body malignant melanomas, should be excluded in patients with unilateral or asymmetric cataracts. Ciliary body tumors can directly impinge on and deform the periphery of the lens and stimulate posterior migration of lens epithelium as well.

Cataract can complicate long-standing glaucoma. In some instances it is related to chronic miotic therapy. Anterior subcapsular vacuoles have been reported in patients receiving topical anticholinesterase agents. Filtering surgery for glaucoma accelerates cataract formation. Scattered focal subcapsular lens opacities called glaukomflecken are observed in some patients who have had a prior attack of acute closed-angle glaucoma. These small, grayish opacities are thought to represent focal areas of lens epithelial necrosis and cortical degeneration and may be caused by hypothetical toxins in the stagnant aqueous humor.

## Sugar Cataracts: Diabetes Mellitus and Galactosemia

The accumulation of sugar alcohol in lens cells is hypothesized to produce osmotic cataracts in patients who have disorders of sugar metabolism such as diabetes mellitus. Rarely, patients with previously undiagnosed diabetes mellitus present with a characteristic type of diabetic cataract caused by markedly elevated levels of serum glucose. Such cataracts may resorb partially when diabetic therapy is instituted. Diabetics are also prone to develop typical senile nuclear and cortical cataracts at a much earlier age than the normal population.

The sugar alcohols that cause osmotic cataracts in patients with diabetes and galactosemia are formed by the enzyme aldose reductase in the alternative hexose monophosphate shunt when the normal glycolytic pathway is overwhelmed by high levels of serum glucose or galactose. Sorbitol, the sugar alcohol of glucose, accumulates in the lens cells of diabetics because it is unable to pass through cellular membranes. Similarly, the sugar alcohol of galactose called galactolol or dulcitol accumulates in the lens cells of galactosemic infants who are deficient in the enzyme galactose 1-phosphate uridyl transferase. Galactosemic cataracts often have a central oil droplet configuration, may be the first clinical manifestation of galactosemia, and are partially reversible if dietary therapy is instituted promptly. Presenile cataracts also occur in patients who are deficient in galactokinase.

## Cataract and Systemic Disease

Patients with myotonic dystrophy develop presenile cataract as well as myotonia, frontal baldness, and testicular atrophy. Myotonic cataracts classically are said to have multiple polychromatic crystals in the anterior and posterior subcapsular cortex.

The sunflower cataract of Wilson's disease (hepatolenticular degeneration) is caused by the deposition of copper in the lens capsule. The familiar Kayser-Fleischer ring in the periphery of the cornea results from an analogous deposition of copper in Descemet's membrane. The central disk of the "sunflower" corresponds to the diameter of the undilated pupil, and the large radial ridges on the back of the iris probably govern the formation of the "petals." An identical cataract may occur in patients who have retained intraocular copper foreign bodies (chalcosis lentis) (see Fig. 3–21). In fact, the similarity between traumatic chalcosis and Wilson's disease led German ophthalmologists to suggest that copper metabolism was abnormal in Wilson's disease.

Posterior spoke-like lens opacities occur in Fabry's disease, an X-linked deficiency of the enzyme $\alpha$-galactosidase A, which causes the storage of ceramide trihexoside in tissues. A vortex pattern of pigment deposition called cornea verticillata occurs in affected males.

It is not surprising that cataracts occur in patients who have certain skin diseases, because the lens and skin are both surface ectodermal derivatives. Most important is the syndermatotic cataract that occurs in atopic dermatitis, an association called Andogsky syndrome. Patients with atopic cataract may do poorly after cataract surgery.

## Traumatic Cataracts

Total opacification of the lens can develop several days after rupture or laceration of the lens capsule. The entire cortex can undergo liquefaction in young individuals, in whom total spontaneous resorption of the lens cortical material occasionally occurs. The iris can seal small lacerations. If the capsule re-forms, only a small focal opacity may result. Severe contusion injuries can rupture the lens. Less severe contusions often produce a superficial type of cataract with a distinctly floral appearance called a petalliform cataract or contusion rosette (see Fig. 3–13). Such cataracts may cause minimal visual loss but are an important clinical marker for prior ocular contusion injury. If a contusion rosette is found during biomicroscopy, gonioscopy should be performed to rule out postcontusion angle deformity, which predisposes to glaucoma.

Vossius' ring is an annulus of pigment on the anterior lens capsule caused by a forceful imprint of the iris pigment epithelium during a contusion injury. Chronically retained intraocular iron foreign bodies can cause siderosis lentis. Siderotic cataract is marked by scattered foci of rust-colored material on the anterior surface of the lens and often is associated with iris heterochromia caused by the deposition of iron pigment in the iris stroma. Histopathology shows subepithelial plaques of lens epithelial cells that contain large quantities of iron pigment. The siderosis or hemosiderosis lentis (iron from intraocular hemorrhage) is evident as a yellowish or yellowish brown discoloration of the anterior lens epithelium in routine sections stained with hematoxylin and eosin. Special iron stains that employ the Prussian blue reaction are used to confirm the presence of iron (see Fig. 3–20). Chalcosis lentis is discussed above.

The crystalline lens is highly sensitive to relatively low doses of ionizing radiation. (Doses as low as 250 cGy can cause cataract.) Hence the lens should be carefully shielded during radiotherapy.

Soemmerring's ring cataract is a donut of residual cortical material that remains in the equatorial part of the lens capsular bag after expulsion of lens nucleus during a perforating corneal or scleral injury. Many eyes that are examined pathologically after planned extracapsular cataract surgery have a Soemmerring's ring of residual lens cortex (Figs. 6–18, 6–19).

Electrical cataracts are caused by lightning strikes or severe electrical injuries. A thin lamella of anterior or posterior subcapsular cortex usually is opacified in this rare type of cataract. Lightning often opacifies the posterior subcapsular cortex because the electrical current passes down the neuraxis. Industrial injuries usually cause anterior opacification because the extremities are the path of the current. The onset of electrical cataract after injury may be delayed.

The blue wavelengths of the argon blue-green laser are absorbed by the yellow urochrome pigment in a nuclear cataract. Focal lenticular burns have occurred during retinal photocoagulation of patients with advanced nuclear sclerosis. This can be avoided by the use of a red laser light, (i.e., krypton red). Absorption of laser energy by the iris pigment epithelium can cause focal thermal opacities in the underlying lens during transpupillary thermotherapy of posterior segment tumors.

## Toxic Cataract

A variety of drugs and toxins can cause cataract. The most important drug-induced cataract is the posterior subcapsular cataract that develops in patients receiving chronic therapy with high doses of systemic corticosteroids. The dose of steroids necessary to produce cataract is uncertain. One study found that cataracts develop in approximately one-third of patients who receive a chronic daily dose of 10 mg prednisolone. The incidence was 20% if the patient received more than 15 mg prednisolone for 2–8 years. Other toxins and drugs that produce cataract include naphthalene, dinitrophenol, mercury, phenothiazine, anticholinesterase agents, triparanol, and cigarette smoke.

## LENS CAPSULAR ABNORMALITIES

True exfoliation of the lens capsule or capsular delamination is marked by a split in the lens capsule that leads to the formation of relucent scrolls on the anterior surface of the lens. True exfoliation is rare. Although it classically is associated with occupational exposure to infrared radiation (e.g., in glass blowers or steel puddlers), most cases are associated with aging. True exfoliation does not predispose to glaucoma.

Pseudoexfoliation of the lens capsule, or exfoliation syndrome, is a relatively common disease that causes a type of secondary open angle glaucoma called capsular glaucoma in about half of affected patients. Dvo-rak-Theobald first used the term pseudoexfoliation to differentiate this disorder from true exfoliation, which does not cause glaucoma.

Clinically, pseudoexfoliation is marked by the deposition of a complex mucoprotein on the anterior lens capsule and on all of the aqueous-bathed surfaces of the anterior segment, including the ciliary processes, zonule, vitreous face, and posterior iris. On the anterior lens capsule, the pseudoexfoliation material forms a central disk of granular white material whose diameter corresponds to that of the undilated pupil (Fig. 6–20). Surrounding the central disk is a clear zone wiped clean of pseudoexfoliation material by the motion of the pupil. A granular zone marked by areas of rarefaction that correspond to radial macroridges on the posterior iridic surface is found peripherally. The pseudoexfoliation may be relatively inconspicuous in an undilated eye. Observation of a few, white, dandruff-like flakes at the pupillary margin should always prompt an examination with dilation.

The pseudoexfoliation material on the anterior surface of the lens is synthesized by the lens epithelium and extruded through the lens capsule, forming clumps of eosinophilic material called Busacca deposits. The light microscopic appearance of these deposits has been likened to magnetized iron filings (Fig. 6–21). Coarser, more irregular clumps of exfoliation material are found on the zonular fibers, ciliary processes, and iris pigment epithelium. Material is also found in the iris stroma, anterior chamber, and trabecular meshwork. Secondary open-angle glaucoma is caused by obstruction of the trabecular meshwork. Electron microscopic studies suggest that some of the pseudoexfoliation material is synthesized within the meshwork. Pseudoexfoliation material has been found in the conjunctiva, orbit, skin, lung, liver, and heart with electron microscopy. The extraocular material is always associated with elastic fibers, and it shows immunoreactivity with antibodies against elastic microfibrils. Such observations suggest that pseudoexfoliation of the lens capsule is the ocular manifestation of a presumably innocuous systemic disorder of elastic tissue.

Involvement of the zonule by pseudoexfoliation predisposes to dislocation of the lens or lens capsular bag after extracapsular cataract surgery. Cataract surgery may also be complicated by poor pupillary dilation and an abnormal leathery consistency of the iris. Histopathologically, one finds "saw-toothing" of the iris pigment epithelium caused by coarsening and coalescence of its circumferential ridges, which are festooned with pseudoexfoliative material (Fig. 6–22). The iris pigment epithelial changes often suggest the diagnosis under low magnification microscopy. Many patients have extensive pigment dispersion, not unlike that found in pigmentary glaucoma.

## ZONULE AND ECTOPIA LENTIS

The lens is suspended in the posterior chamber by zonular fibers, which are composed largely of elastic microfibrils. The zonular fibers arise from the peripheral pars plana and the inner surface of the peripheral retina, and they extend as a sheet anteriorly across the pars plana. At the posterior aspect of the pars plicata, the sheet divides into bundles that pass through the valleys between the ciliary processes. The zonular fibers are attached to the inner surface of the pars plicata, which acts like a fulcrum. Two groups of zonular fibers extend from the ciliary body and insert onto the anterior and posterior surfaces of the lens capsule. They enclose a triangular space called the canal of Hannover.

Trauma (e.g., contusion injury) is the most common cause of lens dislocation. Spontaneous dislocation is also said to occur in patients with tertiary syphilis. Ectopia lentis also occurs in a variety of heritable diseases of connective tissue including Marfan syndrome, homocystinuria, and the Weill-Marchesani syndrome. In most cases the ectopia lentis has been linked to mutations in the gene for the microfibrillar glycoprotein fibrillin-1, located on the long arm of chromosome 15, or by other metabolic disorders that affect the structure of fibrillin secondarily. Fibrillin-1 is a major component of the zonular fibers and is involved also in the formation of elastic tissue throughout the body.

About 70% of cases of heritable ectopia lentis occur in patients with Marfan syndrome, which has been linked to more than 50 mutations in the fibrillin-1 gene. The major manifestations of Marfan syndrome are ocular, skeletal, and cardiovascular. Bilateral lens dislocation occurs in 50–80% of patients and is typically superotemporal in direction. Patients are tall and have arachnodactyly (long spidery fingers and toes), dolichostenomelia, scoliosis, and pectus excavatum or carinatum. Cardiovascular disease is caused by defective elastic tissue and includes fatal dissecting aortic aneurysms and aortic valve defects. Other ocular defects include high myopia, large flat corneas, and a tendency to develop retinal detachment. Fibrillin-1 defects, which presumably are relatively innocuous, also have been identified in families who inherit isolated or simple ectopia lentis as an autosomal dominant trait. The autosomal dominant form of Weill-Marchesani syndrome also has been linked to the fibrillin-1 gene.

The classic manifestations of the Weill-Marchesani syndrome are microspherophakia and brachydactyly. Patients are short and muscular and have short fingers, broad hands, limited joint mobility, and hearing defects. The most debilitating aspects of this syndrome are ocular. Patients typically present with 15–20 diopters of lenticular myopia and often develop axial lens dislocation during their teens (Fig. 6–23). Lens dislocation often causes secondary closed angle glaucoma due to papillary block. The volume of the small, microspherophakic lens is 20–40% less than normal.

The heritable disorders that cause secondary abnormalities in fibrillin-1 are caused by defects in the metabolism of sulfur-containing amino acids. These disorders interfere with the formation of important disulfide bonds that serve to determine the conformation and aggregation of fibrillin-1. They include homocystinuria, sulfite oxidase deficiency, and molybdenum cofactor deficiency.

Many cases of homocystinuria are caused by a deficiency in cystathionine $\beta$-synthase, an enzyme that catalyzes the condensation of homocysteine with serine to form cystathionine, an important precursor of cysteine and cystine. Homocystinuric patients tend to be fair-skinned and blonde and have a tall, marfanoid habitus. About half develop progressive mental retardation, and nearly 75% die by age 30 from venous and arterial thromboses. The latter may be related to the endothelial protein thrombomodulin, which also contains structurally important disulfide bonds. Patients are at increased risk for thromboembolic complications during general anesthesia. Lens dislocation occurs in about 90% of patients. The lens usually dislocates inferiorly or into the anterior chamber. It never dislocates superiorly, as in Marfan syndrome, a clinical feature that differentiates homocystinuric patients who are marfanoid. Patients may present with acute pupillary block glaucoma. High myopia, retinal detachment, and peripheral retinal pigment epithelium (RPE) degeneration are other ocular manifestations. A thick layer of PAS-positive zonular material has been found histopathologically on the surface of the ciliary body.

Sulfite oxidase deficiency usually presents with seizures shortly after birth in infants who have severe neurologic findings. Lens dislocation occurs in about half and typically is found in older infants. Affected patients are unable to convert sulfite to sulfate. This leads to an accumulation of sulfite, which destroys sulfhydryl groups and disulfide bonds. Most patients with sulfite oxidase deficiency have a deficiency in a molybdenum cofactor that is also shared by xanthine dehydrogenase and aldehyde oxidase. The manifestations of the latter two enzyme deficiencies are relatively innocuous.

Ectopia lentis occurs rarely with other hereditary disorders, including hyperlysinemia and Ehlers-Danlos syndrome.

# References

## General References

Eagle RC, Spencer WH: The lens. In Spencer W (ed) Ophthalmic Pathology: An Atlas and Textbook. 4th ed. Vol 1. Philadelphia: Saunders, 1996:372–437.

## Developmental Anomalies

Bellows JG: Phakochronology: the study of dating structural changes in the lens. Br J Ophthalmol 52:540–545, 1968.

Brownell RD, Wolter JR: Anterior lenticonus in familial hemorrhagic nephritis. Arch Ophthalmol 71:481–483, 1964.

Goldberg MF: Persistent fetal vasculature (PFV): an integrated interpretation of signs and symptoms associated with persistent hyperplastic primary vitreous (PHPV): LIV Edward Jackson memorial lecture. Am J Ophthalmol 124:587–626, 1997.

Jampol LM, Kass M, Dueker D, Albert DM: Anterior polar cataracts. Am J Ophthalmol 78:95–97, 1974.

Khalil M, Saheb N: Posterior lenticonus. Ophthalmology 91: 1429–1430, 43A, 1984.

Lambert SR, Drack AV: Infantile cataracts. Surv Ophthalmol 40:427–458, 1996.

Sabates R, Krachmer JH, Weingeist TA: Ocular findings in Alport syndrome. Ophthalmologia 186:204–210, 1983.

Streeten BW, Robinson MR, Wallace RN, et al: Lens capsule abnormalities in Alport syndrome. Arch Ophthalmol 105:1693–1697, 1987.

Yanoff M, Fine BS, Schaffer DB: Histopathology of transient neonatal lens vacuoles. Am J Ophthalmol 76: 363–370, 1973.

## Rubella Cataract

Boniuk M, Zimmerman LE: Ocular pathology in the rubella syndrome. Arch Ophthalmol 17:455–473, 1967.

Roy FH, Fuste F, Hiatt RL, Deutsch AR, Korones SB: The congenital rubella syndrome with virus recovery: ocular pathology and literature review. Am J Ophthalmol 62: 222–232, 1966.

Yanoff M, Schaffer DB, Scheie HG: Rubella ocular syndrome: clinical significance of viral and pathologic studies. Trans Am Acad Ophthalmol Otolaryngol 72: 896–902, 1968.

Zimmerman LE: Histopathologic basis for ocular manifestations of congenital rubella syndrome: the Eighth William Hamlin Wilder memorial lecture. Am J Ophthalmol 65: 837–862, 1968.

## Cataract in Genetic Syndromes

Cogan DG, Kuwabara T: Pathology of cataracts in mongoloid idiocy: a new pathogenesis of cataracts of the coronary-cerulean type. Doc Ophthalmol 16:73–80, 1962.

Curtin VT, Joyce EE, Ballin N: Ocular pathology in the oculo-cerebro-renal syndrome of Lowe. Am J Ophthalmol 64(Part II):533–543, 1967.

Robb RM, Marchevsky A: Pathology of the lens in Down's syndrome. Arch Ophthalmol 96:1039–1042, 1978.

Wadelius C, Fagerholm P, Pettersson U, Anneren G: Lowe oculocerebrorenal syndrome: DNA-based linkage of the gene to Xq24-q26, using tightly linked flanking markers and the correlation to lens examination in carrier diagnosis. Am J Hum Genet 44:241–247, 1989.

Wolter JR, Jones DH: Spontaneous cataract absorption in Hallermann-Streiff syndrome. Ophthalmologica 150: 401–408, 1965.

## Senile Cataract

Benedek GB: Cataract as a protein condensation disease. Invest Ophthalmol Vis Sci 38:1911–1921, 1997.

Boyle DL, Takemoto LJ: Confocal microscopy of human lens membranes in aged normal and nuclear cataracts. Invest Ophthalmol Vis Sci 38:2826–2832, 1997.

Fledelius H: Cataracta ossea and other intraocular ossifications: a case report and a thirty-year Danish material. Acta Ophthalmol (Copenh) 53:790–797, 1975.

Flocks M, Littwin CS, Zimmerman LE: Phacolytic glaucoma: a clinicopathologic study of 138 cases of glaucoma associated with hypermature cataract. Arch Ophthalmol 54:37–45, 1955.

Font RL, Brownstein S: A light and electron microscopic study of anterior subcapsular cataracts. Am J Ophthalmol 78:972–984, 1974.

Henkind P, Prose P: Anterior polar cataract: electron-microscopic evidence of collagen. Am J Ophthalmol 63: 768–771, 1967.

Jensen OA, Laursen AB: Human senile cataract: light- and electron-microscopic studies of the morphology of the anterior lens structures, with special reference of anterior capsular/subcapsular opacity. Acta Ophthalmol (Copenh) 58:481–495, 1980.

Klintworth GK, Garner A: The causes, types, and morphology of cataracts. In Garner A, Klintworth GK (eds), Pathobiology of Ocular Disease: a Dynamic Approach. 2nd ed. Part A. New York: Marcel Dekker, 1994:481–532.

Kluxen G, Wolf E, Kalisch M, Vortkamp ML: Color vision disorders caused by yellow coloration of lenses. Fortschr Ophthalmol 81:180–182, 1984.

Zimmerman LE, Johnson FB: Calcium oxalate crystals within ocular tissues. Arch Ophthalmol 60:372–383, 1958.

## Posterior Capsular Opacification

Apple DJ, Solomon KD, Tetz MR, et al: Posterior capsule opacification. Surv Ophthalmol 37:73–116, 1992.

Green WR, McDonnell PJ: Opacification of the posterior capsule. Trans Ophthalmol Soc UK 104:727–739, 1985.

McDonnell PJ, Zarbin MA, Green WR: Posterior capsular opacification in pseudophakic eyes. Ophthalmology 90: 1548–1553, 1984.

## Posterior Subcapsular Cataract

Greiner JV, Chylack LT Jr: Posterior subcapsular cataracts: histopathologic study of steroid-associated cataracts. Arch Ophthalmol 97:135–144, 1979.

Streeten BW, Eshaghian J: Human posterior subcapsular cataract: a gross and flat preparation study. Arch Ophthalmol 96:1653–1658, 1978.

## Cataracts Caused by Ocular Disease (Complicated Cataracts)

Axelsson U: Glaucoma, miotic therapy and cataract. I. The frequency of anterior subcapsular vacuoles in glaucoma eyes treated with echothiophate (phospholine iodide), pilocarpine or pilocarpine-eserine, and in nonglaucomatous untreated eyes with common senile cataract. Acta Ophthalmol (Copenh) 46:83–98, 1968.

Fagerholm PP, Philipson BT: Cataract in retinitis pigmentosa: an analysis of cataract surgery results and pathological lens changes. Acta Ophthalmol (Copenh) 63:50–58, 1985.

Fisher RF: The lens in uveitis. Trans Ophthalmol Soc UK 101:317–320, 1981.

Loewenfeld IE, Thompson HS: Fuchs's heterochromic cyclitis: a critical review of the literature. I. Clinical characteristics of the syndrome. Surv Ophthalmol 17:394–457, 1973.

## Sugar Cataracts

Beigi B, O'Keefe M, Bowell R, Naughten E, Badawi N, Lanigan B: Ophthalmic findings in classical galactosaemia—prospective study. Br J Ophthalmol 77: 162–164, 1993.

Bron AJ, Sparrow J, Brown NAP, et al: The lens in diabetes. Eye 7:260–275, 1993.

Kinoshita JH: Cataracts in galactosemia. Invest Ophthalmol 4:786–799, 1965.

Stambolian D, Scarpino-Myers V, Eagle RC Jr, et al: Cataracts in patients heterozygous for galactokinase deficiency. Invest Ophthalmol Vision Sci 27:429–433, 1986.

**Cataracts Associated with Systemic Disease**

Bullock JD, Howard RO: Werner syndrome. Arch Ophthalmol 90:53–56, 1973.

Burns CA: Ocular histopathology of myotonic dystrophy: a clinicopathologic case report. Am J Ophthalmol 68: 416–422, 1969.

Dark AJ, Streeten BW: Ultrastructural study of cataract in myotonia dystrophica. Am J Ophthalmol 84:666–674, 1977.

Eshaghian J, March WF, Goossens W, Rafferty NS: Ultrastructure of cataract in myotonic dystrophy. Invest Ophthalmol Vis Sci 17:289–293, 1978.

Fagerholm P, Palmquist BM, Philipson B: Atopic cataract: changes in the lens epithelium and subcapsular cortex. Graefes Arch Clin Exp Ophthalmol 221:149–152, 1984.

Racz P, Kovacs B, Varga L, Ujlaki E, Zombai E, Karbuczky S: Bilateral cataract in acrodermatitis enteropathica. J Pediatr Ophthalmol Strabismus 16:180–182, 1979.

Seland JH: The nature of capsular inclusions in lenticular chalcosis: report of a case. Acta Ophthalmol (Copenh) 54: 99–108, 1976.

Spaeth GL, Frost P: Fabry's disease: its ocular manifestations. Arch Ophthalmol 74:760–769, 1965.

Tso MO, Fine BS, Thorpe HE: Kayser-Fleischer ring and associated cataract in Wilson's disease. Am J Ophthalmol 79:479–488, 1975.

**Traumatic Cataract**

Fraunfelder FT, Hanna C: Electric cataracts. I. Sequential changes, unusual and prognostic findings. Arch Ophthalmol 87:179–183, 1972.

Hanna C, Fraunfelder FT: Electric cataracts. II. Ultrastructural lens changes. Arch Ophthalmol 87:184–191, 1972.

Hanna C, Fraunfelder FT: Lens capsule change after intraocular copper. Ann Ophthalmol 5:9–12 passim, 1973.

Jongebloed WL, Dijk F, Kruis J, Worst JG: Soemmering's ring, an aspect of secondary cataract: a morphological description by SEM. Doc Ophthalmol 70:165–174, 1988.

Masciulli L, Andersen DR, Charles S: Experimental ocular siderosis in the squirrel monkey. Am J Ophthalmol 74: 638–661, 1972.

McCanna P, Chandra SR, Stevens TS, et al. Argon laser induced cataract as a complication of retinal photocoagulation. Arch Ophthalmol 100:1071–1073, 1982.

Rafferty NS, Goossens W, March WF: Ultrastructure of human traumatic cataract. Am J Ophthalmol 78:985–995, 1974.

Talamo JH, Topping TM, Maumenee AE, Green WR: Ultrastructural studies of cornea, iris and lens in a case of siderosis bulbi. Ophthalmology 92:1675–1680, 1985.

**Toxic Cataract**

Hamming NA, Apple DJ, Goldberg MF: Histopathology and ultrastructure of busulfan-induced cataract. Graefes Arch Clin Exp Ophthalmol 200:139–147, 1976.

Hiller R, Sperduto RD, Podgor MJ, et al: Cigarette smoking and the risk of development of lens opacities: the Framingham studies. Arch Ophthalmol 115:1113–1118, 1997.

Kirby TJ: Cataracts produced by triparanol (MER-29). Trans Am Ophthalmol Soc 65:494–543, 1967.

West S, Munoz B, Schein OD, et al: Cigarette smoking and risk for progression of nuclear opacities. Arch Ophthalmol 113:1377–1380, 1995.

**True Exfoliation of the Lens Capsule**

Anderson IL, van Bockxmeer FM: True exfoliation of the lens capsule: a clinicopathological report. Aust NZ J Ophthalmol 13:343–347, 1985.

Brodrick JD, Tate GW Jr: Capsular delamination (true exfoliation) of the lens: report of a case. Arch Ophthalmol 97: 1693–1698, 1979.

Burde RM, Bresnick G, Uhrhammer J: True exfoliation of the lens capsule: an electron microscopic study. Arch Ophthalmol 82:651–653, 1969.

Cashwell LF Jr, Holleman IL, Weaver RG, van Rens GH: Idiopathic true exfoliation of the lens capsule. Ophthalmology 96:348–351, 1989.

**Pseudoexfoliation of the Lens Capsule**

Schlotzer-Schrehardt U, Koca M, Naumann G, et al: Pseudoexfoliation syndrome: ocular manifestation of a systemic disorder? Arch Ophthalmol 110:1752, 1992.

Streeten BW, Dark AJ: Pseudoexfoliation syndrome. In Garner A, Klintworth GK (eds) Pathobiology of Ocular Disease: A Dynamic Approach. 2nd ed. Part A. New York: Marcel Dekker, 1994:591–629.

Streeten BW, Li Zy, Wallace RN, Eagle RC, Keshgegian AA. Pseudoexfoliative fibrillopathy in visceral organs of a patient with pseudoexfoliation syndrome. Arch Ophthalmol 110:1757–1762, 1992.

**Heritable Lens Dislocation (Ectopia Lentis)**

Edwards MJ, Challinor CJ, Colley PW, et al: Clinical and linkage study of a large family with simple ectopia lentis linked to FBN1. Am J Med Genet 53:65–71, 1994.

Fujiwara H, Takigawa Y, Ueno S, Okuda K: Histology of the lens in the Weill-Marchesani syndrome. Br J Ophthalmol 74:631–634, 1990.

Hayward C, Brock DJ: Fibrillin-1 mutations in Marfan syndrome and other type-1 fibrillinopathies. Hum Mutat 10: 415–423, 1997.

Henkind P, Ashton N: Ocular pathology in homocystinuria. Trans Ophthalmol Soc UK 85:21–38, 1965.

Hollister DW, Godfrey M, Sakai LY, Pyeritz RE: Immunohistologic abnormalities of the microfibrillar-fiber system in the Marfan syndrome. N Engl J Med 323:152–159, 1990.

Lueder GT, Steiner RD: Ophthalmic abnormalities in molybdenum cofactor deficiency and isolated sulfite oxidase deficiency. J Pediatr Ophthalmol Strabismus 32: 334–337, 1995.

Maumenee IH: The eye in the Marfan syndrome. Trans Am Ophthalmol Soc 79:684–733, 1981.

Maumenee IH: The Marfan syndrome is caused by a point mutation in the fibrillin gene. Arch Ophthalmol 110: 472–473, 1992.

Maumenee IH: The Weill-Marchesani syndrome. In Beighton P (ed) McCusick's Heritable Disorders of Connective Tissue. St. Louis: Mosby, 1993:179–187.

Pyeritz RE: Homocystinuria. In Beighton P (ed) McCusick's Heritable Disorders of Connective Tissue. St. Louis: Mosby, 1993:137–178.

Schienle HW, Seitz R, Nawroth P, et al: Thrombomodulin and ristocetin cofactor in homocystinuria: a study in two siblings. Thromb Res 77:79–86, 1995.

Shih VE, Abroms IF, Johnson JL, et al. Sulfite oxidase deficiency: biochemical and clinical investigations of a hereditary metabolic disorder in sulfur metabolism. N Engl J Med 297:1022–1028, 1977.

Smith TH, Holland MG, Woody NC: Ocular manifestations of familial hyperlysinemia. Trans Am Acad Ophthalmol Otolaryngol 75:355–360, 1971.

Thomas C, Cordier J, Algan B: Les altérations oculaires de la maladie d'Ehlers-Danlos. Arch Ophtalmol (Paris) 14: 691–697, 1954.

Wirtz MK, Samples JR, Kramer PL, et al: Weill-Marchesani syndrome—possible linkage of the autosomal dominant form to 15q21.1. Am J Med Genet 65:68–75, 1996.

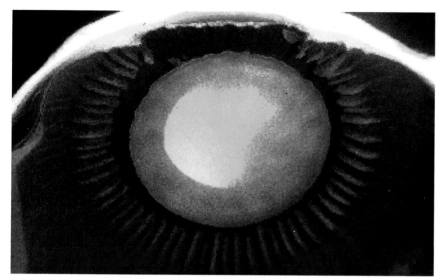

FIGURE 6–1 • **Lens and ciliary body.** The lens is located in the posterior chamber behind the iris and its central aperture, the pupil. The pars plicata of the ciliary body is comprised of a ring of radially oriented ciliary processes, which show mild hyalinization in this specimen.

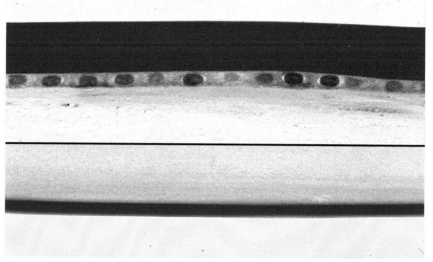

FIGURE 6–2 • **Lens capsule and epithelium.** A monolayer of cuboidal lens epithelial cells is present underneath the anterior lens capsule (*top*), which is much thicker than the posterior capsule (*bottom*). The capsule is a thick basement membrane that stains intensely with the periodic acid-Schiff stain. Periodic acid-Schiff, ×250.

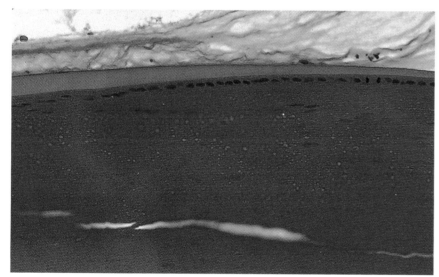

FIGURE 6–3 • **Equatorial lens bow.** The anterior monolayer of cuboidal lens epithelial cells terminates near the lens equator, where cells divide and elongate, forming new lens fiber cells. The nuclei dip into the equatorial cortex, forming a curved pattern called the equatorial bow. As the lens fibers mature, their nuclei degenerate and eventually disappear. Hematoxylin-eosin, ×100.

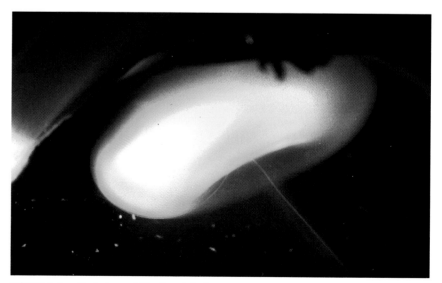

FIGURE 6–4 • **Posterior umbilication, infant eye.** The concave shape of the posterior lens is called posterior umbilication. Posterior umbilication is a fixation artifact that affects the lens in infants. The hyaloid artery persists in this specimen.

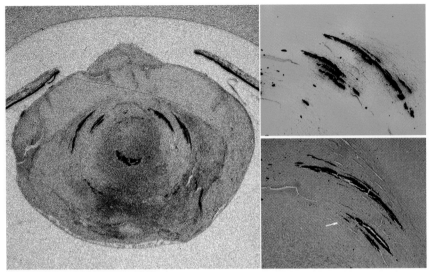

FIGURE 6–5 • **Lamellar cataract, infant eye.** Calcified lamellae of lens fibers surround the lens nucleus. von Kossa, ×5. Positive staining with alizarin red (*top inset*) and von Kossa stains (*bottom inset*) confirms that opacity contains calcium. An anterior subcapsular cataract also is present. Top inset ×25, bottom inset ×25.

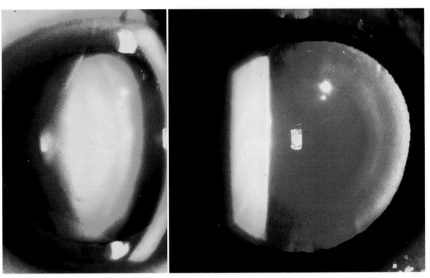

FIGURE 6–6 • **Nuclear sclerosis.** Sclerotic nucleus is evident as an oil droplet in red reflex (*left*). Slit beam discloses yellow urochrome pigment.

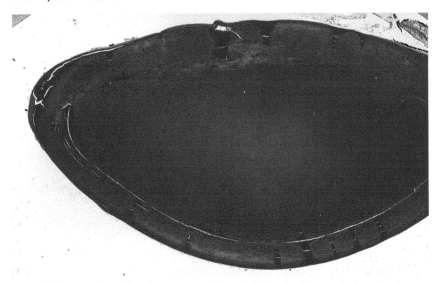

FIGURE 6–7 • **Nuclear sclerosis.** An artifactitious cleft delimits the posterior boundary between the sclerotic nucleus and the cortex. The nucleus is more eosinophilic than the cortex and lacks the artifactitious clefts that normally form when the lens is sectioned. Hematoxylin-eosin, ×5.

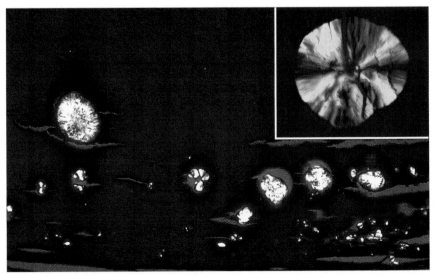

FIGURE 6–8 • **Oxalate crystals, nuclear sclerosis.** Polarization microscopy highlights oval crystals of calcium oxalate in nuclear sclerotic cataract. *Inset:* The crystal exhibits characteristic vivid rainbow-like pattern of birefringence. Hematoxylin-eosin with crossed polarizers. Main figure ×25, inset ×100.

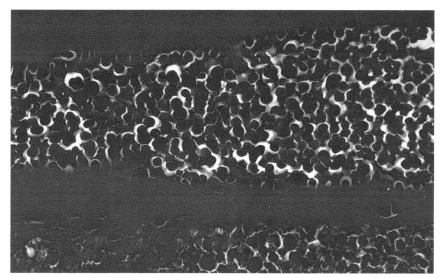

FIGURE 6–9 • **Cortical cataract, morgagnian globules.** Morgagnian globules fill the cleft in a cortical cataract. Morgagnian globules are spherules of degenerated lens cytoplasm that have leaked from fragmented lens fibers. Hematoxylin-eosin, ×50.

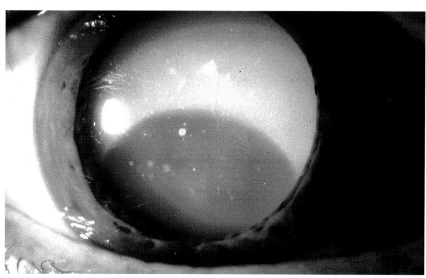

FIGURE 6–10 • **Morgagnian cataract.** Morgagnian cataract results when the lens cortex undergoes total liquefaction. The densely sclerotic nucleus is resistant to liquefaction and sinks to the bottom of the bag of liquefied cortex. Calcium oxalate crystals are evident as lighter spherules in the amber nucleus. (Courtesy of Prof. Dr. med. Wolfgang Lieb, University of Würzburg)

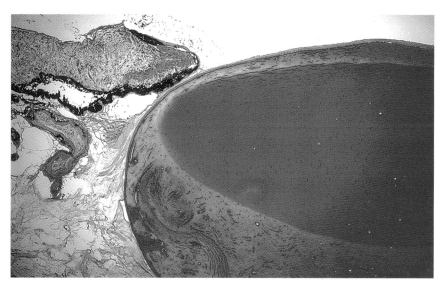

FIGURE 6–11 • **Morgagnian cataract.** Degenerated lens cortex surrounds the intensely eosinophilic sclerotic nucleus. Although most of the cortex has liquefied, a few curved disrupted lens fibers are seen posteriorly. Hematoxylin-eosin, ×10.

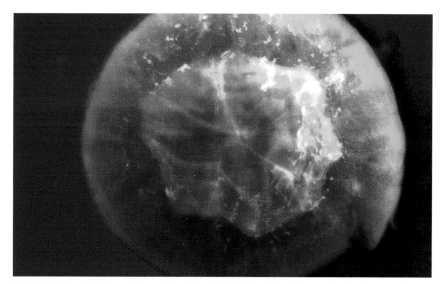

FIGURE 6–12 • **Anterior subcapsular cataract.** The irregular white opacity on the anterior surface of the lens is a plaque of collagen that has been synthesized by lens epithelial cells. The anterior lens capsule is folded, and the lens nucleus is sclerotic.

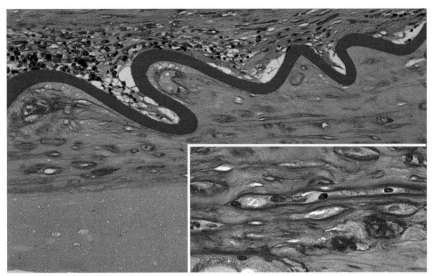

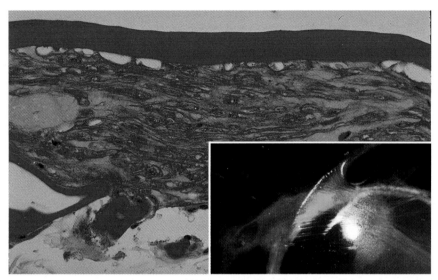

FIGURE 6–13 • **Anterior subcapsular cataract.** Sinuously folded anterior lens capsule covers the anterior surface of a fibrous plaque synthesized by lens epithelial cells irritated by inflammatory membrane in the posterior chamber. *Inset:* Lens epithelial cells within the plaque surrounded by capsules of basement membrane. Periodic acid-Schiff. Main figure ×100, inset ×250.

FIGURE 6–14 • **Capsular fibrosis, post-ECCE.** Lens capsular bag contains a mass of collagenous connective tissue synthesized by residual lens epithelial cells that reside in basement membrane capsules. *Top:* Anterior capsule. *Bottom:* Posterior capsule. *Inset:* Note the capsular folds and opacification near the edge of the intraocular lens. Periodic acid-Schiff, ×100.

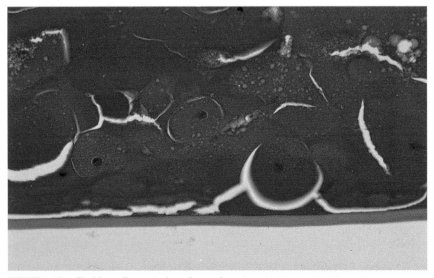

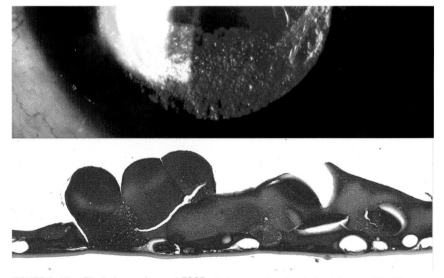

FIGURE 6–15 • **Bladder cells, posterior subcapsular cataract.** Wedl, or bladder, cells represent abortive attempts by lens epithelial cells to form new lens fibers. They develop from aberrantly situated lens epithelial cells that have migrated posteriorly. Several of the bladder cells contain nuclei. The nuclei in the other large cells are not seen in this plane of the section. Hematoxylin-eosin, ×100.

FIGURE 6–16 • **Elschnig pearls, post-ECCE.** Relucent spherules derived from residual lens epithelial cells are seen in the lens capsule after extracapsular cataract extraction. Nuclei of Elschnig pearls on the posterior capsule (below) are not evident in this plane of the section. Hematoxylin-eosin, ×100.

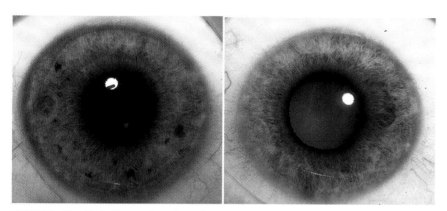

FIGURE 6–17 • **Fuchs' heterochromic cyclitis.** Affected eye (at right) has developed cataract and hypochromic heterochromia iridum.

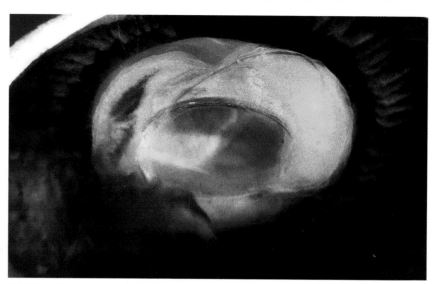

FIGURE 6–18 • **Soemmerring's ring cataract, post ECCE.** Large amounts of residual lens cortex form Soemmerring's ring in the equatorial part of the lens capsular bag.

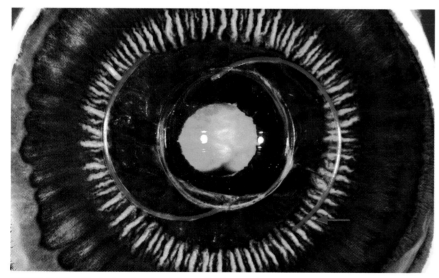

FIGURE 6–19 • **Posterior chamber intraocular lens.** The lens capsule is free of cortex. One of the blue haptics rests on the surface of the hyalinized pars plicata outside the capsular bag (arrow).

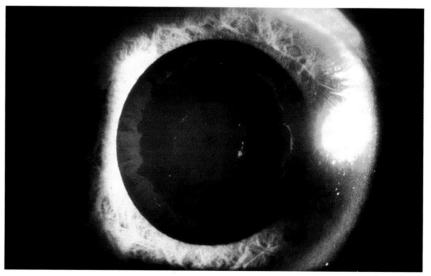

FIGURE 6–20 • **Pseudoexfoliation of the lens capsule.** Grayish white pseudoexfoliative material forms a "target" on the anterior lens capsule. A pseudoexfoliation-free zone wiped clean by the iris surrounds the central bull's eye, whose diameter corresponds to the miotic pupil. The peripheral granular zone contains radial erosions caused by large radial folds on the posterior iris. Focal outward peeling of the margin of the peripheral zone is present.

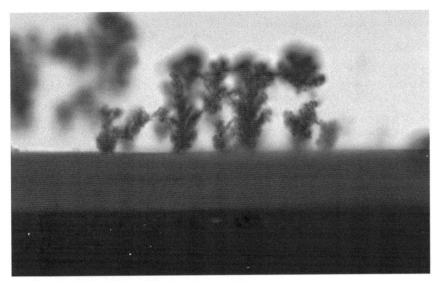

FIGURE 6–21 • **Pseudoexfoliation of the lens capsule.** Eosinophilic bush-like Busacca deposits of pseudoexfoliation material are seen on the anterior lens capsule. The appearance of the material has been likened to iron filings on a magnet. Hematoxylin-eosin, ×250.

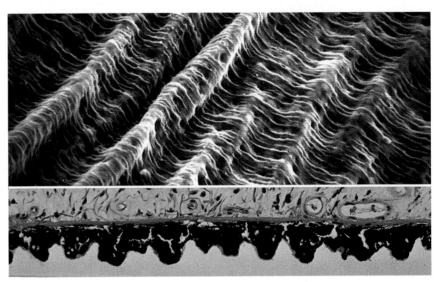

FIGURE 6–22 • **Pseudoexfoliation syndrome, iris pigment epithelium.** Coalescence of circumferential ridges imparts a coarse, "saw-toothed" appearance to the iris pigment epithelium. Pseudoexfoliation material festoons the ridges. Main figure: scanning electron micrograph. Inset: hematoxylin-eosin, ×50.

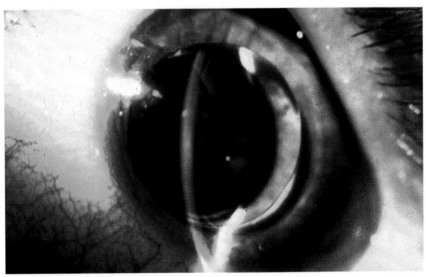

FIGURE 6–23 • **Ectopia lentis, Weill-Marchesani syndrome.** Microspherophakic lens has dislocated into the anterior chamber, causing pupillary block glaucoma. (Courtesy of Dr. Dario Savino-Zari, Caracas, Venezuela)

# CHAPTER 7

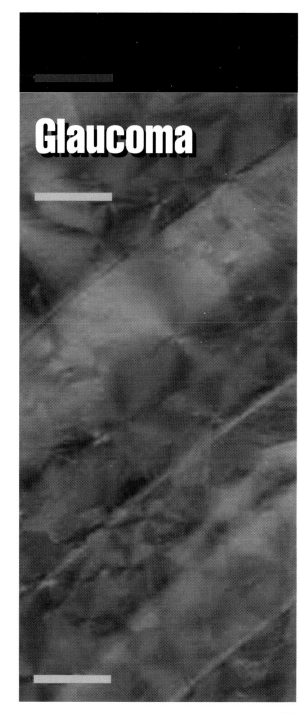

## Glaucoma

isual loss associated with glaucoma is caused by the death of the retinal ganglion cells and their axons that constitute the nerve fiber layer of the retina and the optic nerve (Fig. 7–1). The optic nerve head has a characteristic cupped or excavated configuration in glaucoma (Figs. 7–2, 7–3). Cupping distinguishes glaucomatous optic atrophy from primary optic atrophy, in which loss of retinal ganglion cells and nerve fibers also occurs. Cupping of the optic disk suggests that elevated intraocular pressure is a major risk factor in the pathogenesis of glaucomatous optic atrophy.

How elevated intraocular pressure kills the ganglion cells is not clear. Experimental evidence suggests that it may be related to blockage of axoplasmic flow caused by mechanical compression of axons in the pores of the lamina cribrosa, which are distorted by high levels of intraocular pressure. The blockage of axoplasmic flow may deprive cells of a neurotrophic factor whose absence triggers programmed cell death.

Glaucoma has been defined as "a syndrome characterized by an elevation of intraocular pressure of sufficient degree or chronicity to produce ocular tissue damage" (Yanoff, 1982) or as "an optic neuropathy associated with a characteristic excavation of the optic disc and a progressive loss of visual field sensitivity" (Quigley, 1991). The first definition emphasizes that tissue damage, usually nerve fiber atrophy or optic nerve cupping is a requisite for the diagnosis. The term syndrome indicates that there are many mechanisms that can raise intraocular pressure. The first definition also implies that a single elevated pressure reading is not glaucoma. The second, newer definition does not mention intraocular pressure because authorities recently have stressed that elevation of intraocu-

lar pressure is only one of the risk factors responsible for neuronal loss in glaucoma. The latter definition includes "low tension glaucoma," which develops in patients whose optic nerves seem to be especially vulnerable to damage. Most glaucomatous eyes examined in the ophthalmic pathology laboratory have had elevated intraocular pressure. In nearly all cases of glaucoma, this elevation is caused by obstruction of aqueous outflow.

Intraocular pressure is governed by a delicate balance between the production of aqueous humor by the nonpigmented ciliary epithelial cells and its egress, or outflow, from the eye. Most aqueous humor exits via the traditional aqueous outflow pathway comprised of the trabecular meshwork and the canal of Schlemm, which are located in the anterior chamber in the anterior or corneoscleral part of the angle formed by the cornea and peripheral iris (Figs. 7–4, 7–5, 7–6, 7–7, 7–8). Smaller amounts of aqueous exit through nontraditional pathways, which include iris vessels and posterior uveoscleral outflow via the ciliary body and the vortex veins.

The trabecular meshwork is a sieve-like structure nestled in the anterior crotch of a triangular peninsula of sclera called the scleral spur (Figs. 7–6, 7–7, 7–8). The scleral spur serves as an important anatomic landmark in both clinical and pathologic practice. The longitudinal fibers of the ciliary muscle are firmly attached to the posterior aspect of the scleral spur. During microscopy, the spur is found by following the ciliary muscle fibers to their insertion. Pigment accumulates in the thickest part of the meshwork located directly in front of the spur called the "functioning trabecular meshwork." During gonioscopy, the scleral spur is evident as a white line situated posterior to this pigmented band. If the angle is "wide open," the anterior face of the ciliary body appears as a gray line interposed between the scleral spur and the root of the iris. Descemet's membrane terminates at Schwalbe's line. Schwalbe's line is accentuated in some individuals and forms an elevated ridge of connective tissue. A band of pigment on the posterior cornea anterior to Schwalbe's line is called Sampaolesi's line.

The trabecular meshwork is composed of an interconnected network of small beams or trabeculae. The beams are composed of collagen with a central core of elastic tissue; they are encompassed by trabecular endothelial cells and a thin layer of endothelial basement membrane. The deeper, corneoscleral part of the meshwork is composed of concentrically oriented plates of connective tissue containing pores that are out of register. The interstices of the meshwork do not communicate directly with the lumen of the canal of Schlemm but are separated by a thin layer of extracellular matrix material called the juxtacanalicular connective tissue. Schlemm's canal is a modified vein lined by a continuous layer of endothelial cells. Schlemm's canal runs circumferentially around the chamber angle, giving off branches or collector channels that traverse the sclera and discharge their contents into the epibulbar veins via the aqueous veins of Ascher.

## CLASSIFICATION OF THE GLAUCOMAS

The glaucomas are classified into developmental, primary (or idiopathic), and secondary types. Primary and secondary glaucomas are subclassified into open-angle and closed-angle variants depending on whether the angle is open or closed. Angle closure glaucoma is marked by the apposition or adherence of the peripheral iris to the trabecular meshwork (Figs. 7–9, 7–10). Developmental glaucomas present during infancy or childhood and may be inherited or associated with other ocular anomalies or systemic disorders.

## Developmental Glaucoma

Developmental glaucomas are caused by developmental abnormalities or dysembryogenesis of the aqueous outflow pathways. Primary congenital glaucoma is a bilateral disorder that is often inherited as an autosomal recessive trait. About 40% of cases are present at birth, and 86% become evident during the first year of life. Affected infants often have light sensitivity (photophobia), blepharospasm, and tearing; and they may be misdiagnosed as having nasolacrimal duct obstruction. Ocular enlargement (buphthalmos, or "ox eye") is the clinical hallmark of congenital glaucoma. Elevation of intraocular pressure causes ocular enlargement only during childhood when the sclera is relatively thin and elastic. Corneal enlargement and ectasia of limbal tissues is especially striking (Fig. 7–11). As the cornea stretches, Descemet's membrane may rupture spontaneously causing corneal edema and opacification. Old, healed ruptures in Descemet's membrane in patients with congenital glaucoma are called Haab's striae (Fig. 7–12). Haab's striae usually are oriented horizontally or concentric to the limbus in the peripheral cornea. This distinguishes them from traumatic ruptures caused by obstetric forceps, which usually are oriented obliquely.

Hypothetic mechanisms involved in the pathogenesis of congenital glaucoma include an imperforate mesodermal sheet covering the trabecular meshwork called Barkan's membrane, congenital absence of Schlemm's canal, and persistence of a fetal angle configuration. Histopathologically, the fetal angle is characterized by anterior insertion of the iris root and ciliary processes, the presence of mesenchymal tissue in the angle, and continuity of ciliary muscle fibers with trabecular beams (Fig. 7–13). The anterior chamber usually is quite deep in eyes with congenital glaucoma. The angle is open gonioscopically, and there is high insertion of the iris root.

Developmental glaucoma occasionally occurs in association with other ocular abnormalities or congenital syndromes including aniridia, the Axenfeld-Rieger syndrome, and Peters' anomaly. Glaucoma also complicates von Recklinghausen's neurofibromatosis (NF-I) and Sturge-Weber syndrome, particularly if the upper eyelid is involved by the hamartomatous process; a plexiform or diffuse neurofibroma in NF-1, or a nevus flammeus in Sturge-Weber syndrome. Hamartomatous infiltration of the angle may produce a distinctive gonioscopic appearance in neurofibromatosis. The angle is blanketed by a uniform layer of tan tissue that obscures normal trabecular landmarks. Glaucoma and cataract occur concurrently in Lowe syndrome. Other syndromes that may include congenital glaucoma include Gregg congenital rubella syndrome, Stickler syndrome, Hallerman-Streiff syndrome, Hurler syndrome, Turner syndrome, and trisomies 21 and 13.

## Primary Glaucoma

### Primary Open-Angle Glaucoma

Primary, or idiopathic, open-angle glaucoma is the most common type of glaucoma, affecting an estimated 1–3% of the population. It is an insidious disease that causes asymptomatic painless visual loss. By definition, the angle is open on gonioscopic examination. Primary open-angle glaucoma usually is a bilateral disease, and affected patients frequently have a positive family history.

The cause of aqueous outflow obstruction in primary open angle glaucoma remains uncertain, but the area of obstruction probably is located in the juxtacanalicular connective tissue in the deepest part of the trabecular meshwork bordering Schlemm's canal. Several pathogenetic theories involve obstruction of the meshwork or juxtacanalicular connective tissue by glycosaminoglycans or other abnormal extracellular matrix material. Others have suggested that the disease is caused by abnormalities in the formation of giant vacuoles in the endothelial lining of Schlemm's canal, or that posterior uveoscleral outflow is impeded by age-related sclerosis in the scleral spur. An electron microscopic study found that the density of trabecular endothelial cells is decreased in patients with primary open-angle glaucoma. Loss of endothelial cells could lead to fusion of trabecular beams and decreased porosity of the meshwork (Fig. 7–14). Another study showed that the area of the trabecular cul-de-sacs, which provide a major proportion of normal outflow resistance, are markedly reduced in primary open angle glaucoma (Fig. 7–15).

## Primary Closed-Angle Glaucoma

Primary closed-angle glaucoma (acute angle closure glaucoma or acute congestive glaucoma) is caused by functional apposition or blockage of the trabecular meshwork by the peripheral iris. The resultant acute rise in intraocular pressure produces major symptoms, including severe ocular pain, headache, and gastrointestinal symptoms (nausea and vomiting) caused by a vagal oculogastric reflex. The involved eye is injected and classically has a fixed, dilated pupil during an acute attack of closed-angle glaucoma. The vision usually is diminished by corneal epithelial edema evident clinically as "bedewing," or possibly by posterior segment ischemia. Primary closed-angle glaucoma usually is unilateral and typically occurs in hyperopic ("far-sighted") patients whose small eyes have shallow, crowded anterior chambers. Primary closed-angle glaucoma is rare in myopes (near-sighted individuals) and patients less than age 40. Progressive growth of the lens or development of an intumescent cataract can precipitate an acute attack of closed-angle glaucoma in elderly patients (phacomorphic glaucoma). Acute angle closure glaucoma is more prevalent in certain racial groups (e.g., Inuits) and often occurs in nanophthalmic eyes, which are markedly hyperopic and prone to develop exudative ciliochoroidal detachment.

Functional pupillary block is involved in the pathogenesis of primary closed-angle glaucoma. When the pupil is mid-dilated, the iris pigment epithelium near the pupil is pressed firmly against the anterior surface of the lens, impeding the flow of aqueous humor into the anterior chamber. The pupillary block is functional because adhesions between the iris and lens, called posterior synechias, have not formed. Continual production of aqueous humor behind the iris produces a pressure gradient that bows the peripheral part of the iris forward, obstructing the trabecular meshwork. If this functional papillary block is not relieved expeditiously, permanent adhesions between peripheral iris and trabecular meshwork called peripheral anterior synechias eventually develop. Acute closed-angle glaucoma is cured by making a full-thickness hole in the iris, which equalizes the pressure in the anterior and posterior chambers and allows the iris to fall back into its normal position. The iridotomy usually is performed with a surgical laser.

High intraocular pressure can cause permanent damage to anterior segment structures during an attack of acute closed-angle glaucoma. Ischemic in nature, these changes persist as stigmata of a prior "acute attack" and include permanent dilation and unreactivity of the pupil caused by necrosis of the sphincter muscle, patchy atrophy of the iris stroma, and small grayish anterior subcapsular lens opacities called glaukomflecken. Glaukomflecken probably represent focal areas of lens epithelial necrosis and cortical degeneration.

## Secondary Glaucoma

### Secondary Closed-Angle Glaucoma

Secondary glaucomas are caused by concurrent ocular or systemic disease. Both closed-angle and open-angle varieties of secondary glaucoma occur. Many blind glaucomatous eyes examined in the ophthalmic pathology laboratory have secondary closed-angle glaucoma. Secondary closed-angle glaucoma is characterized by the formation of permanent adhesions between the iris and the trabecular meshwork called peripheral anterior synechias (Figs. 7–9, 7–10). There are many causes of secondary closed-angle glaucoma. Permanent peripheral anterior synechias can form in untreated primary closed-angle glaucoma and often develop in the late stages of retinopathy of prematurity or persistent hyperplastic primary vitreous (PHPV). Posterior segment tumors usually cause secondary closed-angle glaucoma by stimulating iris neovascularization or by a pupillary block mechanism.

The role of functional pupillary block in primary closed-angle glaucoma is discussed above. Pupillary block also is important in several types of secondary closed-angle glaucoma. Inflammatory adhesions between the pupillary part of the iris and the anterior lens capsule called posterior synechias readily form in the sticky, fibrin-rich milieu of iritis or iridocyclitis. The entire circumference of the pupil may become firmly bound to the lens (seclusio pupillae), totally blocking the flow of aqueous humor into the anterior chamber. The elevated pressure in the posterior chamber bows the peripheral part of the iris forward (iris bombé) and blocks the trabecular meshwork secondarily (Fig. 7–16). Cycloplegic medications such as atropine or scopolamine relieve the pain of pupillary and ciliary spasm in uveitis and help prevent posterior synechias by dilating the pupil. The lens or vitreous can also block the pupil. Anterior displacement of the microspherophakic lens in Weill-Marchesani syndrome readily occludes the pupil, causing pupillary block glaucoma (see Fig. 6–23). Pupillary block glaucoma also occurs in patients with traumatic or heritable lens dislocation. Prophylactic peripheral iridectomies were performed routinely during intracapsular cataract surgery to prevent postoperative blockage of the pupil by the anterior face of the vitreous. Pupillary block caused by anterior movement of the lens–iris diaphragm is a common cause of secondary closed-angle glaucoma in eyes that have large posterior segment tumors or extensive bullous retinal detachments.

Several clinically important types of secondary closed-angle glaucoma are caused by the proliferation of cells on anterior chamber structures. These secondary proliferative glaucomas include epithelial downgrowth or ingrowth caused by proliferation of ocular surface epithelium after surgical or nonsurgical trauma, the iridocorneal endothelial syndrome caused by proliferation of abnormal corneal endothelial cells, and neovascular glaucoma caused by iris neovascularization. Epithelial downgrowth is discussed in Chapter 3 (Fig. 7–17; see also Fig. 3–25).

### Neovascular Glaucoma

Many blind, painful eyes accessioned by ophthalmic pathology laboratories have neovascular glaucoma (Figs. 7–18, 7–19, 7–20, 7–21). Peripheral anterior synechia formation in neovascular glaucoma is caused by the proliferation of fibrovascular tissue on the anterior surface of the iris and angle. Angiogenic factors such as vascular endothelial growth factor (VEGF) produced by ischemic parts of the retina or intraocular tumor cells stimulate the iris neovascularization. Clinically, conditions most commonly associated with neovascular glaucoma include retinal vein and artery occlusions, proliferative diabetic retinopathy, and intraocular tumors, particularly retinoblastoma.

Severe iris neovascularization (rubeosis iridis) flattens the anterior surface of the iris, effacing normal architectural details such as contraction furrows. The anterior border layer of the iris normally is a totally avascular site. Any vessels found here during histopathologic examination are abnormal. The new vessels have thin walls and lack the thick mantle of collagen fibers that normally envelops iris stromal vessels. The new vessels are located deep to a flat, delicate sheet of contractile myofibroblasts, which is transparent clinically (Fig. 7–21). The surface layer of myofibroblasts may provide the motive force for synechial closure of the angle and formation of pigment epithelial ectropion (ectropion iridis). In ectropion iridis, the iris pigment epithelium is dragged around the pupillary margin onto the anterior surface of the iris by the contracting sheet of neovascular tissue (Fig. 7–19). An associated ectropion of the pupillary sphincter muscle may also be present.

Fewer eyes with neovascular glaucoma have been enucleated and submitted to ophthalmic pathology laboratories in recent years. This reflects the availability of effective new therapies such as panretinal photocoagulation (PRP) that prevent the development of proliferative retinopathy and iris neovascularization in patients who have diabetes and other ischemic retinopathies. PRP uses hundreds of laser burns to kill outer retinal cells. Hypothetically, it diminishes the production of angiogenic factors by decreasing the demand for oxygen and nutrients or increases the supply of metabolites by disrupting the outer part of the blood–retinal barrier. PRP does not reverse synechias after they have formed. Specialized filtering operations using plastic setons or tube shunts, or transscleral cycloablation procedures that use intense cold or laser energy to reduce aqueous production, can be used to treat established cases of neovascular glaucoma.

### Iridocorneal Endothelial Syndrome

Proliferation of abnormal corneal endothelial cells, possibly transformed by viral infection, causes unilateral closed-angle glaucoma and a characteristic spectrum of iris abnormalities in patients who have the iridocorneal endothelial (ICE) syndrome (Figs. 7–22, 7–23, 7–24). The iris abnormalities include distortion of the pupil, which typically is drawn toward a synechia that develops in the otherwise open angle, marked degrees of iris pigment epithelial ectropion, flattening and effacement of the anterior iridic surface with multiple pigmented iris nodules, and the formation of full-thickness tractional iris holes (Fig. 7–22). The name iridocorneal endothelial syndrome stresses the role of endothelial proliferative in the pathogenesis of the iris abnormalities. Several conditions that form the ICE syndrome are distinguished by the nature of their iris abnormalities. Full-thickness iris holes are a characteristic feature of essential iris atrophy but typically do not develop in the Cogan-Reese or iris nevus syndrome, in which the iris is covered by endothelium and flattened by ectopic Descemet's membrane studded with pigmented nodules. Corneal edema overshadows iris abnormalities in the variant of essential iris atrophy described by Chandler (Chandler syndrome).

Normal corneal endothelium does not proliferate during adult life, but the abnormal endothelial cells in the ICE syndrome are able to multiply and extend across the trabecular meshwork onto the iris where they elaborate large quantities of extracellular matrix material including new Descemet's membrane (Fig. 7–23). The matrix material thickens trabecular beams and welds the flattened iris to the posterior cornea. The iris nodules that characterize Cogan-Reese syndrome and some cases of essential iris atrophy are formed when the sheets of migrating endothelial cells encircle and "pinch off" knuckles of iris stroma (Fig. 7–24). Endothelialization and descemetization of fistulas and filtering blebs leads to failure of glaucoma surgery.

Corneal endothelial abnormalities often are evident on clinical specular microscopy as "dark–light" reversal and the presence of two sharply demarcated populations of endothelial cells that vary in size and shape. What causes the corneal endothelium to transform into a new species of cells capable of proliferation is unclear. Theories include viral transformation of cells, an endothelial neoplasm, or abnormalities in terminal differentiation of neural crest cells.

## Secondary Open-Angle Glaucoma

The angle appears open on gonioscopic examination in patients who have secondary open-angle glaucoma. Causes of secondary open-angle glaucoma include obstruction of the trabecular meshwork by cells, pigment, debris, or other material; damage or scarring of outflow pathways; or systemic or local conditions that elevate the episcleral venous pressure.

Substances that can obstruct the trabecular meshwork include blood, inflammatory cells, particles of lens material, melanin pigment, and an abnormal form of matrix material called pseudoexfoliation that is found in some elderly patients (see Chapter 6). Glaucoma complicates large anterior chamber hemorrhages caused by contusion injuries ("eight-ball" or "black ball" hyphemas). Patients with sickle cell hemoglobinopathies who develop hyphemas are at particular risk for glaucoma because their erythrocytes sickle in a low-oxygen environment; the sickled cells, which are less pliable, then become trapped in the trabecular meshwork.

Infiltration of the trabecular meshwork by inflammatory cells ("trabeculitis") occasionally causes elevated intraocular pressure in eyes with iridocyclitis. Frequently, however, disruption of the blood–aqueous barrier, by the inflammation leads to "shut-down" of aqueous production by the ciliary body.

Several rare types of secondary glaucoma are caused by physical obstruction of the trabecular meshwork by macrophages. Phacolytic glaucoma (Fig. 7–25; see also Fig. 2–10) is caused by macrophages that have ingested degenerated lens material that has leaked through the capsule of a mature cortical cataract. Free high-molecular-weight lens protein also contributes to trabecular blockage. Patients who have phacolytic glaucoma often have undergone successful cataract surgery in their fellow eye and have forgone additional surgery because they are satisfied with uniocular vision. Many eyes with phacolytic glaucoma

were enucleated in the past before the condition was widely recognized. Now most cases respond to lens extraction and anterior chamber lavage.

With hemolytic glaucoma (Fig. 7–26) the trabecular meshwork is obstructed by macrophages laden with blood-breakdown products including globules of the golden-brown pigment hemosiderin and erythrocyte ghost cells. Hemolytic glaucoma usually occurs in patients who have chronic vitreous hemorrhages. Microscopic examination of the khaki or yellow ochre-colored vitreous blood discloses small eosinophilic hemoglobin spherules, macrophages laden with hemosiderin and other blood-breakdown products, and erythrocyte ghost cells. Ghost cells, or erythroclasts, are red blood cells that have lost their hemoglobin. The inner surface of the empty cell membranes is studded with dots called Heinz bodies. All of these blood-breakdown products occasionally are able to enter the anterior segment through defects in the vitreous face or zonule. A relatively pure population of ghost cells blocks the meshwork in the variant of hemolytic glaucoma called ghost cell glaucoma. The clinical findings in ghost cell glaucoma may be subtle; the ghost cells usually form a faint, inconspicuous, khaki-colored layer in the inferior chamber angle.

Macrophages that have ingested melanin pigment released from necrotic pigmented tumors cause melanomalytic glaucoma and melanocytomalytic glaucoma (Figs. 7–27, 7–28). Magnocellular nevi called melanocytomas are particularly prone to undergo spontaneous necrosis. Several cases of melanocytomalytic glaucoma caused by necrosis of iris melanocytomas have been reported. Gonioscopy discloses heavy pigmentation of the trabecular meshwork.

Edematous particles of degenerated lens material dispersed by lens injuries or surgery can cause secondary open-angle glaucoma (lens particle glaucoma). Enzymatic zonulysis used during intracapsular cataract extraction can release zonular fragments and

debris that can temporarily obstruct the trabecular meshwork ($\alpha$-chymotrypsin glaucoma). Secondary trabecular obstruction by photoreceptor outer segments in eyes with chronic rhegmatogenous retinal detachments is called the Schwartz-Matsuo syndrome.

A relatively common type of secondary open-angle glaucoma called glaucoma capsulare occurs in elderly patients who have pseudoexfoliation of the lens capsule (see Chapter 6). Pseudoexfoliation material dispersed by the aqueous physically blocks the trabecular meshwork, and additional material is synthesized within the meshwork by the trabecular endothelial cells. Iris pigment epithelial abnormalities also lead to dispersal of iris pigment epithelial melanin throughout the anterior segment.

Granules of melanin pigment released from the iris pigment epithelium accumulate in the trabecular meshwork and interfere with aqueous outflow in pigmentary glaucoma (Figs. 7–29, 7–30). Pigmentary glaucoma is particularly common in young to middle-aged men who are myopic and have a deep anterior chamber and a tremulous iris (iridodonesis). Campbell suggested that abrasion by bundles of zonular fibers causes release of melanin from the iris pigment epithelium. An inverse pupillary block mechanism appears to bow the peripheral iris against the zonules in some patients. The zonular abrasions cause defects in the pigment epithelium that are evident during transillumination as characteristic radially oriented areas of increased light transmission. Biomicroscopy discloses pigment-laden macrophages (clump cells of Koganei type I) in the superficial iris stroma overlying the defects. Iris pigment phagocytized by the corneal endothelium is seen clinically as a vertically oriented Krukenberg spindle. The orientation of the spindle is governed by convection currents in the aqueous humor. The trabecular meshwork is heavily pigmented. Large, round melanin granules consistent with iris pigment epithelial origin are found within the cytoplasm of the trabecular endothelial cells (Fig. 7–30). Chronic pigmentation is thought to induce trabecular scarring. Only about half of patients with pigment dispersion develop glaucoma.

## TUMORS AND GLAUCOMA

Malignant tumors, particularly malignant melanomas of the ciliary body or iris can cause secondary open-angle glaucoma by diffusely seeding the trabecular meshwork with tumor cells or by proliferating circumferentially around the angle as a "ring melanoma" (Figs. 7–31, 7–32, 7–33). Anterior segment tumors generally cause secondary open-angle glaucoma. Posterior tumors, especially large choroidal melanomas or exophytic retinoblastomas with extensive bullous retinal detachments cause secondary closed-angle glaucoma (Fig. 7–34). Angiogenesis factors produced by tumors can also cause neovascular glaucoma.

Glaucoma often occurs in eyes that have iris melanomas composed of poorly cohesive epithelioid cells. Aqueous dispersion of tumor cells throughout the anterior chamber may cause progressive darkening of the involved iris (hyperchromic heterochromia iridum). Unilateral glaucoma and a subtle change in the color of the iris may be the only indication that a patient harbors a diffuse iris melanoma (Fig. 7–35).

Ocular trauma is another cause of secondary open-angle glaucoma. Chronic inflammation or repeated anterior chamber hemorrhage can cause scarring of the trabecular meshwork. Iron released from retained iron intraocular foreign bodies (siderosis) or recurrent intraocular hemorrhages (hemosiderosis) can have toxic effects on the trabecular endothelial cells and on the retinal photoreceptors. Postcontusion angle recession, a well recognized cause of unilateral glaucoma, is discussed in Chapter 3.

An important factor that determines the outflow of aqueous humor from the eye is the difference between the intraocular pressure and the pressure in the episcleral veins (episcleral venous pressure). Diseases that cause venous obstruction, such as cavernous sinus thromboses or mediastinal syndromes, can cause glaucoma by elevating the episcleral venous pressure. Arterialization of episcleral veins markedly elevates the episcleral venous pressure in some patients with carotid cavernous fistulas. The resultant glaucoma is difficult to manage.

Orbital pathology, (e.g., orbital tumors or the enlarged extraocular muscles of thyroid ophthalmopathy) can raise intraocular pressure by directly compressing the globe.

## OCULAR TISSUE CHANGES IN GLAUCOMATOUS EYES

The histopathologic diagnosis of glaucoma requires the demonstration of ocular tissue damage, typically glaucomatous retinal and optic atrophy. Glaucomatous retinal atrophy is characterized by atrophy of the retinal ganglion and nerve fiber layer, which is comprised of the axons of the ganglion cells (Fig. 7–1). The atrophic nerve fiber layer is often gliotic. Involvement of the inner plexiform layer and the inner part of the inner nuclear layer distinguish inner ischemic retinal atrophy that follows retinal artery occlusion from glaucomatous retinal atrophy. Gliosis typically is absent with ischemic atrophy, and the inner retinal layers may have a hyalinized appearance.

Cupping of the optic disk is the characteristic feature of glaucomatous optic atrophy (Figs. 7–2, 7–3). There is posterior bowing and distortion of the collagenous lamina cribrosa and loss of nerve tissue anterior to the lamina. The pia and pial septa and the subarachnoid space are widened. Schnabel's cavernous optic atrophy occasionally occurs in eyes with severe glaucoma. Clear cavernous spaces filled with hyaluronic acid are found in the retrolaminar part of the nerve (see Figs. 14–14, 14–15).

Focal areas of scleral thinning may develop in eyes with chronically elevated intraocular pressure. These scleral ectasias are called staphylomas if they are lined by uveal tissue (*staphylo* and *uva* mean grape in Greek and Latin, respectively). Corneal changes found in eyes with chronic glaucoma include calcific band keratopathy, vascularization, corneal edema, bullous keratopathy, and degenerative pannus formation. Chronically edematous corneas are at risk for infection. Perforation of corneal ulcers in hypertensive eyes can cause spontaneous expulsive choroidal hemorrhage.

## References

**General Reference**

Spencer WH: Glaucoma. In Spencer W (ed) Ophthalmic Pathology: An Atlas and Textbook. 4th ed. Vol 1. Philadelphia: Saunders, 1996:438–512.

Yanoff M, Fine BS: Ocular Pathology: A Text and Atlas, 2nd ed. Philadelphia, Harper & Row, 1982.

**Optic Nerve Damage**

Anderson DR: Glaucoma: the damage caused by pressure: XLVI Edward Jackson memorial lecture. Am J Ophthalmol 108:485–495, 1989.

Kerrigan LA, Zack DJ, Quigley HA, et al: TUNEL-positive ganglion cells in human primary open-angle glaucoma. Arch Ophthalmol 115:1031–1035, 1997.

Quigley HA, Addicks EM, Green WR: Optic nerve damage in human glaucoma. III. Quantitative correlation of nerve fiber loss and visual field defect in glaucoma, ischemic neuropathy, papilledema, and toxic neuropathy. Arch Ophthalmol 100:135–146, 1982.

Quigley HA, Addicks EM, Green WR, Maumenee AE: Optic nerve damage in human glaucoma. II. The site of injury and susceptibility to damage. Arch Ophthalmol 99: 635–649, 1981.

Quigley HA, Green WR: The histology of human glaucoma and nerve damage: clinicopathologic correlation in 21 eyes. Ophthalmology 86:1803–1827, 1979.

Quigley HA, Brown A, Dorman-Pease ME: Alterations in elastin in the optic nerve in human and experimental glaucoma. Br J Ophthalmol 75:552–557, 1991.

Tripathi RC, Tripathi BJ: Functional anatomy of the anterior chamber angle. In Jakobiec FA (ed) Ocular Anatomy, Embryology and Teratology. Philadelphia: Harper & Row, 1982:197–284.

**Developmental Glaucoma**

Anderson DR: The development of the trabecular meshwork and its abnormality in primary infantile glaucoma. Trans Am Ophthalmol Soc 79:458–485,1981.

Boniuk M: Glaucoma in the congenital rubella syndrome. Int Ophthalmol Clin 12:121–136, 1972.

Broughton WL, Fine B, Zimmerman LE: A histologic study of congenital glaucoma associated with a chromosome defect. Arch Ophthalmol 99:481–486, 1981.

Curtin VT, Joyce EE, Ballin N: Ocular pathology in the oculo-cerebro-renal syndrome of Lowe. Am J Ophthalmol 64(Part II):533–543, 1967.

François J, Hanssens M: Syndrome oculo-cerebro-renal de Lowe: examen histopathogique oculaire. Bull Soc Belge Ophtalmol 135:412–431, 1963.

Furuyoshi N, Furuyoshi M, Futa R, Gottanka J, Lutjen-Drecoll E: Ultrastructural changes in the trabecular meshwork of juvenile glaucoma. Ophthalmologica 211:140–146, 1997.

Grant WM, Walton DS: Distinctive gonioscopic findings in glaucoma due to neurofibromatosis. Arch Ophthalmol 79: 127–134, 1968.

Grant WM, Walton DS: Progressive changes in the angle in congenital aniridia, with development of glaucoma. Trans Am Ophthalmol Soc 72:207–228, 1974.

Honig MA, Barraquer J, Perry HD, Riquelme JL, Green WR: Forceps and vacuum injuries to the cornea: histopathologic features of twelve cases and review of the literature. Cornea 15:463–472, 1996.

Lichter PR: Genetic clues to glaucoma's secrets: the L. Edward Jackson memorial lecture. Part 2. Am J Ophthalmol 117:706–727, 1994.

Maul E, Strozzi L, Munro C, et al: The outflow pathway in congenital glaucoma. Am J Ophthalmol 89:667–675, 1980.

Maumenee AE: The pathogenesis of congenital glaucoma: a new theory. Trans Am Ophthalmol Soc 56:507–570, 1958.

Phelps CD: The pathogenesis of glaucoma in Sturge-Weber syndrome. Trans Am Acad Ophthalmol Otolaryngol 85: 276–286, 1978.

Sarfarazi M: Recent advances in molecular genetics of glaucomas. Hum Mol Genet 6:1667–1677, 1997.

Shaffer RN: Pathogenesis of congenital glaucoma: gonioscopic and microscopic anatomy. Trans Am Acad Ophthalmol Otolaryngol 59:297–300, 1955.

Shields B: Axenfeld-Rieger syndrome: a theory of mechanism and distinctions from the iridocorneal endothelial syndrome. Trans Am Ophthalmol Soc 81:736–784, 1983.

Stoilova D, Child A, Brice G, Crick RP, Fleck BW, Sarfarazi M: Identification of a new "TIGR" mutation in a family with juvenile-onset primary open angle glaucoma. Ophthalmic Genet 18:109–118, 1997.

Traboulsi E, Maumenee IH: Peters' anomaly and associated congenital malformations. Arch Ophthalmol 110: 1739–1742, 1992.

Wiggs JL, Del Bono EA, Schuman JS, Hutchinson BT, Walton DS: Clinical features of five pedigrees genetically linked to the juvenile glaucoma locus on chromosome 1q21-q31. Ophthalmology 102:1782–1789, 1995.

**Primary Open Angle Glaucoma**

Alvarado JA, Murphy CG: Outflow obstruction in pigmentary and primary open angle glaucoma. Arch Ophthalmol 110:1769–1778, 1992.

Alvarado JA, Murphy CG, Juster R: Trabecular meshwork cellularity in primary open-angle glaucoma and nonglaucomatous normals. Ophthalmology 91:564–579, 1984.

Alvarado J, Murphy C, Polansky J, Juster R: Age-related changes in trabecular meshwork cellularity. Invest Ophthalmol Vis Sci 21:714–727, 1981.

Alvarado JA, Yun AJ, Murphy CG: Juxtacanalicular tissue in primary open angle glaucoma and in nonglaucomatous normals. Arch Ophthalmol 104:1517–1528, 1986.

Murphy CG, Johnson M, Alvarado JA: Juxtacanalicular tissue in pigmentary and open angle glaucoma: the hydrodynamic role of pigment and other constituents. Arch Ophthalmol 110:1779–1785, 1992.

**Neovascular Glaucoma**

Aiello LP, Avery RL, Arrigg PG, et al: Vascular endothelial growth factor in ocular fluid of patients with diabetic retinopathy and other retinal disorders N Engl J Med 331: 1519–1520, 1994.

Colosi NJ, Yanoff M: Reactive corneal endothelialization. Am J Ophthalmol 83:219–224, 1977.

Eagle RC Jr: The ocular pathology of diabetes mellitus. In Year Book of Ophthalmology. St. Louis: Mosby-Year Book, 1995:357–364.

John TJ, Sassani JW, Eagle RC Jr: The myofibroblastic component of rubeosis iridis. Ophthalmology 90:721–728, 1983.

Madsen PH: Rubeosis of the iris and hemorrhagic glaucoma in patients with proliferative diabetic retinopathy. Br J Ophthalmol 55:368–371, 1971.

**Iridocorneal Endothelial (ICE) Syndrome**

Alvarado JA, Murphy CG, Juster RP, et al: Pathogenesis of Chandler's syndrome, essential iris atrophy and the Cogan-Reese syndrome. II. Estimated age at disease onset. Invest Ophthalmol Vis Sci 27:873, 1986.

Alvarado JA, Underwood JL, Green WR, et al: Detection of herpes virus simplex viral DNA in the iridocorneal endothelial syndrome. Arch Ophthalmol 112:1601, 1994.

Bourne W, Brubaker R: Decreased endothelial permeability in the iridocorneal endothelial syndrome. Ophthalmology 89:591, 1982.

Bourne WM, Brubaker RF: Progression and regression of partial corneal involvement in the iridocorneal endothelial syndrome. Am J Ophthalmol 114:171, 1992.

Campbell DG, Shields BM, Smith TR: The corneal endothelium and the spectrum of essential iris atrophy. Am J Ophthalmol 86:317–324, 1978.

Chandler P: Atrophy of the stroma of the iris, endothelial dystrophy, corneal edema and glaucoma. Am J Ophthalmol 41:607, 1956.

Cogan D, Reese A: A syndrome of iris nodules, ectopic Descemet's membrane and unilateral glaucoma. Doc Ophthalmol 26:424, 1969.

Eagle RJ, Font R, Yanoff M, Fine B: The iris naevus (Cogan-Reese) syndrome: light and electron microscopic observations. Br J Ophthalmol 64:446, 1980.

Eagle RJ, Font RL, Yanoff M, Fine BS: Proliferative endotheliopathy with iris abnormalities: the iridocorneal endothelial syndrome. Arch Ophthalmol 97:2104–2111, 1979.

Eagle RJ, Shields J: Iridocorneal endothelial syndrome with contralateral guttate endothelial dystrophy. Ophthalmology 94:862, 1987.

Hirst L, Quigley H, Stark W, et al: Specular microscopy of iridocorneal endothelial syndrome. Am J Ophthalmol 89: 11, 1980.

Hirst LW, Bancroft J, Yamauchi K, et al: Immunohistochemical pathology of the corneal endothelium in iridocorneal endothelial syndrome. Invest Ophthalmol Vis Sci 36:820, 1995.

Kramer TR, Grossniklaus HE, Vigneswaran N, et al: Cytokeratin expression in corneal endothelium in the iridocorneal endothelial syndrome. Invest Ophthalmol Vis Sci 33:3581, 1992.

Lee WR, Marshall GE, Kirkness CM: Corneal endothelial cell abnormalities in an early stage of the iridocorneal endothelial syndrome. Br J Ophthalmol 78:624, 1994.

Levy SG, McCartney AC, Baghai MH, et al: Pathology of the iridocorneal-endothelial syndrome: the ICE-cell. Invest Ophthalmol Vis Sci 36:2592, 1995.

Neubauer L, Lund O, Leibowitz H: Specular microscopic appearance of the corneal endothelium in the iridocornal endothelial syndrome. Arch Ophthalmol 101:916, 1983.

Scheie H, Yanoff M: Iris nevus (Cogan-Reese) syndrome: a cause of unilateral glaucoma. Arch Ophthalmol 93:963, 1975.

Shields M: Progressive essential iris atrophy, Chandler's syndrome, and the iris nevus (Cogan-Reese) syndrome: a spectrum of disease. Surv Ophthalmol 24:3, 1979.

Shields M, Campbell D, Simmons R: The essential iris atrophies. Am J Ophthalmol 85:749, 1978.

Yanoff M: Iridocorneal endothelial syndrome: unification of a disease spectrum. Surv Ophthalmol 24:1, 1979.

**Phacolytic Glaucoma**

Flocks M, Littwin CS, Zimmerman LE: Phacolytic glaucoma: a clinicopathologic study of 138 cases of glaucoma associated with hypermature cataract. Am J Ophthalmol 54:37–45, 1955.

Rosenbaum JT, Samples JR, Seymour B, Langlois L, David L: Chemotactic activity of lens proteins and the pathogenesis of phacolytic glaucoma. Arch Ophthalmol 105:1582–1584, 1987.

Smith ME, Zimmerman LE: Contusive angle recession in phacolytic glaucoma. Arch Ophthalmol 74:799–804, 1965.

Volcker HE, Naumann G: Clinical findings in phakolytic glaucoma. Klin Monatsbl Augenheilkd 166:613–618, 1975.

Yanoff M, Scheie HG: Cytology of human lens aspirate: its relationship to phacolytic glaucoma and phacoanaphylactic endophthalmitis. Arch Ophthalmol 80:166–170, 1968.

**Pigmentary Glaucoma**

Campbell DG: Pigmentary dispersion and glaucoma: a new theory. Arch Ophthalmol 97:1667–1672, 1979.

Farrar SM, Shields MB: Current concepts in pigmentary glaucoma. Surv Ophthalmol 37:233–252, 1993.

Fine B, Yanoff M, Scheie H: Pigmentary "glaucoma": a histologic study. Trans Am Acad Ophthalmol Otolaryngol 78:314, 1978.

Potash S, Tello C, Liebmann J, et al: Ultrasound biomicroscopy in pigment dispersion syndrome. Ophthalmology 101:332, 1994.

**Pseudoexfoliation**

Schlotzer-Schrehardt U, Koca M, Naumann G, et al: Pseudoexfoliation syndrome: ocular manifestation of a systemic disorder? Arch Ophthalmol 110:1752, 1992.

Schlotzer-Schrehardt U, Naumann GO: Trabecular meshwork in pseudoexfoliation syndrome with and without open-angle glaucoma: a morphometric, ultrastructural study. Invest Ophthalmol Vis Sci 36:1750–64, 1995.

Streeten BW, Dark AJ: Pseudoexfoliation syndrome. In Garner A, Klintworth GK (eds) Pathobiology of Ocular Disease: A Dynamic Approach. 2nd ed. Part A. New York: Marcel Dekker, 1994:591–629.

Streeten BW, Li Zy, Wallace RN, Eagle RC, Keshgegian AA: Pseudoexfoliative fibrillopathy in visceral organs of a patient with pseudoexfoliation syndrome. Arch Ophthalmol 110:1757–1762, 1992.

**Other Secondary Glaucomas**

Campbell DG: Ghost cell glaucoma following trauma. Ophthalmology 88:1151–1158, 1981.

Campbell DG, Simmons RJ, Grant WM: Ghost cells as a cause of glaucoma. Am J Ophthalmol 81:441–450, 1976.

Fenton RH, Zimmerman LE: Hemolytic glaucoma: an unusual case of acute, open-angle secondary glaucoma. Arch Ophthalmol 70:236–239, 1963.

Lichter PR, Shaffer RN: Interstitial keratitis and glaucoma. Am J Ophthalmol 68:241–248, 1969.

Matsuo T: Photoreceptor outer segments in aqueous humor: key to understanding a new syndrome. Surv Ophthalmol 39:211–233, 1994.

**Tumors and Glaucoma**

Fineman MS, Eagle RC Jr, Shields JA, Shields CL, De Potter P: Melanocytomalytic glaucoma in eyes with necrotic iris melanocytoma. Ophthalmology 105:492–496, 1998.

Shields CL, Shields JA, Shields MB, Augsburger JJ: Prevalence and mechanisms of secondary intraocular pressure elevation in eyes with intraocular tumors. Ophthalmology 94:839–846, 1987.

Teekhasaenee C, Ritch R, Rutnin U, et al: Glaucoma in oculodermal melanocytosis. Ophthalmology 97:562–570, 1990.

Yanoff M, Scheie HG: Melanomalytic glaucoma. Arch Ophthalmol 84:471–473, 1970.

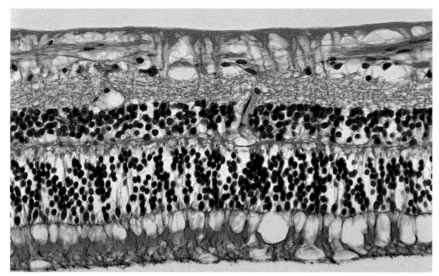

FIGURE 7–1 • **Glaucomatous retinal atrophy.** The ganglion cell and nerve fiber layers of the retina are atrophic. The inner plexiform and inner nuclear layers are well preserved excluding inner ischemic retinal atrophy. Hematoxylin-eosin, ×100.

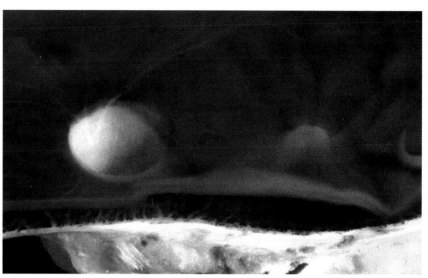

FIGURE 7–2 • **Glaucomatous optic atrophy.** The disk is pale and deeply cupped. Yellow macular pigment is seen temporally.

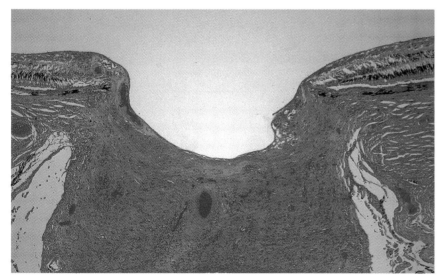

FIGURE 7–3 • **Glaucomatous optic atrophy.** The nerve head is massively cupped, and the lamina cribrosa is bowed posteriorly. The nerve fiber layer of the retina is markedly atrophic. Hematoxylin-eosin, ×10.

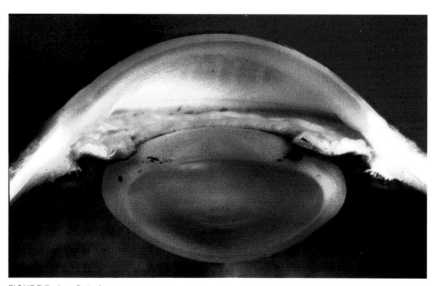

FIGURE 7–4 • **Anterior segment.** The anterior chamber is deep, and the angle is open. The pupil is widely dilated.

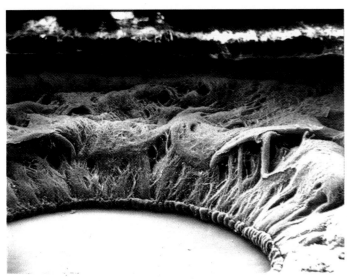

FIGURE 7–5 • **Anterior chamber.** Electronic charging artifact highlights the trabecular meshwork in the periphery of the anterior chamber of this scanning electron micrograph. Crypts of Fuchs pock folded anterior iridic surface. Beaded pigment ruff surrounds the pupil. ×20.

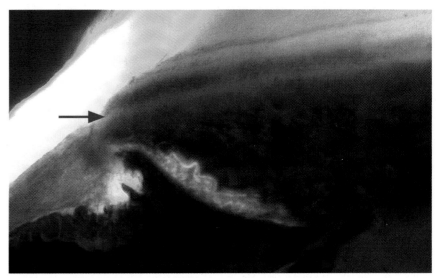

FIGURE 7–6 • **Anterior chamber angle.** Trabecular meshwork is the pigmented band directly in front of the lighter scleral spur, which is marked by an arrow.

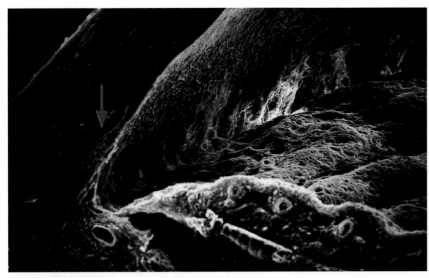

FIGURE 7–7 • **Anterior chamber angle.** Arrow points to the canal of Schlemm in the outer wall of the iridocorneal angle external to the trabecular meshwork. Trabecular beams comprising meshwork are evident in this scanning electron micrograph. The large vessel near iris root is the greater arterial circle of the iris.

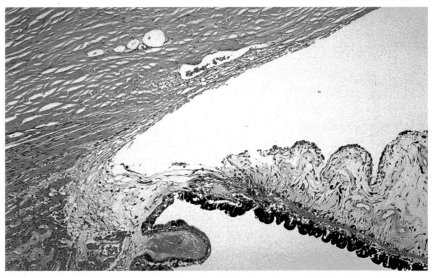

FIGURE 7–8 • **Normal anterior chamber angle.** The trabecular meshwork and canal of Schlemm are nestled in the anterior crotch of the scleral spur. The longitudinal ciliary muscle inserts onto the posterior aspect of the spur. Contraction furrows impart a scalloped configuration to the anterior surface of a lightly pigmented iris. Hematoxylin-eosin, × 25.

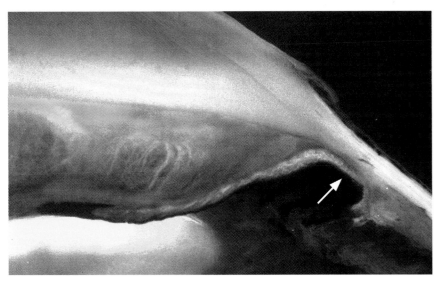

FIGURE 7–9 • **Peripheral anterior synechia.** Arrow points to an area where the peripheral iris adheres to the trabecular meshwork and posterior cornea. The anterior iridic surface is flattened by a subtle neovascular membrane.

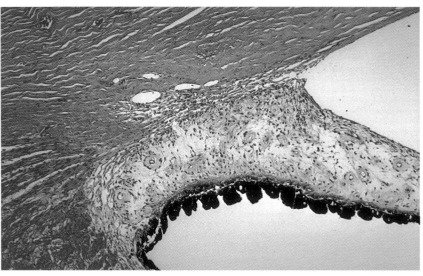

FIGURE 7–10 • **Peripheral anterior synechia.** The peripheral iris adheres to the inner surface of the trabecular meshwork, blocking the outflow of aqueous humor. A neovascular membrane flattens the anterior iridic surface. Hematoxylin-eosin, ×25.

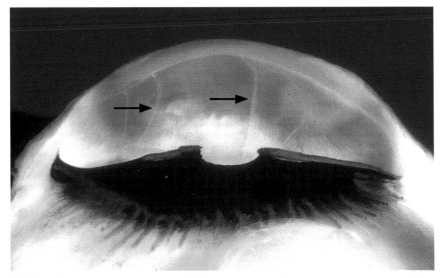

FIGURE 7–11 • **Congenital glaucoma.** Ridges on the back of the cornea (arrows) are healed ruptures in Descemet's membrane (Haab's striae). The cornea is large, the anterior chamber is deep, and the limbal tissues are somewhat ectatic. Depigmentation of the ciliary body was caused by a prior cyclodestructive procedure.

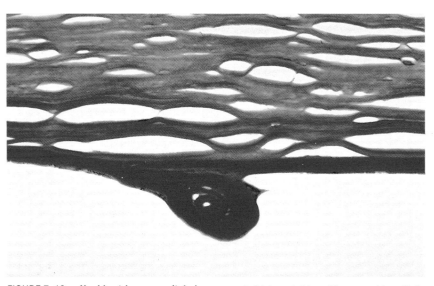

FIGURE 7–12 • **Haab's stria, congenital glaucoma.** A thickened ridge of hypertrophic coiled Descemet's membrane has formed at the site of a rupture caused by corneal enlargement. Intrinsically elastic, Descemet's membrane often coils up when lacerated or ruptured. Periodic acid-Schiff, ×100.

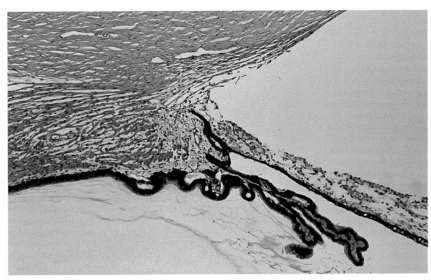

FIGURE 7–13 • **Fetal angle configuration, infant eye.** The iris root and ciliary processes insert anteriorly. Mesenchymal tissue covers the poorly formed scleral spur, and the ciliary muscle fibers are continuous with the trabecular beams. Hematoxylin-eosin, ×25.

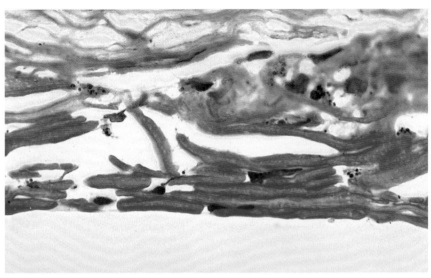

FIGURE 7–14 • **Trabecular meshwork, primary open angle glaucoma.** Trabeculectomy specimen from a patient with primary open-angle glaucoma shows decreased cellularity of the trabecular endothelium and fusion of beams in the inner meshwork. These changes may be artifactitious. Periodic acid-Schiff, ×250.

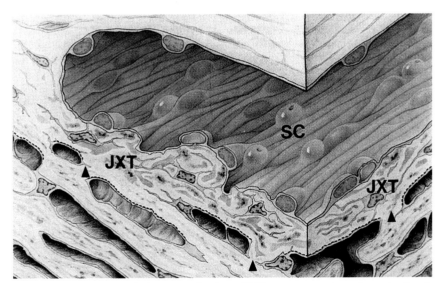

FIGURE 7–15 • **Juxtacanalicular connective tissue (JCT).** Aqueous outflow obstruction in primary open-angle glaucoma probably resides in the JCT, which borders the inner wall of Schlemm's canal. Alvarado has shown that the area of the trabecular cul-de-sacs is markedly reduced in primary open-angle glaucoma. These trabecular cul-de-sacs, which abut the JCT, are responsible for a major proportion of normal outflow resistance. (From Alvarado JA, Murphy CG: Outflow obstruction in pigmentary and primary open angle glaucoma. *Arch Ophthalmol* 110:1769–1778, 1992. Copyright 1992 American Medical Association)

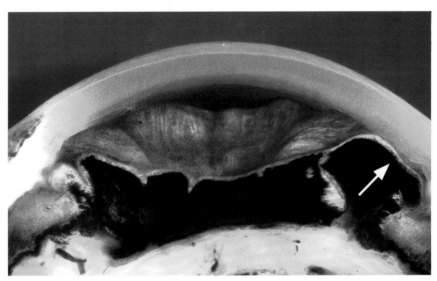

FIGURE 7–16 • **Iris bombé.** Funnel configuration of the iris reflects pupillary seclusion by posterior synechias. The arrow points to a broad peripheral anterior synechia caused by pupillary block.

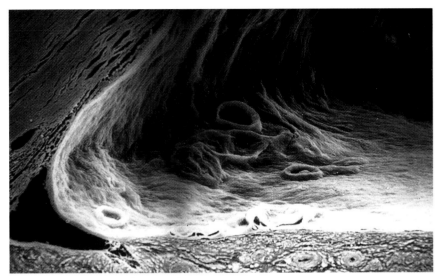

FIGURE 7–17 • **Epithelial downgrowth.** Sheet of surface epithelium introduced by trauma covers the posterior cornea, trabecular meshwork, and iris. The epithelial membrane flattens the anterior surface of the iris. Scanning electron micrograph.

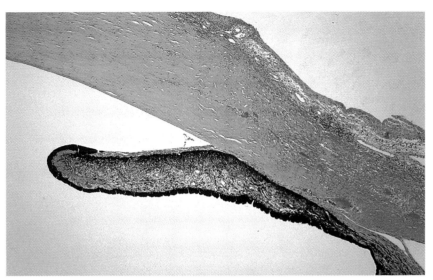

FIGURE 7–18 • **Neovascular glaucoma.** A broad peripheral anterior synechia is present. The free surface of the iris is flattened by a florid neovascular membrane, which is causing ectropion of the iris pigment epithelium and sphincter muscle. Hematoxylin-eosin, ×10.

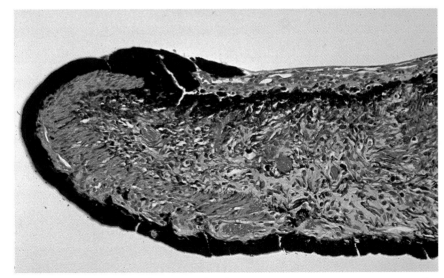

FIGURE 7–19 • **Ectropion iridis, neovascular glaucoma.** A florid fibrovascular membrane flattens the pigmented anterior border layer of the iris, which is normally an avascular site. Traction has pulled the iris pigment epithelium and sphincter muscle onto the front of the iris. Hematoxylin-eosin, ×50.

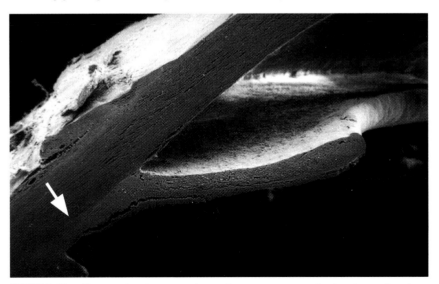

FIGURE 7–20 • **Neovascular glaucoma.** Arrow denotes a compressed trabecular meshwork deep to a broad peripheral anterior synechia in an eye with neovascular glaucoma secondary to central retinal vein occlusion. The anterior surface of the iris is flattened. Scanning electron micrograph, ×20. (From John T, Sassani JW, Eagle RC: The myofibroblastic component of rubeosis iridis. *Ophthalmology* 90:721–728, 1983. Courtesy of *Ophthalmology*)

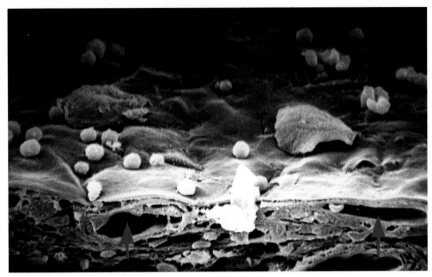

FIGURE 7–21 • **Iris neovascularization.** Arrows point to new vessels on the iris underneath the surface sheet of myofibroblasts. Scanning electron micrograph, ×640. (From John T, Sassani JW, Eagle RC: The myofibroblastic component of rubeosis iridis. *Ophthalmology* 90:721–728, 1983. Courtesy of *Ophthalmology*)

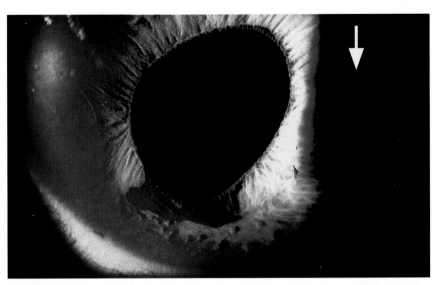

FIGURE 7–22 • **Essential iris atrophy.** Distorted pupil is drawn toward a synechia in the inferior angle. Arrow points to a full-thickness iris hole. Multiple iris nodules are seen in the flattened endothelialized zone of iris bordering the synechia and ectropion iridis. (From Eagle RC Jr: Congenital, developmental and degenerative disorders of the iris and ciliary body. In: Albert DM, Jakobiec FA, eds. *Principles and Practice of Ophthalmology. Clinical Practice.* Vol 1. Philadelphia: Saunders, 1993:367–389)

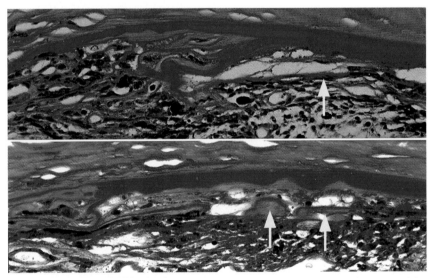

FIGURE 7–23 • **Essential iris atrophy.** Arrows point to ectopic basement membrane material on the iris surface in an area of initial synechial closure. Periodic acid-Schiff, ×100.

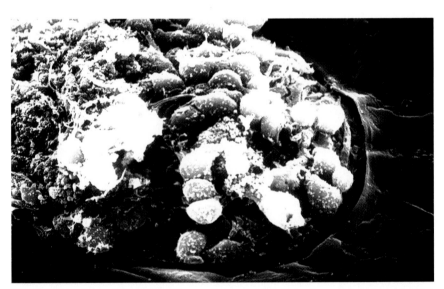

FIGURE 7–24 • **Iris nodule, ICE syndrome.** Sheet of endothelial cells encircles a knuckle of iris stromal melanocytes forming iris nodule. Scanning electron micrograph, ×1216. (From Eagle RC, Font RL, Yanoff M, Fine BS: The iris nevus (Cogan Reese) syndrome: light and electron microscopic observations. *Br J Ophthalmol* 64:446–452, 1980)

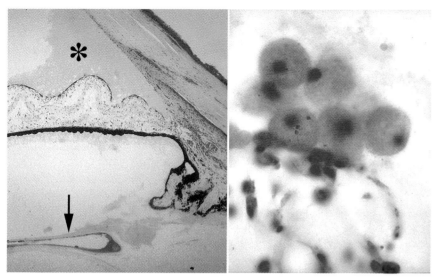

**FIGURE 7–25** • **Phacolytic glaucoma.** Asterisk labels the lens protein-rich fluid in the open angle. Arrow points to the empty lens capsule. Postcontusion angle recession is present. An aggregate of macrophages laden with lens material is seen on the anterior iridic surface (*right*). Hematoxylin-eosin. Left ×10, right ×250.

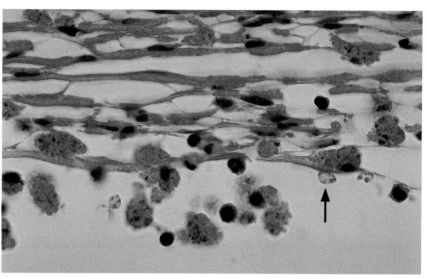

**FIGURE 7–26** • **Hemolytic glaucoma.** Macrophages that have ingested hemosiderin and erythrocyte ghost cells (arrow) infiltrate the trabecular meshwork. Hematoxylin-eosin, ×100.

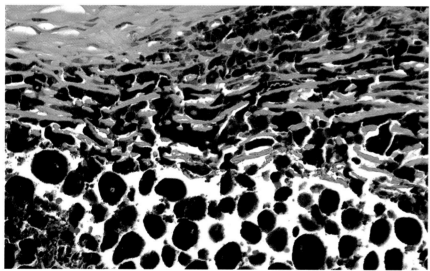

**FIGURE 7–27** • **Melanocytomalytic glaucoma.** Macrophages laden with melanin pigment dispersed by necrotic melanocytoma fill the peripheral anterior chamber and infiltrate the trabecular meshwork. Hematoxylin-eosin, ×100.

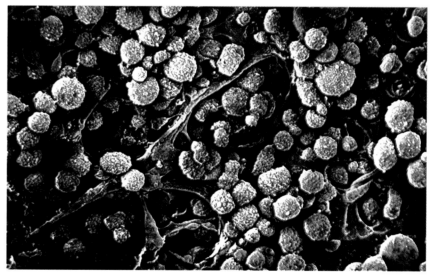

**FIGURE 7–28** • **Melanocytomalytic glaucoma.** False-colorized scanning electron micrograph graphically depicts melanophages obstructing the trabecular meshwork. ×160. (From Fineman MS, Eagle RC Jr, Shields JA, Shields CL, De Potter P: Melanocytomalytic glaucoma in eyes with necrotic iris melanocytoma. *Ophthalmology* 105:492–496, 1998. Courtesy of *Ophthalmology*)

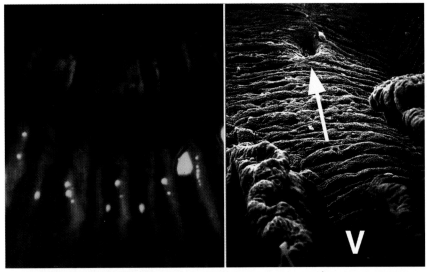

FIGURE 7–29 • **Pigmentary glaucoma.** Depigmented foci on the posterior surface of the iris correspond to erosions in the iris pigment epithelium (arrow), probably caused by zonular bundles, which pass through valleys between ciliary processes (V). Left: macrophotograph; right: false-colorized scanning electron micrograph. (Macrophotograph courtesy of Dr. Myron Yanoff)

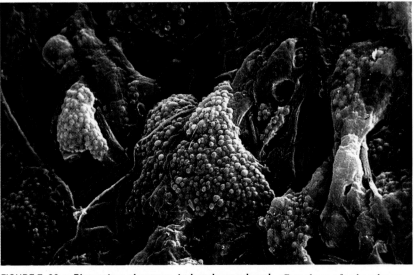

FIGURE 7–30 • **Pigmentary glaucoma, trabecular meshwork.** Cytoplasm of trabecular endothelial cells is replete with large, round to oval granules of iris pigment epithelial melanin. False-colorized scanning electron micrograph, ×1250.

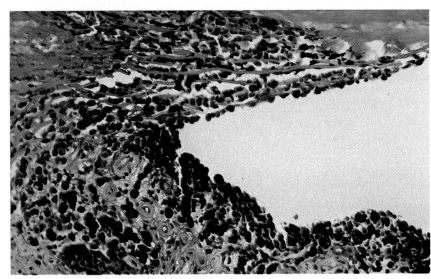

FIGURE 7–31 • **Glaucoma caused by mixed cell iris melanoma.** Melanoma cells blanket the anterior iris and infiltrate the trabecular meshwork. Patient presented with unilateral glaucoma and iris heterochromia. Hematoxylin-eosin, ×25.

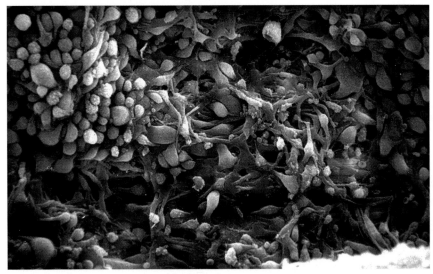

FIGURE 7–32 • **Melanoma cells infiltrating the trabecular meshwork.** Patient had unilateral glaucoma. Round or oval cells are epithelioid melanoma cells. Bipolar spindle cells also are present. Scanning electron micrograph, ×160.

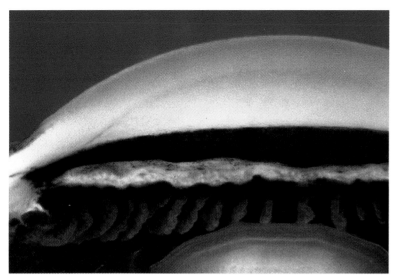

FIGURE 7–33 • **Ring melanoma.** Heavily pigmented tumor has grown circumferentially around the angle, obstructing the trabecular meshwork.

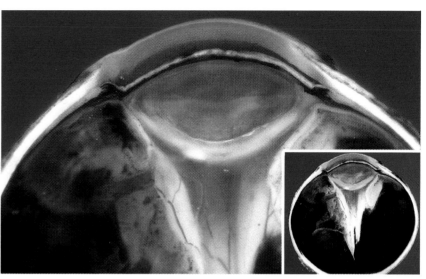

FIGURE 7–34 • **Secondary closed-angle glaucoma, choroidal melanoma.** Anterior displacement of the lens–iris diaphragm has caused secondary closed-angle glaucoma. *Inset:* Large posterior choroidal melanoma and total retinal detachment.

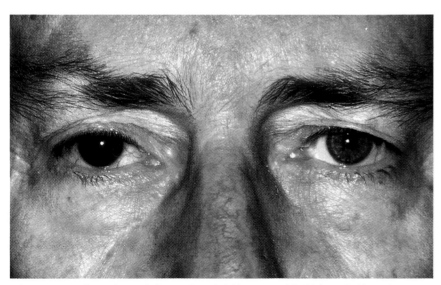

FIGURE 7–35 • **Hyperchromatic heterochromia iridum caused by high-grade iris melanoma.** Patient had uncontrolled unilateral glaucoma.

# CHAPTER 8

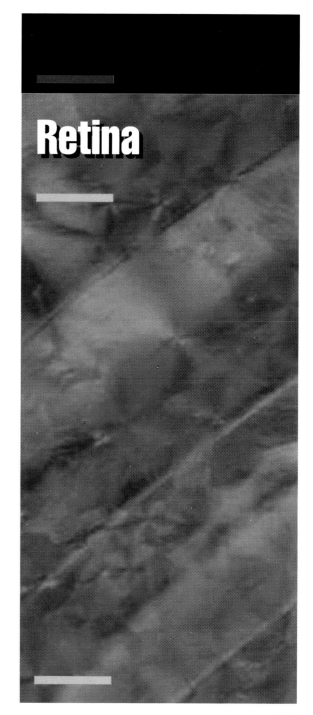

**Retina**

An outpost of the central nervous system (CNS), the retina is a colony of brain cells located in the periphery of the body where it is able to interact with and detect the rather narrow spectrum of electromagnetic radiation called visible light. Death, destruction, or loss of all or part of the retina renders the eye sightless. Visual loss due to the death of retinal cells is permanent and irrevocable because, like brain cells, the cells of the retina are incapable of repair or regeneration.

## RETINAL ANATOMY

The retina is a highly cellular tissue composed of cells arranged in regular layers (Fig. 8–1). Ten retinal layers, including the retinal pigment epithelium, are identified. It is relatively easy to remember the microscopic anatomy of the retina if one recalls that the retina essentially is comprised of three types of cells: photoreceptors and first- and second-order neurons. Regarding orientation, the term *inner* refers to the portion of the retina that is located toward the vitreous cavity or the center of the eye. *Outer* denotes layers that are found closer to the sclera. Cell nuclei are arranged in distinct bands called nuclear layers. The nuclei of the photoreceptors and first order neurons (bipolar cells) form the outer and inner nuclear layers, respectively. The retinal ganglion cells (the second order neurons) make up another layer in the inner retina that varies markedly in thickness. Surrounding the fovea, the ganglion cell layer (GCL) is five or more cells thick. (Multilamination of the GCL is an excellent histologic marker for the macula.) The ganglion cell layer thins rapidly in the more peripheral parts of the retina. A discontinuous monolayer of ganglion cells is present peripheral to the vascular arcades formed by the superior and inferior temporal retinal arterioles.

The retina's plexiform layers are composed of axons and dendrites. The outer plexiform layer (OPL) is interposed between the outer and inner nuclear layers, and the inner plexiform layer separates the inner nuclear layer from the ganglion cell layer. The inner plexiform layer is truly plexiform: Its whole breadth is comprised of an intricately interweaving tangle of ramifying neuronal processes. In contrast, only a narrow inner band of the outer plexiform layer is truly plexiform. Its wider outer part is comprised of an orderly parallel array of photoreceptor axons called Henle's fibers. Although Henle's fibers occur throughout the retina, the eponym generally is applied to the radially oriented photoreceptor axons surrounding the fovea. A line of synaptic connections comprised of cone pedicles, rod spherules, and the dendrites of bipolar cells delimits the outer border of the truly plexiform part of the OPL. This linear row of synapses is often evident light microscopically as the middle limiting membrane (MLM). Like the external limiting membrane, the MLM is not a basement membrane. (The only true basement membrane of the retina is the internal limiting membrane, or ILM.) The MLM delimits the vascularized inner part of the retina; capillaries from the central retinal artery penetrate no deeper than the MLM. External to the MLM, the retina is avascular and depends on the choroidal circulation for oxygen and nutrients. The OPL is a watershed zone between the dual vascular supplies of the retina. This factor contributes to the localization of edema fluid and hard exudates in the OPL.

The inner nuclear layer (INL) contains the nuclei of bipolar, amacrine, horizontal, and Müller cells. Bipolar cells predominate. The horizontal cell nuclei are found in the outer part of the INL and the amacrine cell nuclei in the inner part. The nuclei of the Müller cells can lie at any level of the INL. Accessory glial cells, including fibrous and protoplasmic astrocytes and oligodendrocyte-like cells, are confined to the nerve fiber, ganglion cell, and inner plexiform layers of the retina. Hence gliosis does not occur after retinal arterial occlusion because these cells are killed.

The ILM, which lines the inner surface of the retina, is a true basement membrane synthesized by the basal foot processes of retinal Müller cells. Müller cells are giant glial cells that span the entire thickness of the retina. Intricately interweaving processes of the Müller cells totally fill the interstices between the retinal neurons and serve to segregate their receptive surfaces. There is little or no extracellular space in the retina. The Müller cells are polarized. Electron microscopy discloses microvilli on their apical surfaces, which project into the subretinal space between the photoreceptors. A band of intercellular junctions called the external limiting membrane (XLM) is found in the outer, or apical, part of the neurosensory retina. The XLM is not a true basement membrane; it is composed of permeable adherent junctions (zonulae adherentes) joining the apical part of adjacent Müller cells and photoreceptors. The XLM does not form a barrier to macromolecules because these junctions lack the occluding portion found in the terminal bars of cells such as the retinal pigment epithelium. The XLM has been called the fenestrated membrane of Verhoeff. The inner and outer segments of the rods and cones project through this fenestrated membrane into the subretinal space, where they are encompassed by extracellular matrix material rich in hyaluronidase-resistant acid mucopolysaccharide. Cone cell nuclei are located next to the XLM in the outer nuclear layer.

Rod and cone cells are distinguished light microscopically by the shape of their inner segments. The inner segments of rods are slender rod-like cylinders, whereas extrafoveal cones are conical in shape. Highly specialized cones that resemble rods are densely packed in the cone-rich fovea. The photoreceptor inner segments are packed with mitochondria that provide the energy for the photochemistry of vision.

The inner and outer segments of the photoreceptors are joined by connecting cilia. (Cilia are often found on the apical surface of cells, and photoreceptor outer segments may be highly modified apical cilia.) The photochemistry of vision takes place in the outer segments of the photoreceptors, which contain stacks of narrow cytoplasmic disks encompassed by cell membranes. The stacks of disks are often likened to stacks of coins. Visual pigments such as rhodopsin are incorporated as transmembrane proteins in the disk membranes. Separate disks occur in rods; cone outer segments contain a continuous membrane that is sinuously folded upon itself like "ribbon candy."

The tips of the outer segments abut the apical surface of the retinal pigment epithelium (RPE) (Fig. 8–2). The RPE is a polarized cellular monolayer that is derived embryologically from the outer layer of the neuroectodermal optic cup. Myriad microvilli and cellular processes containing large ellipsoidal granules of melanin project from the surface of the RPE cells and embrace the tips of the outer segments. The RPE cells are firmly joined near their apices by a girdle of intercellular connections called zonulae occludentes. These tight junctions form a barrier to the passage of molecules and constitute the outer part of the blood–retinal barrier. Large ellipsoidal, or football-shaped, granules of melanin pigment measuring approximately 1 $\mu$m in diameter are also found in the apical cytoplasm of the RPE cells. The basal cytoplasm of the RPE cell contains granules of lipofuscin pigment derived from the incomplete digestion of worn-out outer segment tips, which are regularly phagocytized by the RPE. This autofluorescent "wear and tear" pigment accumulates with age.

The RPE rests on a specialized layer of connective tissue called Bruch's membrane, which delimits the inner surface of the choroid. Bruch's membrane separates the RPE from the large fenestrated capillaries of the choriocapillaris, which supply the avascular outer third of the retina. Bruch's membrane consists of collagen and elastic fibrils sandwiched between the basement membranes of the RPE and the choriocapillary endothelial cells. As we age, Bruch's membrane gradually thickens and becomes increasingly periodic acid-Schiff (PAS)-positive. Focal basophilic segments of calcification are often found in the elderly. Such changes are most pronounced posteriorly. Transmission electron microscopy demonstrates that the thickening of Bruch's membrane is due to the gradual accumulation of linear and vesicular structures.

## DEVELOPMENTAL ANOMALIES

Dysplasia of the retina is a characteristic manifestation of trisomy 13 and occurs also in the Walker-Warburg syndrome. Congenital nonattachment of the retina is a rare anomaly caused by faulty invagination of the optic vesicle. Congenitally detached retinas are the cause of leukocoria in male infants with X-linked Norrie's disease, who also are deaf and mentally retarded. The retina lining a choroidal coloboma may be absent, hypoplastic, or dysplastic (see Fig. 1–3).

Aplasia of the fovea occurs in aniridia and albinism. Albinos also have a lightly pigmented albinotic fundus. Tyrosinase-negative albinos lack the enzyme tyrosinase and are unable to synthesize melanin pigment. They have white hair, pink eyes, and pink irides that transilluminate readily. Tyrosinase-positive albinos are able to synthesize melanin pigment but do not package it properly. There are many varieties of tyrosinase-positive albinism. The Hermansky-Pudlak syndrome is common in Puerto Ricans who also have a bleeding diathesis and bruise easily. Parents of affected children have been wrongfully accused of child abuse. Albinos with the rare autosomal recessively inherited Chédiak-Higashi syndrome are subject to bacterial and fungal infection. They have abnormal leukocytes with giant lysosomes and macromelanosomes.

Albinism may affect the skin and eyes (oculocutaneous albinism) or only the eyes primarily (ocular albinism). Ocular albinos may present with decreased vision and nystagmus caused by foveal aplasia. Iris transillumination serves to identify ocular albinos, who have normal skin pigmentation and may have dark hair. Autosomal recessive ocular albinism is most common. Macromelanosomes are found in the RPE and skin in X-linked ocular albinism (Fig. 8–3). Skin biopsy occasionally is used to confirm the diagnosis. Although white female carriers of X-linked ocular albinism have normal vision, iris transillumination is present, and they may have patchy depigmentation of the peripheral RPE.

Focal areas of fundus pigmentation characterize congenital hypertrophy of the RPE (CHRPE) (see Fig. 10–49) and congenital grouped pigmentation of the RPE (see Fig. 10–50).

Myelinated nerve fibers occur in about 1% of the population. Myelination of optic nerve axons normally terminates at the posterior margin of the lamina cribrosa. The patches of aberrant myelination of the nerve fiber layer may or may not be contiguous with the optic disk. Myelinated nerve fibers produce a focal scotoma.

Congenital vascular abnormalities of the retina include retinal arteriovenous communication, cavernous hemangioma of the retina, Leber's miliary retinal aneurysms, Coats' disease (see Figs. 11–34, 11–35, 11–36, 11–37), parafoveal telangiectasis, and retinal capillary hemangioma (see Figs. 1–18, 1–19).

A peripheral retinal fold called Lange's fold occurs at the ora serrata in infant eyes. Lange's fold does not occur in vivo; it is a fixation artifact caused by vitreous traction.

## RETINAL HEMORRHAGES AND EXUDATES

The retinopathies that occur in a variety of systemic and ocular diseases are comprised of six types of retinal hemorrhage and two types of retinal exudate that occur in varying constellations. The clinical appearance of retinal hemorrhages is determined by the location of the blood in the retina (Fig. 8–4). Retinal hemorrhages are categorized as superficial (flame- or splinter-shaped), deep (blot and dot), sub-RPE, sub-ILM, subhyaloid, and vitreous.

Splinter- or flame-shaped hemorrhages are located superficially in the inner nerve fiber layer of the retina. The configuration and feathery margin of these hemorrhages are caused by tracking of the erythrocytes along the axons of the ganglion cells as they arch above and below the fovea. The pattern of hemorrhages can graphically highlight the arcuate distribution of the nerve fibers in patients who have numerous superficial hemorrhages (e.g., after a branch retinal vein occlusion).

Blot-and-dot hemorrhages occur in the deeper layers of the retina where the axons are oriented perpendicular to the plane of the Bruch's membrane. Here, the extravasations of blood have a discrete localized configuration because the erythrocytes are corralled, or fenced-in, by the surrounding axons.

Scaphoid, or boat-shaped, hemorrhages are preretinal hemorrhages that have a fluid level caused by the settling-out of the red blood cells. Two types of scaphoid hemorrhage are recognized histopathologically: sub-ILM and subhyaloid hemorrhages. True subhyaloid hemorrhages are common in patients with proliferative diabetic retinopathy, in whom the blood collects between the ILM and the posterior face of the detached vitreous humor, which may be lined by a sheet of neovascularization (Fig. 8–5). The term hyaloid refers to the hyaloid body, another name for

the vitreous humor. Sub-ILM hemorrhages are hemorrhagic detachments of the ILM. The blood is located between the nerve fiber layer and the outer aspect of the ILM, the retina's single true basement membrane, which is secreted by Müller cells. Occasionally, sub-ILM hemorrhages can be distinguished by the ophthalmoscopic observation of focal relucences called Gunn's dots on their inner surface. The latter correspond to focal concavities on the outer surface of the basement membrane that conform to the foot plates of the Müller cells.

Hemorrhagic detachment of the RPE often occurs in patients who have sub-RPE neovascular membranes. Sub-RPE hemorrhage is an important stage in the evolution of disciform scars in age-related macular degeneration. Sub-RPE hemorrhages typically appear quite dark because the blood is located underneath a layer of pigmented cells. They can be confused clinically with uveal malignant melanoma. However, in contrast to melanomas, sub-RPE hemorrhages block choroidal fluorescence and appear dark during intravenous fluorescein angiography.

Vitreous hemorrhage occurs when blood breaks through the hyaloid membrane into the substance of the formed vitreous. Blood in the formed vitreous can be persistent but gradually undergoes degeneration and assumes a characteristic yellow-ochre color. Nonresorbing vitreous hemorrhage is a common indication for vitrectomy, especially in patients with diabetes mellitus.

The retinal exudates and edema that occur in diabetes, hypertensive retinopathy, and other retinal vascular disorders reflect a breakdown in the blood–retinal barrier (Fig. 8–6). The term blood–retinal barrier refers to structural modifications that protect the retina's delicate neural tissues from fluid overload and osmotic stress. The blood–retinal barrier is analogous to the blood–brain barrier in the CNS. The inner or intraretinal part of the blood–retinal barrier is comprised of the tight junctions that link the endothelial cells that line the retinal vessels. During fluorescein angiography, these impermeable intercellular junctions confine fluorescein dye within the lumens of healthy retinal vessels. The girdle of terminal bars that join the RPE cells near their apices forms the outer part of the blood–retinal barrier. The choriocapillaris, which supplies the avascular outer third of the retina, is composed of fenestrated capillaries that leak fluorescein dye profusely. The RPE serves as the barrier that protects the outer retina from an influx of fluid.

Incompetence of either the inner or outer part of the blood–retinal barrier gives lipid- and protein-rich fluid access to the retinal parenchyma, leading to edema and exudate formation (Fig. 8–7). Hard, yellow, waxy exudates appear histopathologically as pools of eosinophilic proteinaceous fluid (Fig. 8–8). Hard exudates usually are located in the outer plexiform layer, the watershed zone between the retina's dual blood supply. In chronic cases the exudates may be phagocytized by foamy macrophages called gitter cells.

Soft exudates, or cotton wool spots (Figs. 8–9, 8–10, 8–11), are not exudates in the true sense of the word. Cotton wool spots represent focal areas in the nerve fiber layer where the normal flow of axoplasm is blocked. This focal blockage of axoplasmic flow is thought to be a response to focal retinal ischemia and probably is caused by thrombosis of a precapillary arteriole. Cotton wool spots are helpful clinical markers for retinal ischemia. They develop during the preproliferative phase of diabetic retinopathy and also are found with ischemic retinal vein occlusions and severe hypertensive retinopathy. Cotton wool spots occur in relative isolation in patients who have acquired immunodeficiency syndrome (AIDS) or collagen vascular diseases such as systemic lupus erythematosus as a manifestation of intravascular immune complex deposition.

Histopathologic examination of a cotton wool spot shows focal swelling of the nerve fiber layer and cytoid bodies (Figs. 8–10, 8–11). Cytoid bodies are segments of ganglion cell axons ballooned by stagnant axoplasm. They are called cytoid because they superficially resemble cells. They have a nucleoid comprised of aggregated organelles that mimics a cellular nucleus but is eosinophilic rather than basophilic.

## ANGIOID STREAKS

Angioid streaks are linear structures seen on ophthalmoscopy that radiate from the optic disk in an angioid, or vessel-like, fashion (Fig. 8–12). Histopathology has shown that angioid streaks correspond to breaks in Bruch's membrane (Fig. 8–13). They tend to develop in patients who have certain systemic disorders marked by massive calcification of Bruch's membrane. Such diseases include pseudoxanthoma elasticum, Paget's disease of bone, and some cases of sickle hemoglobinopathy. Calcification may impart an egg shell-like fragility to Bruch's membrane predisposing to fracture. The RPE usually is intact overlying the breaks in Bruch's membrane. Sub-RPE neovascularization can complicate angioid streaks and is a major cause of visual loss in affected patients. Unfortunately, when sub-RPE membranes develop, they generally involve the region of the macula for reasons unknown. This fact implies that the development of subretinal neovascularization requires more than a break in Bruch's membrane.

## RETINAL ARTERIAL AND ARTERIOLAR OCCLUSIONS

Interruption of the vascular supply to the inner two-thirds of the retina causes ischemic infarction and coagulative necrosis of its cells. The sequelae of a central or branch retinal artery occlusion are evident histopathologically as a pattern called inner ischemic retinal atrophy (Fig. 8–14). All of the cells nourished by capillaries derived from the central retinal artery are affected, including the nerve fiber layer (NFL) and ganglion cell layers, the inner plexiform layer (IPL), and most of the inner nuclear layer (INL). The outer part of the INL usually persists because its cells are sustained by diffusion from the choriocapillaris. In a long-standing case, the inner retinal layers are paucicellular and have a glassy, hyalinized appearance. Gliosis of the nerve fiber layer is not observed because the fibrous astrocytes and other accessory glial cells that cause NFL gliosis in chronic glaucoma perish in the retinal ictus. The additional involvement of the IPL and the inner part of the INL serve to differentiate inner ischemic retinal atrophy from glaucomatous retinal atrophy. Only the retinal ganglion cells and their axons that form the NFL and optic nerve are atrophic in glaucomatous retinal atrophy.

During the acute stages of a central retinal artery occlusion (CRAO) the retina shows edema, cellular dissolution, and nuclear fragmentation or pyknosis. The normally transparent retina is marked by milky-white opacification clinically (Figs. 8–15, 8–16). A macular cherry red spot is present because the cells comprising the floor of the foveola are normally nourished by the choriocapillaris and remain viable and transparent. Although the foveal photoreceptors persist, central vision is lost because the other cells in the neural pathway are destroyed. Retinal hemorrhages usually are not seen.

Occlusion of the central retinal artery produces a "ministroke" of the entire retina. Only part of the retina is infarcted in hemiretinal or branch retinal arteriolar occlusions (Fig. 8–17). Most branch artery occlusions are caused by emboli that lodge at the bifurcation of an arteriole.

Central retinal artery occlusion is usually a disease of elderly individuals who are often atherosclerotic, hypertensive, and diabetic. Central or branch retinal artery occlusion in a young individual suggests the possibility of a primary cardiac tumor such as a cardiac myxoma, vasculitis, or the presence of anti-cardiolipin (lupus anticoagulant) antibodies. Most CRAOs result from thrombosis or embolization. Thrombosis usually occurs within the optic nerve head and is related to atherosclerosis at this site. Atherosclerosis does not develop in retinal arterioles because those vessels lack a distinct muscularis.

About 60% of retinal emboli are glistening crystals of cholesterol called Hollenhorst plaques, and about 11% are aggregates of platelets and fibrin. Most are shed from the surface of ulcerating atherosclerotic plaques in the internal carotid artery. Calcific emboli originating in the heart are less common.

Giant cell arteritis is an important treatable condition that must be ruled out in any elderly patient who has retinal artery occlusion or ischemic optic neuropathy. The erythrocyte sedimentation rate is typically elevated in affected individuals. Expedient temporal artery biopsy is performed to confirm the diagnosis. Patients who have giant cell arteritis classically have a history of malaise, weight loss, and muscle aches (polymyalgia rheumatica); and they may complain of headache and painful mastication due to jaw claudication. Severely inflamed temporal arteries may be elevated, tender, and cord-like. Biopsy surgery may be relatively bloodless if the arteritis is severe.

An affected segment of artery appears firm, thickened, and opacified grossly. Histopathology discloses compromise or even occlusion of the vascular lumen and chronic inflammation within the thickened arterial wall (Fig. 8–18). The chronic granulomatous inflammatory infiltrate should contain epithelioid histiocytes, but giant cells are *not* particularly common in most positive biopsies and are not necessary for the diagnosis. Inflammation can affect all layers of the artery but classically is concentrated in the vicinity of the internal elastic lamina, which almost invariably shows severe dissolution and segmental loss. Fibrosis and scarring is often seen in the adventitial connective tissue. Signs of old or "healed" giant cell arteritis (e.g., in a patient who has received chronic corticosteroid therapy) include focal atrophy or destruction of the muscularis, extensive segmental destruction of the internal elastic lamina, and perivascular scarring. "Skip lesions" (uninflamed segments in a positive biopsy) do occur but are relatively rare. Hence the biopsied segment of artery should be at least 2 cm long, and bilateral biopsy should be considered if the initial biopsy is negative and clinical suspicion is high.

Prompt diagnosis of giant cell arteritis is critical because bilateral blindness can develop rapidly in untreated cases. High dose systemic corticosteroid therapy should be instituted immediately if giant cell arteritis is suspected. Temporal artery biopsy is done to confirm the diagnosis histopathologically because systemic steroids can have severe side effects in elderly patients.

## RETINAL VENOUS OCCLUSION

Occlusion of the central retinal vein (CRVO) or one of its major branches produces hemorrhagic infarction of the retina. The terms "blood and thunder fundus" or "squashed tomato sign," which have been applied clinically to this retinopathy, reflect the plethora of deep and superficial retinal hemorrhages that develop after venous occlusion (Figs. 8–19, 8–20).

Most retinal venous occlusions (70%) involve branches of the central retinal vein, typically the superotemporal branch vein. Venous occlusions tend to occur in men who are older than 50 years and have diabetes mellitus, hypertension, and arteriosclerosis. Local intraocular conditions that predispose to venous occlusion include elevated intraocular pressure, papilledema, and large drusen of the optic disk. Many CRVOs are thought to be related to arteriosclerosis of the central retinal artery, which shares a common adventitial sheath with the central retinal vein within the lamina cribrosa of the optic nerve (Fig. 8–21). The sclerotic arteriole compresses the vein within the adventitial sheath causing turbulence in the lumen of the vein, which damages the vascular endothelium and predisposes to venous thrombosis.

The early stages of a retinal venous occlusion are characterized histopathologically by diffuse and cystoid edema of the macula. The hemorrhagic retina contains numerous deep, superficial, and full-thickness retinal hemorrhages. Preretinal hemorrhages are found in some cases, and in rare instances blood extends into the subretinal space causing hemorrhagic retinal detachment. Other findings include shallow serous retinal detachment and papilledema. If severe ischemia and capillary nonperfusion are present, focal retinal necrosis and cotton wool spots are noted. The latter are an excellent clinical marker for the ischemic variant of CRVO.

In chronic retinal venous occlusive disease, the histopathology discloses disorganization of the retinal architecture and marked gliosis. The retina often contains macrophages laden with golden brown hemosiderin pigment from blood breakdown, and the retina and other epithelial structures may stain positively for iron (hemosiderosis). Inner ischemic retinal atrophy may be present if the venous occlusion was ischemic. Most eyes requiring enucleation have painful neovascular glaucoma.

Secondary closed-angle glaucoma caused by iris neovascularization (rubeosis iridis) develops in about 20% of patients who have ischemic CRVOs. Profound visual loss, cotton wool spots, and severe nonperfusion of the retinal capillary bed disclosed by fluorescein angiography are clinical signs of ischemic venous occlusion. This type of glaucoma has been called "90 day glaucoma," reflecting its fairly rapid onset.

## HYPERTENSIVE RETINOPATHY

The retinopathy that develops in patients with severe systemic hypertension is caused by vascular incompetence and breakdown of the blood–retinal barrier. Acute, severe elevation of the blood pressure causes retinal arteriolar narrowing and focal vasospasm. If blood pressure levels remain markedly elevated for long periods and vasospasm persists, the muscular and endothelial coats of the vessels eventually become necrotic. Histopathologic studies have revealed changes in the endothelial lining, necrosis of the smooth muscle, and insudation of fibrin-rich plasma in the vessel wall. The endothelial damage causes vascular incompetence with resultant retinal edema, exudation, and occasionally even serous retinal detachment. Small exudates called edema residues may form a stellate pattern around the fovea (macular star figure). This pattern of exudation is governed by the radial orientation of the photoreceptor axons (Henle fibers) in the perifoveal OPL. In the early days of ophthalmoscopy, severe hypertensive retinopathy with a macular star figure was often called hyperalbuminuric retinitis, reflecting the common association between severe hypertension and renal failure. Retinal hemorrhages and papilledema are additional manifestations of hypertensive retinopathy. Retinal hemorrhages are relatively common and occur during the early stages of the disorder. Optic disk edema marks the fourth and final stage of hypertensive retinopathy. It is an important clinical marker for malignant hypertension and potential encephalopathy and an indication for aggressive antihypertensive therapy. Fibrinoid necrosis caused by the insudation and accumulation of plasma proteins in vessel walls may affect retinal and choroidal vessels. Occlusion of small damaged vessels also occurs, causing microinfarctions of the NFL (cotton wool spots) and occasionally infarctions of larger areas of the retina. Focal choroidal infarction with pigmentary change may be evident clinically as Elschnig spots and Seegrist streaks, which were considered to be grave prognostic signs before effective antihypertensive therapy was available. Retinal macroaneurysms occasionally develop in hypertensive patients (Fig. 8–22).

## RETINAL ARTERIOSCLEROSIS

Low grade chronic hypertension induces fibrosis in the walls of retinal arterioles, a process called retinal arteriolar sclerosis (Fig. 8–23). Histopathologically, the sclerotic retinal vessels are encompassed by a thick mantle of collagenous connective tissue. The term "onion skin" often is applied to this change.

Like the surrounding neurosensory retina, the walls of healthy retinal vessels normally are transparent. What one observes ophthalmoscopically as retinal vessels are the columns of pigmented erythrocytes filling the lumina of the vessels. The progressive accumulation of connective tissue in the vessel walls of patients with retinal arteriolarsclerosis gradually obscures the blood column, widening the light reflex and imparting an orange or coppery hue to the arterioles. Eventually, if the process is prolonged and severe, perivascular fibrosis may totally hide the blood column, and the vessels appear as white lines, resembling *silver wires*. Arteriovenous crossing defects (A-V nicking) result when the opaque walls of thickened arterioles obscure part of the underlying venules. In advanced cases there may be deflection or banking of the retinal vein.

## CYSTOID MACULAR EDEMA

Cystoid macular edema (CME) is characterized by the accumulation of serous fluid in cystoid spaces in the parenchyma of the perifoveal retina (Figs. 8–24, 8–25). The intraretinal cysts have a characteristic petalloid appearance on intravenous fluorescein angiopathy. This pattern undoubtedly reflects the radial orientation of the Henle fibers in the perifoveal outer plexiform layer. Fine has suggested that CME may begin as intracellular edema in Müller cells. Cystoid spaces presumably form as a consequence of cellular death in the milieu of chronic edema. Histopathologically, the cystoid spaces appear relatively empty or contain scant amounts of granular or fibrinous material. The latter serves to distinguish them from hard exudates, which are usually pools of eosinophilic hyaline material.

Most cases of cystoid macular edema probably are caused by inflammatory mediators such as prostaglandins that are made in the anterior segment. Vitreous traction on the macula has been incriminated in some instances. Visual loss due to CME may be the presenting clinical manifestation of peripheral lesions including tumors or peripheral uveitis (pars planitis). Cystoid macular edema is an important complication of ocular surgery. The association of CME with cataract surgery is called the Irvine-Gass syndrome. A relatively high incidence of cystoid macular edema occurred in patients who had iris-supported intraocular lenses (IOLs) implanted after intracapsular cataract surgery. The IOL probably stimulated prostaglandin production by the iris, and complete removal of the lens allowed the inflammatory mediator to diffuse readily to the posterior segment. CME can complicate any severe chronic ocular inflammatory disorder. Visual loss may be reversible in early cases.

## AGE-RELATED MACULAR DEGENERATION

Age-related maculopathy, or macular degeneration (ARMD), is a major cause of acquired legal blindness among elderly Americans. (Legal blindness generally is defined as a best-corrected visual acuity of 20/200 or 6/60.) ARMD causes loss of central vision because it involves the fovea, the specialized part of the retina used for high resolution color vision (Figs. 8–26, 8–27, 8–28). Although affected patients have trouble reading and recognizing faces, they retain their peripheral vision and are able to ambulate. Anxious patients may be assured that they will never go totally blind. (This is not entirely true, however, because anticoagulant therapy occasionally does cause massive intraocular hemorrhage in patients with ARMD.)

Atrophic (dry) and exudative (wet) manifestations occur in ARMD. The simultaneous or sequential development of *dry* and *wet* changes in a single patient indicates that these findings are part of a clinical and pathologic spectrum. Dry (atrophic) macular degeneration is characterized by atrophy and death of the subfoveal RPE, which leads to photoreceptor degeneration and outer retinal atrophy.

Drusen are observed ophthalmoscopically in patients with ARMD. Drusen (clinical markers for sick RPE) are mounds or accretions of abnormal extracellular matrix material that form on the inner surface of Bruch's membrane. Drusen probably are synthesized by the RPE. Several types or drusen are recognized clinically and histopathologically. Hard or cuticular drusen are discrete, round or globular mounds of homogeneous, deeply PAS-positive hyaline material (Fig. 8–29). The association of cuticular, or hard, drusen with regional RPE atrophy or the *dry* (atrophic) variant of ARMD has been questioned. Soft drusen, particularly the variety called the basal laminar deposit, play an important role in the pathogenesis of ARMD, especially the severe exudative type, which is complicated by the formation of subretinal neovascular membranes and disciform scar formation.

Basal laminar deposits appear light microscopically as extensive plaques or layers of "soft" granular eosinophilic material that elevate the atrophic RPE from the inner surface of Bruch's membrane (Fig. 8–30).

Transmission electron microscopy has shown that such deposits are located between the plasma membrane and the basement membrane of the RPE and are comprised of extracellular matrix material rich in "curly collagen," or 1000 Å banded basement membrane material. Basal laminar deposits adhere loosely to Bruch's membrane, predisposing to RPE detachments and tears. The deposits theoretically could interfere with biochemical modulation of the choriocapillaries by the RPE and could provide a plane for sub-RPE neovascular invasion. A second, less important variety of diffuse soft drusen, called a basal linear deposit, has been identified electron microscopically. Basal linear deposits are located within Bruch's membrane external to the RPE basement membrane; they are composed of multivesicular phospholipid. It is impossible to distinguish these two varieties of soft drusen with routine light microscopy.

Subretinal neovascular membranes characterize the exudative type of ARMD (Fig. 8–31). Why subretinal neovascularization develops is unclear. Clinically, patients typically present with decreased visual acuity or distorted vision ("metamorphopsia"). Membranes appear as grayish patches on ophthalmoscopy, frequently with associated hemorrhage and overlying subretinal fluid. Intravenous fluorescein angiography is used to confirm the presence of neovascularization. In certain cases, the new vessels can be successfully obliterated by laser photocoagulation.

Untreated subretinal neovascularization occasionally undergoes spontaneous involution. More often, however, the vessels leak or bleed, forming serous or hemorrhagic detachments of the RPE (Fig. 8–32). When the RPE detaches, the plane of the detachment usually is between the inner surface of Bruch's membrane and a basal laminar deposit, which detaches with the RPE. If new vessels have invaded a basal laminar deposit, they are apt to be sheared off during detachment, causing hemorrhagic detachment of the RPE.

Fibrous disciform scar formation, the endstage of exudative ARMD, usually results from the organiza-tion of hemorrhagic RPE detachment. Histopathologically, mature scars are composed of mounds of dense collagenous connective tissue on the inner surface of Bruch's membrane (Fig. 8–33). The collagenous scar usually contains vessels and aggregates of RPE cells. The outer part of the overlying retina undergoes degeneration because the disciform scar is a solid retinal detachment that separates the photoreceptors from their usual source of nourishment. The collagenous part of the scar is derived in part from the fibroblastic component of the granulation tissue that invades and organizes the sub-RPE hemorrhage. The RPE also contributes to scar formation. RPE cells are able to produce large quantities of extracellular matrix material, including drusenoid basement membrane material, collagen, and even bone. Massive fibrous metaplasia of the RPE frequently is observed in eyes with chronic retinal detachment. Bone formation (osseous metaplasia of the RPE) is almost always the rule in phthisical eyes (see Fig. 2–34).

Subretinal neovascular membranes also complicate other conditions, such as angioid streaks. Idiopathic subretinal membranes occasionally occur in relatively young individuals without antecedent cause. Ocular histoplasmosis syndrome (OHS) typically affects patients from the Ohio Valley or other areas where histoplasmosis is endemic. Histopathologically, the disciform scars found in patients with OHS resemble those seen in ARMD, but they typically have a prominent infiltrate of lymphocytes in the underlying choroid (Fig. 8–33). In addition to disciform macular scars, patients with OHS have peripapillary chorioretinal atrophy and multiple white "punched-out" chorioretinal scars (Fig. 8–34). The latter also contain chronic inflammatory cells.

## RETINAL PIGMENT EPITHELIUM

The retinal pigment epithelium (RPE) is vital to the health and survival of the overlying retina (Fig. 8–2).

Responsible for most of the characteristic reddish brown color of the human fundus, the RPE absorbs excess light and prevents intraocular light scattering, similar to the black coating on the inside of a camera (Fig. 8–35). The RPE is also involved in the transport of fluid, nutrients, and vital metabolites such as vitamin A to and from the outer retina. It also appears to plays a major active role in retinal adherence by actively pumping fluid from the subretinal space. The RPE phagocytizes and digests millions of damaged and discarded photoreceptor outer segments every day.

## STARGARDT DISEASE/FUNDUS FLAVIMACULATUS

Striking RPE abnormalities are found in several inherited human retinal diseases. For example, the RPE is markedly abnormal in the inherited macular dystrophy called fundus flavimaculatus. Affected patients lose vision during their teens from an atrophic type of macular degeneration caused by the death of the subfoveal RPE. This type of juvenile macular degeneration was described by Stargardt, and fundus flavimaculatus with juvenile macular degeneration is also called Stargardt's disease. The term fundus flavimaculatus, applied to this disorder by Franceschetti, literally means "yellow-spotted fundus." Ophthalmoscopy discloses pisciform yellow spots at the level of the RPE. The fundus may have a vermilion hue, and a striking clinical abnormality called the dark choroid or the sign of choroidal silence is evident on intravenous fluorescein angiography. This obscuration of the normal choroidal pattern is caused by an opacity at the level of the RPE. Histopathology has shown that this opacification is caused by the massive accumulation of an abnormal lipofuscin-like lipopigment in the cytoplasm of the RPE cells. The surfeit of pigment absorbs excitatory

blue wavelengths during angiography and makes the RPE intensely PAS-positive (Fig. 8–36). The RPE cells are taller than normal and have nuclei that are often displaced toward the apex of the cell. Scanning electron microscopy has revealed markedly enlarged RPE cells that are more numerous in the posterior part of the fundus (Fig. 8–37). Groups of abnormal enlarged RPE cells surrounded by smaller, relatively normal cells may be responsible for the yellow flecked appearance of the fundus. All of the RPE cells contain yellow-brown lipopigment, but the lipofuscin is hidden by a relatively normal complement of apical melanin in the smaller cells. The pisciform aggregates of larger cells appear yellow because these grossly abnormal cells are relatively amelanotic. Macrophages or detached, lipopigment-laden RPE in the subretinal space could also contribute to the flecked retinal appearance. The massive accumulation of pigment probably contributes to RPE dysfunction and death. The death of subfoveal RPE cells in turn leads to photoreceptor degeneration and atrophic macular degeneration.

The gene for autosomal recessive Stargardt disease is located on chromosome 1. Surprisingly, the gene codes for an ATP-binding transport protein (ABCR) that is expressed in rod inner segments, but not the RPE. The nature of the substance normally transported by this protein and how defective transport leads to accumulation of lipofuscin in the RPE remain unclear. Teenagers who have homozygous mutations in the ABCR gene develop fundus flavimaculatus. Heterozygous mutations have been found in adults with the atrophic form of age related macular degeneration.

Lipopigment accumulation may be a relatively stereotyped response of the RPE because excessive amounts of RPE lipopigment have been found in several other disorders. One of these hereditary disorders is Best's disease. This macular dystrophy is also called vitelliform degeneration because a yellowish plaque resembling an egg yolk is observed in the macula during

the early stages of the disorder. Visual loss develops when the egg "scrambles" and chorioretinal scarring develops. Although the early stage of Best's disease has not been examined histopathologically, the egg yolk probably is composed of lipopigment. An abnormal electrooculogram (EOG) incriminates the RPE in Best's disease. An unidentified gene for Best's disease has been found on chromosome 11. A similar disease has been linked to defects in the peripherin/RDS gene.

## RETINITIS PIGMENTOSA

Retinitis pigmentosa (RP) includes a large, complex, diverse group of inherited retinal disorders that have similar characteristic clinical features. Patients with RP usually present with nyctalopia (night blindness) early in life. The electroretinogram typically reveals a marked diminution or total extinction of the retina's electrical responses. A ring-shaped area of blindness called a ring scotoma develops in the patient's equatorial visual field. As the disease progresses, this annular zone of blindness moves posteriorly, progressively encroaching on central vision and producing "tunnel vision."

Ophthalmoscopy discloses RPE atrophy and a characteristic segmental pattern of black intraretinal "bone spicule" pigmentation arranged along retinal vessels (Fig. 8–38). The retinal vessels are usually markedly narrowed, presumably reflecting the atrophic retina's diminished nutritional needs. Although the optic nerve classically displays "waxy pallor," the nerve does not appear to be especially atrophic histopathologically, and this clinical appearance probably is related to decreased vascularity. Macular edema, preretinal membrane formation, and optic disk drusen are also encountered. Patients frequently develop posterior subcapsular cataracts.

Histopathology shows variable degrees of photoreceptor degeneration that initially affects the rods and ultimately the cones (Fig. 8–39). The outer nuclear layer comprising the photoreceptor cell nuclei also becomes atrophic. The extent of involvement depends on both the variant and stage of the disease. The RPE is usually relatively spared compared to the photoreceptors. Presumably, because it is no longer constrained by photoreceptor cell contact inhibition, the RPE proliferates and invades the atrophic retina and grows in the space around retinal vessels, forming perivascular cuffs of intensely pigmented cells, which are evident clinically as bone spicule pigmentation (Fig. 8–40). The intense black pigmentation of the bone spicules is caused by numerous large, round granules of intracytoplasmic melanin, which include macromelanosomes. This pattern of intraretinal pigmentation is not specific for RP; identical findings including macromelanosomes are found in eyes with secondary pigmentary retinopathies related to long-standing retinal detachment. In the latter instance, photoreceptor atrophy caused by chronic retinal detachment presumably facilitates retinal invasion by the RPE.

The retina's response to a wide variety of molecular or enzymatic defects appears to be relatively limited and stereotyped. The constellation of clinical findings called retinitis pigmentosa is now known to be a phenotype associated with disparate defects in at least 25 genes. The specific proteins made by eight of these RP genes have been identified. Four of the proteins such as rhodopsin are involved in rod phototransduction. Others, like peripherin/RDS, are found in rods, but their function is unknown.

Defects in the rod photopigment rhodopsin have been identified in about 20–25% of patients with autosomal dominantly inherited RP. Most are single amino acid (missense) mutations in the opsin part of the molecule. The most common rhodopsin mutation is the substitution of histidine for the normal proline at position 23. This amino acid substitution is caused by a single nucleotide transversion (C to A) in the triplet of nucleotides in the patient's DNA that codes for amino acid 23. Detailed marker studies suggest that all families who have Pro-23-His autosomal dominant (AD) RP are descended from a single individual. AD RP in a few other families is caused by mutations in peripherin/RDS, a protein of unknown function found in the outer rim of rod outer segment disks.

Almost 40% of cases occur sporadically in patients who have no family history of RP. About 37% are autosomal recessively inherited, 20% are autosomal dominantly inherited, and 4% are sex-linked. The disease tends to be more severe and have an earlier onset in patients with sex-linked RP. Autosomal dominantly inherited cases tend to have the most benign course. However, the severity of the disease measured by objective clinical and electrophysiologic criteria in a given kindred of AD RP appears to correlate well with the specific amino acid substitution found in that family (i.e., whether the substituted amino acid occurs in the intradiscal, transmembrane, or cytoplasmic region of the rod outer segment). RP-like changes also occur in a variety of systemic diseases.

## OTHER HERITABLE DISORDERS OF THE RETINA

Specific genetic defects have been discovered in a variety of retinal and vitreous disorders using molecular genetic tools. Ironically, many of these disorders have never been examined histopathologically, or they exhibit relatively nonspecific findings. They include Oguchi disease (mutation in the arrestin gene involved in the shut-off of phototransduction); Sorsby macular degeneration (defect in gene on chromosome 22 encoding tissue inhibitor of metalloproteinase 3, or TIMP3); pattern or butterfly dystrophy (mutations in peripherin/*RDS* gene cause pattern dystrophy in some patients, others have an RP-like picture); choroideremia (X-linked defect in Rab geranylgeranyl trans-

ferase, a protein complex that adds fatty acid side chains to proteins); Norrie's disease, and some forms of familial exudative vitreoretinopathy (defects in Norrie disease gene); gyrate atrophy (autosomal recessive ornithine aminotransferase deficiency); Stickler syndrome (autosomal dominant defect in type II collagen gene); Kearns-Sayre, MERRF, MELAS syndromes (defects in mitochondrial DNA); and Stargardt's disease (defect in outer segment ABCR gene—see above).

The retina and RPE are involved in a wide variety of heritable metabolic storage diseases including the systemic mucopolysaccharidoses, sphingolipidoses, mucolipidoses, neuronal ceroid lipofuscinoses, and disorders of glycoprotein degradation. Retinal pigmentary degeneration resembling that seen in retinitis pigmentosa occurs patients with Hurler (MPS I-H), Scheie (MPS I-S), Hunter (MPS II), Sanfilipo (MPS III), and Morquio (MPS IV) syndromes. Accumulation of GM2 ganglioside in retinal ganglion cells opacifies the ganglion cell-rich perifoveal retina in Tay-Sachs disease (GM2 gangliosidosis type I) (Fig. 8–41). This is evident clinically as a macular cherry red spot because ganglion cells are absent in the floor of the fovea (foveola), which remains transparent. Electron microscopy discloses multimembranous inclusions called zebra bodies within lysosomes. Macular cherry red spots also occur in Sandhoff's disease and the Niemann-Pick group of diseases.

## TOXIC RETINOPATHIES

The chronic administration of certain drugs can cause irreversible visual loss. Some of these chemical compounds are toxic to the RPE. Chloroquine and its hydroxy derivative plaquenil, antimalarial drugs used to treat rheumatoid arthritis and lupus erythematosus, can cause a toxic maculopathy that has a characteristic "bull's eye" appearance. These drugs have an affinity for melanin and are concentrated in the RPE. The macular degeneration appears to be dose-related, and severe visual loss usually develops after patients have received many grams of the drug.

The chronic administration of high doses of phenothiazines, particularly thioridazine (Mellaril), can cause extensive irreversible damage to the RPE and photoreceptors (Fig. 8–42). NP27, a phenothiazine derivative, has been used experimentally as an RPE toxin.

Experimental studies suggest that high levels of the amino acid ornithine are toxic to the RPE. This toxicity appears to be the basis for the widespread chorioretinal atrophy that occurs in patients who have gyrate atrophy. At the molecular level, this rare autosomal recessively inherited disorder is caused by the absence or dysfunction of the mitochondrial matrix enzyme ornithine aminotransferase, which normally converts ornithine to glutamate. The gene is located on chromosome 10. Serum levels of ornithine are elevated 10- to 20-fold in patients with gyrate atrophy. Clinically, gyrate atrophy is characterized by widespread chorioretinal atrophy, which blinds most patients by age 40–50 years.

## PERIPHERAL RETINAL DEGENERATIONS

Peripheral chorioretinal degeneration (commonly called cobblestone or paving stone degeneration) occurs in more than one-fourth of individuals over age 20 years; it is more common in myopes. The lesions appear as yellow-white patches of chorioretinal atrophy that have scalloped, sharply demarcated borders that often are pigmented (Fig. 8–43). Cobblestone degeneration occurs most often in the inferotemporal retina and is separated from the ora serrata by a zone of normal retina. The patches appear white because the overlying sclera is bared by the severe atrophy of the RPE and choriocapillaris. Large choroidal vessels often

persist, however. The pigmented border surrounding many lesions reflects hyperplasia of the adjacent RPE.

Histopathologically, the outer retina is welded to the inner surface of Bruch's membrane, which is devoid of RPE. Replaced by gliosis, the rods and cones are absent in the area of chorioretinal adhesion, and the underlying choriocapillaris is atrophic as well. Unlike lattice degeneration (see below), cobblestone degeneration does not predispose to retinal detachment. In fact, these peripheral chorioretinal scars are similar histopathologically to mature laser burns or cryotherapy scars used to treat retinal disorders. Both therapeutic modalities use thermal effects to induce chorioretinal scarring that firmly binds the outer retina to the denuded inner surface of Bruch's membrane. One sees the typical pattern of outer ischemic retinal atrophy with loss of choriocapillaris, RPE, and outer retina. Retinal breaks do not form because there is no associated vitreoretinal traction. Markedly asymmetric involvement in patients with unilateral ocular ischemia suggest that the cobblestone degeneration might be caused by choroidal vascular insufficiency.

Peripheral microcystoid degeneration is a ubiquitous, generally innocuous degeneration of the peripheral retina found in all adults over age 20. The condition is bilaterally symmetric and most prominent temporally. Clinically or macroscopically, one sees a stippled pattern that corresponds to an array of interconnecting channels or lacunae in the peripheral retina just posterior to the ora serrata (Fig. 8–44). Microscopically, the outer plexiform layer contains multiple cystoid spaces called Blessig-Iwanoff cysts, which are filled with hyaluronic acid and are separated by residual pillars of Müller cells (Fig. 8–45). Zonular traction on the peripheral retina during accommodation may be a cause of peripheral microcystoid degeneration.

Typical degenerative retinoschisis, a split centered in the outer plexiform layer of the retina, is caused by coalescence of the cystoid spaces in peripheral microcystoid degeneration (Fig. 8–46). Degenerative or se-

nile retinoschisis occurs in 1% of adults and usually is located inferotemporally. Although degenerative retinoschisis produces a localized scotoma (a focal area of blindness), the retinal split rarely progresses posteriorly, usually remaining confined to the preequatorial retinal. Rarely, retinal detachment complicates retinoschisis if large holes develop in the outer layer of the retina.

A rarer variant of peripheral microcystoid degeneration, called reticular cystoid degeneration, is said to occur in about 18% of adults; it is bilateral in 41%. Evident as a polygonal patch of delicate tunnels with a finely stippled appearance, reticular cystoid degeneration typically is located posterior to a patch of typical cystoid degeneration. The cysts are located in the nerve fiber layer of the retina (Fig. 8–47). Reticular cystoid degeneration may spawn a corresponding type of retinoschisis called reticular retinoschisis. The split in the retina occurs in the nerve fiber layer.

Juvenile X-linked retinoschisis is an inherited sex-linked disorder. When affected males present with decreased visual acuity during the first decade of life, ophthalmoscopy may disclose a curious stellate pattern of radiating lines or folds in the fovea, which does not leak during fluorescein angiography. These macular changes have never been examined histopathologically. Retinoschisis develops in the periphery of the fundus and can become extensive. The split develops in the nerve fiber layer of the retina (Fig. 8–48). In one case electron microscopy disclosed an accumulation of abnormal vitreous-like material in the retina. Because the vitreous framework is probably synthesized by Müller cells, juvenile X-linked retinoschisis could be a disorder of Müller cells.

Lattice degeneration is a fairly common degenerative condition found in 6–11% of the population. Lattice degeneration is important because it predisposes to the development of rhegmatogenous retinal detachment, particularly in myopic patients. The vitreoretinal degeneration is characterized by the presence of oval areas of retinal thinning, which are sharply demarcated, circumferentially oriented, and located anterior to the equator in the vertical meridians of the eye. The term lattice degeneration is derived from a lattice-like pattern of crisscrossing white lines (sclerotic vessels) that occurs in relatively few (12%) lesions.

Histopathologically, lattice degeneration appears as a focal area of retinal thinning (Fig. 8–49). The inner retinal layers are atrophic, and the internal limiting membrane (ILM) is absent. A pocket of liquefied vitreous overlies the discontinuity in the ILM. Firm vitreoretinal condensations, occasionally fortified by glial cell proliferation, adhere to the margins of the lattice lesions. Thick-walled vessels, which correlate with the white lattice lines seen clinically, are present. Hypertrophy, hyperplasia, and intraretinal migration of the RPE are seen in some cases. The retinal capillary bed is focally occluded.

The firm vitreoretinal adhesions to the margins of the patches of thin atrophic retina predispose to the development of tractional retinal breaks and rhegmatogenous retinal detachment. The tractional breaks typically develop at the posterior or lateral margins of the lesions, and patches of lattice degeneration are often found in the flaps of horseshoe breaks or within small opercula extracted by vitreoretinal traction.

Pars plana cysts usually are innocuous, acquired degenerative lesions that occur in about one-third of normal individuals over age 70 years (Figs. 8–50, 8–51). Most are found incidentally during pathologic examination. Pars plana cysts are formed by detachment of the inner nonpigmented layer of ciliary epithelium from the outer pigmented layer. In normal individuals the cysts contain an acidic glycosaminoglycan presumed to be hyaluronic acid because it is sensitive to digestion with the enzyme hyaluronidase (Fig. 8–51). Multiple pars plana cysts occur in patients with multiple myeloma or other dysproteinemic or hyperproteinemic disorders. Myeloma cysts contain Bence-Jones (myeloma) protein, which is precipitated by fixation and causes milky-white opacification of the cysts (Fig. 8–52).

## RETINAL DETACHMENT

Retinal detachment is a physical separation of the neurosensory retina from the retinal pigment epithelium (the two layers derived, respectively, from the inner and outer layers of the embryonic neuroectodermal optic cup) (Fig. 8–53). Although these two layers normally are closely apposed, they are not joined by intercellular connections; and a potential space called the subretinal space exists between the two. With retinal detachment fluid collects in this potential space. The fluid prevents reapproximation and reattachment of the retina unless it resorbs or is drained. The physical separation deprives the outer, avascular part of the retina of its normal supply of oxygen and nutrients from the choroid, and it precludes vital interactions between the energy-intensive photoreceptors and the RPE. These factors can lead rapidly to permanent visual loss from irreversible degeneration and atrophy of the rods and cones. Hence vision may remain poor after a seemingly successful reattachment operation; that is, surgery can be a technical success but a functional failure.

There are three basic categories of retinal detachment: rhegmatogenous, exudative, and tractional. Rhegmatogenous retinal detachments are caused by holes or breaks (rhegma = break) in the neurosensory retina that provide fluid (usually liquid vitreous) access to the subretinal space (Fig. 8–54). Most retinal holes found in eyes with rhegmatogenous retinal detachment are tears caused by vitreoretinal traction. The vitreous humor's framework of type II collagen fibers is adherent to the internal limiting membrane of the retina. Particularly firm vitreoretinal adhesions occur at the vitreous base, which straddles the ora serrata, the circumference of the optic disk, around the fovea, and along major retinal vessels.

The framework of vitreous humor frequently detaches from the posterior retina in elderly patients or in individuals who have diabetes or other retinal pathology. Anterior movement of the posteriorly detached vitreous caused by eye movements can exert traction on areas where the vitreous and retina remain firmly adherent, causing tears in the retina (that release the traction). Rhegmatogenous retinal detachment is a relatively common complication of intracapsular cataract extraction in which the entire lens is removed within its capsule. Aphakic (no lens) retinal detachment after intracapsular surgery typically is caused by small horseshoe tears located at the posterior vitreous base. Hole formation is related to increased mobility of the posteriorly detached vitreous, which has been deprived of support anteriorly. The apices of horseshoe tears always point posteriorly; that is, the "horse" always walks toward the optic nerve. Posterior vitreous detachment and the mechanics of vitreoretinal traction are responsible for this characteristic orientation.

Rhegmatogenous retinal detachment also is relatively common in patients who are myopic or who have lattice degeneration of the retina. Several factors probably contribute to the development of retinal detachment in those with high myopia. Vitreous degeneration or syneresis is common in myopic eyes. It is evident clinically to most affected persons as vitreous floaters. Most cases of myopia are caused by enlargement of the eye, which usually occurs as the refractive disorder develops toward the end of the first decade. Presumably, the vitreous framework degenerates as the sclera and retina "outgrow" the vitreous. Retinal stretching and attenuation in high myopes also contribute to retinal hole formation. Subretinal neovascularization, macular hemorrhage, and disciform scar formation can complicate pathologic high myopia. Stretching of Bruch's membrane causes splits or ruptures, which are evident clinically as "lacquer cracks" or lightning figures. A central, circular, dark spot called a Förster-Fuchs' spot may develop in the macula during the fourth or fifth decade in association with lacquer cracks. Blood pigment from choroidal hemorrhage and RPE proliferation probably contribute to this spot.

Trauma is another cause of rhegmatogenous retinal detachment. The retina can be torn by severe distortion of the globe during contusion injuries. Lengthy rips in the retina, called giant tears, can result. Giant tears are typically oriented parallel to the limbus and generally extend 90 degrees or more. Contusion injuries can also avulse or physically disinsert the retina from its attachment to the ora serrata. The large peripheral gaps that result are called retinal dialyses. Most retinal dialyses affect the inferotemporal quadrant and occur in young emmetropes.

Tractional retinal detachments are caused by fibrous or fibrovascular vitreoretinal membranes that contract and mechanically pull off the retina (Fig. 8–55). Tractional detachment of the posterior retina, which unfortunately often involves the macula, is a major complication of proliferative diabetic retinopathy. Vitreoretinal traction in diabetics is caused by the contraction of fibrovascular membranes. The neovascular component of such membranes originates within the retina and proliferates on the face of the posteriorly detached vitreous. The organization of vitreous hemorrhage also contributes to vitreoretinal membrane formation and traction. In the past severe fibroplasia and organization of the vitreous in diabetics was termed *retinitis proliferans*. Tractional retinal detachment caused by vitreoretinal neovascularization also complicates sickle cell retinopathy and the retinopathy of prematurity.

Tractional retinal detachment can also follow severe trauma, especially perforating injuries of the globe. The retinal traction is caused by vitreoretinal bands formed by ingrowth of fibrous scar tissue from the wound or by the organization of tracks of hemorrhage in the vitreous. Removal of vitreous hemorrhage after severe injury can help reduce the incidence of this complication.

Severe inflammatory and infectious conditions that stimulate organization of the vitreous are additional causes of tractional retinal detachment. A relatively high incidence of detachment complicates ocular toxocariasis, particularly the peripheral form of the disease. Retinal detachment is also a major problem in AIDS patients who have necrotizing retinitides such as cytomegalovirus (CMV) retinitis (see Chapter 2).

Exudative retinal detachment is caused by the accumulation of fluid in the subretinal space. The subretinal fluid may come from "leaky" vascular lesions in the retina but more often are caused by infiltration of the choroid by tumor or inflammation. Exudative retinal detachments are nonrhegmatogenous; careful clinical examination fails to disclose a hole in the neurosensory retina.

Exudative retinal detachments caused by leaky retinal lesions occur in patients who have Coats' disease or retinal capillary hemangiomas. Coats' disease is discussed in Chapter 11. Retinal capillary hemangiomas (or retinal hemangioblastomas) occur in isolation or may be a manifestation of autosomal dominantly inherited Von Hippel-Lindau disease (see Chapter 1).

Most primary or secondary choroidal tumors usually have some degree of associated exudative retinal detachment. Exudative detachment occurs in most patients who have choroidal malignant melanomas and is often the presenting manifestation of the tumor. Initially, fluid percolates into the space at the margins of the "solid detachment" formed by "tenting-up" and anterior displacement of the retina by the tumor. Degeneration or destruction of the RPE and choriocapillaris overlying the tumor may be additional contributory factors. Extensive exudative retinal detachment typically is found in eyes with carcinoma metastatic to the uvea. The location of the bulk of the subretinal fluid may shift with eye movements (shifting fluid). Exudative retinal detachment is a major cause of visual loss in eyes with choroidal hemangiomas and ultimately can lead to loss of the eye if painful pupillary block glaucoma results. These benign vascular tumors occasionally are treated with radiotherapy to prevent this complication.

Exudative retinal detachment also complicates choroidal inflammatory disease, particularly disorders marked by extensive choroidal infiltration such as sympathetic uveitis or Vogt-Koyanagi-Harada's disease. Exudative retinal detachment complicates toxemia of pregnancy and oxygen toxicity.

## TRUE AND ARTIFACTITIOUS RETINAL DETACHMENTS

Nearly all intact eyes that are fixed routinely by immersion in neutral buffered formalin have an artifactitious detachment of the retina. Several features serve to differentiate true and artifactitious retinal detachments histopathologically. True retinal detachments are characterized by eosinophilic proteinaceous fluid in the subretinal space (*not* present in all cases) and degeneration and atrophy of the photoreceptors, which can involve the outer nuclear layer in long-standing cases. On the other hand, if the retinal detachment is artifactual, the subretinal space is empty, the photoreceptors are well preserved, and ellipsoidal granules of RPE pigment remain attached to the tips of the outer segments.

## SIGNS OF CHRONIC RETINAL DETACHMENT

Findings that indicate a retinal detachment has persisted for some time include budding and papillary and pseudoadenomatous proliferation of the RPE. The RPE has a great capacity for reactive proliferation and migration, which under normal circumstances presumably is held in check by contact inhibition by healthy retinal photoreceptors. Retinal detachment removes this inhibition.

The RPE cells are capable of elaborating enormous quantities of extracellular matrix material including drusenoid basement membrane material, collagen, and even bone. Curious, large, drusen-like structures with a central core of soft granular acellular matrix material enveloped by RPE cells occasionally are found in eyes with long-standing retinal detachments. Osseous metaplasia of the RPE is almost invariably found in blind phthisical eyes with chronic retinal detachment. The intraocular bone always is located on the inner surface of Bruch's membrane and typically occurs at sites of traction near the ora serrata or the optic disk. The bone is mature lamellar bone and often contains fatty marrow.

Chronically detached retinas found in blind, painful eyes typically have a funnel, or "morning glory," configuration (Figs. 8–56, 8–57). This configuration reflects the endstage of proliferative vitreoretinopathy (PVR). It is caused by the growth of cells on both the inner and outer surfaces of the detached retina and on the posterior surface of the detached vitreous, which remains firmly attached to the vitreous base. The cells include RPE cells, glial cells, and myofibroblasts that migrate, proliferate, and elaborate extracellular matrix material and form fibrocellular membranes. Organization of the vitreous and contraction of this scar tissue exerts traction on the inner part of the peripheral retina, drawing it centrally and permanently welding the retina into this floral configuration. Organization of the vitreous also forms cyclitic membranes, which bridge the vitreous cavity behind the lens. The cyclitic membranes exert traction on the vitreous base and detach the ciliary body. PVR is a major cause of inoperable retinal detachment or recurrent detachment after reattachment

surgery. Fibrocellular membranes on its inner and outer surfaces bind adjacent parts of the retina together, forming fixed folds. Other findings in long-standing retinal detachment include gliosis and micro- and macrocystic retinal degeneration (Fig. 8–57).

## OCULAR PATHOLOGY OF DIABETES MELLITUS

The ocular complications of diabetes mellitus are an important cause of acquired visual disability and blindness. In the United States, diabetic retinopathy is the leading cause of new cases of legal blindness between the ages of 20 and 74. Diabetic retinopathy occurs in patients with type I (juvenile-onset or insulin-dependent) or type II (maturity-onset) diabetes mellitus. The prevalence of retinopathy is higher in patients with type I diabetes. Patients with juvenile diabetes also are at greater risk for developing proliferative retinopathy, probably because they generally have more severe hyperglycemia. Overall, however, a significant proportion of the disorder's blinding complications develop in patients with type II diabetes because adult-onset diabetes is more common. The prevalence of retinopathy in both groups is related to the duration of the disease. Retinopathy occurs in about 50% of patients who have had juvenile diabetes mellitus for 15 years. Strict control of blood sugar appears to slow the progression of the disease.

Background, preproliferative, and proliferative forms of diabetic retinopathy are recognized clinically. The initial stage of diabetic retinopathy (background retinopathy) is marked by retinal edema, hemorrhages, and exudates (see above) and capillary microaneurysms. A preponderance of soft exudates or cotton wool spots heralds progressive retinal ischemia as diabetic retinopathy enters the preproliferative phase. Retinal and vitreoretinal neovascularization occur in

proliferative diabetic retinopathy. Neovascularization predisposes to blinding complications: vitreous hemorrhage and tractional retinal detachment.

Diabetic retinopathy is the retinal manifestation of the generalized microangiopathy that occurs throughout the body in diabetes mellitus (Fig. 8–58). Breakdown of the blood–retina barrier is one of the earliest functional lesions in diabetic eyes and contributes to the development of hemorrhages, exudates, and retinal edema. Retinal edema is an important cause of visual loss in diabetic patients. The characteristic retinal vascular abnormalities of diabetic retinopathy can be demonstrated by the trypsin retinal digestion technique. Normal retinal capillaries are comprised of endothelial cells (which form the lining of the capillary) and pericytes or mural cells (which reside in capsules in the perivascular basement membrane) (Fig. 8–59). Pericytes have contractile properties that regulate capillary caliber and the flow within the retinal microcirculation. Normally, endothelial cells and pericytes occur in a 1:1 ratio. Pericytes are lost preferentially during the early stages of diabetic retinopathy (Fig. 8–60).

Pericyte loss appears to be directly related to hyperglycemia. The pericytes may be killed by the intracellular accumulation of sorbitol produced by the enzyme aldose reductase when the normal glycolytic pathway is saturated. Unable to traverse cellular membranes, sorbitol is trapped intracellularly and has a toxic osmotic effect on the cell.

Trypsin digestion of the diabetic retina also discloses capillary microaneurysms and generalized thickening of the capillary basement membranes evident as increased PAS-positive staining. Totally acellular areas of the retinal capillary bed devoid of both endothelial cells and pericytes also are found. The latter correspond to areas of capillary nonperfusion seen on fluorescein angiography. Histopathologic examination of zones of capillary nonperfusion reveals inner ischemic retinal atrophy.

Retinal capillary microaneurysms (Fig. 8–61) are grape-like or spindle-shaped dilatations of retinal capillaries. Many microaneurysms appear cellular, suggesting that capillary endothelial cell proliferation may be involved in their formation. Weakening of the capillary wall secondary to focal pericyte loss may also contribute.

Retinal capillary pericyte loss has several important consequences. Retinal capillaries lose the ability to autoregulate, leading to changes in retinal blood flow. In addition, pericytes appear to have an inhibitory effect on vascular endothelial cell proliferation, which is mediated by transforming growth factor beta (TGFβ). Loss of this inhibitory effect may stimulate endothelial cell proliferation and neovascularization.

Neovascularization occurs in proliferative diabetic retinopathy and is a major factor in the pathogenesis of blinding complications such as vitreous hemorrhage and tractional retinal detachment (Figs. 8–5, 8–55, 8–62, 8–63, 8–64, 8–65). Neovascularization is stimulated by angiogenesis factors produced by the ischemic retina, such as vascular endothelial growth factor (VEGF). VEGF is a potent angiogenesis factor and endothelial cell-specific mitogen whose synthesis is regulated by the level of oxygen in the cellular microenvironment. VEGF has been identified in ocular fluid from patients with active retinal and anterior segment neovascularization associated with several ocular diseases that exhibit retinal ischemia.

Neovascularization begins in the retina where it is evident clinically as intraretinal microvascular abnormalities. The new vessels break through the internal limiting membrane and grow on the inner surface of the retina (Fig. 8–63). Neovascularization cannot invade the formed vitreous, but it readily grows on the posterior face of the detached vitreous (Figs. 8–5, 8-55, 8–64). Neovascularization that originates on the optic disk typically grows into the conical posterior opening of Cloquet's canal, called the area of Martegiani. The neovascularization stimulates fibro-plasia and vitreous fibrosis. Contraction of vitreoretinal membranes and progression of posterior vitreous detachment frequently tears the delicate new vessels, causing subhyaloid and vitreous hemorrhage. Organization of hemorrhage, in turn, engenders a vicious cycle of additional fibrosis, traction, and hemorrhage. Localized tractional detachment of the macula often occurs because the vitreous typically remains adherent to the temporal arcades of the major retinal vessels. The vascularized bridge of detached vitreous contracts, causing retina–retina traction (Fig. 8–65). Anteroposterior traction also contributes to the retinal detachment (Fig. 8–55).

Eyes with proliferative diabetic retinopathy are prone to develop neovascularization of the iris (NVI) and neovascular glaucoma (NVG) (see Figs. 7–18, 7–19, 7–20, 7–21). NVI is caused by the anterior diffusion of angiogenesis factor. NVI (also called rubeosis iridis) may develop or progress markedly after intracapsular cataract extraction, which presumably removes a barrier to diffusion. Iris neovascularization usually starts near the pupillary border and in the angle.

The normal architecture of the iris is flattened and effaced by the fibrovascular membrane on its normally avascular anterior surface. Secondary closed angle glaucoma results when the formation of adhesions between the peripheral iris and the trabecular meshwork called peripheral anterior synechias blocks aqueous outflow.

A more innocuous form of diabetic iridopathy called lacy vacuolization of the iris pigment epithelium occurs in some patients (Figs. 8–66). Lacy vacuolization is marked by an accumulation of glycogen in cystoid spaces within the iris pigment epithelium. The focal glycogenosis of the iris pigment epithelium is thought to be related to chronically elevated levels of blood glucose and may be analogous to an accumulation of glycogen in the renal tubules called Armanni-Ebstein glycogen nephropathy. Transient pig-mentation of aqueous humor observed intraoperatively in some diabetics may reflect pigment epithelial damage caused by lacy vacuolization. Lacy vacuolization may be evident during slit lamp biomicroscopy as a faint moth-eaten pattern of iris transillumination.

Basement membrane thickening occurs throughout the body in diabetic patients. Thickening of the basement membrane of the pigmented ciliary epithelium occurs in many diabetic eyes and is a helpful histologic marker for the disease (Fig. 8–67). Analogous thickening of the glomerular basement membrane is found in the Kimmelstiel-Wilson form of diabetic nephropathy. Thickening of the corneal epithelial basement membrane can predispose to sheet-like desquamation of corneal epithelium during vitreoretinal surgery.

Cataracts complicate diabetes mellitus. A specific form of diabetic cataract may be the presenting manifestation of the disease. Relatively rare, such cataracts are probably caused by the osmotic effect of sorbitol accumulation in the lens. Such opacities may be partially reversible if blood sugar levels are normalized. Diabetics also develop typical senile cataracts at an earlier age. Variable refractive errors in diabetics reflect changes in lens hydration caused by hyperglycemia. Patients usually become more myopic when their blood sugar is elevated.

Diabetics are at increased risk of infection. One of the most serious infections that can complicate diabetes is mucormycosis. Poorly controlled diabetics who are acidotic are particularly at risk for infection by *Mucor*, which normally is a saprophytic fungus. The fungal infection begins in the paranasal sinuses and then invades the orbital tissues secondarily. Usually evident in routine sections stained with hematoxylin-eosin, the large nonseptate fungal hyphae typically invade vessels, producing thrombosis and necrosis (see Fig. 13–4). In rare instances, diabetes mellitus presents with unilateral or even bilateral central retinal artery occlusion caused by mucormycosis.

## SICKLE HEMOGLOBINOPATHY

Vitreoretinal neovascularization is a characteristic finding in patients who have sickle hemoglobinopathy, particularly hemoglobin (Hb) SC disease. Occlusion of peripheral retinal vessels by sickled erythrocytes causes extensive capillary nonperfusion and inner ischemic atrophy of the peripheral retina, especially the longer arc of the temporal retina. Neovascularization develops within the retina just behind the characteristically abrupt junction between its peripheral ischemic nonperfused and posterior perfused parts and then extends into the vitreous. The appearance of the neovascular fronds has been likened to the marine organism *Gorgonia flabellum*, the sea fan. The "sea fans" bleed, causing vitreous hemorrhage. Vitreoretinal traction caused by organization of the vitreous blood produces holes in the retina, which cause rhegmatogenous retinal detachment. Neovascularization is more likely to occur in patients with Hb SC disease because they are less anemic than patients with Hb SS disease; and vascular occlusion is more apt to occur when the hematocrit is higher. Pigmented scars called black sunburst signs caused by chorioretinal hemorrhage are more common in patients with Hb SS disease. The partial resorption of hemorrhages in these patients is evident clinically as salmon patches. Angioid streaks also occur in a small number of patients with sickle hemoglobinopathy. It has been postulated that the deposition of iron in Bruch's membrane somehow predisposes to massive calcification of Bruch's membrane.

## R e f e r e n c e s

### General References

Green W: Pathology of the retina. In Spencer W (ed) Ophthalmic Pathology: An Atlas and Textbook. Vol 2. Philadelphia: Saunders, 1996:667–1331.

### Albinism and Other Developmental Anomalies

Bergsma D, Kaiser-Kupfer M: A new form of albinism. Am J Ophthalmol 77:837, 1974.

Blume R, Wolff S: The Chediak-Higashi syndrome: studies in four patients and a review of the literature. Medicine 51:247, 1972.

Falls H: Sex-linked ocular albinism displaying typical fundus changes in the female heterozygote. Am J Ophthalmol 34:41, 1951.

Forsius H, Eriksson A: Ein neues Augensyndrom mit X-chromosomaler Transmission: eine Sippe mit Fundusalbinismus, Foveahypoplasie, Nystagmus, Myopie, Astigmatismus und Dyschromatopsie. Klin Monatsbl Augenheilkd 144:447, 1964.

Garrod A: Inborn Errors of Metabolism. London: Frowde, 1909.

King R, Creel D, Cervenka J, et al: Albinism in Nigeria with delineation of a new recessive oculocutaneous type. Clin Genet 17:259, 1980.

Mietz H, Green WR, Wolff SM, et al: Foveal hypoplasia in complete oculocutaneous albinism: a histopathologic study. Retina 12:254–260, 1992.

Naumann GOH, Lerche W, Schroeder W: Foveola-Aplasie bei Tyrosinase-positivem oculocutanem Albinismus. Graefes Arch Clin Exp Ophthalmol 200:39–50, 1976.

O'Donnell FJ, Green W, Fleischman J, et al: X-linked ocular albinism in blacks: ocular albinism cum pigmento. Arch Ophthalmol 96:1189, 1978.

O'Donnell FJ, Hambrick GJ, Green W, et al: X-linked ocular albinism: an oculocutaneous macromelanosomal disorder. Arch Ophthalmol 94:1883, 1976.

O'Donnell FJ, King R, WR G, et al: Autosomal recessively inherited ocular albinism: a new form of ocular albinism affecting women as severely as men. Arch Ophthalmol 96:1621, 1978.

Ohrt V: Ocular albinism with changes typical of carriers. Br J Ophthalmol 40:721, 1956.

Read AP, Newton VE: Waardenburg syndrome. J Med Genet 34:656–665, 1997.

Straatsma BR, Foos RY, Heckenlively J, et al: Myelinated retinal nerve fibers. Am J Ophthalmol 91:25–38, 1981.

Straatsma BR, Foos RY, Heckenlively JR, et al: Myelinated retinal nerve fibers associated with ipsilateral myopia, amblyopia and nystagmus. Am J Ophthalmol 88:506–510, 1979.

Traboulsi EI, Green WR, O'Donnell FJ Jr: The eye in albinism. In Tasman W, Jaeger EA (eds) Duane's Clinical Ophthalmology. Vol 4. Chap. 38. Philadelphia: Lippincott-Raven, 1995.

Witkop CJ, Quevedo WJ, Fitzpatrick T: Albinism and other disorders of pigment metabolism. In Stanbury J, Frederickson D, et al (eds) The Metabolic Basic of Inherited Disease. 5th ed. New York: McGraw-Hill, 1985:301.

Wong L, O'Donnell FE Jr, Green WR: Giant pigment granules in the retinal pigment epithelium of a fetus with X-linked ocular albinism. Ophthalmic Paediatr Genet 2: 47–65, 1983.

### Retinal Hemorrhages and Exudates

Ashton N: Pathological and ultrastructural aspect of the cotton-wool spots. Proc R Soc Med 62:1271–1276, 1969.

Ashton N: Pathophysiology of retinal cotton-wool spots. Br Med Bull 26:143–150, 1970.

Ashton N, Harry J: The pathology of cotton-wool spots and cytoid bodies in hypertensive retinopathy and other diseases. Trans Ophthalmol Soc UK 83:91–114, 1963.

Cunha-Vaz JG: The blood-retinal barriers. Doc Ophthalmol 41:287–327, 1976.

Duane TD, Osher RH, Green WR: White centered hemorrhages: their significance. Ophthalmology 87:66–69, 1980.

Wolter JR: Axonal enlargements in the nerve-fiber layer of the human retina. Am J Ophthalmol 65:1–12, 1968.

Wolter JR: Pathology of a cotton-wool spot. Am J Ophthalmol 48:473–485, 1959.

### Angioid Streaks

Dreyer R, Green WR: Pathology of angioid streaks. Trans Pa Acad Ophthalmol Otolaryngol 31:158–167, 1978.

Jampol LM, Acheson R, Eagle RC Jr, Serjeant G, O'Grady R: Calcification of Bruch's membrane in angioid streaks with homozygous sickle cell disease. Arch Ophthalmol 105:93–98, 1987.

### Retinal Artery Occlusion

Arruga J, Sanders MD: Ophthalmologic findings in 70 patients with evidence of retinal embolism. Ophthalmology 89:1336–1347, 1982.

Ball CJ: Atheromatous embolism to the brain, retina, and choroid. Arch Ophthalmol 76:690–695, 1966.

Brownstein S, Font RL, Alper MG: Atheromatous plaques of the retinal blood vessels. Arch Ophthalmol 90:49–52, 1973.

Dahrling BE: The histopathology of early central retinal artery occlusion. Arch Ophthalmol 73:506–510, 1965.

Fineman MS, Savino PJ, Federman JL, Eagle RC Jr: Branch retinal artery occlusion as the initial sign of giant cell arteritis. Am J Ophthalmol 122:428–430, 1996.

Jampol LM, Setogawa T, Rednam KR, Tso MO: Talc retinopathy in primates: a model of ischemic retinopathy. I. Clinical studies. Arch Ophthalmol 99:1273–1280, 1981.

Jampol LM, Wong AS, Albert DM: Atrial myxoma and central retinal artery occlusion. Am J Ophthalmol 75: 242–249, 1973.

Levine SR, Crofts JW, Lesser GR, et al: Visual symptoms associated with the presence of a lupus anticoagulant. Ophthalmology 95:686–692, 1988.

McDonnell PJ, Moore GW, Miller NR, et al: Temporal arteritis: a clinicopathologic study. Ophthalmology 93: 518–530, 1986.

McKibbin DW, Gott VL, Hutchins GM: Fatal cerebral atheromatous embolization after cardiopulmonary bypass. J Thorac Cardiovasc Surg 71:741–745, 1976.

Penner R, Font RL: Retinal embolism from calcified vegetations of aortic valve: spontaneous complications of rheumatic heart disease. Arch Ophthalmol 81:565–568, 1969.

Pfaffenbach DD, Hollenhorst RW: Morbidity and survivorship of patients with embolic cholesterol crystals in the ocular fundus. Trans Am Ophthalmol Soc 70:337–349, 1972.

Pulido JS, Ward LM, Fishman GA, et al: Antiphospholipid antibodies associated with retinal vascular disease. Retina 7:215–218,1987.

Wang FM, Henkind P: Visual system involvement in giant cell (temporal) arteritis. Surv Ophthalmol 23:264–271, 1979.

**Retinal Vein Occlusion**

Frangieh GT, Green WR, Barraquer-Somer E, Finkelstein D: Histopathologic study of nine branch retinal vein occlusions in eight eyes of seven patients. Arch Ophthalmol 100:1132–1140, 1982.

Green WR, Chan CC, Hutchins GM, et al: Central retinal vein occlusion: a prospective histopathologic study of 29 eyes of 28 patients. Trans Am Ophthalmol Soc 79: 371–422, 1981.

Hayreh SS: Pathogenesis of occlusion of the central retinal vessels. Am J Ophthalmol 72:998–1011, 1971.

Rothstein T: Bilateral retinal vein closure as the initial manifestation of polycythemia. Am J Ophthalmol 74: 256–260, 1972.

**Hypertensive Retinopathy**

Garner A, Ashton N: Pathogenesis of hypertensive retinopathy: a review. J R Soc Med 72:362–365, 1979.

Garner A, Ashton N, Tripathi R, Kohner EM, Bulpitt CJ, Dollery CT: Pathogenesis of hypertensive retinopathy: an experimental study in the monkey. Br J Ophthalmol 59: 3–44, 1975.

Hayreh SS, Servais GE, Virdi PS: Fundus lesions in malignant hypertension. VI. Hypertensive choroidopathy. Ophthalmology 93:1383–1400, 1986.

Tso MO, Jampol LM: Pathophysiology of hypertensive retinopathy. Ophthalmology 89:1132–1145, 1982.

Walsh JB: Hypertensive retinopathy: description, classification, and prognosis. Ophthalmology 89:1127–1131, 1982.

**Age-Related Maculopathy**

Allikmets R, Shroyer NF, Singh N et al: Mutation of the Stargardt disease gene (ABCR) in age-related macular degeneration. Science 277:1805–1807, 1997.

Bressler NM, Silva JC, Bressler SB, Fine SL, Green WR: Clinicopathologic correlation of drusen and retinal pigment epithelial abnormalities in age-related macular degeneration. Retina 14:130–142, 1994.

Bressler SB, Silva JC, Bressler NM, Alexander J, Green WR: Clinicopathologic correlation of occult choroidal neovascularization in age-related macular degeneration. Arch Ophthalmol 110:827–832, 1992.

Bynoe LA, Chang TS, Funata M, Del Priore LV, Kaplan HJ, Green WR: Histopathologic examination of vascular patterns in subfoveal neovascular membranes. Ophthalmology 101:1112–1117, 1994.

El Baba F, Jarrett WH, Harbin TS Jr, et al: Massive hemorrhage complicating age-related macular degeneration: clinicopathologic correlation and role of anticoagulants. Ophthalmology 93:1581–1592, 1986.

Green WR: Clinicopathologic studies of treated choroidal neovascular membranes: a review and report of two cases. Retina 11:328–356, 1991.

Green WR, Enger C: Age-related macular degeneration histopathologic studies: the 1992 Lorenz E. Zimmerman lecture. Ophthalmology 100:1519–1535, 1993.

Green WR, McDonnell PJ, Yeo JH: Pathologic features of senile macular degeneration. Ophthalmology 92: 615–627, 1985.

Grossniklaus HE, Hutchinson AK, Capone A Jr, Woolfson J, Lambert HM: Clinicopathologic features of surgically excised choroidal neovascular membranes. Ophthalmology 101:1099–1111, 1994.

Kenyon KR, Maumenee AE, Ryan SJ, Whitmore PV, Green WR: Diffuse drusen and associated complications. Am J Ophthalmol 100:119–128, 1985.

Spraul CW, Lang GE, Grossniklaus HE: Morphometric analysis of the choroid, Bruch's membrane, and retinal pigment epithelium in eyes with age-related macular de-

generation [see comments]. Invest Ophthalmol Vis Sci 37: 2724–2735, 1996.

**Other Macular Degenerations**

Boozalis GT, Schachat AP, Green WR: Subretinal neovascularization from the retina in radiation retinopathy. Retina 7:156–161, 1987.

Dastgheib K, Green WR: Granulomatous reaction to Bruch's membrane in age-related macular degeneration. Arch Ophthalmol 112:813–818, 1994.

Grossniklaus HE, Green WR: Pathologic findings in pathologic myopia. Retina 12:127–133, 1992.

Saxe SJ, Grossniklaus HE, Lopez PF, Lambert HM, Sternberg P Jr, L'Hernault N: Ultrastructural features of surgically excised subretinal neovascular membranes in the ocular histoplasmosis syndrome. Arch Ophthalmol 111:88–95, 1993.

**Toxic Maculopathies**

Bernstein HN: Some iatrogenic ocular diseases from systemically administered drugs. Int Ophthalmol Clin 10: 553–587, 1970.

Henkind P, Rothfield NF: Ocular abnormalities in patients treated with synthetic antimalarial drugs. N Engl J Med 269:433–439, 1963.

Ramsey MS, Fine BS: Chloroquine toxicity in the human eye: histopathologic observations by electron microscopy. Am J Ophthalmol 73:229–235, 1972.

Rosenthal AR, Kolb H, Bergsma D, et al: Chloroquine retinopathy in the rhesus monkey. Invest Ophthalmol Vis Sci 17:1158–1175, 1978.

Smith RS, Berson EL: Acute toxic effects of chloroquine on the cat retina: ultrastructural changes. Invest Ophthalmol Vis Sci 10:237–246, 1971.

Wetterholm DH, Winter FC: Histopathology of chloroquine retinal toxicity. Arch Ophthalmol 71:82–87, 1964.

**Macular Dystrophies**

Allikmets R, Singh N, Sun H, et al: A photoreceptor cell-specific ATP-binding transporter gene (ABCR) is mutated in recessive Stargardt macular dystrophy. Nat Genet 15:236–246, 1997.

Eagle RC, Lucier AC, Bernardino VB, Yanoff M: Retinal pigment epithelial abnormalities in fundus flavimaculatus: a light and electron microscopic study. Ophthalmology 87:1189–1200, 1980.

Frangieh GT, Green WR, Fine SL: A histopathologic study of Best's macular dystrophy. Arch Ophthalmol 100: 1115–1121, 1982.

Lopez PF, Maumenee IH, de la Cruz Z, Green WR: Autosomal-dominant fundus flavimaculatus: clinicopathologic correlation. Ophthalmology 97:798–809, 1990.

Zhang K, Nguyen TH, Crandall A, Donoso LA: Genetic and molecular studies of macular dystrophies: recent developments. Surv Ophthalmol 40:51–61, 1995.

**Gyrate Atrophy**

Kaiser-Kupfer MI, Valle D, Del Valle LA: A specific enzyme defect in gyrate atrophy. Am J Ophthalmol 85:200–204, 1978.

Kuwabara T, Ishikawa Y, Kaiser-Kupfer MI: Experimental model of gyrate atrophy in animals. Ophthalmology 88:331–334, 1981.

Wilson DJ, Weleber RG, Green WR: Ocular clinicopathologic study of gyrate atrophy. Am J Ophthalmol 111:24–33, 1991.

**Retinitis Pigmentosa**

Drack AV, Traboulsi EI: Systemic associations of pigmentary retinopathy. Int Ophthalmol Clin 31:35–59, 1991.

Dryja TP: Doyne lecture: rhodopsin and autosomal dominant retinitis pigmentosa. Eye 6:1–10, 1992.

Dryja TP, Li T: Molecular genetics of retinitis pigmentosa. Hum Mol Genet 4:1739–1743, 1995.

Dryja TP, Hahn LB, Cowley GS, McGee TL, Berson EL: Mutation spectrum of the rhodopsin gene among patients with autosomal dominant retinitis pigmentosa. Proc Natl Acad Sci USA 88:9370–9374, 1991.

Dryja TP, Hahn LB, Kajiwara K, Berson EL: Dominant and digenic mutations in the peripherin/RDS and ROM1 genes in retinitis pigmentosa. Invest Ophthalmol Vis Sci 38:1972–1982, 1997.

Dryja TP, McGee TL, Hahn LB, et al: Mutations within the rhodopsin gene in patients with autosomal dominant retinitis pigmentosa. N Engl J Med 323:1302–1307, 1990.

Huang SH, Pittler SJ, Huang X, Oliveira L, Berson EL, Dryja TP: Autosomal recessive retinitis pigmentosa caused by mutations in the alpha subunit of rod cGMP phosphodiesterase. Nat Genet 11:468–471, 1995.

Li ZY, Possin DE, Milam AH: Histopathology of bone spicule pigmentation in retinitis pigmentosa. Ophthalmology 102:805–816, 1995.

Luckenbach MW, Green WR, Miller NR, Moser HW, Clark AW, Tennekoon G: Ocular clinicopathologic correlation of Hallervorden-Spatz syndrome with acanthocytosis and pigmentary retinopathy. Am J Ophthalmol 95:369–382, 1983.

Sandberg MA, Weigel-DiFranco C, Dryja TP, Berson EL: Clinical expression correlates with location of rhodopsin mutation in dominant retinitis pigmentosa. Invest Ophthalmol Vis Sci 36:1934–1942, 1995.

**Choroideremia**

Cameron JD, Fine BS, Shapiro I: Histopathologic observations in choroideremia with emphasis on vascular changes of the uveal tract. Ophthalmology 94:187–196, 1987.

MacDonald IM, Chen MH, Addison DJ, Mielke BW, Nesslinger NJ: Histopathology of the retinal pigment epithelium of a female carrier of choroideremia. Can J Ophthalmol 32:329–333, 1997.

Rodrigues MM, Ballintine EJ, Wiggert BN, Lee L, Fletcher RT, Chader GJ: Choroideremia: a clinical, electron microscopic, and biochemical report. Ophthalmology 91:873–883, 1984.

Seabra MC, Brown MS, Goldstein JL: Retinal degeneration in choroideremia: deficiency of rab geranylgeranyl transferase. Science 259:377–381, 1993.

**Other Heritable Disorders**

Bergsma DR Jr, Chen CJ: The Mizuo phenomenon in Oguchi disease. Arch Ophthalmol 115:560–561, 1997.

Carrero-Valenzuela RD, Klein ML, Weleber RG, Murphey WH, Litt M: Sorsby fundus dystrophy: a family with the Ser181Cys mutation of the tissue inhibitor of metalloproteinases 3. Arch Ophthalmol 114:737–738, 1996.

Nakazawa M, Wada Y, Fuchs S, Gal A, Tamai M: Oguchi disease: phenotypic characteristics of patients with the frequent 1147delA mutation in the arrestin gene. Retina 17:17–22, 1997.

Nichols BE, Drack AV, Vandenburgh K, Kimura AE, Sheffield VC, Stone EM: A 2 base pair deletion in the RDS gene associated with butterfly-shaped pigment dystrophy of the fovea. Hum Mol Genet 2:601–603, 1993.

Shastry BS, Hejtmancik JF, Trese MT: Identification of novel missense mutations in the Norrie disease gene associated with one X-linked and four sporadic cases of familial exudative vitreoretinopathy. Hum Mutat 9:396–401, 1997.

Sieving PA, Boskovich S, Bingham E, Pawar H: Sorsby's fundus dystrophy in a family with a Ser-181-CVS mutation in the TIMP-3 gene: poor outcome after laser photocoagulation. Trans Am Ophthalmol Soc 94:275–294; discussion 295–297, 1996.

Wong F, Goldberg MF, Hao Y. Identification of a nonsense mutation at codon 128 of the Norrie's disease gene in a male infant. Arch Ophthalmol 111:1553–1557, 1993.

**Peripheral Retinal Degenerations**

Foos RY: Senile retinoschisis: relationship to cystoid degeneration. Trans Am Acad Ophthalmol Otolaryngol 74:33–51, 1970.

Foos RY, Feman SS: Reticular cystoid degeneration of the peripheral retina. Am J Ophthalmol 69:392–403, 1970.

O'Malley PF, Allen RA: Peripheral cystoid degeneration of the retina: incidence and distribution in 1,000 autopsy eyes. Arch Ophthalmol 77:769–776, 1967.

O'Malley PF, Allen RA, Straatsma BR, et al: Pavingstone degeneration of the retina. Arch Ophthalmol 73:169–182, 1965.

Straatsma BR, Foos RY: Typical and reticular degenerative retinoschisis: XXVI Francis I. Proctor memorial lecture. Am J Ophthalmol 75:551–575, 1973.

Zimmerman LE, Spencer WH: The pathologic anatomy of retinoschisis: with a report of two cases diagnosed clinically as malignant melanoma. Arch Ophthalmol 63:10–19, 1960.

**Juvenile Retinoschisis**

Condon GP, Brownstein S, Wang NS, Kearns JA, Ewing CC: Congenital hereditary (juvenile X-linked) retinoschisis: histopathologic and ultrastructural findings in three eyes. Arch Ophthalmol 104:576–583, 1986.

Harris GS, Yeung J: Maculopathy of sex-linked juvenile retinoschisis. Can J Ophthalmol 11:1–10, 1976.

Manschot WA: Pathology of hereditary juvenile retinoschisis. Arch Ophthalmol 88:131–138, 1972.

Yanoff M, Kertesz Rahn E, Zimmerman LE: Histopathology of juvenile retinoschisis. Arch Ophthalmol 79:49–53, 1968.

**Lattice Degeneration**

Straatsma BR, Allen RA: Lattice degeneration of the retina. Trans Am Acad Ophthalmol Otolaryngol 66:600–613, 1962.

Straatsma BR, Zeegan PD, Foos RY, et al: Lattice degeneration of the retina. Trans Am Acad Ophthalmol Otolaryngol 78:87–113, 1974.

Streeten BW, Bert M: The retina surface in lattice degeneration of the retina. Am J Ophthalmol 74:1201–1209, 1972.

**Pars Plana Cysts**

Baker T, Spencer W: Ocular findings in multiple myeloma. Arch Ophthalmol 91:110, 1974.

Gärtner J: Fine structure of pars plana cysts. Am J Ophthalmol 73:971, 1972.

Johnson B: Proteinaceous cysts of the ciliary epithelium. II. Their occurrence in nonmyelomatous hypergammaglobulinemic conditions. Arch Ophthalmol 84:171, 1970.

Johnson B, Storey J: Proteinaceous cysts of the ciliary epithelium. I. Their clear nature and immunoelectrophoretic analysis in a case of multiple myeloma. Arch Ophthalmol 84:166, 1970.

Zimmerman L, Fine B: Production of hyaluronic acid by cysts and tumors of the ciliary body. Arch Ophthalmol 72: 365, 1964.

**Diabetic Retinopathy**

Aiello LP: Vascular endothelial growth factor: 20th-century mechanisms, 21st-century therapies. Invest Ophthalmol Vis Sci 38:1647–1652, 1997.

Aiello LP, Avery RL, Arrigg PG, et al. Vascular endothelial growth factor in ocular fluid of patients with diabetic retinopathy and other retinal disorders. N Engl J Med 331: 1480–1487, 1994.

Cogan DG, Toussaint D, Kuwabara T: Retinal vascular patterns. IV. Diabetic retinopathy. Arch Ophthalmol 66: 366–378, 1961.

D'Amore PA. Mechanisms of retinal and choroidal neovascularization. Invest Ophthalmol Vis Sci 35:3974–3979, 1994.

DCCT Research Group: The effect of intensive treatment of diabetes in the development and progression of long-term complications in insulin-dependent diabetes. N Engl J Med 329:977–986, 1993.

Engerman RL, Kern TS: Experimental galactosemia produces diabetic-like retinopathy. Diabetes 33:97–100, 1984.

Gabbay KH: The sorbitol pathway and the complications of diabetes mellitus. N Engl J Med 288:831–836, 1973.

Fine BS, Berkow JW, Helfgott JA: Diabetic lacy vacuolization of the iris pigment epithelium. Am J Ophthalmol 69: 197–200, 1970.

Frank RN: Etiologic mechanisms in diabetic retinopathy. In Ryan SJ (ed) Retina. Vol 2. St. Louis: Mosby, 1994: 1243–1276.

Jampol LM, Ebroon DA, Goldbaum MH: Peripheral proliferative retinopathies: an update on angiogenesis, etiologies and management. Surv Ophthalmol 38:519–540, 1994.

Kador PF, Akagi Y, Takahashi Y, et al: Prevention of retinal vessel changes associated with diabetic retinopathy in galactose-fed dogs by aldose reductase inhibitors. Arch Ophthalmol 108:1301–1309, 1990.

Klein R, Klein BEK, Moss SE, et al: The Wisconsin epidemiologic study of diabetic retinopathy. II. Prevalence and risk of diabetic retinopathy when age of diagnosis is less than 30 years. Arch Ophthalmol 102:520–526, 1984.

Klein R, Klein BEK, Moss SE, et al: The Wisconsin epidemiologic study of diabetic retinopathy. III. Prevalence and risk of diabetic retinopathy when age of diagnosis is 30 or more years. Arch Ophthalmol 102:527–532, 1984.

Kuwabara T, Cogan DG: Studies of retinal vascular patterns. I. Normal architecture. Arch Ophthalmol 64:904–911, 1960.

Yanoff M: Diabetic retinopathy. N Engl J Med 274: 1344–1349, 1966.

Yanoff M, Fine BS, Berkow JW: Diabetic lacy vacuolization of iris pigment epithelium. Am J Ophthalmol 69:201–210, 1970.

**Sickle Retinopathy**

Eagle RC Jr, Yanoff M, Fine BS: Hemoglobin SC retinopathy and fat emboli to the eye: a light and electron microscopical study. Arch Ophthalmol 92:28–32, 1974.

Goldberg MF: Classification and pathogenesis of proliferative sickle retinopathy. Am J Ophthalmol 71:649–665, 1971.

Romayananda N, Goldberg MF, Green WR: Histopathology of sickle cell retinopathy. Trans Am Acad Ophthalmol Otolaryngol 77:652–676, 1973.

**Macular Holes**

Frangieh GT, Green WR, Engel HM: A histopathologic study of macular cysts and holes. Retina 1:311–336, 1981.

Gass JD: Idiopathic senile macular hole: its early stages and pathogenesis. Arch Ophthalmol 106:629–639, 1988.

Gass JD: Reappraisal of biomicroscopic classification of stages of development of a macular hole. Am J Ophthalmol 119:752–759, 1995.

Yooh HS, Brooks HL Jr, Capone A Jr, L'Hernault NL, Grossniklaus HE: Ultrastructural features of tissue removed during idiopathic macular hole. Am J Ophthalmol 122:67–75, 1996.

**Retinal Detachment and Proliferative Vitreoretinopathy**

Aaberg TM: Management of anterior and posterior proliferative vitreoretinopathy. XLV. Edward Jackson memorial lecture. Am J Ophthalmol 106:519–532, 1988.

Elner SG, Elner VM, Diaz-Rohena R, Freeman HM, Tolentino FI, Albert DM: Anterior proliferative vitreoretinopathy: clinicopathologic, light microscopic, and ultrastructural findings. Ophthalmology 95:1349–1357, 1988.

Elner SG, Elner VM, Freeman HM, Tolentino FI, Albert DM: The pathology of anterior (peripheral) proliferative vitreoretinopathy. Trans Am Ophthalmol Soc 86: 330–353, 1988.

Lean JS, Stern WH, Irvine AR, Azen SP: Classification of proliferative vitreoretinopathy used in the silicone study: the Silicone Study Group. Ophthalmology 96:765–771, 1989.

Lewis H, Aaberg TM, Abrams GW, McDonald HR, Williams GA, Mieler WF: Subretinal membranes in proliferative vitreoretinopathy. Ophthalmology 96: 1403–1414; discussion 1414–1415, 1989.

Lewis H, Burke JM, Abrams GW, Aaberg TM: Perisilicone proliferation after vitrectomy for proliferative vitreoretinopathy. Ophthalmology 95:583–591, 1988.

Lopez PF, Grossniklaus HE, Aaberg TM, Sternberg P Jr, Capone A Jr, Lambert HM: Pathogenetic mechanisms in anterior proliferative vitreoretinopathy. Am J Ophthalmol 114:257–279, 1992.

Machemer R: Proliferative vitreoretinopathy (PVR): a personal account of its pathogenesis and treatment. Proctor lecture. Invest Ophthalmol Vis Sci 29:1771–1783, 1988.

Machemer R, Aaberg TM, Freeman HM, Irvine AR, Lean JS, Michels RM: An updated classification of retinal detachment with proliferative vitreoretinopathy. Am J Ophthalmol 112:159–165, 1991.

Mazure A, Grierson I: In vitro studies of the contractility of cell types involved in proliferative vitreoretinopathy. Invest Ophthalmol Vis Sci 33:3407–3416, 1992.

Schwartz D, de la Cruz ZC, Green WR, Michels RG: Proliferative vitreoretinopathy: ultrastructural study of 20 retroretinal membranes removed by vitreous surgery. Retina 8:275–281, 1988.

Wiedemann P, Weller M: The pathophysiology of proliferative vitreoretinopathy. Acta Ophthalmol Suppl 189:3–15, 1988.

Wilkes SR, Mansour AM, Green WR: Proliferative vitreoretinopathy: histopathology of retroretinal membranes. Retina 7:94–101, 1987.

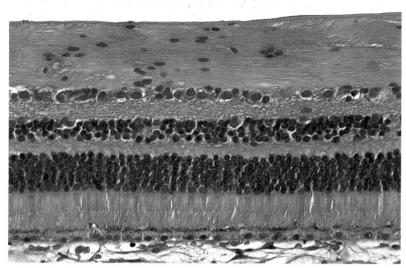

FIGURE 8–1 • **Retinal histology.** The retina's 10 layers include nuclear layers comprised of nuclei and plexiform layers comprised of axons and dendrites. "Inner" refers to layers toward the vitreous; "outer" refers to layers toward the sclera. Hematoxylin-eosin, ×100.

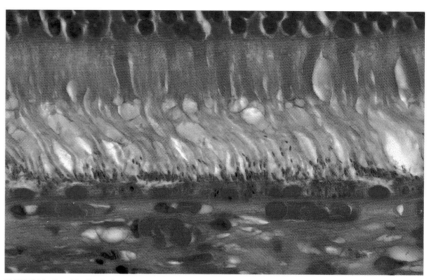

FIGURE 8–2 • **Retinal pigment epithelium and choroid.** The RPE rests on the inner surface of Bruch's membrane. Large ellipsoidal granules of melanin are present in the apical cytoplasm of the RPE cells. The large fenestrated capillaries of the choriocapillaris, that supply the outer retinal layers, are present underneath Bruch's membrane. Hematoxylin-eosin, ×250.

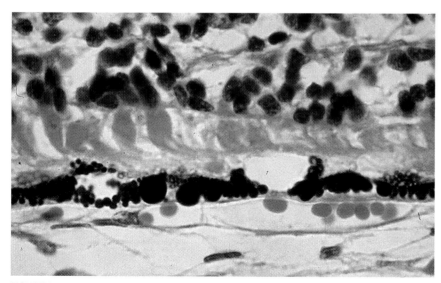

FIGURE 8–3 • **X-linked ocular albinism.** The RPE contains large spherical macromelanosomes. Hematoxylin-eosin, ×250. (Courtesy of Dr. W.R. Green. From Eagle RC Jr: Congenital, developmental and degenerative disorders of the iris and ciliary body. In: Albert DM, Jakobiec FA, eds. *Principles and Practice of Ophthalmology. Clinical Practice.* Vol 1. Philadelphia: Saunders, 1993:367–389)

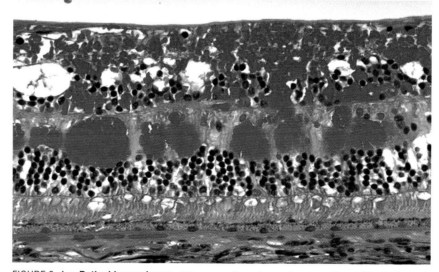

FIGURE 8–4 • **Retinal hemorrhages.** Flame or splinter hemorrhages are located in the inner nerve fiber layer of the retina. Blot and dot hemorrhages are located in the deeper retinal layers. Hematoxylin-eosin, ×100.

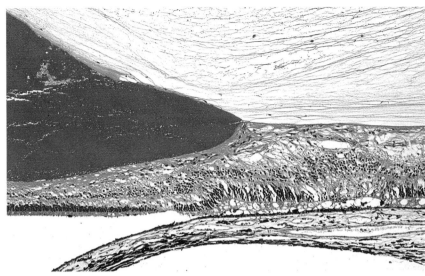

FIGURE 8–5 • **Subhyaloid hemorrhage, proliferative diabetic retinopathy.** The blood is located between the internal limiting membrane and the posterior surface of the detached vitreous. Hematoxylin-eosin, ×25.

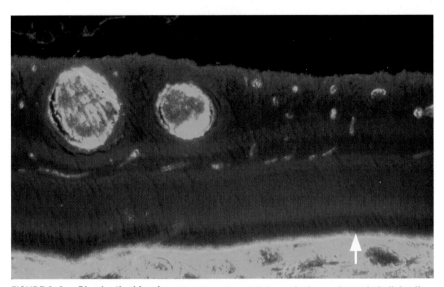

FIGURE 8–6 • **Blood retinal barrier.** Tight junctions joining retinal vascular endothelial cells constitute the inner part of the blood–retinal barrier, which confines fluorescein dye within lumina of retinal vessels. Occluding junctions joining apices of RPE cells comprise the outer part of the barrier. Choriocapillaris is composed of leaky fenestrated capillaries. Arrow denotes yellow band of autofluorescent lipofuscin in the RPE. Freeze-dried preparation, fluorescent microscopy, ×100. (From Eagle RC: Mechanisms of maculopathy. *Ophthalmology* 91:613–625, 1984, Courtesy of *Ophthalmology*).

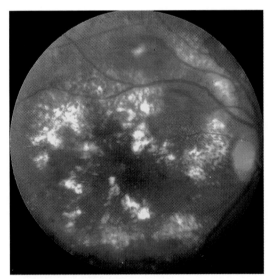

FIGURE 8–7 • **Retinal hard exudates.** Posterior pole contains numerous hard exudates. A cotton wool spot is seen superiorly.

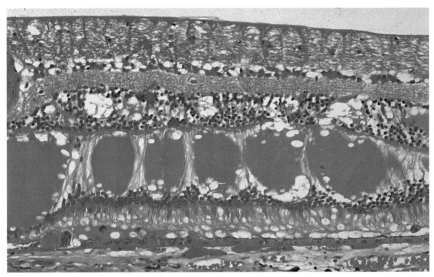

FIGURE 8–8 • **Retinal hard exudates.** The pools of eosinophilic protein-rich fluid in the outer plexiform layer (OPL) are hard exudates. Hard exudates typically occur in the OPL because that layer is the watershed zone between the retina's two blood supplies. Hematoxylin-eosin, ×100.

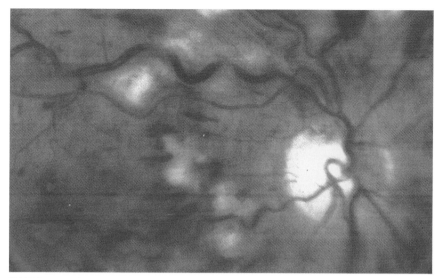

FIGURE 8–9 • **Cotton wool spots.** Cotton wool spots represent focal areas where axoplasmic flow is blocked in the nerve fiber layer. They are a clinical marker for retinal ischemia.

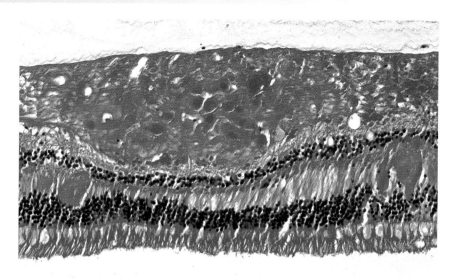

FIGURE 8–10 • **Cotton wool spot.** The nerve fiber layer is focally thickened by eosinophilic axoplasm. Several cytoid bodies with prominent eosinophilic nucleoids are evident. Small, hard exudates are seen in the outer plexiform layer. Hematoxylin-eosin, ×100.

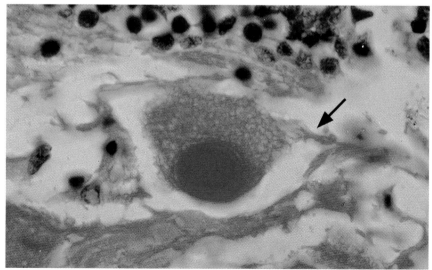

FIGURE 8–11 • **Cytoid body, cotton wool spot.** Cytoid bodies resemble cells but actually are focal areas of axonal swelling. Eosinophilic staining distinguishes the nucleoid in the cytoid body from a nucleus. Several axons are greatly distended with frothy pink axoplasm. An axon enters the cytoid body (arrow). Hematoxylin-eosin, ×250.

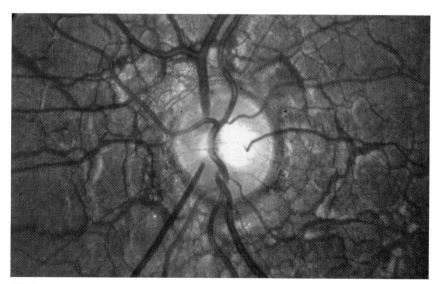

FIGURE 8–12 • **Angioid streaks.** The gray linear structures radiating from the optic disk in an *angioid*, or vessel-like, pattern are angioid streaks. They occur in several systemic disorders marked by massive calcification of Bruch's membrane.

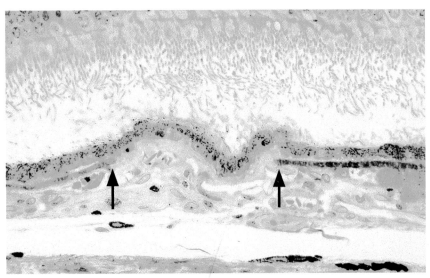

FIGURE 8–13 • **Angioid streak.** Arrows denote margins of a break in Bruch's membrane. Heavily calcified Bruch's membrane appears as a thick, dark band underneath the RPE. The RPE is intact overlying the break in Bruch's membrane. The patient had sickle cell anemia. Toluidine blue, ×150. (From Jampol LM, Acheson R, Eagle RC Jr, Serjeant G, O'Grady R. Calcification of Bruch's membrane in angioid streaks with homozygous sickle cell disease. *Arch Ophthalmol* 105:93–98, 1987. Copyright 1987 American Medical Association)

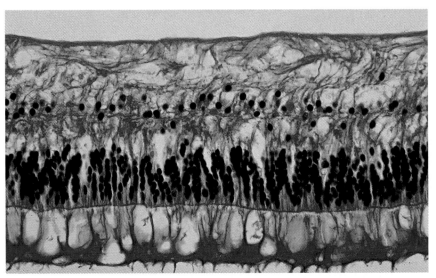

FIGURE 8–14 • **Inner ischemic retinal atrophy, central retinal artery occlusion.** All of the inner layers of the retina supplied by the central retinal artery are atrophic, including the inner plexiform and nuclear layers, which are spared in glaucomatous atrophy. A few nuclei persist in the outer part of the inner nuclear layer. Hematoxylin-eosin, ×100.

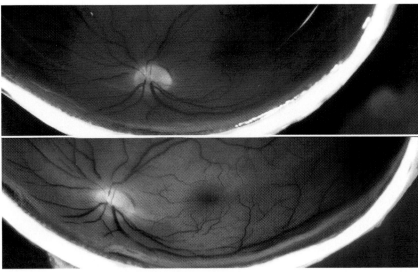

FIGURE 8–15 • **Retinal opacification.** The retina of freshly enucleated unfixed eye (*top*) is transparent. Fixation causes retinal opacification (*bottom*). Cellular death caused by ischemia causes similar retinal opacification after central retinal artery occlusion.

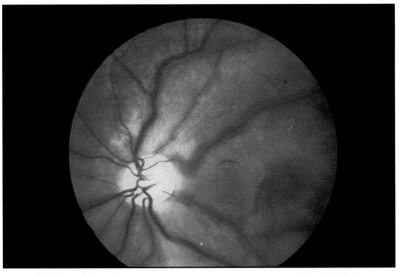

FIGURE 8–16 • **Central retinal artery occlusion.** Foveola appears as a cherry red spot in opacified, infarcted retina.

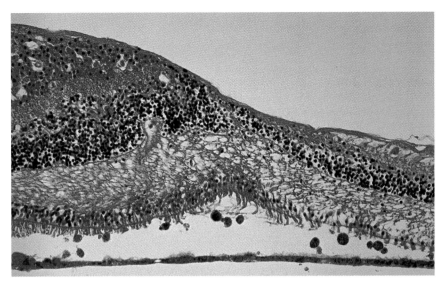

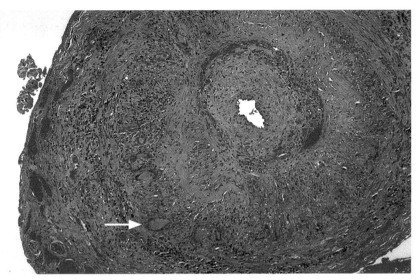

FIGURE 8–17 • **Branch retinal artery occlusion, fovea.** The fovea is seen centrally. The layers of the perfused parafoveal retina at left are well preserved. The retina supplied by the obstructed arteriole (at right) shows marked inner ischemic atrophy. The ganglion cell layer is absent, and the inner nuclear layer is reduced in caliber. Photoreceptor atrophy was caused by a shallow detachment of the macula. Hematoxylin-eosin, ×50.

FIGURE 8–18 • **Giant cell arteritis, temporal artery biopsy.** The lumen of the chronically inflamed artery is largely occluded. Chronic inflammatory cells including epithelioid histiocytes, giant cells, and lymphocytes infiltrate the vessel wall. There is extensive destruction of the lamina and the muscularis and fibrosis of the adventitia. Giant cell arteritis is an important cause of artery occlusion and ischemic optic neuropathy in elderly patients. Hematoxylin-eosin, ×25.

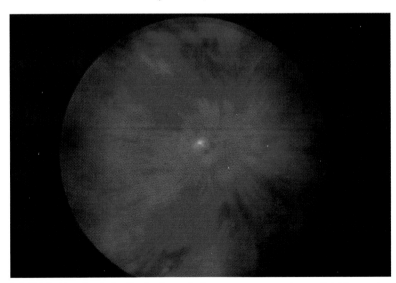

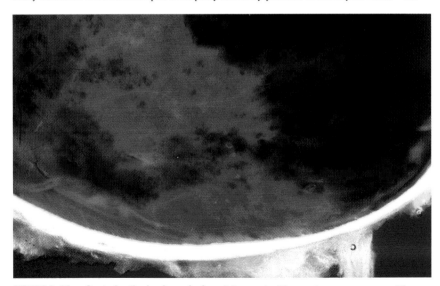

FIGURE 8–19 • **Central retinal vein occlusion.** Many deep and superficial hemorrhages are present. Retinal veins are dilated and tortuous. Cotton wool spots surrounding the swollen optic nerve indicate ischemia.

FIGURE 8–20 • **Central retinal vein occlusion.** Many retinal hemorrhages are present. The eye was enucleated for neovascular glaucoma.

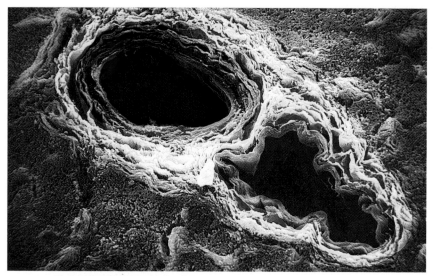

FIGURE 8–21 • **Central retinal artery and vein.** Common adventitial sheath (yellow) surrounds a central retinal artery (red) and vein (blue) in a transverse section of the optic nerve. Sclerosis of the artery is a factor in the pathogenesis of many cases of CRVO. False-colorized scanning electron micrograph.

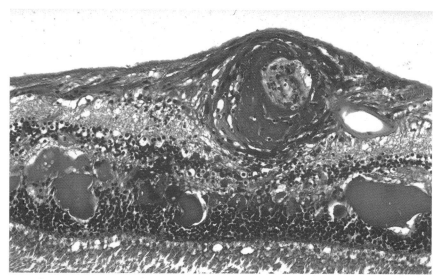

FIGURE 8–22 • **Retinal arterial macroaneurysm.** Proteinaceous material surrounds the thrombosed macroaneurysm in the inner retina. Pools of proteinaceous fluid comprising hard exudates are seen in the outer nuclear and outer plexiform layers. Hematoxylin-eosin, ×100.

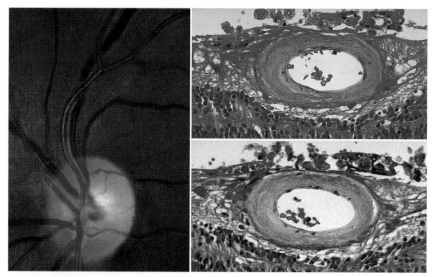

FIGURE 8–23 • **Retinal arteriolar sclerosis.** Copper-hued sclerotic arterioles and A-V crossing defects are seen in the fundus. Photomicrographs show a sclerotic vessel surrounded by a thick mantle of collagenous connective tissue. Blue staining with Masson trichrome (*bottom*) confirms the presence of collagen. Top inset: hematoxylin-eosin, ×100; bottom: Masson trichrome, ×100.

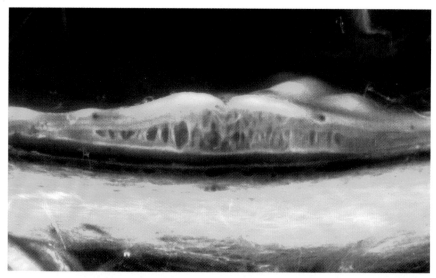

FIGURE 8–24 • **Cystoid macular edema.** The parafoveal retina is thickened by small intraretinal cysts. Most of the cysts are located in the outer layers of the retina. A small foveal pit persists. The gray cysts appear empty.

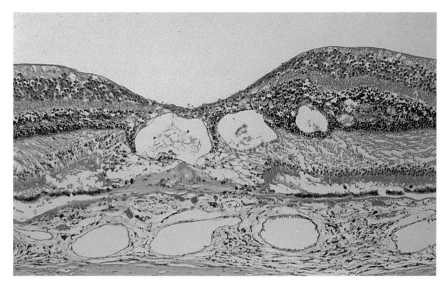

FIGURE 8–25 • **Cystoid macular edema.** Large cystoid spaces filled with granular protein-aceous fluid are seen in the outer plexiform and inner nuclear layers. A small subfoveal disci-form scar also is present. Hematoxylin-eosin, ×50.

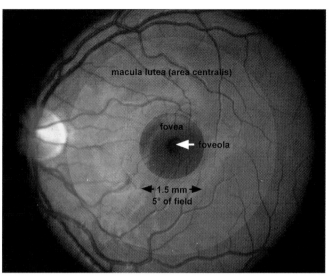

FIGURE 8–26 • **"Macula."** The foveola is located in the center of the 1.5 mm wide fovea, or pit. The area centralis is delimited by the temporal vascular arcades. The imprecise term macula (from macula lutea, "yellow spot") is often applied clinically to this region.

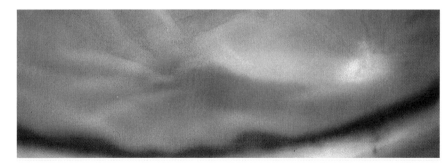

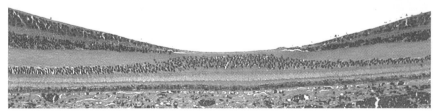

FIGURE 8–27 • **Macula lutea and fovea.** Retina of the posterior pole contains an irregular yellow spot of carotenoid xanthophyll pigment, which encompasses the fovea. Thin foveolar retina in the floor of the foveal pit, seen below, is comprised only of the photoreceptor and outer nuclear layers and part of the outer plexiform layers. Bottom: hematoxylin-eosin, ×25.

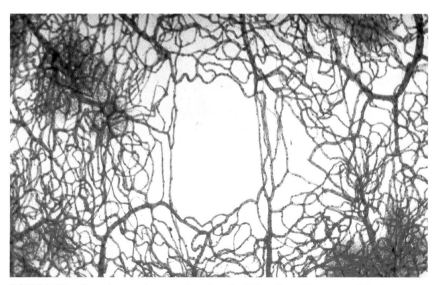

FIGURE 8–28 • **Foveal avascular zone, trypsin retinal digestion.** The center of the fovea is avascular because the retinal arterial capillaries penetrate only to the middle limiting membrane in the inner part of the outer plexiform layer. The inner retinal layers are absent in the foveola. Periodic acid-Schiff, ×20.

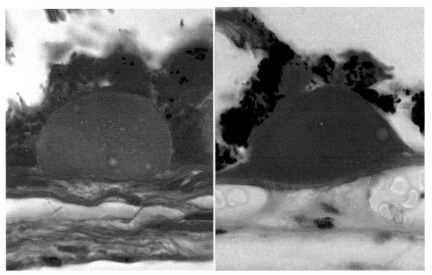

FIGURE 8–29 • **Cuticular drusen, Bruch's membrane.** Cuticular drusen are excrescences of homogeneous abnormal basement membrane material on the inner surface of Bruch's membrane. Drusen are synthesized by the RPE. Left: hematoxylin-eosin, ×250; right: periodic acid-Schiff, ×250.

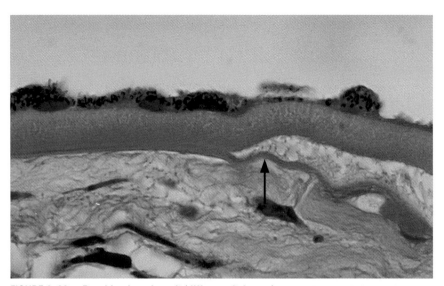

FIGURE 8–30 • **Basal laminar deposit (diffuse soft drusen).** A thick band of abnormal basement membrane material elevates the retinal pigment epithelium off the inner surface of Bruch's membrane. Part of the deposit has detached artifactitiously from Bruch's membrane (arrow). The RPE cells are flattened and atrophic. Basal laminar deposits predispose to RPE detachment and age-related macular degeneration. Hematoxylin-eosin, ×250.

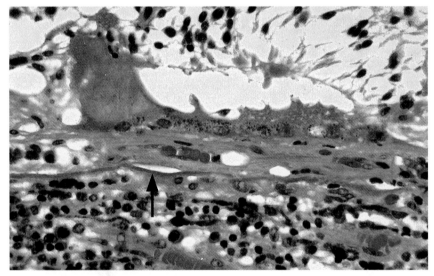

FIGURE 8–31 • **Subretinal neovascular membrane.** A thin layer of fibrous tissue containing capillaries elevates the atrophic RPE from the inner surface of Bruch's membrane. The atrophic outer retina shows extensive photoreceptor loss. Bruch's membrane (arrow) is fractured and focally calcified. The choroid contains an incidental focus of chronic inflammatory cells. Hematoxylin-eosin, ×100.

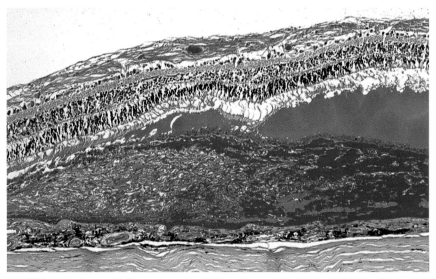

FIGURE 8–32 • **Age-related macular degeneration.** The retinal pigment epithelium is detached by blood and vascularized connective tissue. A collagenous disciform scar is forming on the inner surface of Bruch's membrane as the hemorrhagic RPE detachment undergoes organization. Hematoxylin-eosin, ×25.

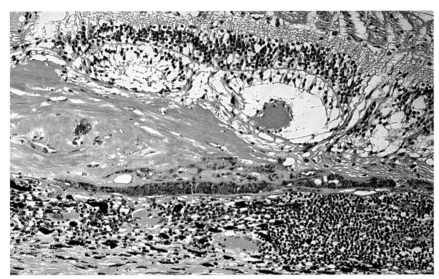

FIGURE 8–33 • **Disciform scar, ocular histoplasmosis syndrome.** A mound of connective tissue containing vessels and RPE cells rests on Bruch's membrane and focally detaches the retina. The photoreceptors are atrophic. Chronic inflammation is seen in the underlying choroid. Hematoxylin-eosin, ×100.

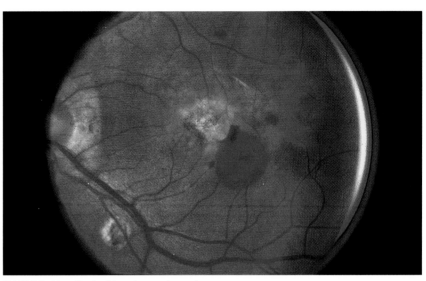

FIGURE 8–34 • **Ocular histoplasmosis syndrome.** The triad of hemorrhagic disciform macular scar, peripapillary chorioretinal atrophy, and "punched-out" chorioretinal scars are seen in the fundus.

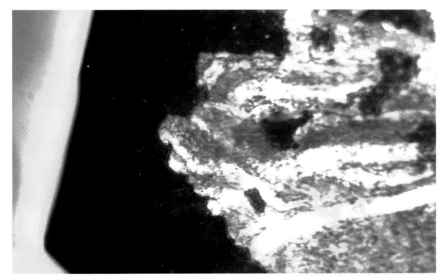

FIGURE 8–35 • **RPE and choroid.** RPE has been wiped-off Bruch's membrane (at right), disclosing large choroidal vessels. A concentration of dendritiform melanocytes between vessels in the heavily pigmented choroid causes a tigroid appearance. The reddish-brown RPE is largely responsible for the color of the fundus.

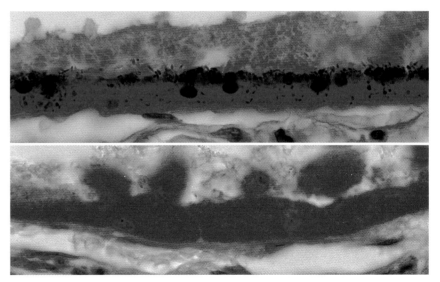

FIGURE 8–36 • **Fundus flavimaculatus.** RPE cells are packed with granules of PAS-positive material thought to be an abnormal form of lipofuscin. Nuclei in small peripheral RPE cells (*top*) are displaced apically. Posterior cells are abnormally large and amelanotic. The abnormal pigment in the RPE blocks normal choroidal fluorescence during intravenous fluorescein angiography, producing a dark choroid. Periodic acid-Schiff, ×250.

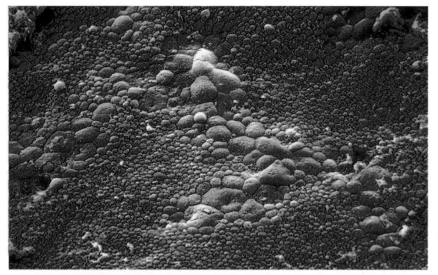

FIGURE 8–37 • **Abnormal RPE, fundus flavimaculatus.** False-colorized scanning electron micrograph shows aggregates of markedly enlarged RPE cells in the posterior part of the eye obtained postmortem from a patient with autosomal recessive fundus flavimaculatus. Hypothetically, the groups of large cells may appear as yellow spots clinically because they have less apical melanin pigment that the surrounding smaller, more normal cells. ×120. (From Eagle RC, Lucier AC, Bernardino VB, Yanoff M: Retinal pigment epithelial abnormalities in fundus flavimaculatus: a light and electron microscopic study. *Ophthalmology* 87:1189–1200, 1980. Courtesy of *Ophthalmology*)

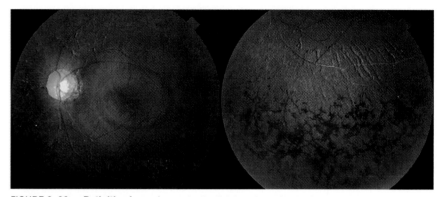

FIGURE 8–38 • **Retinitis pigmentosa.** Optic disk is pale and retinal vessels are attenuated (at left). Patchy bone spicule pigmentation ensheaths atrophic vessels in the peripheral retina.

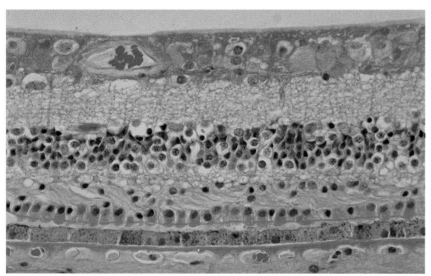

FIGURE 8–39 • **Autosomal dominant retinitis pigmentosa.** Only an interrupted monolayer of cone nuclei persists as the outer nuclear layer in the posterior part of the retina. The inner segments of the residual cones are grossly abnormal and outer segments are not seen. The RPE and the inner retinal layers are well preserved. (Case presented by Dr. David G. Cogan, Verhoeff Society, 1989)

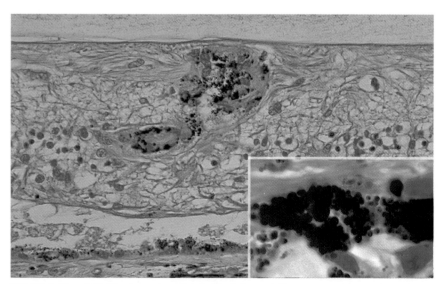

FIGURE 8–40 • **Retinitis pigmentosa, intraretinal pigmentation.** Focus of bone spicule pigmentation is comprised of perivascular proliferation of RPE cells. *Inset:* Macromelanosomes in hyperplastic RPE. Hematoxylin-eosin. Main figure ×100, inset ×250.

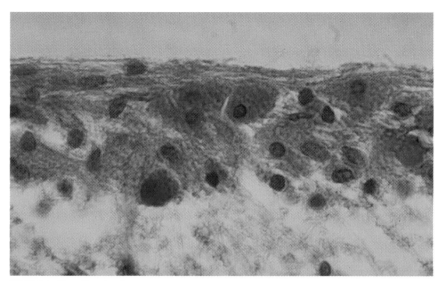

FIGURE 8–41 • **Tay-Sachs disease.** PAS-positive GM-2 ganglioside fills the cytoplasm of reti-nal ganglion cells. Opacification of thick perifoveal ganglion cell layer causes cherry red spot clinically. Periodic acid-Schiff, ×250.

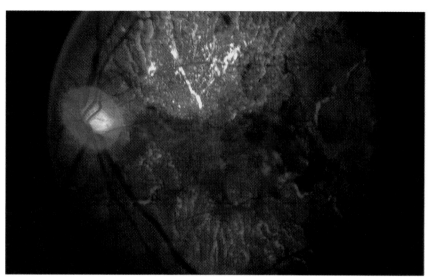

FIGURE 8–42 • **Thioridazine toxicity, RPE.** This psychiatric patient had received high doses of thiorizadine (Mellaril).

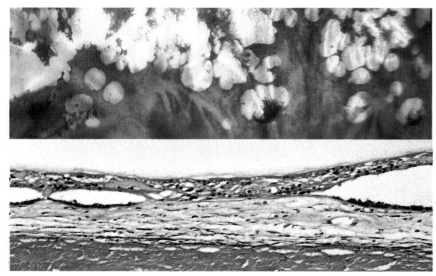

FIGURE 8–43 • **Peripheral chorioretinal atrophy (cobblestone or paving stone degeneration).** Photograph (*top*) shows yellow-white patches of chorioretinal atrophy with scalloped, sharply demarcated borders. Photomicrograph (*bottom*) shows firm chorioretinal adhesion binding the atrophic outer retina to the denuded segment of Bruch's membrane. The peripheral retina is thin and atrophic. Hematoxylin-eosin, ×25.

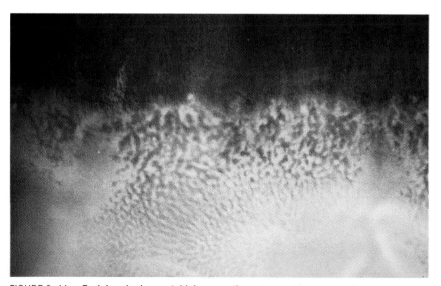

FIGURE 8–44 • **Peripheral microcystoid degeneration.** Array of interconnecting cystoid chan-nels is evident grossly as a stippled pattern in the peripheral retina bordering the ora serrata. Pe-ripheral microcystoid degeneration is almost a universal finding in the peripheral retina after age 8 years.

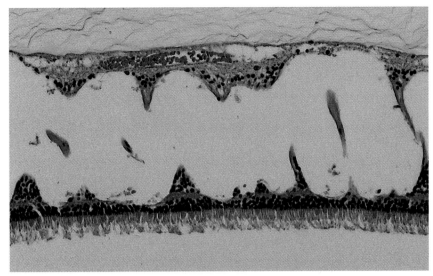

FIGURE 8–45 • **Peripheral microcystoid degeneration.** Cystoid spaces called Blessig-Iwanoff cysts are located in the mid-retina. The cysts contain hyaluronidase-sensitive acid mucopolysaccharide. Coalescence of the cysts causes typical degenerative retinoschisis. Early schisis formation is evident in this photomicrograph. Hematoxylin-eosin, ×50.

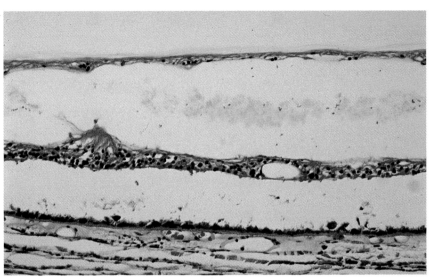

FIGURE 8–46 • **Typical degenerative retinoschisis.** Coalescence of Blessig-Iwanoff cysts has caused a split in the mid-retina. Hematoxylin-eosin, ×50.

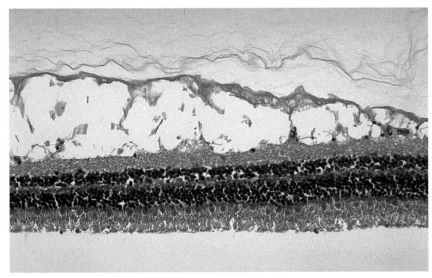

FIGURE 8–47 • **Reticular cystoid degeneration.** The cystoid spaces are located in the nerve fiber layer of the retina. Reticular cystoid degeneration always occurs posterior to a focus of typical peripheral microcystoid degeneration. It can evolve into reticular retinoschisis. Hematoxylin-eosin, ×50.

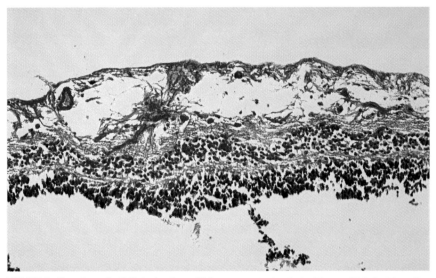

FIGURE 8–48 • **Juvenile X-linked retinoschisis.** The retinal split in this rare X-linked hereditary disorder is located in the nerve fiber layer. Many affected patients have stellate folds in the macula. Periodic acid-Schiff, ×50.

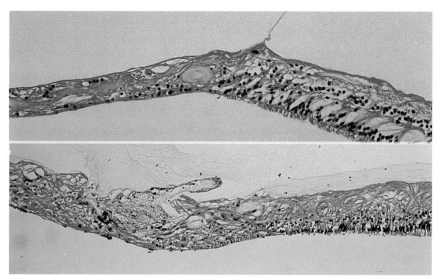

FIGURE 8–49 • **Lattice degeneration of the retina.** The involved part of the retina (*left*) is diffusely atrophic and disorganized. A sclerotic vessel is seen in the lesion above and an intraretinal focus of pigment below. Vitreous strands adhere to the margin of both foci. Tractional retinal breaks caused by vitreoretinal traction predispose to retinal detachment in patients with lattice degeneration. Pools of liquefied vitreous typically are found overlying lattice lesions, and the internal limiting membrane of the retina is focally absent. Both figures: hematoxylin-eosin, ×50.

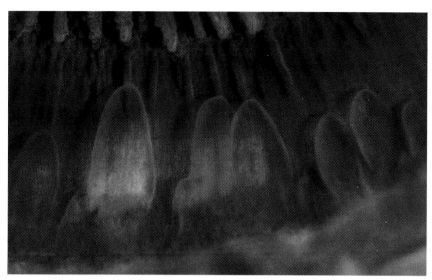

FIGURE 8–50 • **Pars plana cysts.** Cysts of the pars plana occasionally are found in eyes from elderly patients.

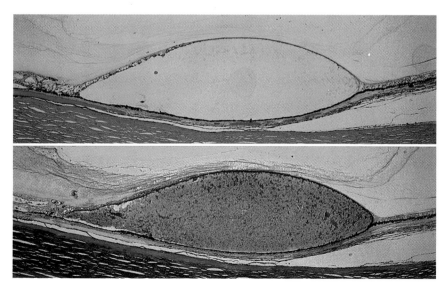

FIGURE 8–51 • **Pars plana cysts.** The inner nonpigmented layer of the ciliary epithelium has detached from the outer pigmented layer, which remains attached to the choroid. The blue substance in the cyst below is acid mucopolysaccharide, which was sensitive to hyaluronidase digestion. Top: hematoxylin-eosin, ×10; bottom: Hale's colloidal iron for AMP, ×10.

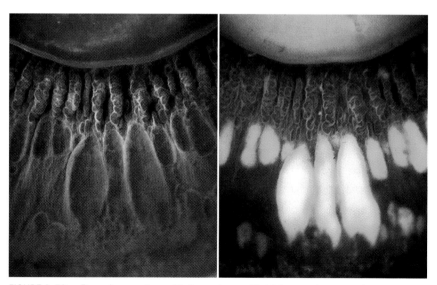

FIGURE 8–52 • **Pars plana cysts, multiple myeloma.** Multiple pars plana cysts in an eye obtained postmortem from a patient with multiple myeloma are seen before (*left*) and after (*right*) fixation. Fixation precipitates the myeloma protein filling the cysts, causing milky-white opacification. The cysts are clear *in vivo*.

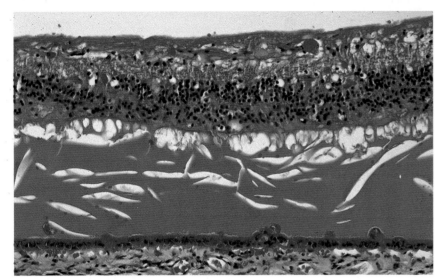

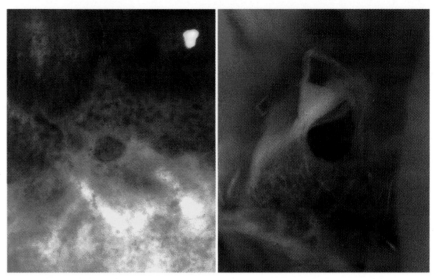

FIGURE 8–53 • **Chronic retinal detachment.** Eosinophilic proteinaceous fluid fills the subretinal space. The photoreceptors are totally absent, and the outer nuclear layer is mildly atrophic. The RPE shows focal budding. The subretinal fluid contains cholesterol clefts. Hematoxylin-eosin, ×100.

FIGURE 8–54 • **Retinal holes.** Peripheral microcystoid degeneration surrounds a round atrophic hole near the nasal ora serrata (at left). A tractional break that developed within a patch of perivascular lattice degeneration is seen at right.

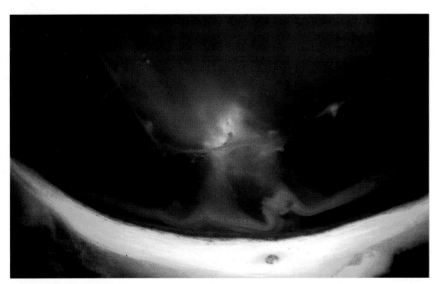

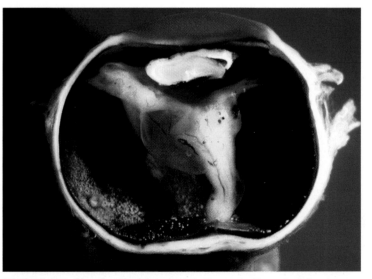

FIGURE 8–55 • **Tractional retinal detachment, proliferative diabetic retinopathy.** New vessels bridge the subretinal space and arborize on the posterior face of the detached vitreous. The organized vitreous is exerting anteroposterior traction on the retina, causing focal retinal detachment.

FIGURE 8–56 • **Chronic retinal detachment.** Long-standing retinal detachments typically have a funnel or morning glory configuration caused by proliferative vitreoretinopathy. Retinal macrocysts are an indicator of chronicity.

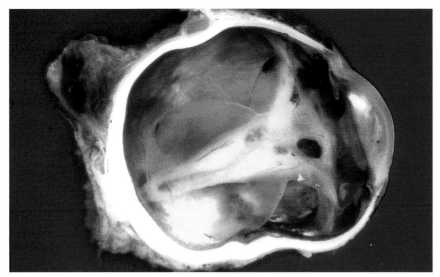

**FIGURE 8–57 • Chronic retinal detachment wtih macrocystic degeneration.** Large cyst arises from the stalk of a chronic funnel-shaped retinal detachment. Extensive PVR is present. The eye has had prior surgery for retinal detachment.

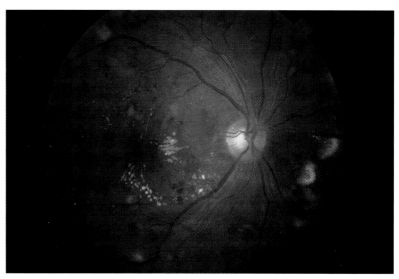

**FIGURE 8–58 • Background diabetic retinopathy.** Retinal hemorrhages, hard yellow waxy exudates, cotton wool spots, and retinal edema are present.

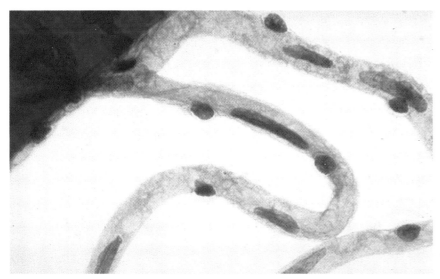

**FIGURE 8–59 • Normal retinal capillaries, trypsin retinal digestion.** Normal retinal capillaries are comprised of approximately equal numbers of endothelial cells and pericytes. The nuclei of the endothelial cells are cigar-shaped. The pericyte nuclei are round. The pericytes are embedded in the basement membrane of the capillary wall. Periodic acid-Schiff, ×250.

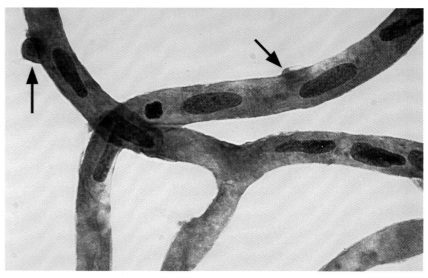

**FIGURE 8–60 • Retinal capillaries in diabetes mellitus, trypsin retinal digestion.** A preferential loss of pericytes occurs during the early stages of diabetic retinopathy, disturbing the normal 1:1 ratio between pericytes and endothelial cells. Arrows denote pericyte ghosts in the capillary basement membrane. Diabetic thickening of the basement membrane causes intense staining with PAS stain. Periodic acid-Schiff, ×250.

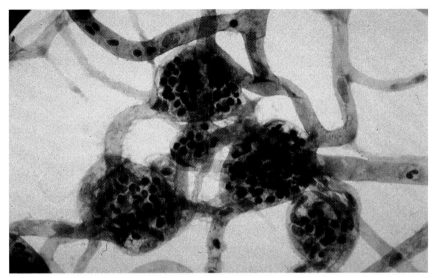

FIGURE 8–61 • **Diabetic microaneurysms, trypsin retinal digestion.** Periodic acid-Schiff, ×100.

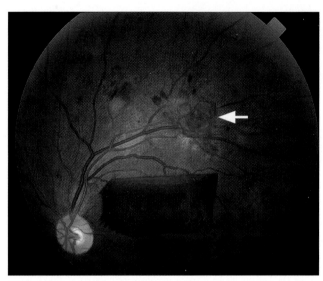

FIGURE 8–62 • **Proliferative diabetic retinopathy.** Arrow points to a large frond of vitreoretinal neovascularization above a flat-topped subhyaloid hemorrhage. Fluorescein retinopathy disclosed extensive retinal capillary nonperfusion.

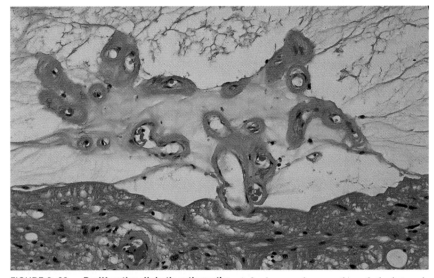

FIGURE 8–63 • **Proliferative diabetic retinopathy.** A feeder vessel passes through the internal limiting membrane and enters the base of the neovascular frond. The new vessels are encompassed by collagen. Hematoxylin-eosin, ×100.

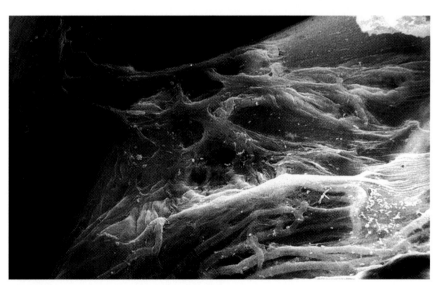

FIGURE 8–64 • **Proliferative diabetic retinopathy.** Scanning electron microscopy discloses new vessels proliferating on a scaffold of posteriorly detached vitreous.

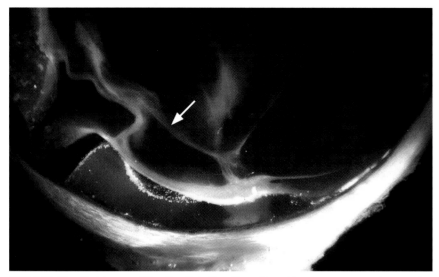

FIGURE 8–65 • **Endstage proliferative diabetic retinopathy.** Fibrosis accentuates the posterior face of the organized and partially detached vitreous (arrow), which remains focally adherent to the retina. Anteroposterior traction lines are evident. Blood fills the subhyaloid space where the organized posterior hyaloid face bridges the retina. The formed vitreous contains blood. Gelatinous subretinal fluid detaches the posterior retina. The glistening white particles in the subretinal fluid are lipid histiocytes.

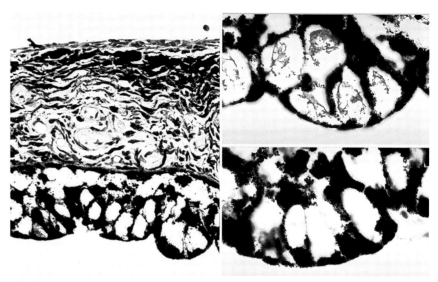

FIGURE 8–66 • **Diabetic iridopathy.** A fibrovascular membrane flattens the anterior iridic surface. Multiple vacuoles impart a lacy appearance to the thickened iris pigment epithelium. The vacuoles are filled with PAS-positive granules of glycogen (*top inset*) which are digested by diastase (*bottom inset*). Main figure: hematoxylin-eosin, ×50; top inset: periodic acid-Schiff (PAS), ×250; bottom inset: PAS with diastase, ×250.

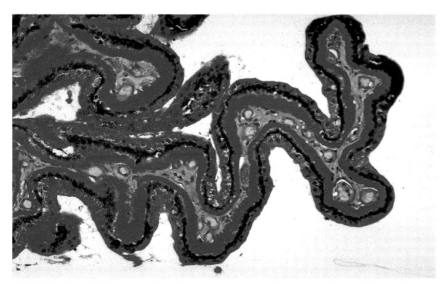

FIGURE 8–67 • **Thickening of ciliary body basement membrane, diabetes mellitus.** PAS stain accentuates massive thickening of the basement membrane of the pigmented pars plicata ciliary epithelium in an eye from a relatively young diabetic patient. Periodic acid-Schiff, ×100.

# CHAPTER 9

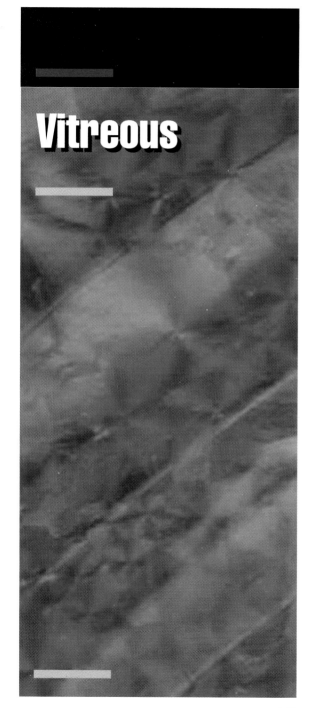

# Vitreous

The transparent gelatinous vitreous humor fills most of the interior of the eye. The vitreous humor is the most delicate connective tissue in the body. It is composed of a framework of thin, randomly oriented, unbranched fibrils of type II collagen, and it is rich in hyaluronic acid, an extremely large, negatively charged, hydrophilic polysaccharide. Hyaluronic acid is named after the hyaloid body, an older term for the vitreous humor. (Both *hyaloid* and *vitreous* mean *glassy*.)

The collagenous framework of the vitreous humor adheres to the internal limiting membrane of the retina, the periphery of the optic disk, and most firmly to the 2 mm wide vitreous base that straddles the ora serrata. The anterior attachment of the vitreous is particularly firm. Relatively severe trauma that typically disrupts the ciliary epithelium is required to detach or avulse the vitreous from the vitreous base. In contrast, the posterior attachments of the vitreous are tenuous. Posterior vitreous detachment affects many individuals after age 55 years and is found in more than 60% of the population during the eighth decade (Fig. 9–1). Patients usually complain of the abrupt onset of floaters and occasionally light flashes, which signify vitreoretinal traction. The peripapillary condensation of the vitreous framework may be evident clinically or macroscopically after detachment as a Weiss ring (Fig. 9–2).

The vitreous humor contributes to visual loss in two basic ways. First, the vitreous framework serves as a growth scaffold for cellular proliferation, and resultant vitreoretinal traction plays an important role in the pathogenesis of many retinal detachments. Second, under pathologic conditions the transparent medium may be opacified by the accumulation of materials, including blood, acute or chronic inflammatory or tumor cells, iridescent particles, and amyloid.

Vitreoretinal adhesions and traction cause retinal holes or breaks that predispose to rhegmatogenous retinal detachment. New blood vessels, cells, and fibrous tissue also proliferate on exposed surfaces of the vitreous framework. Tractional retinal detachment is caused by subsequent organization and contraction of the vitreous. The organization of vitreous hemorrhage or inflammation also stimulates vitreous traction.

Detachment of the vitreous and retina exposes new surfaces that can serve as a substrate for cellular growth. The contraction of delicate glial membranes on the inner retinal surface causes sinuous folds in the internal limiting membrane (surface wrinkling or cellophane retinopathy) that distort vision (Figs. 9–3, 9–4). Proliferation of myofibroblasts, retinal pigment epithelial (RPE) cells, and glial cells forms fibrocellular membranes on retinal surfaces exposed by retinal detachment. These membranes can bind the detached retina into a folded mass that may be impossible to reattach surgically. Analogous cellular proliferation can also occur on the detached posterior face of the vitreous, inducing fibrosis. Somewhat analogous to "*in vivo* tissue culture," this process is called proliferative vitreoretinopathy (PVR). PVR is an important cause of inoperable retinal detachment, or recurrent detachment after reattachment surgery (Fig. 9–5).

The most common substance that opacifies the vitreous is blood. Common sources of vitreous hemorrhage include trauma, proliferative diabetic retinopathy and other disorders with vitreoretinal neovascularization, tractional retinal tears, and posterior vitreous detachment. Rarer causes include intraocular tumors, exudative age-related macular degeneration, and subarachnoid hemorrhage (Terson syndrome).

Vitreous hemorrhage is a major indication for vitreous surgery. Blood and other opacities in the vitreous are removed by a surgical procedure called vitrectomy. This procedure employs miniaturized cutting and aspiration instruments, intraocular illuminators, and laser photocoagulators, which are inserted through small incisions in the pars plana. The excised vitreous is replaced with saline, introduced through an infusion port.

Vitrectomy specimens are processed for histopathology by Millipore filtration or cytocentrifugation. The filter and its entrapped fragments of ocular tissue are stained and mounted on a microslide. If particulates are numerous, the fluid can be centrifuged and the pellet embedded in paraffin as a cell block for histologic study.

Microscopic examination of a vitrectomy specimen from a case of chronic vitreous hemorrhage discloses blood and blood-breakdown products including erythroclasts or erythrocyte ghost cells, hemoglobin spherules, and macrophages laden with ghost cells and golden-brown granules of the blood pigment hemosiderin (Figs. 9–6, 9–7). In chronic cases the blood-breakdown products occasionally stimulate a granulomatous inflammatory foreign body response. Hemoglobin spherules may be quite large if the vitreous blood originates from the choroid. Clinically and macroscopically, chronic vitreous hemorrhage typically is yellow-ochre and may appear as an "ochre membrane" (Fig. 9–8). If the anterior face of the vitreous is ruptured, ghost cells and hemosiderin-laden macrophages may enter the anterior chamber and block the trabecular meshwork, causing secondary open-angle glaucoma (ghost cell or hemolytic glaucoma).

The vitreous is rapidly opacified by an intense influx of polymorphonuclear leukocytes and macrophages in acute purulent endophthalmitis (see Fig. 2–19). A vitreous abscess comprised of polymorphonuclear neutrophils (polys) forms in neglected cases or virulent infections. Some of the inflammatory cells in a vitreous abscess may be arranged in a linear fashion, reflecting the alignment of the cells along the fibrils of the collagenous vitreous framework. A large solitary vitreous abscess characterizes bacterial endophthalmitis. Fungal endophthalmitis, which is generally a more indolent infection, typically is marked by the presence of multiple small vitreous microabscesses (see Figs. 2–21, 2–22). Digestive enzymes released from degenerating polys in a vitreous abscess cause extensive necrosis of intraocular tissues including retinal destruction. Vitrectomy is used to "drain" the vitreous abscess surgically in some patients with endophthalmitis. If vitrectomy is not performed, the vitreous may be organized by an ingrowth of granulation tissue from the ciliary body and choroid. Eventually, a dense collagenous scar elaborated by fibroblasts and metaplastic RPE cells fills the vitreous cavity.

Remnants of the embryonic hyaloid vascular system are seen by patients as innocuous vitreous opacities called floaters, or muscae volitantes ("flying flies"). Patients frequently complain that they see a spot like a moving insect in their peripheral visual field. Floaters are especially prevalent in myopes and are caused by syneresis or degeneration of the vitreous framework in the enlarging myopic eye. When light flashes accompany floaters, vitreoretinal traction is present and retinal holes must be excluded by a careful ophthalmoscopic examination.

Iridescent particles accumulate in the vitreous humor in two disorders: asteroid hyalosis and synchysis scintillans. Asteroid hyalosis (Benson's disease) is relatively common, occurring in about 1% of the population (Figs. 9–9, 9–10, 9–11). Asteroid hyalosis was once called asteroid hyalitis, but the name was changed when it became apparent that the disorder is degenerative, not inflammatory, in nature.

Clinical examination with the slit lamp biomicroscope or ophthalmoscope discloses a starry array of white iridescent particles in the vitreous (Fig. 9–9). The asteroid bodies are firmly attached to the vitreous framework; they move with the vitreous and do not sink to the bottom of the eye. The iridescent particles are tiny spherules of calcium soap in the form of phospholipid liquid crystals. The spherules stain gray with hematoxylin-eosin (H&E), are moderately periodic acid-Schiff (PAS)-positive, and show a positive histochemical reaction for calcium (Fig. 9–10). They show a vivid "Maltese cross" pattern of birefringence on polarization microscopy (Fig. 9–11). How and why the spherules form is uncertain. Asteroid hyalosis has been reported to be more common in patients who have coronary artery disease and gout.

Synchisis scintillans is a rare disorder marked by the accumulation of sparkling crystals of cholesterol in the vitreous (Fig. 9–12). It is said to occur bilaterally in young patients, who are blind from a chronic degenerative disorder. Although intraocular cholesterol (cholesterolosis bulbi) is not that uncommon, involvement of the vitreous is unusual. Cholesterol crystals typically are found in the subretinal fluid of chronic exudative detachments caused by retinal vascular abnormalities (e.g., Coats' disease, diabetes, or radiation retinopathy), or less often in the anterior chamber. Blood breakdown is a major source of intraocular cholesterol. Erythrocyte cell membranes are an excellent source of the lipid. The cholesterol crystals in synchisis scintillans are not attached to the vitreous framework, and they sink to a dependent position when the eye is at rest.

The first therapeutic vitrectomy was performed for vitreous amyloidosis (Figs. 9–13, 9–14). This rare form of vitreous opacification occurs in patients who have several types of primary familial amyloidosis (familial amyloidotic polyneuropathy) that are caused by autosomal recessively inherited allelic missense mutations in the gene for transthyretin, a plasma transport protein for vitamin A and thyroid hormone. Many patients who present with vitreous involvement are elderly women who have the Portuguese variant (methionine 30 substitution) of familial amyloidosis. The family history is typically negative, and vitreous amyloidosis is often the initial manifestation of the disease.

Tumors cells can infiltrate or seed the vitreous humor. Primary lymphoma of the central nervous system

(CNS) and retina characteristically involves the vitreous. This rare form of primary CNS lymphoma should be suspected in elderly patients who have chronic vitritis that does not respond to therapy. Cytologic examination of diagnostic vitrectomy specimens reveals a highly cellular and extensively necrotic infiltrate that contains atypical lymphocytes with prominent nucleoli and protrusions of the nuclear membrane (Fig. 9–15). The lymphoma cells also infiltrate the retina and typically collect between Bruch's membrane and the retinal pigment epithelium, forming solid yellowish RPE detachments. If vitreous lymphoma is diagnosed, imaging studies and spinal fluid examination should be performed to exclude CNS involvement. The vitreous usually is spared when disseminated, non-CNS, visceral lymphomas involve the eye secondarily. Such lymphomas usually involve the uvea. Many patients who undergo diagnostic vitrectomy to exclude lymphoma are found to have a form of granulomatous vitritis termed idiopathic senile vitritis. Cytologically, the latter lacks necrosis and contains a mixture of well-differentiated lymphocytes and epithelioid histiocytes with a spindled or dendritiform configuration. Careful cytologic screening and follow-up are warranted in such cases, however, because vitreous lymphoma occasionally presents with chronic inflammation.

Uveitis and vitritis occur rarely in Whipple's disease. PAS-positive macrophages filled with bacterial cell walls and degenerating *Tropheryma whippelii* bacteria comprise the retinal and vitreal infiltrate in Whipple's disease (Fig. 9–16). Endophytic or diffuse infiltrating retinoblastomas often cause vitreous seeding (Fig. 9–17).

# R e f e r e n c e s

## General References

Brucker AJ, Michels RG, Green WR: Pars plana vitrectomy in the management of blood-induced glaucoma with vitreous hemorrhage. Ann Ophthalmol 10:1427–1437, 1978.

Chess J, Sebag J, Tolentino FI, et al: Pathologic processing of vitrectomy specimens: a comparison of findings with celloidin bag and cytocentrifugation of 102 vitrectomy specimens. Ophthalmology 90:1560–1564, 1983.

Eagle RC Jr: Specimen handling in the ophthalmic pathology laboratory. Ophthalmol Clin North Am 8:1–15, 1995.

Eagle RC Jr: The pathology of vitrectomy specimens. In Cohen EJ (ed) The Year Book of Ophthalmology, 1996. St. Louis: Mosby, 1996:353–368.

Engel H, de la Cruz ZC, Jiminiz-Abalihin LD, et al: Cytopreparatory techniques for eye fluid specimens obtained by vitrectomy. Acta Cytol 26:551–560, 1982.

Engel HM, Green WR, Michels RG, et al: Diagnostic vitrectomy. Retina 1:121–149, 1981.

Green WR: Diagnostic cytopathology of ocular fluid specimens. Ophthalmology 91:726–749, 1984.

Spencer WH: The vitreous. In Spencer WH (ed) Ophthalmic Pathology: An Atlas and Textbook. 3rd ed. Philadelphia: Saunders, 1985:548–588.

Streeten BAW, Wilson DJ: Disorders of the vitreous. In Garner A, Klintworth GK (eds) Pathobiology of Ocular Disease: A Dynamic Approach. 2nd ed. Part A. New York: Marcel Dekker, 1994:701–742.

## Posterior Vitreous Detachment

Foos RY: Posterior vitreous detachment. Trans Am Acad Ophthalmol Otolaryngol 76:480–497, 1972.

Foos RY, Wheeler NC: Vitreoretinal juncture synchysis senilis and posterior vitreous detachment. Ophthalmology 89:1502–1512, 1982.

Foos RY, Kreiger AE, Forsythe AB, Zakka KA: Posterior vitreous detachment in diabetic subjects. Ophthalmology 87:122–128, 1980.

Linder B: Acute posterior vitreous detachment and its retinal complications: a clinical biomicroscopic study. Acta Ophthalmol (Scand) Suppl 87:1–108, 1966.

## Vitreoretinal Membranes and Proliferative Vitreoretinopathy

Clarkson JG, Green WR, Massof D: A histopathologic review of 168 cases of preretinal membrane. Am J Ophthalmol 84:1–17, 1977.

Elner SG, Elner VM, Diaz-Rohena R, Freeman HM, Tolentino FI, Albert DM: Anterior proliferative vitreoretinopathy: clinicopathologic, light microscopic, and ultrastructural findings. Ophthalmology 95:1349–1357, 1988.

Elner SG, Elner VM, Freeman HM, Tolentino FI, Albert DM: The pathology of anterior (peripheral) proliferative vitreoretinopathy. Trans Am Ophthalmol Soc 86:330–353, 1988.

Kampik A, Kenyon KR, Michels RG, et al: Epiretinal and vitreous membranes: a comparative study of 56 cases. Arch Ophthalmol 99:1445–1453, 1981.

Lopez PF, Grossniklaus HE, Aaberg TM, Sternberg P Jr, Capone A Jr, Lambert HM: Pathogenetic mechanisms in anterior proliferative vitreoretinopathy. Am J Ophthalmol 114:257–279, 1992.

Machemer R, Aaberg TM, Freeman HM, Irvine AR, Lean JS, Michels RM: An updated classification of retinal detachment with proliferative vitreoretinopathy. Am J Ophthalmol 112:159–165, 1991.

Michels RG: A clinical and histopathologic study of epiretinal membranes affecting the macula and removed by vitreous surgery. Trans Am Ophthalmol Soc 80:580–656, 1980.

Peczon BD, Wolfe JK, Gipson IK, Hirose T, et al: Characterization of membranes removed during open-sky vitrectomy. Invest Ophthalmol Vis Sci 24:1382–1389, 1983.

Schwartz D, de la Cruz ZC, Green WR, Michels RG: Proliferative vitreoretinopathy: ultrastructural study of 20 retroretinal membranes removed by vitreous surgery. Retina 8:275–281, 1988.

Wilkes SR, Mansour AM, Green WR: Proliferative vitreoretinopathy: histopathology of retroretinal membranes. Retina 7:94–101, 1987.

## Vitreous Hemorrhage

Campbell DG: Ghost cell glaucoma following trauma. Ophthalmology 88:1151–1158, 1981.

Campbell DG, Simmons RJ, Grant WM: Ghost cells as a cause of glaucoma. Am J Ophthalmol 81:441–450, 1976.

Grossniklaus HE, Frank E, Fahri DC, et al: Hemoglobin spherulosis in the vitreous cavity. Arch Ophthalmol 106:961–962, 1988.

Meredith TA, Gordon PA: Pars plana vitrectomy for severe penetrating injury with posterior segment involvement. Am J Ophthalmol 103:549–554, 1987.

Ryan SJ: Penetrating ocular trauma and pars plana vitrectomy. Trans New Orleans Acad Ophthalmol 31:129–136, 1983.

Spraul CW, Grossniklaus HE: Vitreous hemorrhage. Surv Ophthalmol 42:3–39, 1997.

## Asteroid Hyalosis

Bergren RL, Brown GC, Duker JS: Prevalence and association of asteroid hyalosis with systemic diseases. Am J Ophthalmol 111:289–293, 1991.

Eagle RC, Yanoff M: Cholesterolosis of the anterior chamber. Graefes Arch Ophthalmol 193:121, 1975.

Miller H, Miller B, Rabinowitz H, Zonis S, Nir I: Asteroid bodies—an ultrastructural study. Invest Ophthalmol Vis Sci 24:133–136, 1983.

Renaldo DP: Pars plana vitrectomy for asteroid hyalosis. Retina 1:252–254, 1981.

Safir A, Dunn SN, Martin RG, Tate GW, Mincey GJ: Is asteroid hyalosis ocular gout? Ann Ophthalmol 22:70–77, 1990.

Streeten BW: Vitreous asteroid bodies: ultrastructural characteristics and composition. Arch Ophthalmol 100:969–975, 1982.

Topilow HW, Kenyon KR, Takahashi M, Freeman HM, Tolentino FI, Hanninen LA: Asteroid hyalosis: biomicroscopy, ultrastructure, and composition. Arch Ophthalmol 100:964–968, 1982.

## Vitreous Amyloidosis

Benson MD: Hereditary amyloidosis—disease entity and clinical model. Hosp Pract 23:165–72, 177, 181, 1988.

Ciulla TA, Tolentino F, Morrow JF, Dryja TP: Vitreous amyloidosis in familial amyloidotic polyneuropathy: report of a case with the Val30Met transthyretin mutation. Surv Ophthalmol 40:197–206, 1995.

Doft BH, Machemer R, Skinner M, et al: Pars plana vitrectomy for vitreous amyloidosis. Ophthalmology 94:607–611, 1987.

Sandgren O, Holmgren G, Lundgren E: Vitreous amyloidosis associated with homozygosity for the transthyretin methionine-30 gene. Arch Ophthalmol 108:1584–1586, 1990.

## Vitreous Lymphoma

Barr CC, Green WR, Payne JW, et al: Intraocular reticulum cell sarcoma: clinical pathological study of 4 cases and review of the literature. Surv Ophthalmol 19:224–239, 1975.

Carroll DM, Franklin RM: Vitreous biopsy in uveitis of unknown cause. Retina 1:245–251, 1981.

Char DH, Ljung B-M, Miller T, Phillips T: Primary intraocular lymphoma (ocular reticulum cell sarcoma), diagnosis and management. Ophthalmology 95:625–630, 1988.

Dean JM, Novak MA, Chan CC, Green WR: Tumor detachments of the retinal pigment epithelium in ocular/central nervous system lymphoma. Retina 16:47–56, 1996.

Rankin GA, Jakobiec FA, Hidayat AA: Intraocular lymphoproliferations simulating uveitis. In Albert DM, Jakobiec FA (eds) Principles and Practice of Ophthalmology: Clinical Practice. Vol 1. Philadelphia: Saunders, 1994:524–548.

Vogel MH, Font RL, Zimmerman LE, et al: Reticulum cell sarcoma of the retina and uvea: report of six cases and review of the literature. Am J Ophthalmol 66:205–215, 1968.

Whitcup SM, de Smet MD, Rubin BI, et al: Intraocular lymphoma: clinical and histopathologic diagnosis. Ophthalmology 100:1399–1406, 1993.

## Whipple's Disease

Avila MP, Jalkh AE, Feldman E, Trempe CL, Schepens CL: Manifestations of Whipple's disease in the posterior segment of the eye. Arch Ophthalmol 102:384–390, 1984.

Durant WJ, Flood T, Goldberg MF, Tso MO, Pasquali LA, Peyman GA: Vitrectomy and Whipple's disease. Arch Ophthalmol 102:848–851, 1984.

Font RL, Rao NA, Issarescu S, et al: Ocular involvement in Whipple's disease. Arch Ophthalmol 96:1431–1436, 1978.

Knox DL, Green WR, Troncoso JC, Yardley JH, Hsu J, Zee DS: Cerebral ocular Whipple's disease: a 62-year odyssey from death to diagnosis. Neurology 45:617–625, 1995.

Rickman LS, Freeman WR, Green WR, et al. Uveitis caused by Tropheryma whippelii (Whipple's bacillus) N Engl J Med 332:390–392, 1995.

Selsky EJ, Knox DL, Maumenee AE, Green WR: Ocular involvement in Whipple's disease. Retina 4:103–106, 1984.

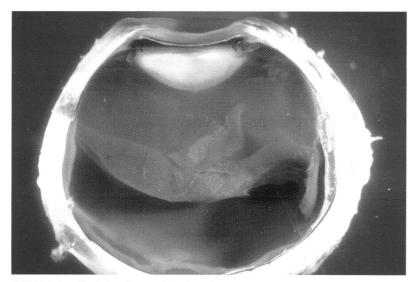

FIGURE 9–1 • **Posterior vitreous detachment.** Mild opacification by protein accentuates the vitreous. The vitreous framework has detached from the inner retina posteriorly. It remains attached to the anterior vitreous base, which straddles the ora serrata. The attachment there is very strong. The anterior chamber is flat, and part of the retina is shallowly detached by gelatinous exudate rich in lipid.

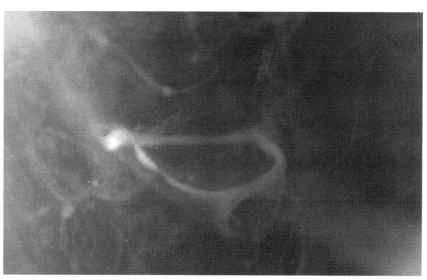

FIGURE 9–2 • **Weiss ring, posterior vitreous detachment.** The white ring represents the peripapillary condensation of the vitreous framework, which has separated from the optic disk during a posterior vitreous detachment.

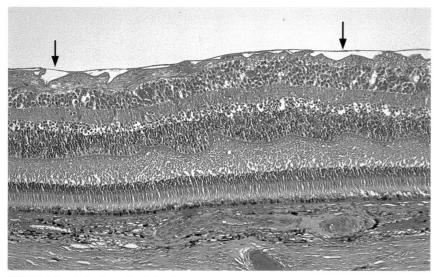

FIGURE 9–3 • **Epiretinal gliosis (surface wrinkling retinopathy).** Arrows denote delicate membrane of glial cells on the inner retinal surface after posterior vitreous detachment. Contraction of the membrane has caused folds in the internal limiting membrane. Hematoxylin-eosin, ×50.

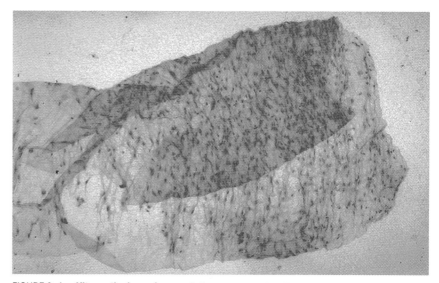

FIGURE 9–4 • **Vitreoretinal membrane.** Cells presumed to be glial cells form a subconfluent membrane on the surface of a condensed sheet of vitreous. The cells have bland spindled nuclei. The indication for vitrectomy was macular pucker. Millipore filter preparation, hematoxylin-eosin, ×50.

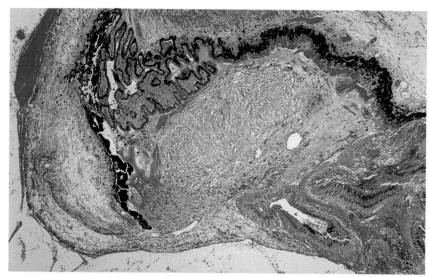

FIGURE 9–5 • **Anterior variant of proliferative vitreoretinopathy.** Fibrosis of residual vitreous overlying the ciliary body exerts traction on the retina and produces anterior loop retinal detachment. Hematoxylin-eosin, ×10.

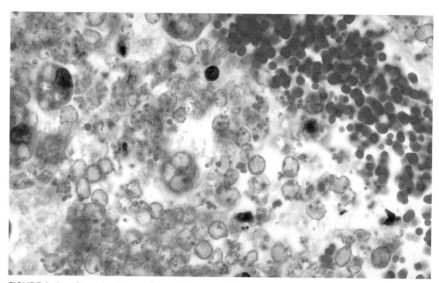

FIGURE 9–6 • **Chronic vitreous hemorrhage.** Numerous erythrocyte ghost cells or erythroclasts are seen below. Ghost cells are the empty cell membranes of erythrocytes that have lost their hemoglobin-rich cytoplasm. The eosinophilic bodies above are hemoglobin spherules. Macrophages that have ingested ghost cells, and other blood-breakdown products also are present. Hematoxylin-eosin, ×250.

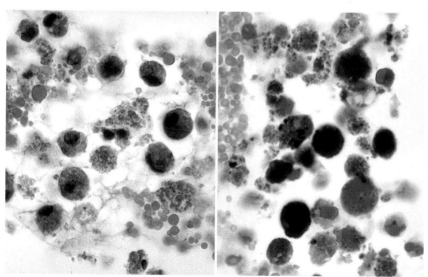

FIGURE 9–7 • **Hemosiderin-laden macrophages, chronic vitreous hemorrhage.** The yellow brown pigment in the macrophages is the blood break-down product hemosiderin. The pigment in some of the macrophages in this chronic vitreous hemorrhage stains positively (blue) for iron (*right*). Many hemoglobin spherules are present. Left: hematoxylin-eosin, ×250; right: Perls' stain for iron, ×250.

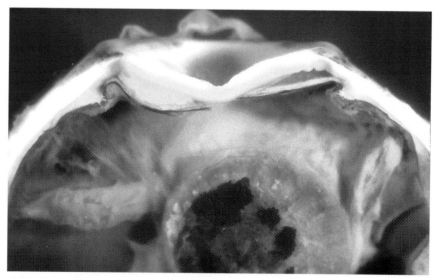

FIGURE 9–8 • **Ochre membrane, chronic vitreous hemorrhage.** The degenerated blood in the anterior chamber and posteriorly detached vitreous has a characteristic yellow-ochre color. The brunescent lens was dislocated during sectioning.

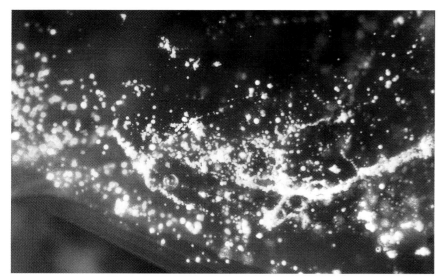

FIGURE 9–9 • **Asteroid hyalosis.** Numerous calcified spherules impart a starry sky appearance to the posteriorly detached vitreous. The asteroid hyalosis was an incidental finding in an eye enucleated for uveal melanoma.

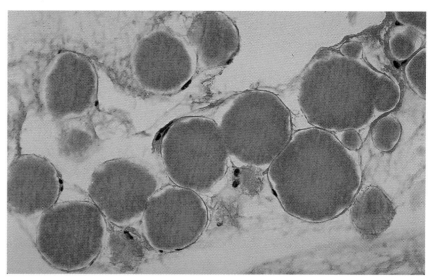

FIGURE 9–10 • **Asteroid hyalosis.** Asteroid bodies appear as grayish blue spherules in routine H&E sections. They are attached to the vitreous framework. Hematoxylin-eosin, ×250.

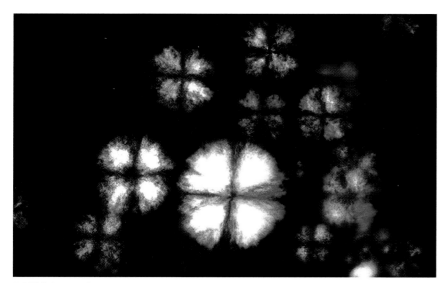

FIGURE 9–11 • **Asteroid hyalosis.** Intact asteroid bodies are vividly birefringent during polarization microscopy, showing a characteristic Maltese cross pattern. Millipore filter preparation, hematoxylin-eosin with crossed polarizers, ×250.

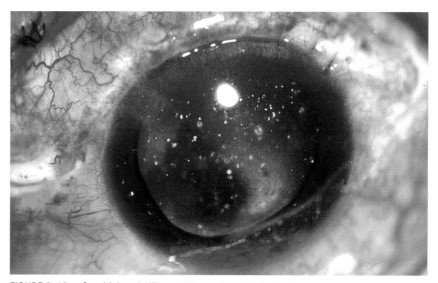

FIGURE 9–12 • **Synchisis scintillans.** Vitreous in a blind aphakic eye contains blood and glistening polychromatic crystals of cholesterol.

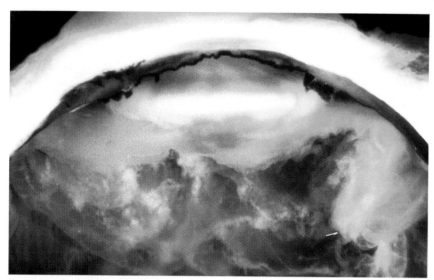

FIGURE 9–13 • **Vitreous amyloidosis.** Amyloid comprised of mutant transport protein transthyretin opacifies the vitreous in an eye obtained postmortem from a patient with the Indiana (SER 84) type of hereditary amyloidosis. A vitrectomy has been performed previously. (Specimen submitted by Dr. Merrill Benson, Indianapolis, IN)

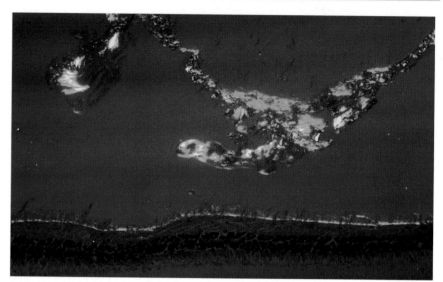

FIGURE 9–14 • **Vitreous amyloidosis.** The vitreous amyloid shows apple green birefringence during polarization microscopy. Amyloid also lines the inner retinal surface. Congo red with crossed polarizers, ×25.

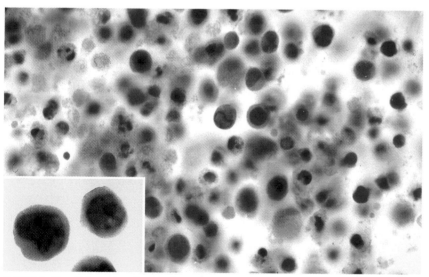

FIGURE 9–15 • **Primary lymphoma, vitreous.** Infiltrate obtained during diagnostic vitrectomy contains large atypical lymphocytes, necrotic lymphoid cells, and nuclear debris. *Inset:* Lymphoma cells have nuclear membrane protrusions and prominent nucleoli. Main figure: Millipore filter, hematoxylin-eosin ×250.

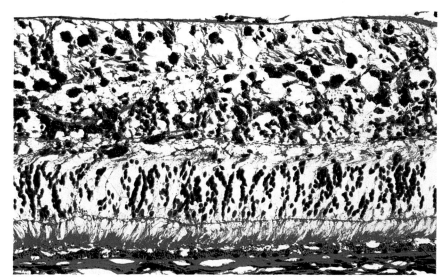

FIGURE 9–16 • **Whipple's disease.** PAS-positive macrophages that have phagocytized *Tropheryma whippelii* bacteria infiltrate the inner retina and cortical vitreous. Periodic acid-Schiff, × 250. (Courtesy of Dr. Ramon L. Font, Houston, TX)

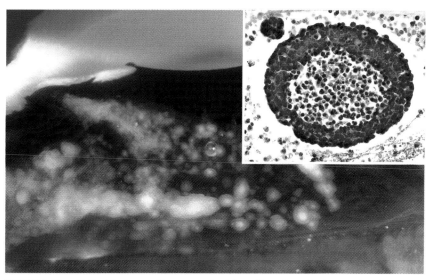

FIGURE 9–17 • **Retinoblastoma, vitreous seeds.** The white spheres in the anterior vitreous are seeds of retinoblastoma shed by an endophytic tumor in the posterior segment. Many of the seeds have a whiter center, reflecting central necrosis. *Inset:* A seed with central necrosis. Inset: hematoxylin-eosin, ×100.

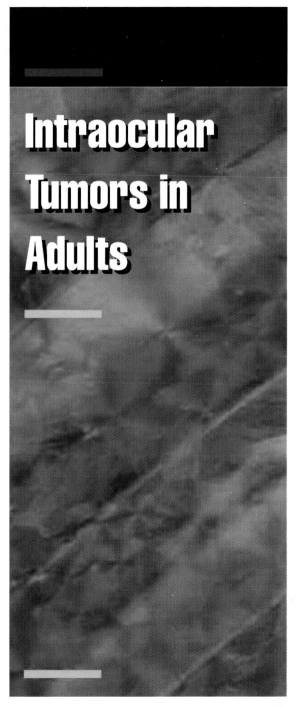

# CHAPTER 10

# Intraocular Tumors in Adults

Intraocular tumors have the potential to cause loss of life as well as loss of vision. Primary intraocular tumors in adults generally involve the uveal tract. Most are malignant melanomas and melanocytic nevi. Secondary intraocular tumors probably are more common than primary tumors, but many are not detected clinically. Most are metastases to the choroid from breast or lung carcinomas. Other rarer primary intraocular tumors in adults include choroidal hemangiomas, leiomyomas, schwannomas and ciliary or retinal pigment epithelial tumors.

## UVEAL MALIGNANT MELANOMA

Uveal malignant melanoma is the most common primary intraocular tumor of adults. These melanomas arise from the dendritic melanocytes of the uvea, the middle pigmented and vascularized coat of the eye that includes the iris, ciliary body, and choroid (Figs. 10–1, 10–2, 10–3). Choroidal melanomas are most common. Uveal melanomas are relatively rare tumors; about 1500 tumors occur in the United States yearly.

Uveal melanoma generally affects older patients. The median age at diagnosis is 53 years. Although pediatric and even congenital cases have been reported, fewer than 1.6% of uveal melanomas occur in patients less than 20 years of age. Older patients tend to have larger tumors and are more likely to die from their tumors after enucleation. Race is a major predisposing factor. Uveal malignant melanoma has a predilection for Europeans with lightly colored eyes. In the United States the incidence of uveal melanoma in white patients is 8.5 times greater than the incidence in African Americans. The tumor is also relatively uncommon in Latin America and Asia.

Caucasian patients who have congenital ocular or oculodermal melanocytosis (nevus of Ota) (see Figs. 4–46, 4–47, 4–48, 4–49) are especially at risk to develop uveal malignant melanoma. These patients have a diffuse nevus of the uvea that is evident clinically as hyperchromic heterochromia iridum. White patients who have uveal melanoma have a 25 fold greater incidence of ocular melanocytosis than to white patients without melanoma. Nevus of Ota is more common in blacks and Asians, but malignant transformation generally occurs in Caucasians. Uveal melanomas occasionally arise from localized uveal nevi, but the estimated incidence of malignant transformation is quite low. Uveal melanoma has been reported in patients with neurofibromatosis type I and the dysplastic nevus or familial atypical mole-melanoma syndrome. The tumor's propensity for blue-eyed individuals and the inferior exposed part of the iris suggests that exposure to ultraviolet light could be a predisposing factor.

Most posterior uveal melanomas present with painless visual loss. Visual symptoms are caused most often by serous or solid detachment of the retina (or both). Other mechanisms of visual loss include physical obscuration of the fovea, cystoid macular edema, cataracts caused by expanding ciliary body tumors, and rarely vitreous hemorrhage, which usually develops when tumors erode through the retina. Melanomas occasionally are found in asymptomatic patients during routine ophthalmologic examinations (Figs. 10–4, 10–5). Iris melanomas may present as an enlarging pigmented blemish or a change in eye color (heterochromia iridum). Other tumors present with unilateral glaucoma. Anterior segment melanomas cause secondary glaucoma by directly seeding or infiltrating the aqueous outflow pathways. Posterior segment tumors usually cause secondary closed-angle glaucoma by a pupillary block mechanism or by stimulating iris neovascularization. Infarcted or extensively necrotic tumors can cause prominent inflammatory signs. Advanced cases with extrascleral tumor extension into the orbit may present with ocular proptosis. Unsuspected melanomas occasionally are found when blind, painful glaucomatous eyes with opaque media are examined pathologically. Distant metastases usually are not evident when the tumor is first detected and treated.

Choroidal melanomas are classified as small, medium, and large based on the tumor's largest basal diameter (LTD). Small choroidal melanomas measure 10 mm or less in LTD and appear as a focal discoid or oval area of choroidal thickening. Medium-sized melanomas measure 11–15 mm, and large tumors are more than 15 mm in LTD. Actively growing choroidal melanomas frequently rupture through Bruch's membrane into the subretinal space and assume a characteristic collar button or mushroom configuration (Figs. 10–5, 10–6, 10–7). If a choroidal tumor has a mushroom configuration, one can be reasonably certain it is a uveal melanoma. There are exceptions to this rule, but they are rare. Dilated blood vessels typically are found in the mushrooming head of the tumor (Fig. 10–8). The ruptured ends of Bruch's' membrane exert a compressive cinch-like effect on the waist of the tumor causing vascular congestion in its apex. Malignant melanomas occasionally diffusely thicken the choroid without forming an elevated mass. These diffuse melanomas usually are less differentiated cytologically and have a poorer prognosis. They have a tendency to extend extraocularly and may invade the optic nerve (Fig. 10–9).

Choroidal melanomas typically cause an exudative serous detachment of the overlying and adjacent retina. Large tumors may cause total retinal detachment (Fig. 10–7). The detached retina typically shows photoreceptor atrophy and microcystoid retinal degeneration. The retinal pigment epithelium on the surface of the tumor undergoes atrophy and proliferation,

forming drusenoid material and occasionally a plaque of metaplastic fibrous tissue. Many tumors infiltrate the overlying retina. The melanoma may perforate the retina in exceptional cases, causing vitreous hemorrhage and tumor seeding of the vitreous and the inner retinal surface. Large tumors may totally fill the globe. Eventually some melanomas extend extraocularly through the sclera and invade the orbit. Secondary glaucoma is often present in eyes with advanced or neglected tumors. Uveal malignant melanomas vary markedly in their pigment content. Some tumors are totally amelanotic. Other maximally pigmented tumors appear jet-black grossly and must be bleached before they can be interpreted histopathologically. Varying degrees of pigmentation are typically found within a single tumor. The cut surface of some tumors has a marbleized appearance. Clumps of orange pigment are found on the surface of many melanomas (Fig. 10–10). The orange pigment is composed of aggregates of macrophages that have ingested lipofuscin pigment and melanin from the damaged retinal pigment epithelium (Fig. 10–11). The pigment generally is thought to be a clinical marker for an actively growing tumor.

Ciliary body melanomas are less common than choroidal tumors and tend to have a more spherical shape (Fig. 10–12). They typically are larger when first detected because they have been hidden behind the iris. Occasionally, ciliary body melanomas that have invaded the anterior chamber present with iris heterochromia and secondary glaucoma. The glaucoma is caused by seeding of the trabecular meshwork by tumor cells or by circumferential growth around the angle (ring melanoma) (see Figs. 7–31, 7–32. 7–33).

Most melanocytic lesions of the iris are benign nevi or low grade spindle cell tumors (Figs. 10–13, 10–14, 10–15). About half of the adult population has small, nonprogressive iris nevi called freckles (Figs. 10–16, 10–17). Larger pigmented iris lesions initially should be observed for growth. Only 6.5% enlarge during a 5

year observation period. Clinical features suggesting that a pigmented iris tumor is a melanoma include large size, documented growth, elevated intraocular pressure, hyphema, and tumor vascularity. The development of acquired hyperchromic iris heterochromia and unilateral glaucoma in an eye with an iris tumor strongly suggests that the tumor is a high grade lesion that contains dyscohesive malignant epithelioid cells that are readily dispersed by the aqueous humor (Fig. 10–18; see also Fig. 7–35). Pigmented tumors of the iris pigment epithelium are rare (Fig. 10–19).

Two major categories of cells are found when uveal melanomas are examined histopathologically: spindle cells and epithelioid cells. Spindle cells are bipolar fusiform cells that have long, tapering processes and grow as parallel fascicles. They typically form a syncytium; the cytoplasmic margins of individual cells are indistinct. Two subcategories of spindle cells, spindle A and spindle B, are distinguished by nuclear characteristics. Spindle A cells have bland, slender, cigarshaped nuclei with finely dispersed chromatin and indistinct nucleoli (Fig. 10–20). A longitudinal fold in the nuclear membrane is seen as a chromatin stripe or line in many spindle A cells. Spindle B melanoma cells are less differentiated than spindle A cells. Spindle B nuclei are plumper and oval, and they have a distinct nucleolus and a coarser chromatin pattern (Fig. 10–21).

The epithelioid cell is the least differentiated type of uveal melanoma cell (Fig. 10–22). Tumors that are rich in epithelioid cells have a poorer prognosis. Epithelioid melanoma cells have abundant cytoplasm and are polyhedral. They have distinct cytoplasmic margins and are poorly cohesive. The epithelioid cell nucleus usually is large and round or oval. Epithelioid cells typically have large reddish purple nucleoli. The nucleus is often vesicular. The chromatin is coarse and clumps along the inner side of the nuclear membrane (peripheral margination of chromatin). Variants of epithelioid cells include relatively uniform small epithelioid cells (Fig. 10–23). and highly anaplastic tumor giant cells (Fig. 10–24). Melanoma cell type is determined by careful assessment of nuclear characteristics. Spindle shaped epithelioid cells occasionally are encountered.

Four types of uveal melanoma are recognized on the basis of cytology. A tumor composed entirely of nevus cells or benign spindle A cells is a spindle cell nevus. Spindle melanomas are composed of malignant spindle A cells, spindle B cells, or a mixture of A and B cells. Melanomas of the mixed cell type contain a mixture of spindle and epithelioid melanoma cells (Fig. 10–25). Most larger tumors treated by enucleation are mixed cell melanomas. Epithelioid melanomas are composed predominantly of epithelioid cells. Purely epithelioid tumors are rare and have the poorest prognosis. Totally necrotic melanomas occasionally are encountered (Fig. 10–26). They behave like mixed tumors. In many instances the cell type of a necrotic tumor can be determined by careful oil immersion microscopy. The fascicular category, which was part of the original Callender classification, is no longer used because it is based on a histologic pattern, not cytologic criteria (Fig. 10–27).

About half of patients with uveal melanoma eventually die from their tumors. The two most important factors that help the pathologist predict survival are cell type and tumor size. The association between tumor mortality and the cytologic characteristics of uveal melanoma (cell type) is called the Callender classification. Callender's cell type, as modified at the Armed Forces Institute of Pathology, remains one of the most reliable prognosticators of mortality from uveal melanoma. Tumor mortality is greater if uveal melanomas contain epithelioid cells (epithelioid melanomas or mixed epithelioid/spindle cell type). The 5-year mortality of uveal melanomas that contain epithelioid cells is 42%. At 15 years death from metastatic melanoma increases to 63%. The prognosis of patients with spindle cell tumors is much better: 90% survive 5 years, and 72% survive 15 years. Al-

though rare, fatal spindle A melanomas have been reported; most tumors composed entirely of spindle A cells are thought to be benign spindle cell nevi.

Large melanomas have a poorer prognosis than small and medium-sized melanomas. Tumor size generally is recorded as the LTD measured at the base. The 5-year survival of patients with small ($< 10$ mm), medium (10–15 mm), and large ($> 15$ mm) melanomas are 86%, 66%, and 56%, respectively. These survival rates drop to 76%, 51%, and 41% at 10 years and 70%, 43%, and 35% at 15 years. Small melanomas are more likely to be spindle cell tumors.

The presence of certain vascular patterns in the tumor, most notably vascular loops and networks of loops, is associated with a poorer prognosis (Fig. 10–28). Other prognostic factors shown by multivariate statistical analysis to be less important are mitotic activity, extraocular tumor extension (Fig. 10–29), necrosis, pigmentation, anterior location, and lymphocytic infiltration. Paradoxically, the prognosis of heavily pigmented tumors may be slightly poorer. The presence of lymphocytic infiltration in the tumor also seems to have a adverse effect on survival because hematogenous dissemination of tumor cells may be a requisite for stimulation of the immune system. Mitotic activity seems to be a better predictor in spindle cell tumors. Mitoses are relatively rare in most uveal melanomas. The mitoses are counted during pathologic examination and reported as the number found in 40 high-power (dry) fields. Experimental studies suggest that melanoma cells that co-express vimentin and cytokeratins 8 and 18 are more likely to metastasize.

Unlike retinoblastoma, uveal melanoma rarely invades the optic nerve (Figs. 10–9, 10–29). Melanomas typically extend out of the eye through the emissarial canals of vessels and nerves in the sclera or via the lumina of the vortex veins (Fig. 10–30).

Hematogenous metastasis is the most important cause of death in patients with uveal melanoma. Metastases rarely are detected when the patient ini-

tially presents or is treated. Uveal melanoma has a predilection for metastatic spread to the liver (Fig. 10–31). Hepatic metastases occur in more than 90% of patients with metastatic melanoma and are the first metastases detected in 80%. For this reason liver enzymes are used clinically to monitor patients for recurrence. Current therapy for metastatic uveal melanoma is unsatisfactory; more than 50% of patients die within 1 year.

Many posterior uveal melanomas are diagnosed by direct ophthalmoscopic visualization of the tumor. Adjunctive studies, including A and B scan ultrasonography, intravenous fluorescein angiography, and computed tomography or magnetic resonance imaging, frequently are used to confirm the clinical impression and may be particularly important if the ocular media are opacified. Transvitreal fine needle aspiration biopsy (FNAB) performed under direct ophthalmoscopic visualization occasionally is performed if the diagnosis remains uncertain after routine tests. The choice of therapy requires an accurate diagnosis. Examples include the patient with a history of breast cancer who presents with a solitary amelanotic choroidal tumor that could be a secondary primary amelanotic melanoma, or the patient who is thought to have a choroidal metastasis but has no history of cancer.

The therapy of uveal malignant melanoma remains somewhat controversial. Part of this controversy stems from Zimmerman's hypothesis that enucleation of an eye with uveal melanoma may increase tumor deaths by disseminating tumor cells (Fig. 10–32). Never proved or disproved, this hypothesis spurred interest in alternative treatment methods, particularly plaque brachyradiotherapy. This treatment employs radioactive plaques comprised of radioisotopes such as iodine 125 ($^{125}$I). The plaques are surgically affixed to the sclera external to uveal tumors and left in place for a period of time calculated to deliver a lethal dose of radiation. Currently, most melanomas are treated by enucleation (removal of the eye) or brachyradiotherapy. Enucleation remains the treatment of choice for large tumors. Small pigmented uveal tumors generally are observed for growth before initiating therapy, as it may be impossible to distinguish large benign nevi from melanomas by all other clinical criteria. External beam radiotherapy employing focused beams of charged particles (protons or helium ions) is available in a few localities. Other therapeutic modalities used occasionally include local resection, cryotherapy, and laser photocoagulation.

Evaluation of nonrandomized data suggests that survival after plaque radiotherapy and enucleation are similar. A multicenter randomized clinical trial called the Collaborative Ocular Melanoma Study (COMS) comparing enucleation and $^{125}$I plaque therapy in small and medium-sized tumors is under way. It is hoped that the results of this study will provide new information about the natural history and pathology of uveal melanoma as well as treatment recommendations.

Other disorders included in the differential diagnosis of uveal malignant melanoma are benign melanocytic nevi, choroidal hemangiomas, and metastases from distant nonocular primary neoplasms, as well as simulating nonneoplastic lesions such as posterior scleritis and the disciform scars of age-related macular degeneration. Other rare primary intraocular tumors include choroidal schwannomas and leiomyomas as well as adenomas and adenocarcinomas of the retinal pigment epithelium (RPE) and the pigmented and nonpigmented ciliary epithelia.

## CHOROIDAL HEMANGIOMAS

Choroidal hemangiomas are benign vascular tumors composed of large thin-walled, endothelial-lined vascular channels (Fig. 10–33). Choroidal hemangiomas occur sporadically or in association with the Sturge-Weber syndrome (encephalotrigeminal angiomatosis).

Sporadic cases appear as discrete orange-red tumefactions, often with an associated exudative serous retinal detachment (Fig. 10–34). In contrast, the hemangiomas of Sturge-Weber syndrome typically are diffuse lesions that obscure normal choroidal landmarks and impart a tomato-ketchup appearance to the fundus on ophthalmoscopy (see Fig. 1–20). Choroidal hemangiomas are often complicated by exudative retinal detachment, secondary glaucoma, or both. Glaucoma in Sturge-Weber syndrome usually occurs ipsilateral to the facial port wine stain and is caused by iris neovascularization, elevated episcleral venous pressure, or maldevelopment of the angle. Because choroidal hemangioma is a benign tumor, treatment is intended to control retinal detachment, which can lead to blindness or the loss of the eye. Treatment modalities include delimiting laser photocoagulation and low dose plaque radiotherapy. Clinically, choroidal hemangioma and melanoma are differentiated using intravenous fluorescein angiography and ultrasonography. Hemangiomas appear acoustically solid on B-scan ultrasonography because their constituent vascular channels form multiple acoustic interfaces. Uveal melanomas usually exhibit acoustic hollowness.

## UVEAL METASTASES

Although ocular oncologists see more patients with uveal melanoma, cancer metastatic to the uvea is widely believed to be the most prevalent intraocular malignant tumor. It has been estimated that 4% of patients dying from all types of carcinoma have ocular metastases. Most of these secondary ocular tumors occur in terminally ill patients but are not detected clinically.

Most tumors that metastasize to the uvea are carcinomas; sarcomas rarely metastasize to the eye. Although all parts of the uveal tract including the iris are affected, almost 90% of metastases affect the choroid.

Most choroidal metastases occur posteriorly in the macular area (12%) or between the macula and the equator (80%). Choroidal metastases typically appear as yellow, nummular or plateau-shaped masses with associated subretinal fluid (Fig. 10–35). Diffuse choroidal infiltration is the rule; although exceptional cases have been reported, metastases almost never have the mushroom-like configuration that characterizes uveal melanoma (Fig. 10–36). Some patients have multiple metastases that may be bilateral; about 30% of affected eyes have two or more metastatic foci. Visual loss usually results from exudative retinal detachment with shifting subretinal fluid. Ocular metastases from cutaneous melanoma often cause vitreous seeding by pigmented tumor cells. Metastases to the retina are rare.

Breast and lung carcinomas are the primary cancers that metastasize to the uvea most often. In a series of 420 patients with uveal metastases, the primary cancer was in the breast in 196 (47%), lung in 90 (21%), gastrointestinal tract in 18 (4%), kidney in 9 (2%), skin in 9 (2%), prostate in 9 (2%), and other sites in 16 (4%). Women with metastases from breast carcinoma usually have a history of mastectomy. Lung carcinoma is common in men, in whom it may be the initial manifestation of an occult primary tumor. Overall, about one-third of patients who present with uveal metastases have no history of cancer. Systemic evaluation fails to disclose a primary tumor in half of these patients.

Histopathologically, the affected uvea is thickened and replaced by nests, cords, and sheets of malignant tumor cells (Fig. 10–37). Larger metastases are often extensively necrotic. Mucin stains such as alcian blue and mucicarmine are used in the laboratory to determine if the primary tumor is a mucin-secreting adenocarcinoma. Carcinomas are distinguished immunohistochemically from melanomas by positive immunoreactivity for cytokeratins and other epithelial antigens. In rare instances (e.g., prostate or thyroid cancer) immunohistochemical staining can identify a specific primary tumor. Occasionally, diagnostic FNAB is used to distinguish between amelanotic uveal melanoma, metastatic carcinoma, and other simulating lesions that require different therapies.

Relatively few eyes with metastatic carcinoma are received in the ophthalmic pathology laboratory. Although painful glaucoma occasionally is an indication for enucleation, most eyes with metastatic carcinoma are treated with radiotherapy or chemotherapy (or both).

## NEVI

Uveal nevi are proliferations of atypical but benign-appearing melanocytes that are incapable of metastasis (Fig. 10–38). Choroidal nevi typically appear as flat patches of increased choroidal pigmentation with feathery margins; they measure 1–2 mm in diameter. Malignant melanomas rarely arise from uveal nevi; the rate of malignant transformation is estimated to be only 1/10,000 to 1/15,000 per year. Large choroidal nevi may be impossible to differentiate from small malignant melanomas clinically because they can cause RPE degeneration, a scotoma, and localized serous retinal detachment. Observed growth is the only clinical criterion that is helpful in this regard. Choroidal nevi are comprised of variable mixtures of slender or plump spindle cells, dendritic cells, plump polyhedral cells filled with melanin pigment, and lipidized cells with foamy cytoplasm called balloon cells.

A melanocytoma is type of intensely pigmented uveal nevus. It is composed of plump polyhedral nevus cells that have copious quantities of maximally pigmented cytoplasm. Melanocytomas classically involve the optic disk but can arise from any part of the uvea including the iris and ciliary body (Fig. 10–39). The large quantity of pigment usually obscures nuclear details in melanocytoma cells requiring depigmented

sections for proper evaluation (Fig. 10–40). When depigmented sections are examined, the tumor cells are found to have a low nuclear/cytoplasmic ratio and bland nuclei with inconspicuous nucleoli. Melanocytomas are especially common in black patients. Transformation into malignant melanoma occurs rarely. Melanocytomas often undergo spontaneous necrosis. Macrophages that have ingested melanin pigment released by partially necrotic iris melanocytomas can cause secondary glaucoma by physically obstructing aqueous outflow pathways (see Figs. 7–27, 7–28).

## OTHER INTRAOCULAR TUMORS

Primary intraocular tumors occasionally arise from the RPE and the ciliary epithelium. They include rare adenomas and adenocarcinomas of the RPE and the pigmented and nonpigmented ciliary epithelia. Primary neoplasms of the RPE are rare. This fact is somewhat surprising because the RPE readily undergoes reactive hyperplasia and metaplasia, forming extensive amounts of fibrous tissue and bone. Although they occasionally are amelanotic, RPE tumors classically are jet black and have abruptly elevated margins (Fig. 10–41). They are located on the inner surface of the choroid. RPE carcinomas may show an infiltrative growth pattern but do not metastasize.

Ciliary epithelial tumors can be predominantly pigmented or nonpigmented (Figs. 10–42, 10–43, 10–44). Both types arise from the epithelium on the inner surface of the ciliary body and spare its stroma. The cytoplasm of many pigmented ciliary epithelial tumors contains multiple small cystoid spaces (Fig. 10–42). Nonpigmented tumors are white or yellowish white and often produce focal cataract or lens dislocation (Figs. 10–43, 10–44). In contrast to melanoma, ciliary epithelial tumors arise from the inner surface of the ciliary body and usually do not involve its stroma. Local resection usually is curative.

Congenital hypertrophy of the RPE (CHRPE) appears ophthalmoscopically as a flat, round or oval pigmented spot (Fig. 10–45). The lesions are surrounded by a depigmented halo and usually develop depigmented lacunae with time. CHRPE occasionally were confused with melanomas before the advent of the modern binocular indirect ophthalmoscope. Microscopy discloses patches of tall RPE cells packed with large, round melanosomes. Congenital grouped pigmentation ("bear tracks") is a variant of CHRPE (Fig. 10–46). Multiple bilateral pigmented RPE lesions that bear a superficial resemblance to CHRPE have been reported to be an ocular marker for the heritable cancer diathesis Gardner syndrome (familial adenomatous polyposis with extracolonic manifestations).

Leiomyomas are rare nonpigmented ciliary body tumors that usually affect young women. Most are situated in the supraciliary space, and they characteristically transmit light during transillumination. Compared to melanomas, leiomyomas are paucicellular and their cells have fibrillar eosinophilic cytoplasm (Fig. 10–47). Positive immunoreactivity for smooth muscle actin and other muscle markers differentiates leiomyoma from uveal melanoma and rare neurogenic tumors (Fig. 10–48). The term mesectodermal leiomyoma has been applied to leiomyomas that have a distinctly neural appearance on routine light microscopy.

Choroidal osteoma, or osseous choristoma, is another rare primary uveal tumor that chiefly affects young women (Fig. 10–49). These interesting lesions are often bilateral, peripapillary in location, and yellow-orange with characteristic scalloped margins. The bone in osseous choristomas is located within the choroid, not on its inner surface like the osseous metaplasia of the RPE found in phthisical eyes. Ultrasonography or computed tomography readily establishes the diagnosis.

Iris pigment epithelial cysts are easily confused clinically with anterior uveal malignant melanomas because they are heavily pigmented and may cause focal shallowing of the anterior chamber. Histopathologically, these cysts are comprised of polarized iris pigment epithelium that is one or more layers thick. The lumen contains clear fluid.

Reactive lymphoid hyperplasia of the uvea probably is a form of lymphoma (Fig. 10–50). The uveal stroma may be affected during the late stages of a systemic lymphoma or by leukemia. Primary lymphoma of the central nervous system involves the vitreous and retina but generally spares the uveal tract (see Fig. 9–16). Visceral lymphoma rarely involves the vitreous secondarily.

# References

## General References

Margo CE, McLean IW: Malignant melanoma of the choroid in black patients. Arch Ophthalmol 102:77–79, 1984.

McLean I: Uveal nevi and malignant melanomas. In Spencer W (ed) Ophthalmic Pathology: An Atlas and Textbook. 4th ed. Vol 3. Philadelphia: Saunders, 1996:2121.

Singh AD, Shields CL, Shields JA, Eagle RC, De Potter P: Uveal melanoma and familial atypical mole and melanoma (FAM-M) syndrome. Ophthalmic Genet 16: 53–61, 1995.

Zimmerman LE: Melanocytic tumors of interest to the ophthalmologist. Ophthalmology 87:497–501, 1980.

## Ocular and Oculodermal Melanocytosis

Gonder J, Ezell P, Shields J: Ocular melanocytosis: a study to determine the prevalence rate of ocular melanocytosis. Ophthalmology 88:372, 1981.

Gonder J, Shields J, Albert D: Malignant melanoma of the choroid associated with oculodermal melanocytosis. Ophthalmology 88:372, 1981.

Gonder J, Shields J, Shakin J, et al: Bilateral ocular melanoma of the choroid associated with ocular melanocytosis. Br J Ophthalmol 65:843, 1981.

Nik N, Glew W, Zimmerman L: Malignant melanoma of the choroid in the nevus of Ota in a black patient. Arch Ophthalmol 100:1641, 1982.

Singh AD, De Potter P, Fijal BA, et al: Lifetime prevalence of uveal melanoma in white patients with oculo(dermal) melanocytosis. Ophthalmology 105:195–198, 1998.

## Posterior Uveal Melanoma

Affeldt JC, Minckler DS, Azen SP, Yeh L: Prognosis in uveal melanoma with extraocular extension. Arch Ophthalmol 98:1975–1979, 1980.

Callender GR: Malignant melanotic tumors of the eye: a study of histologic types in 111 cases. Trans Am Acad Ophthalmol Otolaryngol 36:131–142, 1931.

Callender GR, Wilder HC, Ash JE: Five hundred melanomas of the choroid and ciliary body followed five years or longer. Am J Ophthalmol 25:562–567, 1942.

Collaborative Ocular Melanoma Study Group: Mortality in patients with small choroidal melanoma. COMS Report No. 4. Arch Ophthalmol 115:886–893, 1997.

De Potter P, Shields CL, Eagle RC Jr, Shields JA, Lipkowitz JL: Malignant melanoma of the optic nerve. Arch Ophthalmol 114:608–612, 1996.

Folberg R, Rummelt V, Parys-Van Ginderdevren R, et al: The prognostic value of tumor blood vessel morphology in primary uveal melanoma. Ophthalmology 100: 1389–1398, 1993.

Gamel JW, McLean IW: Modern developments in histopathologic assessment of uveal melanomas. Ophthalmology 91:679–684, 1984.

Gass JDM: Observation of suspected choroidal and ciliary body melanomas for evidence of growth prior to enucleation. Ophthalmology 87:523–528, 1980.

Hendrix MJC, Seftor EA, Seftor REB, et al: Biologic determinants of uveal melanoma metastatic phenotype: role of intermediate filaments as predictive markers. Lab Invest 78:153–163, 1998.

McLean IW: Prognostic features of uveal malignant melanoma. Ophthalmol Clin North Am 8:143–153, 1995.

McLean IW, Foster WD, Zimmerman LE: Modifications of Callender's classification of uveal melanoma at the Armed Forces Institute of Pathology. Am J Ophthalmol 96:502–509, 1983.

McLean IW, Foster WD, Zimmerman LE: Prognostic factors in small malignant melanomas of the choroid and ciliary body. Arch Ophthalmol 95:48–58, 1977.

McLean IW, Foster WD, Zimmerman LE: Uveal melanoma: location, size, cell type and enucleation as risk factors in metastasis. Hum Pathol 13:123–132, 1982.

McLean IW, Zimmerman LE, Evans RM: Reappraisal of Callender's spindle A type of malignant melanoma of the choroid and ciliary body. Am J Ophthalmol 86:557–564, 1978.

Mooy CM, De Jong PTVM: Prognostic parameters in uveal melanoma: a review. Surv Ophthalmol 41:215–228, 1996.

Saornil MA, Fisher MR, Campbell RJ, et al: Histopathologic study of eyes after iodine I 125 episcleral plaque irradiation for uveal melanoma. Arch Ophthalmol 115: 1395–400, 1997.

Shammas HF, Blodi FC: Orbital extension of choroidal and ciliary body melanomas. Arch Ophthalmol 95: 2002–2005, 1977.

Shields JA, Shields CL: Current management of posterior uveal melanoma. Mayo Clin Proc 68:1196–1200, 1993.

Whelchel JC, Farah SE, McLean IW, Burnier MN: Immunohistochemistry of infiltrating lymphocytes in uveal malignant melanoma. Invest Ophthalmol Vis Sci 34: 2603–2606, 1993.

Wilder HC, Paul EV: Malignant melanoma of the choroid and ciliary body: a study of 2,535 cases. Milit Surg 109: 370–378, 1951.

Zimmerman LE: Diffuse malignant melanoma of the uveal tract: a clinicopathologic report of 54 cases. Trans Am Acad Ophthalmol Otolaryngol 72:877–894, 1968.

Zimmerman LE, McLean IW: Metastatic disease from untreated uveal melanomas. Am J Ophthalmol 88:524–534, 1979.

Zimmerman LE, McLean IW: The Montgomery lecture, 1975: changing concepts of the prognosis and management of small malignant melanomas of the choroid. Trans Ophthalmol Soc UK 95:487–494, 1975.

Zimmerman LE, Sobin LH: Histologic typing of tumours of the eye and its adnexa. In International Histological Classification of Tumours No. 24. Geneva: World Health Organization, 1980.

## Iris Melanoma

Arentsen JJ, Green WR: Melanoma of the iris: report of 72 cases treated surgically. Ophthalmic Surg 6:23–37, 1975.

Grossniklaus HE, Oakman JH, Cohen C, Calhoun FP Jr, DeRose PB, Drews-Botsch C: Histopathology, morphometry, and nuclear DNA content of iris melanocytic lesions. Invest Ophthalmol Vis Sci 36:745–750, 1995.

Harbour JW, Augsburger JJ, Eagle RC Jr: Initial management and follow-up of melanocytic iris tumors. Ophthalmology 102:1987–1993, 1995.

Jakobiec FA, Silbert G: Are most iris "melanomas" really nevi? Arch Ophthalmol 99:2117–2132, 1981.

Rones B, Zimmerman L: The production of heterochromia and glaucoma by diffuse malignant melanoma of the iris. Trans Am Acad Ophthalmol Otolaryngol 61:447, 1957.

Rones B, Zimmerman LE: The prognosis of primary tumors of the iris treated by iridectomy. Arch Ophthalmol 60: 193–205, 1958.

**Choroidal Hemangiomia**

Shields JA, Zimmerman LE: Lesions simulating malignant melanoma of the posterior uvea. Arch Ophthalmol 89:466–471, 1973.

Spraul CW, Kim D, Fineberg E, Grossniklaus HE: Mushroom-shaped choroidal hemangioma. Am J Ophthalmol 122:434–436, 1996.

Witschel H, Font RL: Hemangioma of the choroid: a clinicopathologic study of 71 cases and a review of the literature. Surv Ophthalmol 20:415–431, 1976.

**Uveal Metastasis**

Ferry AP, Font RL: Carcinoma metastatic to the eye and orbit: a clinicopathologic study of 227 cases. Arch Ophthalmol 92:276–286, 1974.

Nelson CC, Herzberg BS, Klintworth GK: A histopathologic study of 716 unselected eyes in patients with cancer at the time of death. Am J Ophthalmol 95:788–793, 1983.

Shields CL, Shields JA, Gross NE, Schwartz GP, Lally SE: Survey of 520 eyes with uveal metastases. Ophthalmology 104:1265–1276, 1997.

**Fine Needle Aspiration Biopsy**

Augsburger JJ: Fine needle aspiration biopsy of suspected metastatic cancers to the posterior uvea. Trans Am Ophthalmol Soc 86:499–560, 1988.

Shields JA, Shields CL, Ehya H, et al: Fine-needle aspiration biopsy of suspected intraocular tumors: the 1992 Urwick lecture. Ophthalmology 100:1677–1684, 1993.

Spraul CW, Martin DF, Hagler WS, Grossniklaus HE: Cytology of metastatic cutaneous melanoma to the vitreous and retina. Retina 16:328–332, 1996.

**Choroidal Nevi**

Gass JDM: Problems in the differential diagnosis of choroidal nevi and malignant melanomas: the XXXIII Edward Jackson memorial lecture. Am J Ophthalmol 83: 299–323, 1977.

Joffe L, Shields JA, Osher RH, Gass JDM: Clinical variations and follow-up studies of melanocytomas of the optic disc. Ophthalmology 86:1067–1083, 1979.

Naumann GOH, Hellner K, Naumann LR: Pigmented nevi of the choroid: clinical study of secondary changes in the overlying tissue. Trans Am Acad Ophthalmol Otolaryngol 75:110–123, 1971.

**Ciliary Epithelial Tumors**

Grossniklaus HE, Lim JI: Adenoma of the nonpigmented ciliary epithelium. Retina 14:452–456, 1994.

Lieb WE, Shields JA, Eagle RC Jr, Kwa D, Shields CL: Cystic adenoma of the pigmented ciliary epithelium: clinical, pathology, and immunohistopathologic findings. Ophthalmology 97:1489–1493, 1990.

Shields JA, Eagle RC Jr, Shields CL, De Potter P: Acquired neoplasms of the nonpigmented ciliary epithelium (adenoma and adenocarcinoma). Ophthalmology 103: 2007–2016, 1996.

**RPE Tumors**

Font RL, Zimmerman LE, Fine BS: Adenoma of the retinal pigment epithelium. Am J Ophthalmol 73:544–554, 1972.

Garner A: Tumors of the retinal pigment epithelium. Br J Ophthalmol 54:715–723, 1970.

Spraul CW, d'Heurle D, Grossniklaus HE: Adenocarcinoma of the iris pigment epithelium. Arch Ophthalmol 114: 1512–1517, 1996.

**Congenital Hypertrophy of the RPE**

Kasner L, Traboulsi EI, Delacruz Z, Green WR: A histopathologic study of the pigmented fundus lesions in familial adenomatous polyposis. Retina 12:35–42, 1992.

Lloyd WC III, Eagle RC Jr, Shields JA, Kwa DM, Arbizo W: Congenital hypertrophy of the retinal pigment epithelium: electron microscopic and morphometric observations. Ophthalmology 97:1052–1060, 1990.

Regillo CD, Eagle RC Jr, Shields JA, Shields CL, Arbizo VV: Histopathologic findings in congenital grouped pigmentation of the retina. Ophthalmology 100:400–405, 1993.

Traboulsi EI, Apostolides J, Giardiello FM, et al: Pigmented ocular fundus lesions and APC mutations in familial adenomatous polyposis. Ophthalmic Genet 17:167–174, 1996.

Traboulsi EI, Murphy SF, de la Cruz ZC, Maumenee IH, Green WR: A clinicopathologic study of the eyes in familial adenomatous polyposis with extracolonic manifestations (Gardner's syndrome). Am J Ophthalmol 110: 550–561, 1990.

**Other Primary Intraocular Tumors**

Jakobiec FA, Font RL, Tso MOM, Zimmerman LE: Mesectodermal leiomyoma of the ciliary body: a tumor of presumed neural crest origin. Cancer 39:2102–2113, 1977.

Ryan SJ Jr, Zimmerman LE, King FM: Reactive lymphoid hyperplasia: an unusual form of intraocular pseudotumor. Trans Am Acad Ophthalmol Otolaryngol 76:652–671, 1972.

Shields CL, Shields JA, Augsburger JJ: Choroidal osteoma. Surv Ophthalmol 33:17–27, 1988.

Shields JA, Hamada A, Shields CL, De Potter P, Eagle RC Jr: Ciliochoroidal nerve sheath tumor simulating a malignant melanoma. Retina 17:459–460, 1997.

Shields JA, Sanborn GE, Kurz GH, et al: Benign peripheral nerve sheath tumor of the choroid. Ophthalmology 88:1322–1329, 1983.

Shields JA, Shields CL, Eagle RC Jr, DePotter P: Observations on seven cases of intraocular leiomyoma: the 1993 Byron Demorest lecture. Arch Ophthalmol 112:521–528, 1994.

**Iris Cysts**

Augsburger J, Affel L, Benarosh D: Ultrasound biomicroscopy of cystic lesions of the iris and ciliary body. Trans Am Ophthalmol Soc 94:259, 1996.

Azuara-Blanco A, Spaeth G, Araujo S, et al: Plateau iris syndrome associated with multiple ciliary body cysts: report of three cases. Arch Ophthalmol 114:666, 1996.

Shields J: Primary cysts of the iris. Trans Am Ophthalmol Soc 79:772, 1981.

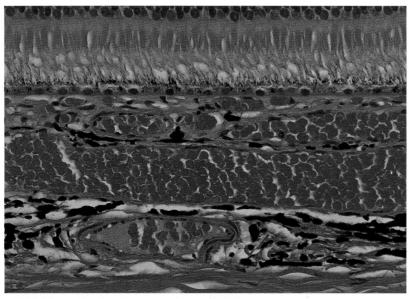

FIGURE 10–1 • **Choroid.** The choroid is the posterior part of the uveal tract. Its stroma contains dendritiform melanocytes and vessels. The latter include the choriocapillaris, which is located directly underneath Bruch's membrane, and Sattler's and Haller's layers comprised of progressively larger vessels.

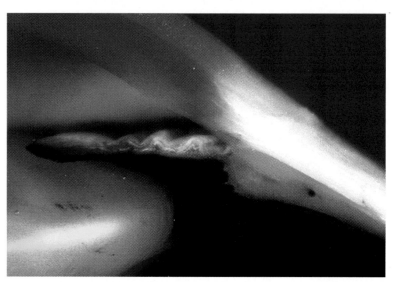

FIGURE 10–2 • **Ciliary body and iris.** The ciliary body has two parts: the anterior pars plicata composed of ciliary processes and the flat pars plana. Smooth muscle occupies most of the ciliary body's stroma. The ciliary stroma has a triangular configuration in this meridional section.

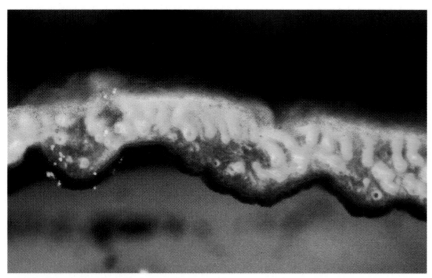

FIGURE 10–3 • **Iris.** Thick mantle of collagen highlights vessels in the iris stroma. The pigment of the light brown iris is concentrated in melanocytes of the anterior border layer. Posterior iris pigment epithelium is maximally pigmented.

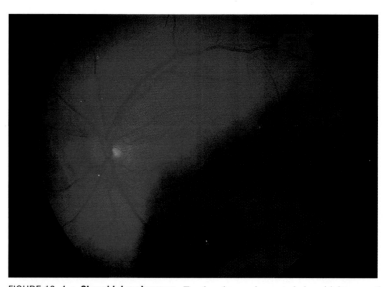

FIGURE 10–4 • **Choroidal melanoma.** Fundus shows pigmented choroidal tumor elevating the inferotemporal retina.

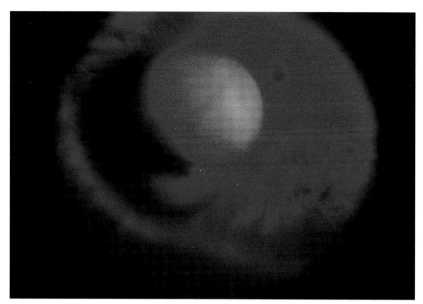

FIGURE 10–5 • **Choroidal melanoma.** Tumor seen in this wide angle photograph has broken through Bruch's membrane and has assumed a characteristic mushroom configuration.

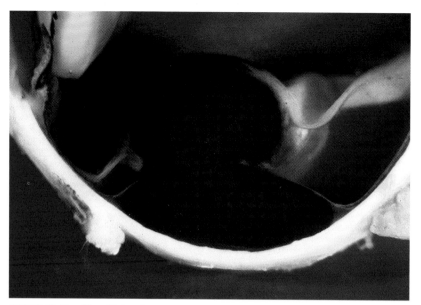

FIGURE 10–6 • **Choroidal melanoma.** A heavily pigmented melanoma has arisen from the equatorial choroid and has ruptured through Bruch's membrane. The tumor has a characteristic mushroom or collar-button configuration. Infiltration of the retina is seen at the tumor's apex. Posterior to the tumor, the retina is detached by serous fluid.

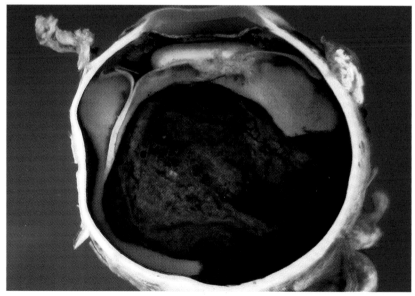

FIGURE 10–7 • **Large choroidal melanoma.** A large, heavily pigmented mushroom-shaped melanoma has produced total retinal detachment and secondary glaucoma.

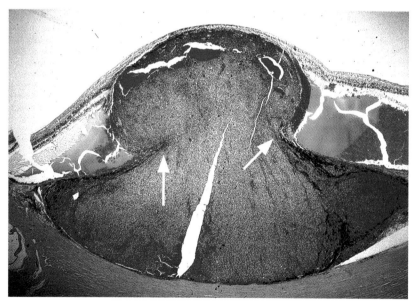

FIGURE 10–8 • **Choroidal melanoma.** Arrows point to the edge of a rupture in Bruch's membrane. Dilated vessels in the mushrooming head of the tumor are caused by the compressive cinch-like effect of the ends of Bruch's membrane on the waist of the tumor. The retina is detached by serous fluid. Hematoxylin-eosin, ×5.

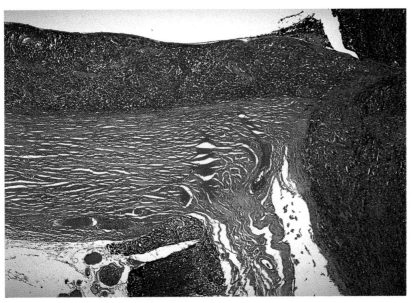

FIGURE 10–9 • **Diffuse choroidal melanoma.** Melanoma diffusely thickens the choroid. This highly aggressive tumor has massively invaded the optic nerve and has extended extraocularly along posterior emissarial canal. Hematoxylin-eosin, ×25.

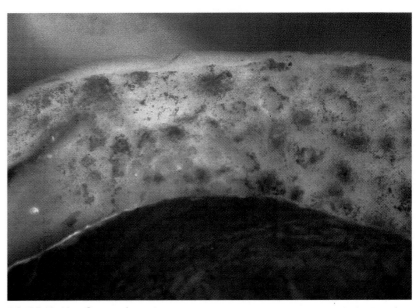

FIGURE 10–10 • **Orange pigment.** Clumps of orange pigment are seen on the back surface of the detached retina overlying an actively growing melanoma.

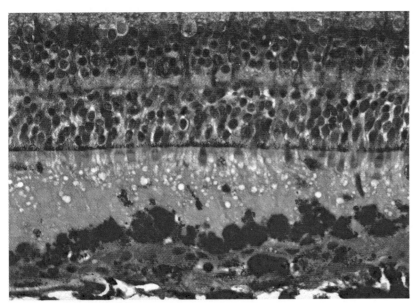

FIGURE 10–11 • **Orange pigment.** Orange pigment is comprised of aggregates of macrophages that have phagocytized PAS-positive lipofuscin and melanin pigment released by RPE cells that have been disrupted by the actively growing tumor. Periodic acid-Schiff, ×100.

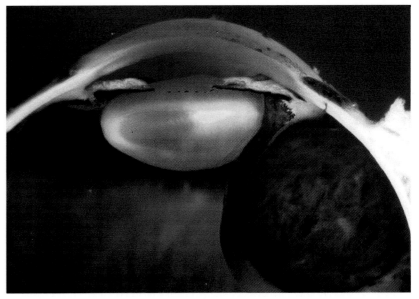

FIGURE 10–12 • **Ciliary body melanoma.** Oval ciliary body melanoma impinges on the lens equator and causes focal shallowing of the anterior chamber.

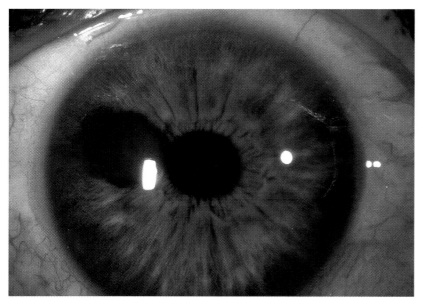

FIGURE 10–13 • **Iris nevus.** Most pigmented tumors of the iris are benign nevi. Very few enlarge when observed.

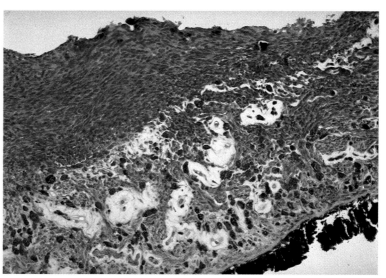

FIGURE 10–14 • **Low-grade spindle cell melanoma of the iris.** Moderately pigmented spindle cells infiltrate and thicken the stroma; they form typical plaque on the anterior iridic surface. The nuclei of the tumor cells are quite bland. Hematoxylin-eosin, ×50.

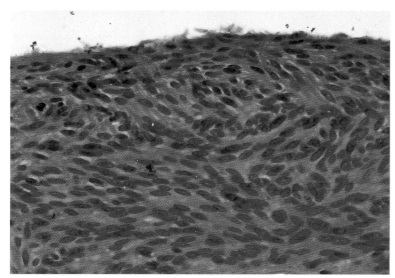

FIGURE 10–15 • **Low-grade spindle cell tumor of the iris.** Bland oval nuclei of a low-grade amelanotic spindle cell tumor lack nucleoli and contain finely dispersed chromatin. Hematoxylin-eosin, ×100.

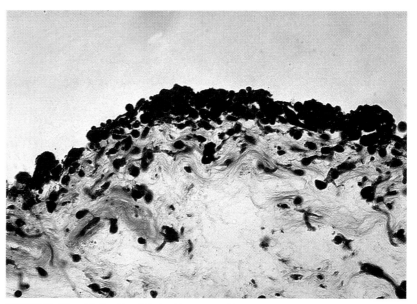

FIGURE 10–16 • **Iris freckle.** Iris freckles are small, nonprogressive nevi that occur in nearly half the adult population. Their constituent cells have rounded cellular processes that are densely packed with large melanosomes. Epon section, PD, ×100.

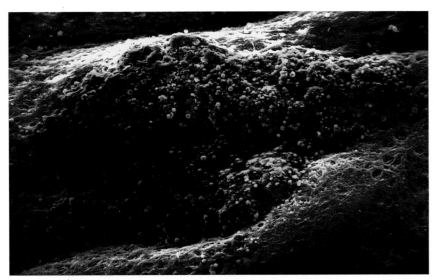

FIGURE 10–17 • **Iris freckle.** Sharply delimited colony of nevus cells is located anterior to the plane of the surrounding iris stroma. Round cellular processes decorate the surface of the nevus. False-colorized scanning electron micrograph, ×160. (Modified from Eagle RC Jr: Congenital, developmental and degenerative disorders of the iris and ciliary body. In Albert DM, Jakobiec FA, eds. *Principles and Practice of Ophthalmology. Clinical Practice.* Vol 1. Philadelphia: Saunders, 1993:367–389)

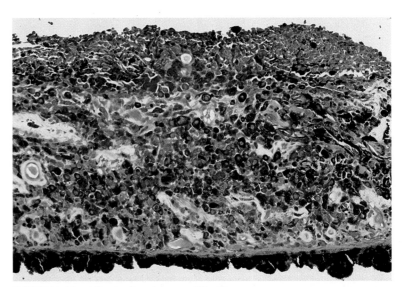

FIGURE 10–18 • **Mixed cell melanoma of the iris.** This heavily pigmented tumor is comprised of a mixture of spindle and epithelioid melanoma cells. The epithelioid cells in the stroma are distinguished by their round cytoplasmic profiles and round nuclei with prominent nucleoli. The tumor cells form a plaque on the anterior surface of the iris. Hematoxylin-eosin, ×25.

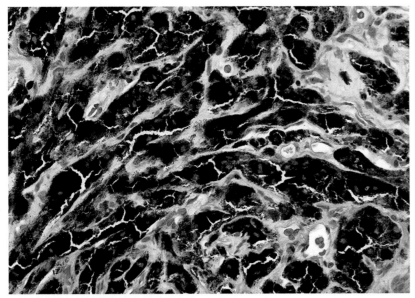

FIGURE 10–19 • **Adenoma of the iris pigment epithelium.** Cords of heavily pigmented epithelial cells comprise this iris tumor. Hematoxylin-eosin, ×100.

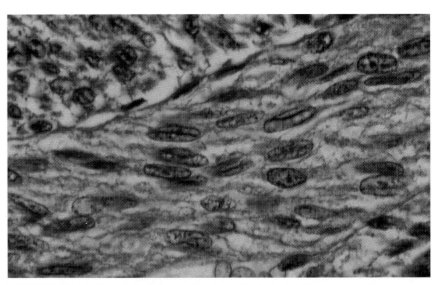

FIGURE 10–20 • **Spindle A melanoma cells.** Several spindle A cells are seen at the center of the figure. They have bland, slender, cigar-shaped nuclei with finely dispersed chromatin and indistinct nucleoli. Longitudinal folds in the nuclear membrane are apparent microscopically as a chromatin stripe or line. A few spindle B nuclei also are present. The latter have distinct nucleoli. Hematoxylin-eosin, ×250.

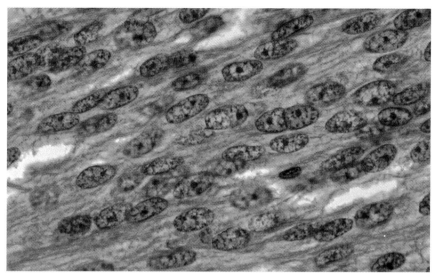

FIGURE 10–21 • **Spindle B melanoma cells.** Most of the cells in this field are spindle B melanoma cells. They have oval nuclei and an obvious nucleolus. Compared to spindle A cells, their chromatin is more coarsely clumped. The spindle cells form a syncytium and have indistinct cytoplasmic margins. Hematoxylin-eosin, ×250.

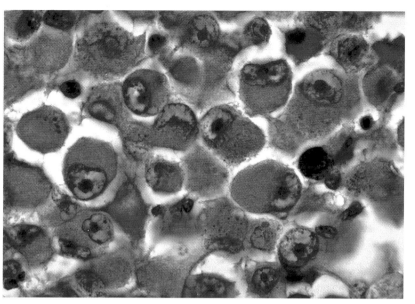

FIGURE 10–22 • **Epithelioid melanoma cells.** The cytoplasmic margins of these large, poorly cohesive epithelioid melanoma cells are easily discernible. Epithelioid cell nuclei are typically round and have peripheral margination of coarsely clumped chromatin. Epithelioid cells usually have prominent reddish purple nucleoli. They typically are polyhedral in shape and have copious amounts of cytoplasm. Hematoxylin-eosin, ×250.

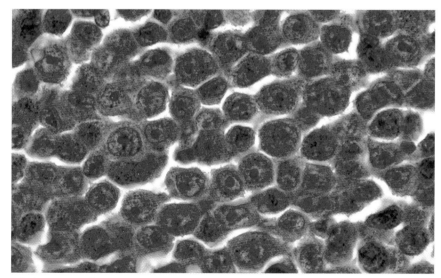

FIGURE 10–23 • **Small epithelioid cells.** Although these cells are relatively small, they are definitely epithelioid in character. They are polyhedral in shape and have distinct cytoplasmic outlines. The round or oval nuclei have prominent nucleoli. Clones of small epithelioid cells are encountered occasionally in uveal melanomas. Hematoxylin-eosin, ×250.

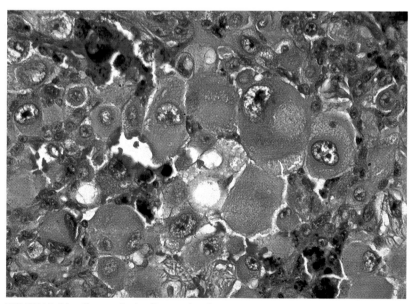

FIGURE 10–24 • **Tumor giant cells, uveal melanoma.** Tumor giant cells are highly anaplastic epithelioid cells. They are relatively rare, and their prognostic significance is uncertain. Hematoxylin-eosin, ×100.

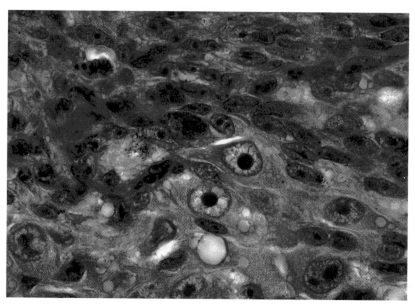

FIGURE 10–25 • **Uveal melanoma, mixed cell type.** Mixed cell melanomas are comprised of a mixture of spindle cells (above) and epithelioid cells (below). Hematoxylin-eosin, ×250.

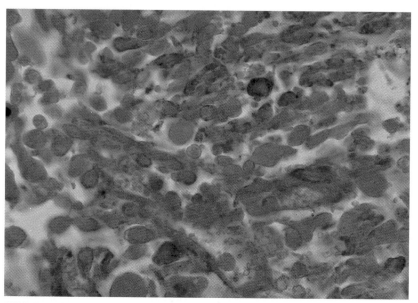

FIGURE 10–26 • **Necrotic uveal melanoma.** The cells of this necrotic melanoma are eosinophilic because they have lost their basophilic nuclear DNA. The cell type of a necrotic melanoma often can be ascertained if careful microscopy with an oil-immersion lens is performed. Necrotic uveal melanomas tend to behave clinically like mixed-cell type melanomas.

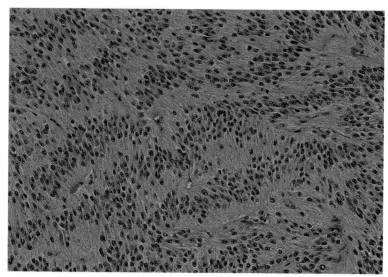

FIGURE 10–27 • **Fascicular melanoma.** The fascicular category of uveal melanoma has been removed from the modern revision of Callender's classification because cellular arrangement does not appear to affect the prognosis. This amelanotic melanoma has a striking fascicular appearance. The nuclei of its constituent spindle cells form rows that resemble the Antoni A pattern seen in schwannomas. Hematoxylin-eosin, ×50.

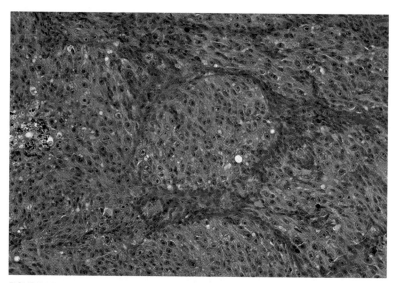

FIGURE 10–28 • **Vascular loops, uveal melanoma.** Fibrovascular septa divide parts of this predominantly epithelioid melanoma into roughly circular zones called vascular loops. Vascular networks are composed of adjacent vascular loops. Uveal melanomas that contain vascular loops and networks have a poorer prognosis. Hematoxylin-eosin, ×50.

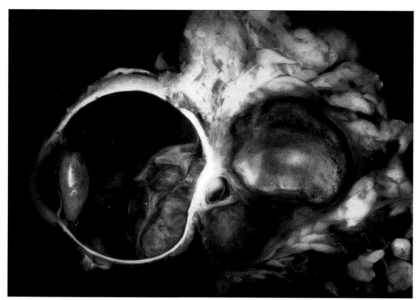

FIGURE 10–29 • **Massive extrascleral extension, uveal melanoma.** Posterior choroidal melanoma has extended extrasclerally, forming a large pigmented orbital mass that dwarfs the intraocular tumor. Optic nerve invasion is present. The patient presented with ocular proptosis.

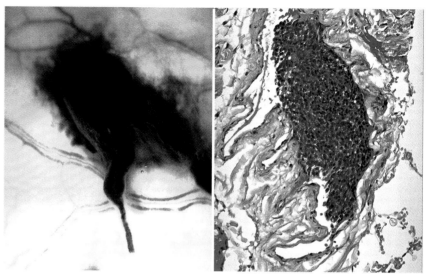

FIGURE 10–30 • **Vortex vein invasion by uveal melanoma.** *Left:* The vortex vein is massively distended by heavily pigmented tumor. *Right:* Photomicrograph shows melanoma in the lumen of the vessel. Hematoxylin-eosin, ×100.

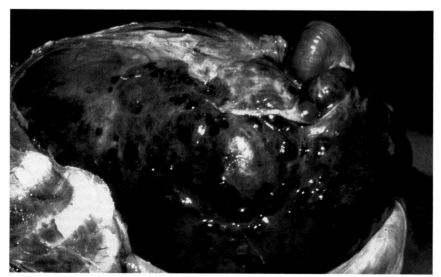

FIGURE 10–31 • **Liver metastases, uveal melanoma.** Postmortem examination of a patient who died from metastatic uveal melanoma shows massive replacement of liver by tumor. (Slide courtesy of Dr. Daniel M. Albert)

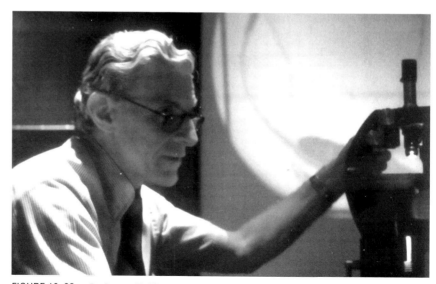

FIGURE 10–32 • Dr. Lorenz E. Zimmerman, conducting an ophthalmic pathology conference at the Armed Forces Institute of Pathology in Washington, DC circa 1978. A short time later "Zimm" formulated his hypothesis concerning the effect of enucleation on the dissemination of uveal melanoma.

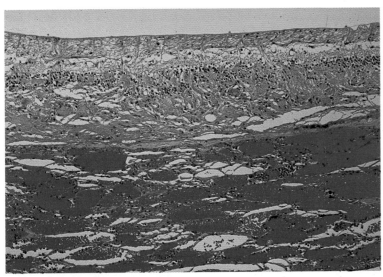

FIGURE 10–33 • **Choroidal hemangioma.** Benign vascular tumor in the choroid is composed of large thin-walled vessels. The scarred outer part of the retina adheres to the apex of the tumor. Hematoxylin-eosin, ×50.

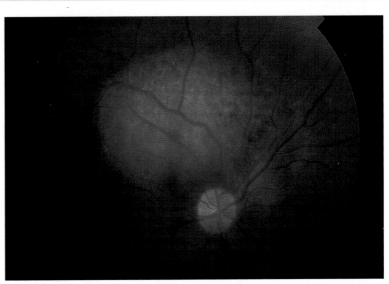

FIGURE 10–34 • **Sporadic choroidal hemangioma.** Discrete orange-red tumor is located underneath the superotemporal vascular arcade. The patient did not have Sturge-Weber syndrome.

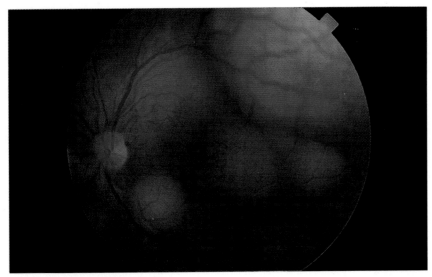

FIGURE 10–35 • **Metastatic carcinoma.** The posterior pole contains multiple nodules of amelanotic tumor. The patient was known to have metastatic mammary carcinoma. (Courtesy of Dr. Carol L. Shields, Wills Eye Hospital)

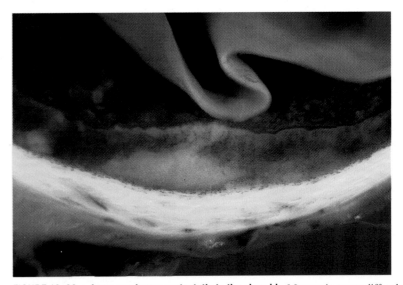

FIGURE 10–36 • **Lung carcinoma metastatic to the choroid.** Metastatic tumor diffusely thickens the choroid. Bruch's membrane is intact. The retina is detached, and the RPE is focally disrupted. The apparent pigmentation of the cut surface of the extensively necrotic tumor was caused by dispersal of uveal pigment.

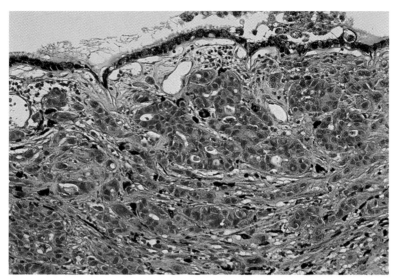

FIGURE 10–37 • **Choroidal metastasis, lung carcinoma.** Nests and islands of metastatic pulmonary adenocarcinoma infiltrate the choroidal stroma. The tumor is forming glands and is producing mucin. The detached retina is not seen. Uveal metastasis may herald an occult lung cancer. Hematoxylin-eosin, ×50.

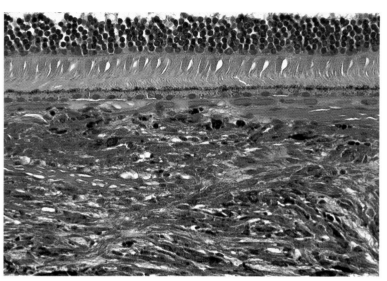

FIGURE 10–38 • **Choroidal nevus.** Pigmented spindle cells with bland nuclei infiltrate the choroid. The RPE is intact, and the overlying retina remains attached. Hematoxylin-eosin, ×100.

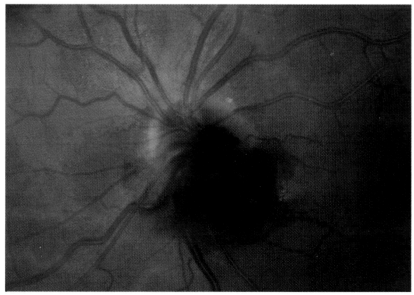

FIGURE 10–39 • **Melanocytoma, optic nerve.** The intensely pigmented magnocellular nevus partially obscures the optic nerve. Melanocytomas classically affect the optic nerve, but they may involve any part of the uvea.

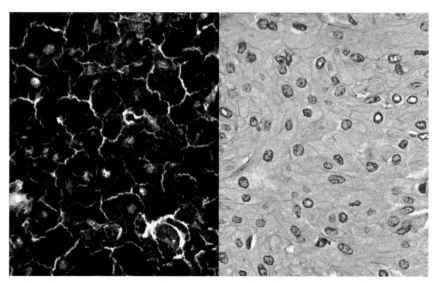

FIGURE 10–40 • **Melanocytoma.** *Left:* Copious quantities of melanin pigment obscure nuclear details. *Right:* Bleaching of melanin pigment discloses bland nuclei and a low nuclear/cytoplasmic ratio, consistent with benign magnocellular nevus. Left: hematoxylin-eosin, ×100; right: bleach, ×100.

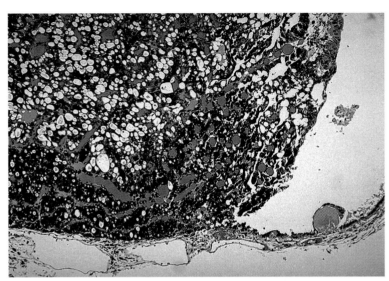

FIGURE 10–41 • **RPE adenoma.** Heavily pigmented, highly vascular tumor arises abruptly from the RPE. The tumor is located on the inner surface of Bruch's membrane and does not involve the choroidal stroma. It contains many small cystoid spaces. Hematoxylin-eosin, ×50.

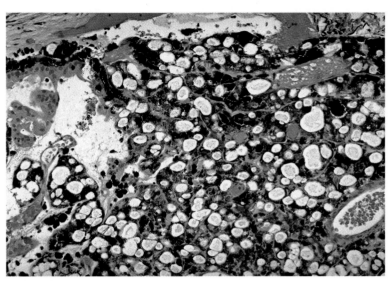

FIGURE 10–42 • **Adenoma of pigmented ciliary epithelium.** The tumor contains many small cystoid spaces. Continuity with the ciliary epithelium is seen at top left. Hematoxylin-eosin, ×100.

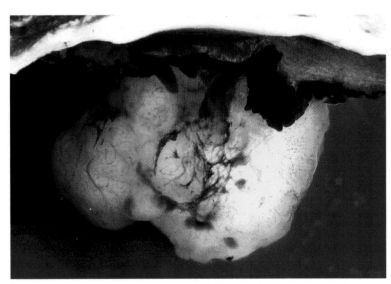

FIGURE 10–43 • **Adenoma of nonpigmented ciliary epithelium.** Nonpigmented ciliary epithelial tumor rests on the inner surface of the ciliary body and does not involve its stroma.

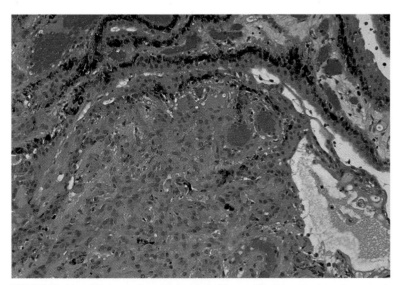

FIGURE 10–44 • **Adenoma of nonpigmented ciliary epithelium.** Benign adenoma arises from ciliary epithelium on the inner surface of the pars plicata. Its constituent epithelial cells are largely nonpigmented. Hematoxylin-eosin, ×100.

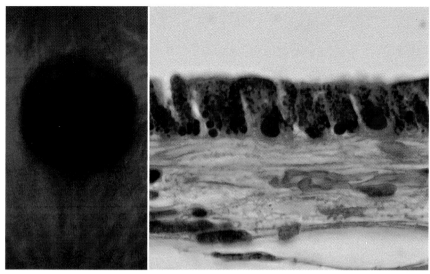

FIGURE 10–45 • **Congenital hypertrophy of the RPE (CHRPE).** Round lesion (*Inset*) lacks lacunae. Histopathology of a similar lesion shows tall, hypertrophic RPE cells that are intensely pigmented. The pigment includes many large, round macromelanosomes. Hematoxylin-eosin, ×250.

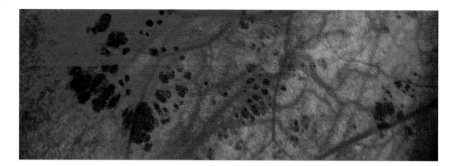

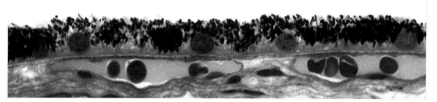

FIGURE 10–46 • **Congenital grouped pigmentation of the RPE ("bear tracks").** *Top:* Note the numerous flat, well demarcated pigmented lesions that have been likened to animal tracks. *Bottom:* Photomicrograph shows increased numbers of ellipsoidal melanin granules filling the cytoplasm of the RPE cells. Melanosomes are confined to the apical cytoplasm in normal RPE cells.

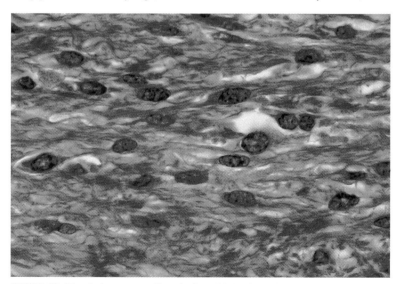

FIGURE 10–47 • **Leiomyoma, ciliary body.** This benign spindle cell tumor of smooth muscle derivation is relatively paucicellular compared to an amelanotic spindle cell melanoma. The spindle cells have bland nuclei and finely fibrillar cytoplasm. Immunohistochemical stains for smooth muscle actin were strongly positive. Some uveal leiomyomas have a distinctly neural appearance. Hematoxylin-eosin, ×250.

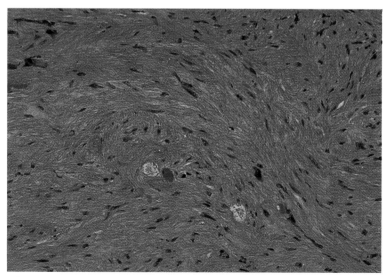

FIGURE 10–48 • **Benign peripheral nerve sheath tumor, choroid.** The cytology of this bland, paucicellular choroidal tumor is consistent with a schwannoma. Schwannomas are rare intraocular tumors. Immunohistochemical staining or electron microscopy is necessary to confirm the diagnosis. Hematoxylin-eosin, ×50.

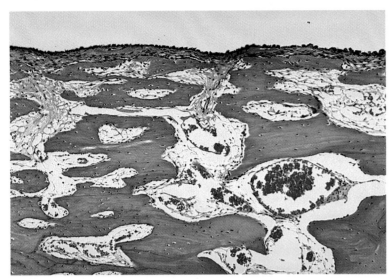

FIGURE 10–49 • **Choroidal osteoma.** The tumor is composed of irregular spicules of bone surrounded by an areolar stroma containing large vascular channels. The bone is found within the choroid, deep to Bruch's membrane, the choriocapillaris, and an intact layer of RPE. The intrachoroidal location of the bone distinguishes choroidal osteoma from the bone formed by osseous metaplasia of the RPE in blind phthisical eyes. Metaplastic bone typically is located on the inner surface of Bruch's membrane. Hematoxylin-eosin, ×25.

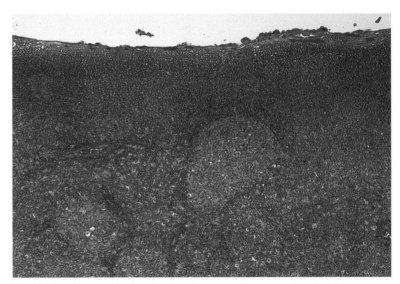

FIGURE 10–50 • **Reactive lymphoid hyperplasia of the uvea.** The choroid is massively thickened by an infiltrate of lymphocytes. The lighter foci are germinal centers. Additional foci of lymphoid cells were present on the epibulbar surface of the eye. An exudative retinal detachment is present. Reactive lymphoid hyperplasia of the uvea is now thought to be a low-grade lymphoid neoplasm. Hematoxylin-eosin, ×25.

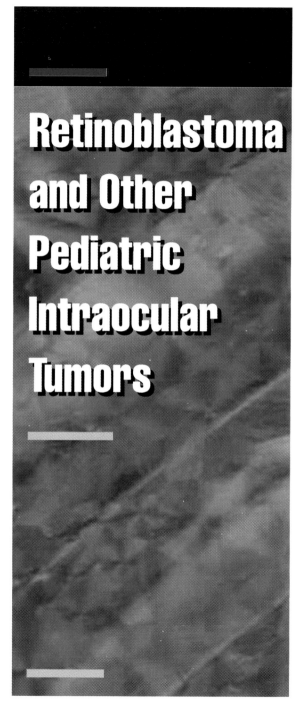

# CHAPTER 11

# Retinoblastoma and Other Pediatric Intraocular Tumors

R etinoblastoma is the most common intraocular tumor of childhood, although it is relatively rare: Only 250 cases occur yearly in the United States. Retinoblastoma has no racial or sexual predilection. The tumor is diagnosed at a mean age of 18 months, and about 90% of cases are diagnosed before 3 years of age. Rare cases that occur in older children and adults are often misdiagnosed.

Retinoblastoma typically presents clinically with a white pupillary reflex called leukocoria (Figs. 11–1, 11–2). In fact, 90% of cases present with leukocoria in the United States and Europe. Strabismus or ocular misalignment is found in about one-third of cases. For this reason, careful ophthalmoscopy should be performed in all children with strabismus to exclude retinoblastoma or some other significant retinal pathology. Rarer presentations include neovascular glaucoma, which may cause secondary buphthalmos, and iris heterochromia. Pseudohypopyons composed of tumor cells may develop when endophytic or diffuse infiltrating retinoblastomas seed the anterior chamber (Fig. 11–3). Children who have intraocular infarction caused by tumor-induced neovascular glaucoma occasionally present with an orbital cellulitis-like picture. Late stages of the disease are often encountered in underdeveloped countries. There, retinoblastoma typically presents as a massive orbital tumor (Fig. 11–4).

Macroscopically, retinoblastoma has a white encephaloid or brain-like appearance, which is not unexpected as the tumor arises from the retina, a peripheral colony of brain cells (Figs. 11–5, 11–6, 11–7). Lighter flecks of calcification are often evident grossly in the tumor.

Tumors with endophytic, exophytic, mixed, and diffuse infiltrating growth patterns occur. Endophytic retinoblastomas arise from the inner layers of the retina (Fig. 11–5). The retina remains attached, and seeding of the vitreous and anterior chamber often occurs. Tumors with a predominantly endophytic growth pattern may be confused clinically with inflammatory disorders such as uveitis or ocular toxocariasis. Exophytic retinoblastomas arise from the outer layers of the retina and cause retinal detachment (Fig. 11–6). Exophytic retinoblastomas are usually confused clinically with simulating lesions, such as Coats' disease, which cause an exudative retinal detachment. Strictly endo- or exophytic retinoblastomas are relatively uncommon; most tumors have a mixed endophytic–exophytic growth pattern. About 1.4% of retinoblastomas diffusely thicken the retina without forming a distinct mass (Fig. 11–7). This rare diffuse infiltrating growth pattern usually is found in older children (mean age 6 years) who often present with pseudoinflammatory signs and invariably have unilateral sporadic tumors (Figs. 11–3, 11–8).

Histopathologically, the retinoblastoma arises from and destroys the retina (Fig. 11–9). Under low magnification retinoblastoma appears blue, pink, and purple (Fig. 11–10). The blue areas represent viable parts of the tumor, which are composed of poorly differentiated neuroblastic cells that have basophilic nuclei and scanty cytoplasm (Fig. 11–11). Retinoblastoma cells readily outgrow their blood supply and undergo necrosis. Sleeves or cuffs of viable cells that measure about 90–100 $\mu$m in radius generally persist around vessels (Fig. 11–10, 11–12). The necrotic tumor cells lose their basophilic nuclear DNA and become pink or eosinophilic. Dystrophic calcification, which appears reddish purple in hematoxylin-eosin (H&E)-stained sections, often develops in the necrotic parts of the tumor (Fig. 11–10). The calcified foci are readily detected with ultrasonography or computed tomography (CT) scans and help establish the clinical diagnosis. Retinoblastomas contain many mitoses. Intensely basophilic DNA released from necrotic tumor cells may deposit in vessel walls, the iris stroma, the trabecular meshwork and walls of Schlemm's canal, and the lens capsule and retinal internal limiting membrane (Fig. 11–13). Iris neovascularization is found in about 50% of enucleated eyes, which may have peripheral anterior synechias and neovascular glaucoma. Tumors cells also typically collect on the inner surface of Bruch's membrane, forming focal retinal pigment epithelial (RPE) detachments. The tumor infiltrates and destroys the retina, which is usually partially detached. Extensive seeding may involve the vitreous and the inner and outer surfaces of the retina (see Fig. 9–18). The prevalence of intraocular seeding makes it difficult to diagnose multifocal retinoblastoma.

Varying degrees of retinal differentiation occur in retinoblastoma. This includes the formation of Wright and Flexner-Wintersteiner rosettes and photoreceptor differentiation (fleurettes) (Figs. 11–14, 11–15, 11–16, 11–17).

Wright rosettes (named after James Homer Wright) indicate neuroblastic differentiation (Fig. 11–14). They lack a central lumen, and their constituent cells encompass a central tangle of neural filaments. Wright rosettes are relatively nonspecific. They also occur in neuroblastoma and medulloblastoma.

Flexner-Wintersteiner rosettes (Fig. 11–15) represent early retinal differentiation and are a characteristic histopathologic feature of retinoblastoma. They have a central lumen that corresponds to the subretinal space and is filled with hyaluronidase-resistant glycosaminoglycan analogous to the interphotoreceptor matrix material. A girdle of intercellular connections (zonulae adherentes) analogous to the retina's external limiting membrane joins the apices of the cells forming the Flexner-Wintersteiner rosette. Cilia with the 9+0 doublet pattern found in the central nervous system (CNS) project into the lumen. (Photoreceptor outer segments are thought to be derived from cilia.) Although highly characteristic of retinoblastoma, Flexner-Wintersteiner rosettes are not pathognomonic: They do occur in malignant medulloepitheliomas and some pineal tumors.

Fleurettes (Fig. 11–16) represent photoreceptor differentiation. Photoreceptor differentiation typically is found is areas of viable tumor that appear relatively eosinophilic under low magnification (Fig. 11–17). The cells have prominent eosinophilic cellular processes filled with mitochondria that represent neoplastic photoreceptor inner segments. Transmission electron microscopy occasionally reveals foci of abortive outer segment disks. Some fleurettes are composed of a small bouquet of tumor cells aligned along a segment of neoplastic external limiting membrane.

Retinal tumors composed entirely of fleurettes are thought to be benign tumors called retinocytomas or retinomas. Accordingly, their constituent cells appear relatively bland compared to those of retinoblastoma, with a low nuclear/cytoplasmic ratio, finely dispersed chromatin, few mitoses, and absent necrosis. Calcification is found in viable parts of the tumor.

Clinically, retinocytomas once were thought to be retinoblastomas that had undergone spontaneous regression (Fig. 11–18). They have a "fish flesh" appearance and contain abundant amounts of calcification that has been likened to cottage cheese. An annulus of RPE depigmentation typically surrounds the tumor. Retinocytomas are relatively resistant to radiation, like other benign tumors. It is therefore not surprising that foci of photoreceptor differentiation are found more often in enucleated eyes with a history of external beam radiotherapy or chemoreduction. Retinocytomas rarely undergo malignant transformation.

Retinoblastomas occasionally regress spontaneously. In such cases histopathologic examination shows a degenerated, phthisical eye that contains foci of calcified tumor cells in a matrix of glial scar tissue and evidence of extensive intraocular necrosis (Fig. 11–19). Spontaneous necrosis occurs unilaterally in patients with bilateral tumors, making an immunologic mechanism unlikely. Tumor infarction caused by severe neovascular glaucoma is the probable cause of both the regression and phthisis.

Untreated retinoblastoma is invariably fatal. The growing tumor progressively fills the eye and then extends extraocularly to form an orbital mass. Optic nerve invasion is a characteristic feature of the retinoblastoma (Fig. 11–20). Prognosis is directly related to the depth of optic nerve invasion. The tumor may travel along the optic nerve to the brain, or tumor cells may be dispersed along the neuraxis if they gain access to the cerebrospinal fluid (CSF).

Four routes of extraocular extension or metastasis are possible. The tumor can reach the brain by direct infiltration along the optic nerve, or it can pass through orbital bones or foramina from areas of orbital involvement. Retinoblastoma cells can be carried to the subarachnoid space of the brain and spinal cord by the CSF. Distant blood-borne metastasis to the lung, bones, and brain generally occurs in patients who have extrascleral extension or massive invasion of the uvea. The tumor can also spread to preauricular or cervical lymph nodes if it gains access to lymphatics in the conjunctiva. Metastasis from retinoblastoma typically occurs within 2 years of treatment. Retained tumor cells in the orbit or in the residual optic nerve are responsible for most recurrences.

The most important prognostic factors of retinoblastoma are the presence and extent of optic nerve invasion, extraocular extension into the orbit, and probably extensive uveal invasion (Figs. 11–21, 11–22). Unlike uveal melanoma, the size of the retinoblastoma does not appear to be an important prognostic factor for life.

The depth of optic nerve invasion is important. In one series only 8% of patients without histologic evidence of optic nerve invasion died. The mortality rate was 15% if the tumor had invaded to the lamina cribrosa and rose to 44% with retrolaminar invasion; 64% died if the retinoblastoma had extended to the surgical margin. Therefore a long segment of optic nerve should always be obtained when an eye that is known or suspected to contain a retinoblastoma is enucleated. The pathologist must carefully examine the surgical margin, marking it and removing a transverse section of optic nerve before opening the globe. The optic nerve section should be wrapped in tissue and submitted in a separate cassette to avoid contamination.

## RETINOBLASTOMA GENE

Familial, chromosomal deletion and sporadic variants of retinoblastoma occur. About 5–10% of retinoblastomas are familial. Familial retinoblastoma is often bilateral and is transmitted to offspring as an apparent autosomal dominant trait that is recessive at the molecular level (Figs. 11–2, 11–23). The average age of patients with familial retinoblastoma is about 1 year. Most retinoblastomas (85%) are sporadic tumors that arise in patients who have no family history of the tumor. About 75% of these sporadic tumors are caused by somatic mutations. Somatic sporadic retinoblastomas are always unilateral, unifocal tumors that cannot be passed on to progeny. They tend to occur in slightly older infants (mean age 2 years). The remaining one-fourth of sporadic cases are caused by germinal mutations and represent new familial cases that can be passed on to progeny. Fewer than 5% of retinoblastomas are associated with deletions in the long arm of chromosome 13 that are evident in karyotypic analysis. Patients with the 13Q− deletion have a syndrome that in addition to retinoblastoma includes mental retardation, imperforate anus, genital anomalies, and facial anomalies such as low-set ears, a thin upper lip, and broad nasal bridge. The association of retinoblas-

toma with the 13Q− syndrome initially suggested that the retinoblastoma gene was located on chromosome 13.

The paradigmatic recessive oncogene, the retinoblastoma (Rb) gene is located in the 1–4 band of the long arm of chromosome 13. The gene sequence contains more than 180,000 basepairs and encodes a protein product comprised of 928 amino acids that is found in the nucleus of cells. There the Rb protein interacts with other transcription factors to control the cell cycle. During the resting ($G_1$) phase of the cell cycle, Rb protein forms a complex with the E2F transcription factor. Phosphorylation of the Rb protein causes it to separate from E2F, which then is able to activate a variety of other genes that activate DNA synthesis. Absence of Rb protein causes continual cell division and lack of terminal differentiation, (i.e., cancer).

Normal individuals have two functional copies of the Rb gene (Fig. 11–24). Sporadic somatic retinoblastomas are caused by the loss or inactivation of both copies of the Rb gene in a single retinal cell. Carriers of familial retinoblastoma are heterozygous for the Rb gene (Fig. 11–25). A retinoblastoma develops when the single remaining or functional gene is lost or inactivated in a retinal cell leading to loss of Rb protein (Fig. 11–26). Genes usually are lost during cellular division. The spontaneous mutation rate for the Rb gene is $10^{-7}$ or higher. It has been estimated that $10^8$ mitoses are involved in the growth and development of the retina, a number that is greater than the spontaneous mutation rate for the Rb gene. Hence it is probable that a retinal tumor will arise in a heterozygous carrier of the Rb gene (Fig. 11–27). It is also probable that bilateral tumors will arise because $10^8$ mitoses are involved in the formation of *each* retina. These figures are also compatible with multiple tumors in a single retina.

Bilateral tumors occur in about two-thirds of cases of familial retinoblastoma (Fig. 11–28). If bilateral

retinoblastomas are found, it is certain that the affected patient is a carrier of familial retinoblastoma who can transmit the tumor to half of his or her progeny. Unfortunately, the opposite is not true. Patients with unilateral sporadic tumors still may harbor transmissible sporadic germline mutations.

Sporadic somatic retinoblastomas are caused by the loss or inactivation of both Rb genes in a single retinal cell in a patient whose genotype is normal. Sporadic somatic tumors invariably are unilateral and unifocal and are diagnosed on average at age 24 months because two gene inactivations, or "hits," presumably are required (Fig. 11–29). Familial tumors require only a single "hit" and occur a year earlier.

Familial retinoblastoma appears to be an autosomal dominant trait but is recessive at the molecular level. When a heterozygous carrier of the Rb gene (Rbrb) mates with a normal individual (RbRb) 50% of the offspring will be new carriers prone to develop retinoblastoma and 50% will be normal, a ratio that perfectly mimics autosomal dominant inheritance (Fig. 11–30). Most retinoblastomas occur before age 3 years because genes are inactivated during cellular division and mitotic activity in the retina has largely ceased at birth.

It is not surprising that the Rb gene has been incriminated in other nonocular cancers, as it plays such a central role in the control of the cell cycle. Heterozygous carriers of familial retinoblastoma have a 20–50% chance of developing a second nonocular neoplasm in 20 years. Tumors, including osteogenic and other sarcomas, are especially prone to develop in the orbit after external beam radiotherapy. The risk of developing osteogenic sarcoma outside the field of radiation is also increased 500-fold. Retinoblastoma-like tumors of the pineal gland may develop in carriers of the Rb gene, an association called trilateral retinoblastoma. Rb gene inactivation has been found in some breast and lung cancers. Certain tumor viruses, such as human papilloma virus (HPV) and some strains of adenovirus, cause cancer by producing proteins that bind to and inactivate Rb protein.

## DIFFERENTIAL DIAGNOSIS OF RETINOBLASTOMA

Retinoblastoma must be differentiated clinically from several benign childhood disorders that cause leukocoria. The three most common conditions confused with retinoblastoma are ocular toxocariasis, persistent hyperplastic primary vitreous, and Coats' disease.

Ocular toxocariasis (nematode endophthalmitis) is a localized ocular manifestation of visceral larva migrans caused by larvae of the nematode *Toxocara canis*. Ocular toxocariasis usually is unilateral and occurs in children toward the end of the first decade of life. Diffuse nematode endophthalmitis, retinal detachment, or an eosinophilic abscess located anteriorly in the vitreous can cause leukocoria. Subfoveal granulomas occasionally present with visual loss in eyes with clear media. Histopathology discloses necrotic larval fragments surrounded by granulomatous inflammation containing many eosinophils (Fig. 11–31). Serial sections may be necessary to demonstrate the parasite in a presumptive eosinophilic abscess. Clinically, an enzyme-linked immunosorbent assay (ELISA) for *Toxocara* antigen excludes the diagnosis if it is negative. A positive ELISA does not exclude retinoblastoma, however, because antibodies to *T. canis* are common in some populations.

Persistent hyperplastic primary vitreous (PHPV) (Figs. 11–32, 11–33, 11–34). is a congenital anomaly that is present at birth and classically found in a microophthalmic eye. Affected patients have leukocoria caused by a fibrovascular plaque behind the lens, which initially is clear. The fibrovascular plaque is derived from the embryonic primary vitreous and is supplied by a persistent hyaloid artery and anterior components of the embryonic vasculature. The tips of the ciliary process adhere to the margins of the retrolental plaque, and the processes are drawn centrally by ocular growth (Fig. 11–32). The elongated processes are readily seen when the pupil is dilated and help to establish the diagnosis clinically. Shunt vessels are also seen traversing the anterior iridic surface. Intralenticular adipose tissue and even bone have been reported in PHPV (Fig. 11–33). Persistent fetal vasculature (PFV) may be a more appropriate term for this disorder.

Coats' disease is a congenital disorder of the retinal vasculature that typically presents with massive exudative retinal detachment (Figs. 11–35, 11–36). Coats' disease usually is unilateral and has a peak incidence toward the end of the first decade. Two-thirds of cases occur in boys. Congenital retinal vascular anomalies occur, including dilated telangiectatic vessels, microaneurysms, and dilated veins that resemble light bulbs fluorangiographically. Fluorescein angiography typically discloses areas of capillary nonperfusion in the adjacent retina. The retinal vascular abnormalities leak profusely, causing an exudative retinal detachment with lipid-rich, densely proteinaceous subretinal fluid. Histopathology shows abnormal vessels in the detached retina (Fig. 11–37). The outer layers of the retina usually are massively thickened by eosinophilic exudates. The subretinal fluid contains rhomboidal cholesterol crystals evident in sections as empty clefts and lipid-laden histiocytes with foamy vacuolated cytoplasm (Fig. 11–38). Eyes with Coats' disease frequently are enucleated when they become blind and painful. Most have secondary closed-angle glaucoma caused by the bullous retinal detachment.

Glial neoplasms, especially the retinal astrocytomas that occur in patients with tuberous sclerosis, can be difficult to distinguish clinically from retinoblastoma. Retinal astrocytomas in tuberous sclerosis can exhibit progressive growth and become quite large (Fig. 1–15). A reactive proliferation of retinal glial cells can reach tumor-like proportions after trauma or surgery. This reaction is called massive gliosis of the retina.

Retinopathy of prematurity (ROP), once called retrolental fibroplasia, classically develops in premature infants who have received supplemental oxygen therapy. ROP is characterized by vitreoretinal neovascularization that may progress to tractional retinal detachment. The retinal neovascularization probably is caused by the effect of increased oxygen levels on the immature vasculature of the peripheral retina. ROP is often bilateral; it is not present at birth but develops sometime afterward, features it shares with retinoblastoma. The retinopathy typically develops in the longer temporal part of the retina that is less likely to be completely vascularized. Capillary proliferation begins in the retina after an initial vasoconstrictive phase induced by high levels of oxygen. The capillaries break through into the vitreous, forming a band of vitreoretinal neovascularization located between the peripheral avascular and the posterior vascularized parts of the retina (Figs. 11–39). Vitreous hemorrhage, fibrosis, and organization usually complicate severe untreated cases. Tractional retinal detachment forms an opaque white retrolental mass that may be difficult to differentiate from retinoblastoma (Figs. 11–40, 11–41). The fovea and optic disk are dragged temporally as the retina is incorporated into the peripheral mass. The endstage of ROP is marked by total retinal detachment, leukocoria, closed angle glaucoma, phthisis bulbi, and blindness.

Relatively rare causes of leukocoria include Norrie's disease, the Bloch-Sulzberger type of incontinentia pigmenti, retinal dysplasia, and embryonal medulloepithelioma.

Norrie's disease is an X-linked recessive heritable disorder marked by mental retardation or deterioration, progressive sensorineural deafness, and bilateral congenital blindness caused by intraocular tumor-like masses of detached malformed retina (pseudogliomas). Mutations in the norrin gene have been found in patients with other heritable retinal disorders including X-linked exudative vitreoretinopathy.

Incontinentia pigmenti is a heritable disorder carried on the X chromosome; it occurs only in girls and probably is lethal in males. Some affected females develop peripheral vitreoretinal neovascular proliferation, which is related to retinal capillary nonperfusion and can progress to retinal detachment, mimicking retinoblastoma. Shortly after birth, infants with incontinentia pigmenti develop vesiculobullous skin lesions rich in eosinophils. A marbleized pattern of skin pigmentation subsequently develops. Other manifestations of incontinentia pigmenti include retinal pigment epithelial mottling, foveal hypoplasia, strabismus, loss of eyelashes and brow hair, dental anomalies, mental retardation, and seizures.

Most cases of retinal dysplasia are associated with trisomy 13 (see Fig. 1–3). Dysplastic retinal rosettes are composed of multiple retinal layers and are larger than the Flexner-Wintersteiner rosettes of retinoblastoma. Patients with trisomy 13 often have other severe ocular abnormalities, including colobomas, PHPV, and microphthalmia. Anophthalmos, and cyclopia-synophthalmos can also occur. Microphthalmic eyes with trisomy 13 often contain islands of hyaline cartilage in a coloboma.

Medulloepithelioma (diktyoma) is the second most common intraocular tumor of childhood (Figs. 11–42, 11–43, 11–44, 11–45, 11–46). Medulloepitheliomas are thought to arise from an anlage of the primitive medullary epithelium that lines the forebrain and optic vesicle during early embryonic life. Although usually considered an embryonal tumor, medulloepithelioma typically becomes symptomatic at around age 4 years and is diagnosed a year later. Misdiagnosis is frequent, and tumors occasionally are discovered when blind, painful eyes are examined in the laboratory. Most medulloepitheliomas are nonpigmented tumors that arise from the inner surface of the ciliary body (Fig. 11–43). The optic nerve head is affected rarely. Many tumors contain cystic areas. Clinically, medulloepithelioma often causes a secondary coloboma of the lens (lens notching) and a retrolental cyclitic membrane. Neovascular glaucoma develops in many eyes.

Histologically, medulloepitheliomas are composed of cords and sheets of polarized neuroepithelial cells that form elongated tubules and cystic structures (Fig. 11–44). Many tumors contain abundant, loose mesenchymal stroma rich in hyaluronic acid, analogous to primitive vitreous (Fig. 11–45). Medulloepitheliomas are classified as benign or malignant and teratoid or nonteratoid. About two-thirds of medulloepitheliomas are malignant. Some malignant tumors harbor undifferentiated areas that resemble retinoblastoma and may contain Flexner-Wintersteiner rosettes. Others contain sarcomatous stroma. Invasiveness and extraocular extension are other important histologic criteria for malignancy. Teratoid tumors, which account for about 37.5% of cases, contain foci of heterologous tissue including hyaline cartilage, rhabdomyoblasts or striated muscle, and brain (Fig. 11–46). Fatalities can result from direct intracranial extension in cases with orbital invasion. Eyes containing medulloepitheliomas should be enucleated because the tumor almost always recurs after local resection.

Other rare intraocular tumors of childhood include glioneuroma, melanogenic neuroectodermal tumor of the retina, intraocular ectopic lacrimal gland tissue, rhabdomyosarcomas of the iris and ciliary body, and juvenile xanthogranuloma (JXG). JXG of the iris is a cause of spontaneous hyphema and secondary glaucoma.

# References

## General References

Abramson DH, Gombos DS: The topography of bilateral retinoblastoma lesions. Retina 16:232–239, 1996.

Burnier MN, McLean IW, Zimmerman LE, Rosenberg SH: Retinoblastoma: the relationship of proliferating cells to blood vessels. Invest Ophthalmol Vis Sci 31:2037–2040, 1990.

Eagle RC Jr: Retinoblastoma and pseudoglioma. In Duane TD, Jaeger EA (eds) Biomedical Foundations of Ophthalmology. Vol 3. Philadelphia: Harper & Row, 1986:1–29.

Kyritsis AP, Tsokos M, Triche TJ, Chader GJ: Retinoblastoma: a primitive tumor with multipotential characteristics. Invest Ophthalmol Vis Sci 27:1760–1764, 1986.

McLean IW: Retinoblastomas, retinocytomas and pseudoretinblastomas. In Spencer W (ed) Ophthalmic Pathology: An Atlas and Textbook. 4th ed. Vol 2. Philadelphia: Saunders, 1996:1332–1380.

Mietz H, Hutton WL, Font RL: Unilateral retinoblastoma in an adult: report of a case and review of the literature [see comments]. Ophthalmology 104:43–47, 1997.

Morgan G: Diffuse infiltrating retinoblastoma. Br J Ophthalmol 55:600–606, 1971.

Mullaney J: Retinoblastomas with DNA precipitation. Arch Ophthalmol 82:454–456, 1969.

Nork TM, Millecchia LL, de Venecia GB, Myers FL, Vogel KA: Immunocytochemical features of retinoblastoma in an adult. Arch Ophthalmol 114:1402–1406, 1996.

Nork TM, Schwartz TL, Doshi HM, Millecchia LL: Retinoblastoma: cell of origin. Arch Ophthalmol 113:791–802, 1995.

Rubenfeld M, Abramson DH, Ellsworth RM, Kitchin FD: Unilateral vs. bilateral retinoblastoma: correlations between age at diagnosis and stage of ocular disease. Ophthalmology 93:1016–1019, 1986.

Schofield PB: Diffuse infiltrating retinoblastoma. Br J Ophthalmol 44:35–41, 1960.

Shields CL, Shields JA, Shah P: Retinoblastoma in older children. Ophthalmology 98:395–399, 1991.

Tso MOM, Fine BS, Zimmerman LE: The Flexner-Wintersteiner rosettes in retinoblastoma. Arch Pathol 88:665–671, 1969.

Tso MOM, Zimmerman LE, Fine BS: The nature of retinoblastoma: photoreceptor differentiation: a clinical and histopathological study. Am J Ophthalmol 69:339–349, 1970.

Tsokos M, Kyritsis AP, Chader GJ, Triche TJ: Differentiation of human retinoblastoma in vitro into cell types with characteristics observed in embryonal or mature retina. Am J Pathol 123:542–552, 1986.

Vrabec T, Arbizo V, Adamus G, McDowell JH, Hargrave PA, Donoso LA: Rod cell-specific antigens in retinoblastoma. Arch Ophthalmol 107:1061–1063, 1989.

## Retinoma/Retinocytoma

Eagle RC Jr, Shields JA, Donoso L, et al: Malignant transformation of spontaneously regressed retinoblastoma, retinoma/retinocytoma variant. Ophthalmology 96:1389–1395, 1989.

Gallie BL, Ellsworth RM, Abramson DH, Phillips RA: Retinoma: spontaneous regression of retinoblastoma or benign manifestation of the mutation? Br J Cancer 45: 513–521, 1982.

Lueder GT, Heon E, Gallie BL: Retinoma associated with vitreous seeding. Am J Ophthalmol 119:522–523, 1995.

Margo C, Hidayat A, Kopelman J, Zimmerman LE: Retinocytoma: a benign variant of retinoblastoma. Arch Ophthalmol 101:1519–1531, 1983.

**Prognostic Factors**

Khelfaoui F, Validire P, Auperin A, et al: Histopathologic risk factors in retinoblastoma: a retrospective study of 172 patients treated in a single institution. Cancer 77: 1206–1213, 1996.

Kopelman JE, McLean IW, Rosenberg SH: Multivariate analysis of risk factors for metastasis in retinoblastoma treated by enucleation. Ophthalmology 94:371–377, 1987.

MacKay CJ, Abramson DH, Ellsworth RM: Metastatic patterns of retinoblastoma. Arch Ophthalmol 102:391–396, 1984.

Magramm I, Abramson DH, Ellsworth RM: Optic nerve involvement in retinoblastoma. Ophthalmology 96: 217–222, 1989.

McLean IW, Rosenberg SH, Messmer EP, et al: Prognostic factors in cases of retinoblastoma: analysis of 974 patients from Germany and the United States treated by enucleation. In Bornfeld N, Gragoudas ES, Lommatzsch PK (eds) Tumors of the Eye. Proceedings of the International Symposium on Tumors of the Eye. Amsterdam: Kugler Publications, 1991:69–72.

Rootman J, Hofbauer J, Ellsworth RM, Kitchin D: Invasion of the optic nerve by retinoblastoma: a clinicopathological study. Can J Ophthalmol 11:106–114, 1976.

Shields CL, Shields JA, Baez K, Cater JR, De Potter P: Optic nerve invasion of retinoblastoma: metastatic potential and clinical risk factors. Cancer 73:692–698, 1994.

**Retinoblastoma Gene**

Cavenee WK, Dryja TP, Phillips RA, et al: Expression of recessive alleles by chromosomal mechanisms in retinoblastoma. Nature 305:779–784, 1983.

McGee TL, Yandell DW, Dryja TP: Structure and partial genomic sequence of the human retinoblastoma susceptibility gene. Gene 80:119–128, 1989.

Murphree AL: Molecular genetics of retinoblastoma. Ophthalmol Clin North Am 8:155–166, 1995.

Weichselbaum RR, Zakov ZN, Albert DM, et al. New findings in the chromosome 13 long-arm deletion syndrome and retinoblastoma. Ophthalmology 86:1191–201, 1979.

**Second Tumors**

Abramson DH, Ellsworth RM, Zimmerman LE: Nonocular cancer in retinoblastoma survivors. Trans Am Acad Ophthalmol Otolaryngol 81:454–457, 1976.

Bader JL, Meadows AT, Zimmerman LE, et al: Bilateral retinoblastoma with ectopic intracranial retinoblastoma: trilateral retinoblastoma. Cancer Genet Cytogenet 5: 203–213, 1982.

Holladay DA, Holladay A, Montebello JF, Redmond KP: Clinical presentation, treatment, and outcome of trilateral retinoblastoma. Cancer 67:710–715, 1991.

Pesin SR, Shields JA: Seven cases of trilateral retinoblastoma. Am J Ophthalmol 107:121–126, 1989.

Roarty JD, McLean IW, Zimmerman LE: Incidence of second neoplasms in patients with bilateral retinoblastoma. Ophthalmology 95:1583–1587, 1988.

**Differential Diagnosis of Retinoblastoma**

Shields JA, Shields CL: Differential diagnosis of retinoblastoma. In Intraocular Tumors: A Text and Atlas. Philadelphia: Saunders, 1992:341–362.

Shields JA, Shields CL, Parsons HM: Differential diagnosis of retinoblastoma. Retina 11:232–243, 1991.

Yanoff M: Pseudogliomas: differential diagnosis of retinoblastoma. Ophthalmol Dig 34:9, 1972.

**Toxocariasis**

Ashton N: Larval granulomatosis of the retina due to Toxocara. Br J Ophthalmol 44:129–148, 1960.

Brown DH: Ocular Toxocara canis. J Pediatr Ophthalmol 7: 182–191, 1970.

Shields JA, Shields CL, Eagle RC Jr, Barrett J, De Potter P: Endogenous endophthalmitis simulating retinoblastoma: the 1993 David and Mary Seslen endowment lecture. Retina 15:213–219, 1995.

Wilder HC: Nematode endophthalmitis. Trans Am Acad Ophthalmol Otolaryngol 54:99–109, 1950.

**Coats' Disease**

Ergerer I, Tasman W, Tomer T: Coats' disease. Arch Ophthalmol 92:109–112, 1974.

Patel HK, Augsburger JJ, Eagle RC Jr: Unusual presentation of advanced Coats' disease. J Pediatr Ophthalmol Strabismus 32:120–122, 1995.

Shields JA, Eagle RC Jr, Fammartino J, Shields CL, De Potter P: Coats' disease as a cause of anterior chamber cholesterolosis [letter]. Arch Ophthalmol 113:975–977, 1995.

**PHPV**

Font RL, Yanoff M, Zimmerman LE: Intraocular adipose tissue and persistent hyperplastic primary vitreous. Arch Ophthalmol 82:43–50, 1969.

Goldberg MF: Persistent fetal vasculature (PFV): an integrated interpretation of signs and symptoms associated with persistent hyperplastic primary vitreous (PHPV): LIV Edward Jackson memorial lecture. Am J Ophthalmol 124:587–626, 1997.

Haddad R, Font RL, Reeser F: Persistent hyperplastic primary vitreous: a clinicopathologic study of 62 cases and review of the literature. Surv Ophthalmol 23:123–134, 1978.

**Retinopathy of Prematurity**

De Juan E Jr, Machemer R, Flynn JT, Green WR: Surgical pathoanatomy in stage 5 retinopathy of prematurity. Birth Defects 24:281–286, 1988.

Green WR: Retrolental fibroplasia (RLF). In Spencer WH (ed) Ophthalmic Pathology: An Atlas and Textbook. Vol 2. 3rd ed. Philadelphia: Saunders, 1985:647–651.

Tasman W: Vitreoretinal changes in cicatricial retrolental fibroplasia. Trans Am Ophthalmol Soc 68:548–594, 1970.

**Medulloepithelioma**

Broughton WL, Zimmerman LE: A clinicopathologic study of 56 cases of intraocular medulloblastoma. Am J Ophthalmol 85:407–418, 1978.

Canning CR, McCartney ACE, Hungerford JL: Medulloepithelioma (diktyoma). Br J Ophthalmol 72:764–767, 1988.

Green WR, Iliff WJ, Trotter RR: Malignant teratoid medulloepithelioma of the optic nerve. Arch Ophthalmol 91: 451–454, 1974.

Shields JA, Eagle RC Jr, Shields CL, Marcus S, DePotter P, Riegel EM: Fluorescein angiography and ultrasonography of malignant intraocular medulloepithelioma. J Pediatr Ophthalmol Strabismus 33:193–196, 1996.

Shields JA, Eagle RC Jr, Shields CL, Potter PD: Congenital neoplasms of the nonpigmented ciliary epithelium (medulloepithelioma). Ophthalmology 103:1998–2006, 1996.

Zimmerman LE: Verhoeff's "terato-neuroma": a critical reappraisal in light of new observations and current concepts of embryonic tumors: the fourth Frederick H. Verhoeff lecture. Am J Ophthalmol 72:1039–1057, 1971.

**Astrocytoma**

Jakobiec FA, Brodie SE, Haik B, Iwamoto T: Giant cell astrocytoma of the retina: a tumor of possible Mueller cell origin. Ophthalmology 90:1565–1576, 1983.

Nork TM, Ghobrial MW, Peyman GA, Tso MO: Massive retinal gliosis: a reactive proliferation of Müller cells. Arch Ophthalmol 104:1383–1389, 1986.

Robertson DM: Ophthalmic manifestations of tuberous sclerosis. Ann NY Acad Sci 615:17–25, 1991.

Ulbright TM, Fulling KH, Helveston EM: Astrocytic tumors of the retina: differentiation of sporadic tumors from phakomatosis-associated tumors. Arch Pathol Lab Med 108:160–163, 1984.

**Juvenile Xanthogranuloma**

Chang MW, Frieden IJ, Good W: The risk intraocular juvenile xanthogranuloma: survey of current practices and assessment of risk. J Am Acad Dermatol 34:445–449, 1996.

Shields JA, Eagle RC Jr, Shields CL, Collins ML, DePotter P: Iris juvenile xanthogranuloma studied by immunohistochemistry and flow cytometry. Ophthalmic Surg Lasers 28:140–144, 1997.

Zimmerman LE: Ocular lesions of juvenile xanthogranuloma, nevoxanthoendothelioma. Trans Am Acad Ophthalmol Otolaryngol 69:412–439, 1965.

**Other Simulating Lesions**

Apple DJ, Fishman GA, Goldberg MF: Ocular histopathology of Norrie's disease. Am J Ophthalmol 78:196–203, 1974.

Freitag SK, Eagle RC Jr, Shields JA, Duker JS, Font RL: Melanogenic neuroectodermal tumor of the retina (primary malignant melanoma of the retina). Arch Ophthalmol 115:1581–1584, 1997.

Goldberg MF, Custis PH: Retinal and other manifestations of incontinentia pigmenti (Bloch-Sulzberger syndrome). Ophthalmology 100:1645–1654, 1993.

Hoepner J, Yanoff M: Ocular anomalies in trisomy 13–15. Am J Ophthalmol 74:729–737, 1972.

Lahav M, Albert DM, Wyand S: Clinical and histopathologic classification of retinal dysplasia. Am J Ophthalmol 75:648–667, 1973.

Leonardy NJ, Rupani M, Dent G, Klintworth GK: Analysis of 135 eyes for ocular involvement in leukemia. Am J Ophthalmol 109:436–444, 1990.

Shields JA, Eagle RC Jr, Shields CL, De Potter P, Poliak JG: Natural course and histopathologic findings of lacrimal gland choristoma of the iris and ciliary body. Am J Ophthalmol 119:219–224, 1995.

Wong F, Goldberg MF, Hao Y. Identification of a nonsense mutation at codon 128 of the Norrie's disease gene in a male infant. Arch Ophthalmol 111:1553–1557, 1993.

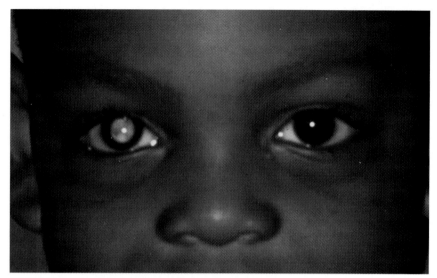

FIGURE 11–1 • **Leukocoria. Unilateral sporadic retinoblastoma.** About 90% of patients with retinoblastoma in the United States present with a white pupillary reflex. (Courtesy of Dr. Jerry A. Shields, Wills Eye Hospital)

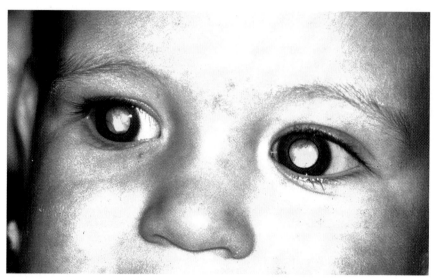

FIGURE 11–2 • **Bilateral leukocoria, familial retinoblastoma.** Bilateral tumors occur in about two-thirds of patients with familial retinoblastoma. The presence of bilateral tumors indicates that the affected patient is a carrier of familial retinoblastoma who can transmit the tumor to progeny. (Courtesy of Dr. Jerry A. Shields, Wills Eye Hospital)

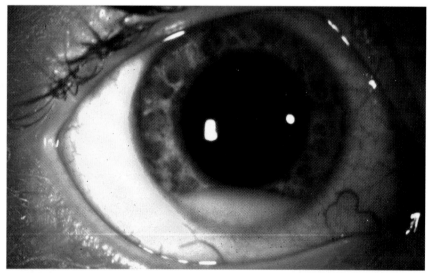

FIGURE 11–3 • **Pseudohypopyon, retinoblastoma.** A layered deposit of tumor cells in the anterior chamber of this quiet eye was the presenting manifestation of diffuse infiltrating retinoblastoma in this older child.

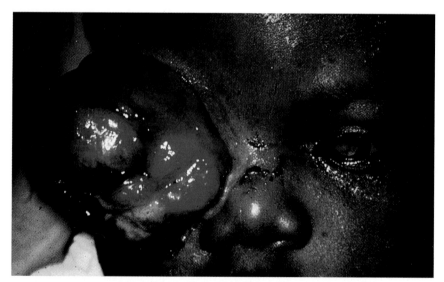

FIGURE 11–4 • **Neglected case of bilateral retinoblastoma from the United States.** Retinoblastoma frequently presents as an orbital tumor in underdeveloped countries. Note the presence of leukocoria in the fellow eye. (From Zimmerman LE: Retinoblastoma, including a report of illustrative cases. *Med Ann DC* 38:366–374, 1969)

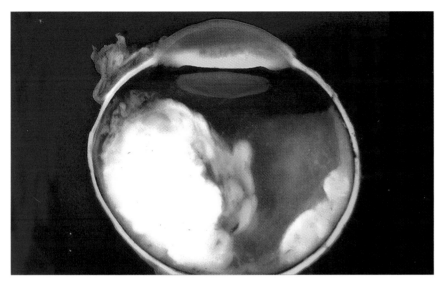

FIGURE 11–5 • **Endophytic retinoblastoma.** The bulk of the tumor in this eye is located internal to the retina in the vitreous cavity. The retina remains largely attached. Fine seeding of the vitreous is present.

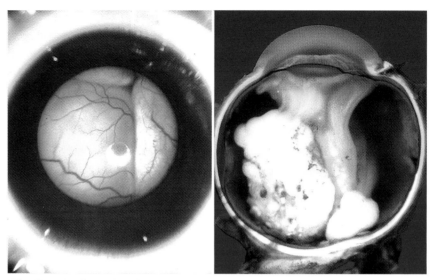

FIGURE 11–6 • **Exophytic retinoblastoma.** *Left:* Exophytic retinoblastomas arise from the outer layers of the retina and cause retinal detachment. Retinal vessels are seen directly behind the lens. *Right:* Enucleated eye with exophytic retinoblastoma shows an encephaloid tumor in the subretinal space and total bullous retinal detachment, which adheres to the back of the lens. The lens-iris diaphragm is displaced anteriorly, causing secondary closure of the angle.

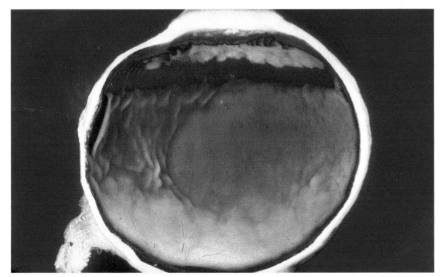

FIGURE 11–7 • **Diffuse infiltrating retinoblastoma.** The neoplasm diffusely infiltrates, thickens, and opacifies part of the retina but does not form a distinct mass. Tumor is present on the pars plana. The unilateral sporadic tumor was found in a 7-year-old boy who presented with anterior chamber seeding.

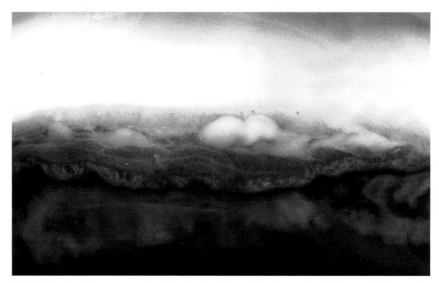

FIGURE 11–8 • **Anterior chamber seeding by diffuse infiltrative retinoblastoma.** White seeds of viable retinoblastoma rest on the anterior surface of the iris. Tumor is also seen in the posterior chamber between ciliary processes.

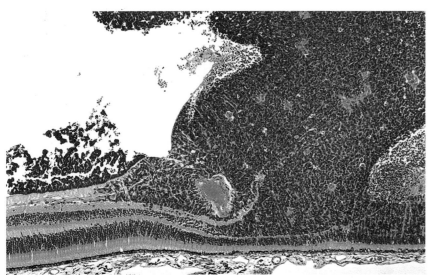

FIGURE 11–9 • **Endophytic retinoblastoma.** This poorly differentiated basophilic neoplasm arises from and destroys the retina. The retina remains attached as the endophytic tumor invades the vitreous cavity. Rosettes are not seen. Hematoxylin-eosin, ×25.

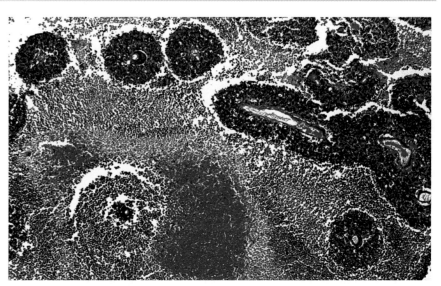

FIGURE 11–10 • **Retinoblastoma.** Low magnification photomicrograph of a retinoblastoma showing basophilic areas of viable tumor, eosinophilic zones of necrosis, and purple foci of dystrophic calcification within the necrotic zones. The viable cells form characteristic sleeves around vessels. Hematoxylin-eosin, ×5.

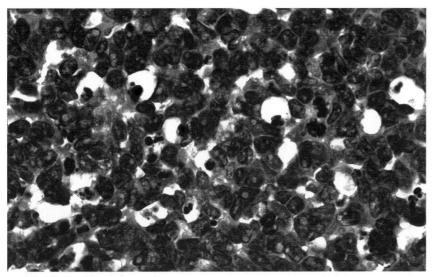

FIGURE 11–11 • **Retinoblastoma, poorly differentiated neuroblastic cells.** Viable parts of a retinoblastoma appear blue in H&E-stained sections because the tumor is composed of cells with scanty cytoplasm and prominent basophilic nuclei. Mitoses and patchy cellular necrosis are common. Hematoxylin-eosin, ×250.

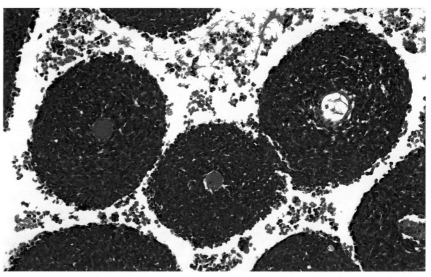

FIGURE 11–12 • **Retinoblastoma, perivascular sleeves of viable tumor.** Retinoblastoma typically outgrows its blood supply and undergoes necrosis. It usually occurs when its cells have grown approximately 90–100 $\mu$m away from a vessel. The necrotic cells appear eosinophilic because they have lost nuclear DNA. Hematoxylin-eosin, ×50.

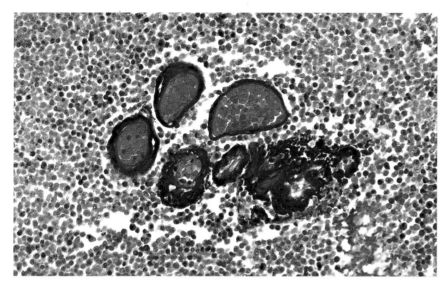

FIGURE 11–13 • **Retinoblastoma, DNA deposition around vessels.** Basophilic material surrounding vessels is nuclear DNA released by necrotic cells. The surrounding tumor cells are necrotic. Hematoxylin-eosin, ×100.

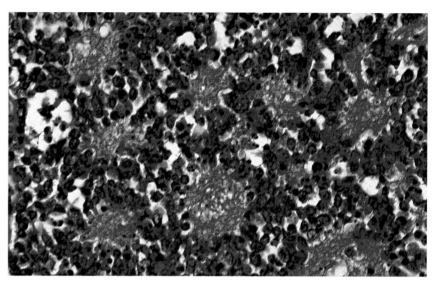

FIGURE 11–14 • **Retinoblastoma, Homer Wright rosettes.** Each ring of cells surrounds a central tangle of neural processes. A central lumen is not present. Homer Wright rosettes are indicative of neuroblastic differentiation. They are the least differentiated form of rosette found in retinoblastoma and occur also in other tumors such as neuroblastoma. Hematoxylin-eosin, ×250.

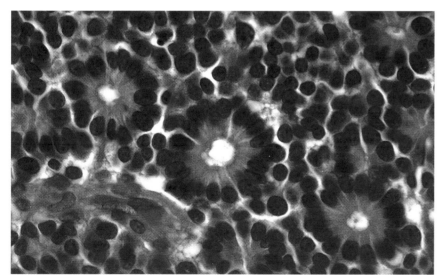

FIGURE 11–15 • **Retinoblastoma, Flexner-Wintersteiner rosettes.** Flexner-Wintersteiner rosettes represent differentiation toward primitive retina. The central lumen corresponds to the subretinal space. The tumor cells surrounding the lumen are joined near their apices by cellular connections that are analogous to the external limiting membrane. Hematoxylin-eosin, ×250.

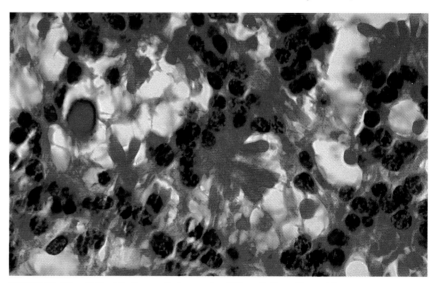

FIGURE 11–16 • **Retinoblastoma, photoreceptor differentiation.** Several fleurettes are present. Neoplastic photoreceptor inner segments form bouquets of pink "flowers." The photoreceptors project through a segment of neoplastic external limiting membrane. The nuclei are bland, and mitoses and necrosis are not evident. Tumors composed entirely of fleurettes are considered to be benign variants of retinoblastoma called retinomas or retinocytomas. Hematoxylin-eosin, ×250.

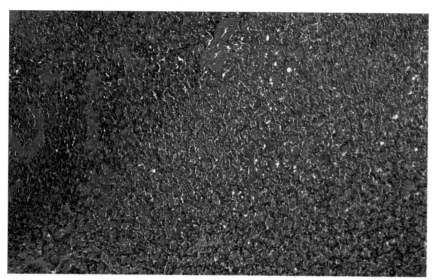

FIGURE 11–17 • **Retinoblastoma, photoreceptor differentiation.** Part of a tumor containing photoreceptor differentiation (at right) is relatively eosinophilic compared to poorly differentiated retinoblastoma. Hematoxylin-eosin, ×25.

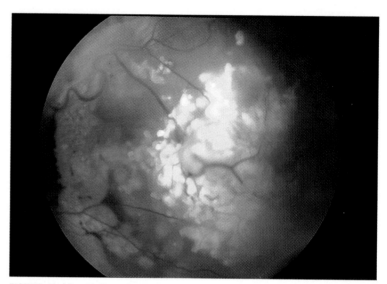

FIGURE 11–18 • **Retinocytoma.** The tumor has a translucent "fish flesh" appearance and contains large amounts of calcification that has been likened to cottage cheese. An annulus of RPE depigmentation typically surrounds the tumor. The tumor shown here was detected at preschool vision screening and was observed unchanged for several years before undergoing malignant transformation. (From Eagle RC Jr, Shields JA, Donoso L: Malignant transformation of spontaneously regressed retinoblastoma, retinoma/retinocytoma variant. *Ophthalmology* 96: 1389–1395, 1989. Courtesy of *Ophthalmology*)

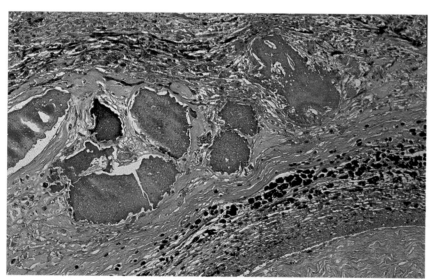

FIGURE 11–19 • **Spontaneously regressed retinoblastoma, phthisical eye.** Basophilic foci of necrotic calcified tumor cells are the only remnants of retinoblastoma in this phthisical eye. The calcified tumor is encased by scar tissue that contains strands of hyperplastic RPE. The choroid is scarred and shows evidence of necrosis. Hematoxylin-eosin, 25.

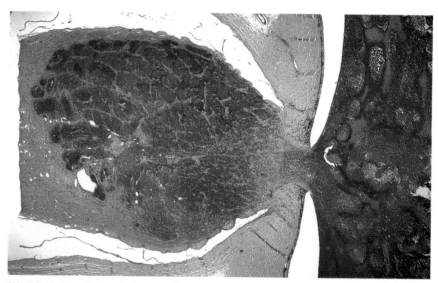

FIGURE 11–20 • **Retinoblastoma, optic nerve invasion.** There is massive replacement of the retrolaminar parenchyma of the optic nerve by basophilic tumor. Tumor is seen in close proximity to the cut surface of the nerve. A cross section of nerve containing the true surgical margin was excised and submitted for sections before the eye was opened. Hematoxylin-eosin, ×5.

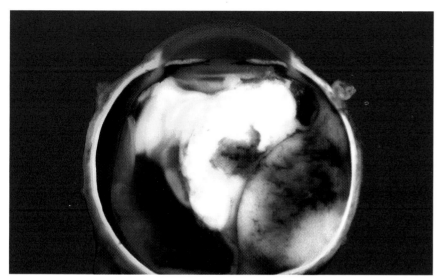

FIGURE 11–21 • **Retinoblastoma, massive choroidal invasion.** The right half of the choroid is massively thickened by invasive retinoblastoma. The area of choroidal invasion contains hemorrhagic foci. Careful examination disclosed no extraocular extension. The patient developed metastases after the parents declined prophylactic chemotherapy.

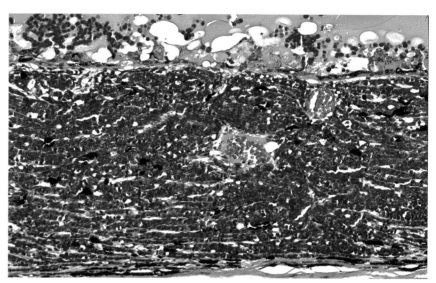

FIGURE 11–22 • **Retinoblastoma, choroidal invasion.** A basophilic infiltrate of poorly differentiated, viable retinoblastoma cells diffusely thickens the choroid. No necrosis is evident in the richly vascular choroid. The RPE is variably pigmented, and the retina is detached. Hematoxylin-eosin, ×50.

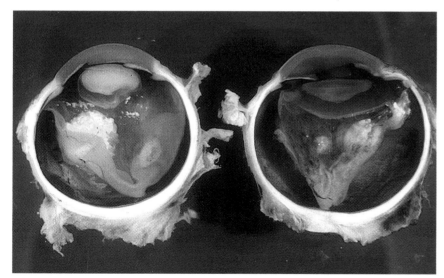

FIGURE 11–23 • **Bilateral retinoblastoma.** Both eyes had to be enucleated after therapy failed to control the tumors. Bilateral involvement indicates that the patient has a potentially transmissible germ-line mutation in the *Rb* gene.

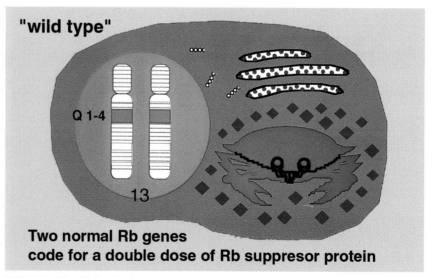

FIGURE 11–24 • **Retinoblastoma gene.** Normal individuals have two copies of the retinoblastoma gene, which is located on the long arm of chromosome 13. The gene encodes Rb protein, which suppresses tumor formation.

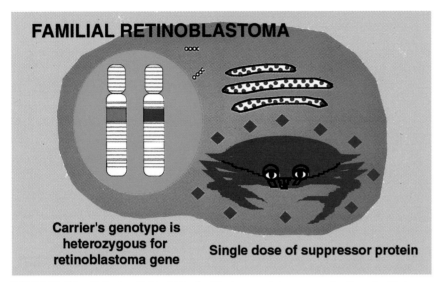

FIGURE 11–25 • Patients with familial retinoblastoma are heterozygous for the retinoblastoma gene.

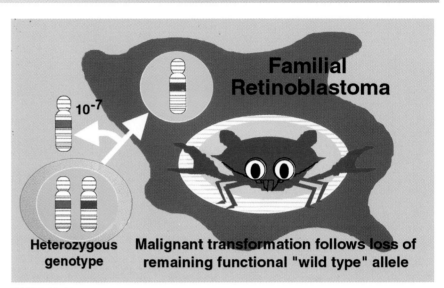

FIGURE 11–26 • Retinoblastoma develops when both copies of the retinoblastoma gene in a retinal cell are lost or inactivated.

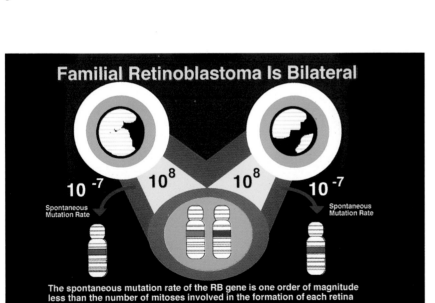

FIGURE 11–27 • The spontaneous mutation rate of the Rb gene is less than the number of mitoses required for the formation of each retina. This is the basis for bilateral and multifocal tumors in heterozygous carriers.

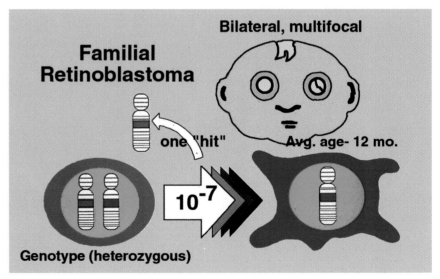

FIGURE 11–28 • Familial retinoblastomas typically are bilateral and multifocal. They occur earlier than tumors caused by sporadic somatic mutations because only a single "hit" or gene inactivation is required.

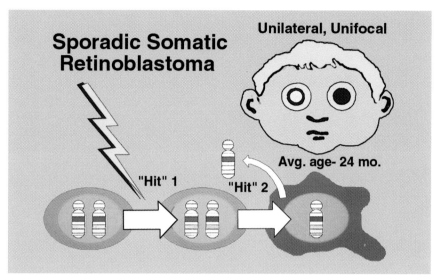

FIGURE 11–29 • Retinoblastomas caused by sporadic somatic mutations are most common. They are always unilateral and typically occur at about age 2 years.

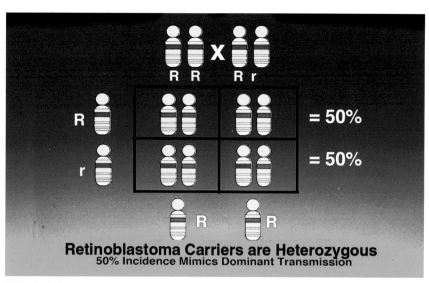

FIGURE 11–30 • Familial retinoblastoma appears to be an autosomal dominant trait, but the gene is recessive at the molecular level.

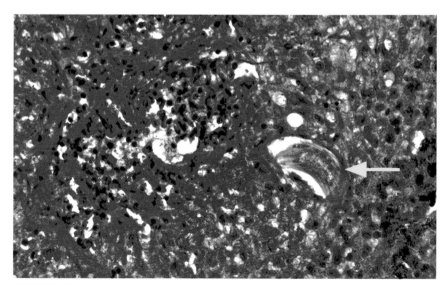

FIGURE 11–31 • **Ocular toxocariasis.** Arrow points to a fragment of nematode in an eosinophilic abscess. Hematoxylin-eosin, ×100.

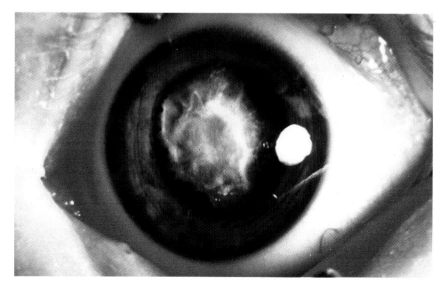

FIGURE 11–32 • **Persistent hyperplastic primary vitreous (PHPV).** Inwardly drawn ciliary processes adhere to the margin of vascularized retrolental fibrous plaque. The lesion was present at birth, and the affected eye was microphthalmic.

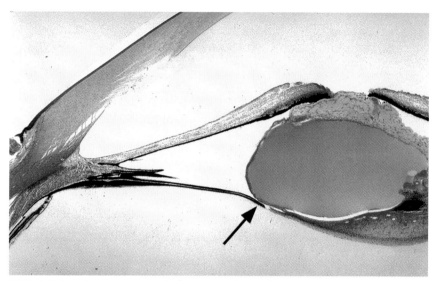

FIGURE 11–33 • **Persistent hyperplastic primary vitreous (PHPV).** A long, attenuated ciliary process (arrow) attaches to the margin of a fibrous plaque on the posterior surface of the lens. An anterior subcapsular cataract also is present. Hematoxylin-eosin, ×5.

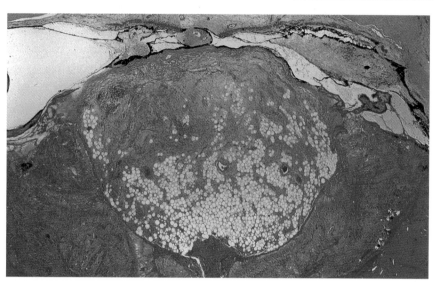

FIGURE 11–34 • **Intraocular adipose tissue, PHPV.** Totally detached retina adheres to the back of the lens, which contains mature adipose tissue. Hematoxylin-eosin, ×10.

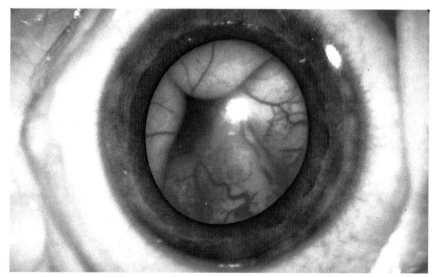

FIGURE 11–35 • **Coats' disease.** Abnormal telangiectatic vessels are evident in the detached retina directly behind the lens. These leaky vessels have caused an exudative retinal detachment. The subretinal space contains yellowish fluid rich in lipid. Coats' disease may simulate an exophytic retinoblastoma.

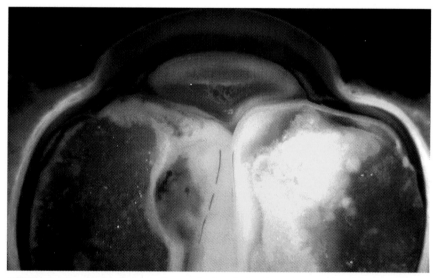

FIGURE 11–36 • **Coats' disease.** The totally detached retina adheres to the back of the lens and the pars plana. The lens iris diaphragm is displaced forward, obliterating the anterior chamber and closing the angle. The yellow subretinal exudate contains cholesterol crystals and aggregates of lipid-laden histiocytes. The glaucomatous eye was enucleated because it was blind and painful, and there was concern about a possible retinoblastoma.

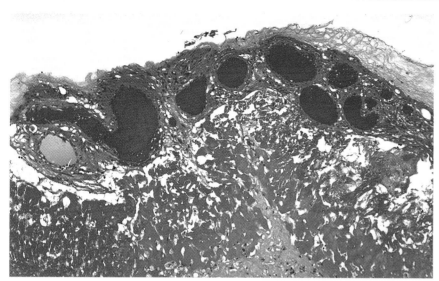

FIGURE 11–37 • **Coats' disease.** An increased number of large abnormal retinal vessels is present. The outer two-thirds of the retina is massively thickened by eosinophilic exudates. Hematoxylin-eosin, ×50.

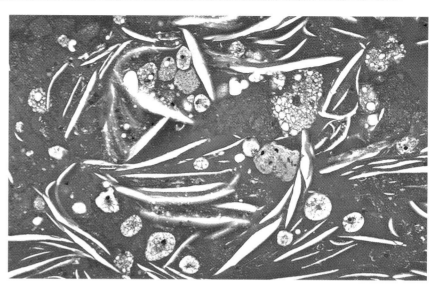

FIGURE 11–38 • **Coats' disease.** The eosinophilic, densely proteinaceous subretinal fluid contains slit-like cholesterol clefts and foamy histiocytes that have ingested lipid. Hematoxylin-eosin, ×100

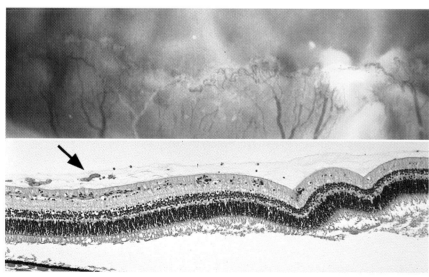

FIGURE 11–39 • **Retinopathy of prematurity.** *Top:* Note the band of vitreoretinal neovascularization bordering the nonvascularized temporal periphery of the retina. *Bottom:* Arrow points to new vessels in this photomicrograph. The peripheral part of the retina (at right) is avascular. Hematoxylin-eosin, ×25.

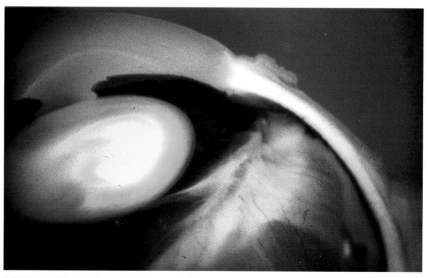

FIGURE 11–40 • **Retinopathy of prematurity.** Fibrovascular proliferation has led to the formation of a mass of folded retina in the temporal periphery behind the lens. The eye was obtained postmortem from a premature infant who had received supplemental oxygen.

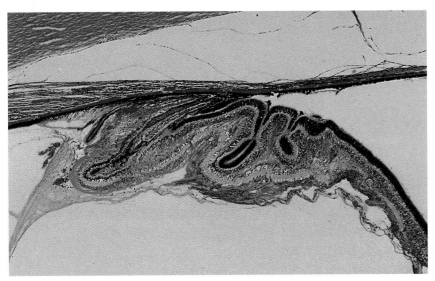

FIGURE 11–41 • **Retinopathy of prematurity.** Photomicrograph shows folded retina comprising a mass shown grossly in Figure 11–39. Hematoxylin-eosin, ×10.

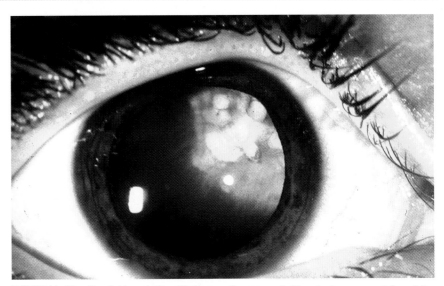

FIGURE 11–42 • **Teratoid medulloepithelioma.** Superonasal ciliary body mass contains white foci of hyaline cartilage. A delicate cyclitic membrane is present. (From Shields JA, Eagle RC Jr, Shields CL: Fluorescein angiography and ultrasonography of malignant intraocular medulloepithelioma. *J Pediatr Ophthalmol Strabismus* 33:193–196, 1996)

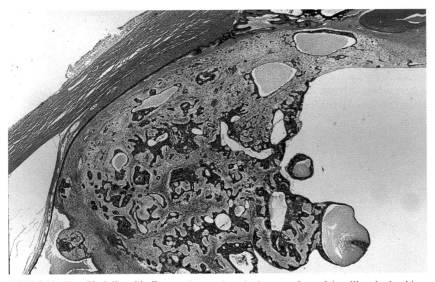

FIGURE 11–43 • **Medulloepithelioma.** Centered on the inner surface of the ciliary body, this medulloepithelioma is composed of cords of neuroepithelial cells resembling the primitive medullary epithelium. The epithelial elements are surrounded by loose stroma resembling embryonal mesenchyme. Several tumor cysts are present. A sheet of tumor extends anteriorly to envelop the lens at right. Hematoxylin-eosin, ×5.

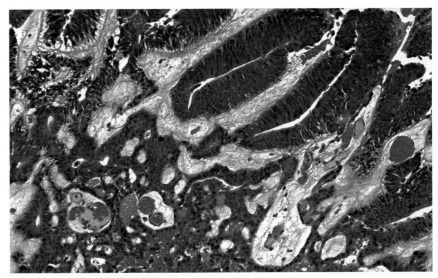

FIGURE 11–44 • **Medulloepithelioma.** Nonteratoid medulloepithelioma contains thick bands of polarized neuroepithelium that resemble embryonic medullary epithelium. Hematoxylin-eosin, ×50.

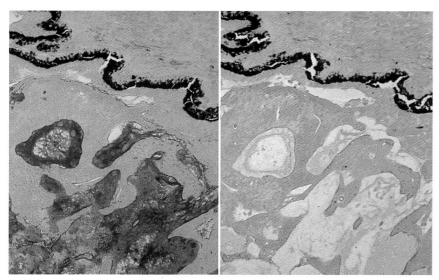

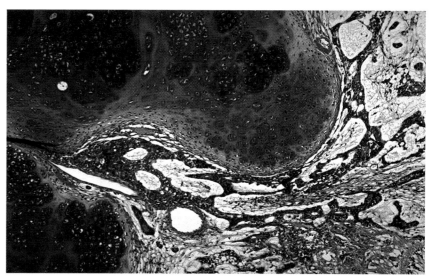

FIGURE 11–45 • **Medulloepithelioma.** The tumor contains pools of vitreous-like material that stain vividly (blue) for acid mucopolysaccharide (*left*). Pretreatment with hyaluronidase abolishes positive staining, indicating that the mucin is hyaluronic acid, a major component of the vitreous humor. The medulloepithelioma rests on the inner surface of the ciliary epithelium above. Both figures: Hale's colloidal iron for AMP, ×50.

FIGURE 11–46 • **Teratoid medulloepithelioma containing hyaline cartilage.** Teratoid medulloepitheliomas contains heteroplastic elements including hyaline cartilage, striated muscle, rhabdomyoblasts, and brain. This tumor contains prominent lobules of neoplastic cartilage. Cords and ribbons of neuroepithelial cells are seen in the myxoid stroma at right. Hematoxylin-eosin, ×25.

# CHAPTER 12

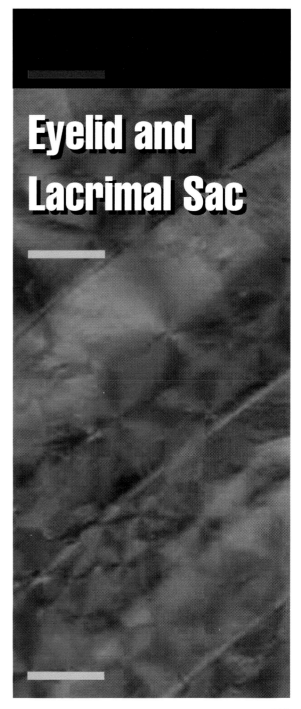
The eyelids are flaps of modified skin with highly modified epidermal appendages that cover and protect the eye. The eyelids form a moist chamber lined by mucous membrane (conjunctiva) that is absolutely essential for the maintenance of corneal transparency. The importance of the eyelids in the maintenance of corneal health and transparency becomes evident when facial paralysis or stupor prevent normal eyelid closure and produce corneal exposure or lagophthalmos (rabbit eye). If congenital defects in the eyelid called colobomas (coloboma = "a defect") are not corrected expeditiously, corneal ulceration or opacification caused by epidermalization invariably results. The corneal epithelium literally turns to skin if it is not continuously moistened.

## EYELID ANATOMY AND HISTOLOGY

The anterior surface of the eyelid is covered by skin, and its posterior surface is lined by a mucous membrane, the palpebral conjunctiva, which is closely applied to the tarsal plate (Figs. 12–1, 12–2, 12–3, 12–4). The tarsal plate is a curved plate of dense connective tissue that serves as the lid's internal skeleton. Striated fibers of the orbicularis muscle are found between the skin and the anterior surface of the tarsus. The orbicularis muscle encircles the eyelid fissure, forming a large sphincter that functions during eyelid closure. The bundles of the orbicularis are sectioned transversely in standard histologic sections. A mucocutaneous junction between eyelid skin and conjunctiva occurs near the eyelid margin. Here, the epidermis is mildly thickened and has small rete ridges. Just anterior to the lid margin, slit lamp biomicroscopy discloses a line of tiny meibomian gland orifices. The meibomian glands are large sebaceous glands that occupy almost the entire length of the tarsal plate and are oriented perpendicular to the lid margin (Fig. 12–5). The oily secretion of the meibomian glands helps retard evaporation of the tear film. About 25 meibomian glands are present in the upper lid and 20 in the lower lid. The meibomian glands in the upper lid are much longer, reflecting the greater length of the upper tarsal plate (11 mm). The upper lid is identified grossly and in tissue sections by the length of the tarsal plate and the lid's roughly rectangular shape (Fig. 12–1, 12–3). The shape of the lower lid is roughly triangular (Figs. 12–2, 12–4). The greater mass of meibomian gland tissue in the upper tarsus probably explains why sebaceous carcinoma occurs most often in the upper lid. The eyelid fissure is encircled by a protective ring of cilia (eyelashes). The hair bulbs of the cilia are located deep within the lid next to the tarsal plate. Malignant tumors such as sebaceous gland carcinoma that arise deep in the substance of the lid often produce loss of lashes (madarosis).

Other eyelid glands bear eponyms. The sebaceous glands of the eyelashes are the glands of Zeis. Sebaceous glands are holocrine glands. The glandular secretion called sebum is composed of entire cells (*holos* = whole). Cellular division occurs in the peripheral germinative layer of sebaceous gland lobules. As new cells form, the older cells are pushed toward the center of the glandular lobule. The cells degenerate as they mature. Their nuclei become karyorrhectic and pyknotic, and the cytoplasm becomes intensely lipidized and foamy (Fig. 12–5).

The glands of Moll are apocrine sweat glands (Fig. 12–6). Their dilated lumina are lined by tall, eosinophilic cells capped with the "apical snouts" that characterize apocrine decapitation secretion. Eccrine sweat glands, which bear no eponym, also are found. Glandular epithelial cells remain intact during eccrine secretion. The glands of Wolfring or Ciaccio are small accessory lacrimal glands located at the proximal margins of the tarsal plates. There are two to five glands of Wolfring at the upper margin of the superior tarsal plate and two glands at the lower margin of the lower tarsus. Other accessory lacrimal glands, called the glands of Krause, are found near the conjunctival fornix. The accessory lacrimal glands are responsible for baseline tear secretion. The main lacrimal gland releases copious amounts of watery secretion (endogenous irrigating fluid) in response to emotional stimuli or severe ocular irritation.

## TERMS USED IN SKIN PATHOLOGY

The external surface of the eyelid is covered by one of the thinnest, most delicate layers of skin in the body (Fig. 12–7). The epidermis of the eyelid skin is generally only five or six cells in thickness and is covered by a thin layer of surface keratinization. Unlike skin elsewhere, eyelid epidermis lacks rete ridges. The basal cell, or germinative layer, of the epidermis, where cellular division normally occurs, rests on a delicate basement membrane. Compared to the squamous cells of the overlying epidermis, the basal cells have relatively little cytoplasm. Hence lesions comprised of basal cells (e.g., basal cell carcinoma) appear blue or basophilic on low power microscopy. Most of the epidermis is composed of the prickle cells of the stratum spinosum, or malpighian layer. These cells are polygonal and are joined by bundles of tonofilaments evident on light microscopy as intercellular bridges. Squamous cell lesions appear pink or eosinophilic under low power microscopy because the cells have abundant eosinophilic cytoplasm.

Thickening of the prickle cell layer is termed acanthosis (from Greek *acantha*, a thorn). As basal cells mature and approach the surface of the skin, they become flattened and squamoid. The nuclei undergo apoptosis as the cells near the surface, releasing intensely basophilic granules of nucleoprotein that form the granular cell layer. The dead, desiccated, anucleate cellular remnants form a thin, horny layer of keratin called the stratum corneum (from Latin *cornu*, a horn). Abnormal thickening of this normally thin surface layer of keratin is called hyperkeratosis (Fig. 12–8). Hyperkeratosis, commonly found on the surface of benign squamous papillomas, is responsible for the greasy or scaly character of seborrheic keratoses. Colonies of yeast or bacteria frequently are found in the thick layer of keratin.

Retention of nuclei in the stratum corneum is termed parakeratosis (Fig. 12–9). Parakeratosis generally occurs in pathologic states when the epidermis is rapidly proliferating. When parakeratosis is present, there is no granular cell layer in the underlying epidermis. Parakeratosis is relatively rare and should alert one that he or she may be dealing with a premalignant lesion such as actinic keratosis.

Dyskeratosis refers to the keratinization of single cells within the prickle cell layer. Dyskeratotic cells are round and intensely eosinophilic and have pyknotic nuclei. Dyskeratosis is particularly striking in the conjunctival lesions of hereditary benign intraepithelial dyskeratosis (see Fig. 4–40).

## CONGENITAL AND DEVELOPMENTAL LESIONS

Developmental anomalies of the eyelids include ablepharon, cryptophthalmos, colobomas, microblepharon, ankyloblepharon, euryblepharon, blepharophimosis, congenital ectropion, epicanthal folds, and dystopia canthorum. An intact sheet of skin covers the eye in cryptophthalmos. Affected patients may have Fraser syndrome, which includes syndactyly, renal agenesis, and aural and genital malformations. Colobomas are partial- or full-thickness defects in the lid that affect the lid margin. Lid colobomas are common in Goldenhar syndrome and mandibulofacial dysostosis. Isolated strands of skin bridge the palpebral fissure in ankyloblepharon filiforme adnatum and are related to the fusion of the upper and lower lids that normally occurs in utero. Dystopia canthorum, iris heterochromia, a white forelock, synophrys, and deafness comprise Waardenburg syndrome. An accessory row of eyelashes arises from the meibomian glands in distichiasis. Phakomatous choristoma (Zimmerman's tumor) is a rare congenital neoplasm that involves the lower medial eyelid or anterior orbit. The ultimate choristoma, Zimmerman's tumor, is composed of extraocular eye lens tissue including lens epithelium, neoplastic lens capsule, and bladder cells like those found in posterior subcapsular cataract (Fig. 12–10).

## AGING CHANGES

Aging produces atrophy and laxity of eyelid skin (dermatochalasis), loss of orbital fat and subcutaneous tissue, and relaxation of eyelid ligaments. Folds of redundant skin overhang the upper lid margin, and the orbital fat protrudes through the attenuated orbital septum, producing bags under the eyes. Chronic light damage (senile or actinic elastosis) is evident histologically as basophilic degeneration of dermal collagen.

Laxity of eyelid tissues predisposes to senile entropion or ectropion. Entropion occurs when the preseptal part of the orbicularis muscle overrides the pretarsal part. The lateral canthal tendon is lax in senile ectropion, and the exposed conjunctiva becomes inflamed and undergoes epidermalization. The floppy eyelid syndrome occurs in obese men who have eyelids with a rubbery tarsus that are easily everted. Spontaneous eversion of the eyelids or loss of eyelid contact occurs during sleep, causing chronic papillary conjunctivitis.

## COMMON INFLAMMATORY LESIONS OF THE EYELID

Hordeolums (styes) and chalazia are common inflammatory lesions of the eyelid. Hordeolums are acute purulent infections of eyelash follicles (external hordeolums) or meibomian glands (internal hordeolums) usually caused by staphylococci (Fig. 12–11). Internal hordeolums are more painful because the inflammation is localized within a confined space. Hordeolums usually respond to conservative therapy (e.g., hot compresses) and therefore are rarely examined histopathologically.

Chalazia typically appear as mildly tender nodules, or areas of localized nodular thickening on the eyelid (Fig. 12–12). Inflammatory signs such as pain and redness are not especially prominent because chalazia are chronic inflammatory lesions. They are chronic lipogranulomas (i.e., "endogenous foreign body reactions" to the lipid-rich secretions of the meibomian and Zeis glands). When sebum escapes from its normal confines in these sebaceous glands, it is extremely irritating and stimulates chronic granulomatous inflammation. Histopathology discloses epithelioid histiocytes and inflammatory giant cells that typically surround empty spaces (lipid vacuoles) (Fig. 12–13). *In vivo* the vacuoles contained lipid. During tissue processing solvents such as alcohol and xylene dissolve the lipid. Other chronic inflammatory cells, such as lymphocytes and plasma cells, contribute to the chronic inflammatory infiltrate in chalazion specimens. If the chalazion has ruptured spontaneously or if prior incision and drainage has been performed, granulation tissue is often found. Although granulation tissue typically is nongranulomatous, that associated with chalazion may contain epithelioid cells or giant cells, which are residua of the lipogranulomatous response. Chalazion curettings often include fragments of tarsal plate.

Sebaceous carcinoma, which also arises in zeis and meibomian glands, can be confused with chronic chalazia clinically. It is imperative that recurrent or atypical chalazia be submitted for histopathologic examination to exclude the possibility of this potentially fatal eyelid malignancy. The author personally has seen several cases of sebaceous carcinoma that were initially misdiagnosed as chalazia. These lesions were treated with incision and drainage and were not examined histopathologically. When the correct diagnosis was finally made, extensive pagetoid involvement of the conjunctiva by tumor cells necessitated orbital exenteration. Other unusual neoplasms such as sweat gland carcinomas, Merkel cell tumors, and carcinoma metastatic to the eyelid have been misdiagnosed clinically as chalazia.

## VIRAL LESIONS

Verruca vulgaris, a benign papillomatous skin lesion caused by human papilloma virus type 2 (HPV-2), a DNA papovavirus, occasionally occurs on the eyelid. These viral papillomas are distinguished by elongated spire-shaped papillary fronds and rete ridges that bend inwardly toward the center of the lesion (Fig. 12–14). Vertical tiers of parakeratosis occur on the crests of papillomatous elevations and overlie foci of vacuolated cells that contain eosinophilic intranuclear and intracytoplasmic viral inclusions. The viral inclusions, which are necessary for definitive diagnosis, are found only in early lesions. Verruca vulgaris is diagnosed infrequently in the ophthalmic pathology laboratory.

Molluscum contagiosum is a fairly common viral tumor with a distinctive histopathologic appearance. Caused by a pox virus, molluscum contagiosum often is associated with poor hygiene, and lesions may occur in crops on the face and eyelids of children as the result of autoinoculation. Massive involvement of eyelids and adnexal skin has been reported in patients with acquired immunodeficiency syndrome (AIDS). Clinically, molluscum contagiosum appears as either an elevated smooth nodule with a central umbilication or a larger pore enclosing multiple flattened papillae. Histopathologically, molluscum contagiosum typically has an elevated cup-shaped or crateriform configuration and is composed of lobules of markedly acanthotic benign epithelium (Fig. 12–15). The epithelial cells contain large intracytoplasmic inclusion bodies called Henderson-Patterson corpuscles (Fig. 12–16). The inclusions are eosinophilic near the base of the epithelium where they form, and they become denser and more basophilic as they mature and migrate toward the surface where they discharge virus particles. The individual virus particles are quite large and can be resolved with the oil immersion objective of the light microscope in 1 $\mu$m thick plastic-embedded sections. Molluscum contagiosum on the eyelid margin can incite unilateral chronic follicular conjunctivitis by dispersing viral particles into the conjunctival sac. The lids of any patient who has chronic follicular conjunctivitis should be inspected carefully for molluscum contagiosum (or the presence of pubic, or "crab," lice whose waste can incite a similar reaction).

Molluscum contagiosum is one of three cup-shaped or crateriform lesions commonly found on eyelid skin. Basal cell carcinoma and keratoacanthoma also are often umbilicated or have a central area of ulceration. Both tend to be larger than molluscum contagiosum.

Other viral lesions that affect eyelid skin include the vesicular eruptions caused by the herpes simplex and varicella-zoster viruses. Herpes simplex infection causes fluid-filled intraepidermal vesicles marked by profound epidermal degeneration and acantholysis (Fig. 12–17). Round acantholytic balloon cells and multinucleated giant cells that contain eosinophilic intranuclear viral inclusions are found.

## BENIGN CYSTIC LESIONS

Eyelid cysts are commonly accessioned by ocular pathology laboratories. Most are epidermal inclusion cysts or sweat ductal cysts.

Epidermal inclusion cysts are round or oval, are unilocular (have a single lumen), and are filled with cheesy, foul-smelling keratin debris. They are lined by keratinizing stratified squamous epithelium that resembles normal epidermis (Figs. 12–18, 12–19). By definition, the epithelial lining has no epidermal appendages such as pilosebaceous units or sweat glands. (If epidermal appendages are present, and hair shafts are found mixed with the keratin filling the lumen, the cyst probably should be classified as a cystic dermoid, a developmental lesion caused by entrapment of epidermis in bony sutures). Many epidermal inclusion cysts are caused by the cystic dilatation of hair follicles by keratin debris. "Follicular cyst, infundibular type" is the dermatopathologic term applied to this type of cyst. In such cases, the lining of the cyst may communicate with the skin through a pore. Clinically, epidermal inclusion cysts are often inappropriately called sebaceous cysts.

Sweat ductal cysts, sudoriferous cysts, or hidrocystomas are caused by blockage of a sweat duct. These cysts are soft, smooth, and fluctuant and are filled with watery fluid. Some are transparent or translucent, and they readily transilluminate. Some patients have multiple cysts that may involve the skin of both medial or lateral canthi (Fig. 12–20).

Histopathologically, sweat ductal cysts are often multilocular, and their lumens appear empty or contain scant amounts of granular eosinophilic material consistent with serous fluid. The epithelial lining, which is often attenuated, is composed of a dual layer of cells that resembles the normal lining of an eccrine sweat duct (Fig. 12–21). Although most sudoriferous cysts are eccrine hidrocystomas, the epithelial lining occasionally shows apocrine differentiation. Apocrine hidrocystomas are recognized by their epithelial lining, which is composed of tall cells with eosinophilic cytoplasm and the apical snouts of decapitation secretion (Fig. 12–22). The cytoplasm of the apocrine cells may contain golden-brown granules of lipofuscin pigment that are periodic acid-Schiff (PAS)-positive. Apocrine hidrocystomas often contain brown fluid stained by this pigment and may be misdiagnosed preoperatively as primary melanocytic lesions (Fig. 12–23).

## BENIGN EPIDERMAL LESIONS

Benign tumors that arise from the epidermis generally are located anterior to the plane of the surrounding normal skin because they are composed of cells that are unable to invade or infiltrate the dermis or deeper structures of the lid as can malignant lesions (Figs. 12–24, 12–25). The redundant epidermis formed by the proliferation of these benign cells typically forms a branching tree-shaped lesion comprised of fronds, or finger-like projections, that have cores of fibrovascular tissue analogous to dermis. A lesion that exhibits this growth pattern is called a papilloma (Fig. 12–26). Papillomas can be elevated and exophytic or relatively squat and sessile. A variety of lesions show a papillomatous growth pattern including some malignant tumors, (e.g., papillary squamous cell carcinoma of the conjunctiva).

Benign papillomatous lesions of eyelid skin, such as seborrheic keratoses and squamous cell papillomas, frequently are submitted for histopathologic evaluation. In most instances the correct diagnosis is suspected preoperatively, and cosmesis is a major indication for excisional biopsy.

Seborrheic keratoses usually occur in elderly patients. They are sharply demarcated, superficial lesions that sit anterior to the plane of surrounding epidermis like a button on the surface of the skin (Fig. 12–27). They typically have a greasy or scaly appearance caused by hyperkeratosis and are often pigmented. Approximately one-third of black adults have multiple, small, pigmented seborrheic keratoses on their facial skin, a condition called dermatosis papulosa nigra (Fig. 12–28).

Seborrheic keratoses are an upward papillomatous proliferation of basaloid cells that resemble normal epidermal basal cells. Therefore under low magnification seborrheic keratoses often appear "blue" and are situated "above" the plane of the surrounding skin (signifying a benign lesion of basal cells) (Fig. 12–24). In contrast to "garden variety" squamous papillomas, acrochordons (or skin tags), that are often exophytic and pedunculated, seborrheic keratoses are often sessile. A thick surface layer of keratin usually is present, and circular spaces filled with keratin called "horn cysts," or pseudohorn cysts, are found within the acanthotic epithelium. Most probably represent invaginations of surface keratin (Fig. 12–29).

Interweaving bands composed of benign cells are found in the dermis in the adenoid variant of seborrheic keratosis (Fig. 12–30), which should not be confused with the highly infiltrative morpheaform variant of basal cell carcinoma. Inverted follicular keratosis (IFK) is considered by some to be an irritated form of seborrheic keratosis. IFK typically has an inverted cup-shaped configuration and surface invaginations that have been interpreted as hair follicles (Figs. 12–31, 12–32). Other characteristic histopathologic features include acantholysis (widening of intercellular spaces between squamous cells ) and small foci of squamous differentiation called squamous eddies.

Many benign eyelid papillomas do not fulfill all of the diagnostic criteria for seborrheic keratosis. Such lesions tend to be small and pedunculated, and their epidermal component is not particularly basaloid; it resembles normal or only slightly acanthotic skin with minimal hyperkeratosis (Fig. 12–33). The dermal component often contains a sparse to moderate infiltrate of chronic inflammatory cells. Such lesions usually are diagnosed as squamous papillomas and are also called skin tags or acrochordons. Some are viral in origin.

# KERATOACANTHOMA

Keratoacanthoma is a crater-shaped squamous cell lesion that classically arises rapidly in elderly patients and then undergoes spontaneous involution (Fig. 12–34). Although keratoacanthoma has been classified as a benign pseudoepitheliomatous hyperplasia in the past, some authorities now believe that it may be a "deficient squamous cell carcinoma" that tends to involute spontaneously. Rare cases invade deeply, like squamous cell carcinomas.

Histopathology discloses a central crater filled with a mass of keratin enclosed by markedly acanthotic squamous epithelium that typically extends like a lip or buttress over the side of the crater (Fig. 12–35). The base of a well developed lesion appears regular and well demarcated, and the margin is relatively smooth and "pushing " rather than infiltrative (Fig. 12–36). An intense band of inflammation usually is present in the underlying dermis. The overall configuration of the lesion is important from a diagnostic standpoint. It is usually impossible to differentiate keratoacanthoma from squamous cell carcinoma in a small incisional biopsy because keratoacanthoma frequently harbors

atypical cells and mitotic figures. Keratoacanthomas should be totally excised.

# MALIGNANT TUMORS OF THE EYELID

## Basal Cell Carcinoma

Basal cell carcinoma is the most common malignant tumor affecting the periocular skin. Basal cell carcinomas tend to affect fair-skinned adults but can occur in younger persons. They arise in sun-exposed skin and are thought to be caused by actinic damage.

Several variants of basal cell carcinoma are recognized clinically. Noduloulcerative basal cell carcinomas are firm, elevated, pearly nodules whose surface initially may be marked by telangiectatic vessels (Fig. 12–37). Ulceration often develops centrally as the nodules increase in size. More advanced lesions appear as slowly enlarging ulcers with prominent rolled pearly borders. Noduloulcerative basal cell carcinomas usually have relatively distinct margins.

In contrast, the sclerosing or morpheaform variant of basal cell carcinoma frequently has relatively indistinct margins and does not tend to ulcerate until late. (The term morpheaform alludes to the lesion's similarity to morphea, a circumscribed type of scleroderma.) Widespread superficial multicentric involvement occurs in some patients. Extensive areas of ulceration called "rodent ulcers" are found in neglected cases. Patients who are cancerphobic, are afraid of doctors, or manifest excessive denial may present late in the course of the disease with ghastly disfiguring facial destruction (Fig. 12–38).

Basal cell carcinoma occurs 15–40 times more often than squamous cell carcinoma on the eyelids. The tumor arises most frequently in the lower eyelid, followed by the inner canthus, upper lid, and outer canthus. Considering its frequency, it is fortunate that

basal cell carcinoma rarely metastasizes. The unusual cases that do metastasize usually are of the metatypical or basosquamous type. Rare fatalities can result, however, when deeply infiltrative, ulcerative lesions invade the orbital bones and meninges and cause secondary meningitis.

Basal cell carcinoma appears "blue" and "below" on low power light microscopy. The neoplastic basaloid cells of basal cell carcinoma typically form large masses or fields, or smaller nests, islands, or cords (Figs. 12–25, 12–39). Peripheral palisading of nuclei and contraction artifact are seen at the periphery of the tumor lobules (Fig. 12–40). Peripheral palisading refers to an arrangement of peripheral nuclei perpendicular to the margin of a tumor lobule, which has been likened to the logs in a colonial fort or palisade. Shrinkage of the mucin-rich stroma during processing causes retraction artifact, an empty space or cleft between the tumor lobule and the surrounding stroma.

The fibrous stroma that separates the lobules of neoplastic epithelial cells in basal cell carcinoma is generally is more fibrotic and much denser than the adjacent normal dermis. The stimulation of fibrosis by the tumor is called desmoplasia.

Several histopathologic variants of basal cell carcinoma are recognized. In these variants the tumor appears to be undergoing differentiation toward various epidermal appendages. Mucin production is evident as intralobular pools of foamy, lucent, slightly basophilic material in the adenoid variant of basal cell carcinoma. Keratotic basal cell carcinomas contain small keratinized horn cysts that may represent abortive pilar differentiation. Sebaceous differentiation is rare and should raise concern about an internal malignancy (see Muir-Torre syndrome, below). Pigmented basal cell carcinomas contain melanin pigment and may be confused clinically with malignant melanomas or nevi. Pseudocystic basal cell carcinomas are formed by necrobiosis in the center of a large mass of tumor cells, which is somewhat analogous to holocrine secretion. Morpheaform basal cell carcinomas are comprised of slender cords or tendrils of tumor cells embedded in a densely fibrotic stroma (Fig. 12–41). Morpheaform tumors can widely and deeply infiltrate the tissues of the eyelid and orbit, and they have indistinct margins. Excision may be incomplete unless frozen section control of margins or Mohs surgery is performed.

Optimally, basal cell carcinomas of the eyelid and periocular skin are excised with frozen section control of surgical margins. Frozen sections probably are unnecessary for some small noduloulcerative lesions that have clinically distinct margins. The time-consuming modified Mohs technique is best suited for extensive and deeply infiltrative lesions arising in areas such as the inner canthus, where the danger of orbital invasion is great. Basal cell carcinoma does not invariably recur after incomplete excision. We frequently find no residual basal cell carcinoma histopathologically when re-excision is performed on tumors that were reported as having been incompletely excised. The initial trauma of surgery or postoperative inflammation may destroy the residual tumor in such cases.

In approximately 0.7% of cases, multiple basal cell carcinomas occur on the face and body of young patients who inherit an autosomal dominantly inherited syndrome that includes a predisposition to the tumor. Patients with the basal cell nevus or Gorlin-Goltz syndrome also have odontogenic keratocysts of the jaw, skeletal anomalies such as bifid ribs, neurologic abnormalities, and endocrine disorders. Basal cell carcinomas from patients with the basal cell nevus syndrome may contain spicules of bone.

## Actinic Keratosis and Squamous Cell Carcinoma

Actinic keratosis is a premalignant squamous cell lesion that develops on the sun-exposed skin of fair-skinned middle-aged individuals. Clinically, these keratoses appear as scaly, keratotic, flat-topped lesions or erythematous nodules. Microscopy reveals thickened epidermis that is partially replaced by atypical squamous cells (Fig. 12–42). Parakeratosis usually is present, and the granular cell layer is absent. Irregular buds of atypical keratinocytes extend into the papillary dermis at the base of some lesions. The disease spares the openings of the pilosebaceous units. The underlying dermis characteristically shows solar elastosis (elastotic degeneration) similar to that seen in pinguecula and pterygium. The elastotic degeneration stains positively with the Verhoeff-van Gieson stain for elastic tissue.

Squamous cell carcinoma of the eyelid is relatively rare compared to basal cell carcinoma. Squamous cell carcinoma typically affects elderly, fair-skinned individuals. Although the lower lid margin is typically involved, squamous cell carcinoma is said to be more common than basal cell carcinoma in the upper lid and outer canthus.

Histopathologically, squamous cell carcinomas are composed of nests, cords, and islands of malignant squamous cells that have abundant eosinophilic cytoplasm and appear "pink" under low power (Figs. 12–43, 12–44). Reflecting the tumor's invasive malignant potential, tumor cells are seen deep to the plane of the epidermis. More differentiated tumors produce keratin. Squamous cell carcinomas of the eyelid rarely metastasize. Metastatic disease is particularly uncommon if the squamous cell carcinoma has arisen from a preexisting actinic keratosis (Fig. 12–45). Approximately 12% of patients who had actinic keratosis in one series developed a nonaggressive form of squamous cell carcinoma that had an excellent prognosis compared to squamous cell carcinoma that arose *de novo*. The incidence of metastatic disease was only 0.5%. A larger study from Australia found a much lower incidence (0.1%) of progression to squamous cell carcinoma. Many actinic keratoses in that series underwent spontaneous regression.

## Sebaceous Carcinoma and Other Sebaceous Tumors

Sebaceous carcinoma is about as common as squamous cell carcinoma of the eyelid. Rarely encountered before age 40, sebaceous carcinoma typically occurs in elderly patients and is more common in women and Asians. Sebaceous carcinoma has a definite predilection for the sebaceous glands of the eyelid but is rare elsewhere in the body. It can arise from the meibomian glands, the glands of Zeis, or rarely the sebaceous glands in the caruncle.

Sebaceous carcinoma is an important tumor that can confound both ophthalmologists and pathologists. Lesions that arise deep in the substance of the lid (e.g., meibomian carcinomas) typically cause no abnormalities in the overlying skin until late in the course of the disease. Meibomian gland carcinomas can be confused with chalazia, which typically arise within the tarsal plate. Recurrent or atypical chalazia should be submitted for histopathologic examination.

Rarely, sebaceous carcinoma presents as a chronic unilateral keratoconjunctivitis that is unresponsive to therapy. This "masquerade syndrome" is caused by the intraepithelial spread of tumor that has replaced the conjunctival epithelium in a pagetoid fashion. Any elderly patient who has unilateral chronic keratoconjunctivitis that does not respond to treatment should be biopsied.

Two-thirds of sebaceous carcinomas arise in the upper eyelid, undoubtedly reflecting the greater mass of meibomian gland tissue in the upper lid (Fig. 12–46). Sebaceous carcinoma grows, forming lobules and sheets whose size and shape are somewhat reminiscent of normal sebaceous glands (Fig. 12–47). Meibomian glands in the tarsus are often completely replaced by tumor. The tumor lobules lack peripheral palisading, and the nuclei of the cells tend to be larger, pleomorphic, hyperchromatic, and more atypical than those in basal cell carcinoma. Mitotic figures are common and may be abnormal. In well-differentiated cases, the cytoplasm of the tumor cells has a frothy or foamy appearance caused by lipid vacuoles. Special fat stains such as oil red O can document the presence of lipid but must be performed on frozen sections because the solvents used in normal tissue processing and paraffin embedding dissolve fat (Fig. 12–48). If sebaceous carcinoma is suspected clinically, the surgeon should inform the pathologist so wet tissue can be reserved for possible fat stains. Experienced ocular pathologists generally perform fat stains only on exceptional cases with equivocal sebaceous differentiation. Large lobules of sebaceous carcinoma frequently are necrotic centrally, a feature called the comedocarcinoma pattern, which recapitulates the necrobiosis that occurs during normal holocrine secretion. Another characteristic and important feature of sebaceous carcinoma is the tumor's ability to invade and replace eyelid skin and conjunctival epithelium in a pagetoid fashion (Fig. 12–49). The term pagetoid derives from the similarity of this process to Paget's disease of the nipple, which is marked by replacement of the skin by breast carcinoma cells. The observation of pagetoid involvement of the skin or conjunctiva helps to confirm the diagnosis of sebaceous carcinoma. The ability to invade and replace the conjunctival epithelium is one of the tumor's most insidious features. A relatively small eyelid tumor can give rise to extensive intraepithelial spread. Histopathologically, the affected segments of conjunctival epithelium are thickened and often are totally replaced by tumor cells. The infiltrated epithelium is often poorly adherent and may be lost or desquamated, leading to nondiagnostic biopsies.

Sebaceous carcinoma can spread by direct extension and can metastasize to regional lymph nodes and distant sites such as lung, liver, brain, and skull. Mortality due to the tumor was estimated to be about 15% in a large series by Rao et al. from the Armed Forces Institute of Pathology that included many advanced lesions. Factors associated with poor prognosis include origin from the upper eyelid, tumor diameter larger than 10 mm, origin from meibomian glands, duration of symptoms before diagnosis more than 6 months, an infiltrative growth pattern, poor sebaceous differentiation, extensive pagetoid invasion, and invasion of lymphatics, vessels, and the orbit.

Early diagnosis and treatment are important. No fatal tumors were reported in recent series, reflecting increased awareness of sebaceous carcinoma by ophthalmologists. Wide local excision should be performed with frozen section control of surgical margins. Radiation should be reserved for palliation of advanced cases in patients who refuse or cannot tolerate radical surgery. Orbital exenteration is performed in many institutions if there is orbital invasion or extensive pagetoid replacement of the conjunctiva. Some have questioned whether exenteration is excessive therapy for the latter, which essentially is an *in situ* disease process. Cryotherapy of conjunctival disease has been advocated to treat this diffuse, yet relatively localized form of the disease.

Senile sebaceous gland hyperplasia and sebaceous adenoma are other sebaceous lesions that occur on facial and eyelid skin. Relatively common, senile sebaceous gland hyperplasia appears as a nodule that may be umbilicated and often is misdiagnosed as basal cell carcinoma. Histopathology shows mature sebaceous gland lobules surrounding a central dilated duct (Fig. 12–50).

Sebaceous adenomas are rare tumors composed of irregular lobules of incompletely differentiated sebaceous glands comprised of foamy sebaceous cells, nonlipidized germinative cells, and intermediate cells (Fig. 12–51). The lobules are not arranged around a duct. Multiple sebaceous gland neoplasms, especially sebaceous adenomas, are associated with a visceral cancer, especially colon carcinoma, in the Muir Torre syndrome.

## Melanocytic Lesions

Melanocytic nevi are relatively common eyelid lesions. They are often misdiagnosed preoperatively when they are amelanotic or papillary in configuration. Nevi are classified as junctional, intradermal, or compound. Junctional nevi are flat, pigmented, and relatively rare. The nevus cells in junctional nevi are confined to the junction between the epidermis and the dermis. Junctional activity is much more common in young patients. As we age, nevus cells tend to leave the epidermal–dermal junction and migrate into the underlying dermis. Most nevi submitted to ophthalmic pathology laboratories are intradermal (or dermal) nevi (Fig. 12–52). They are often papillomatous, pedunculated, or dome-shaped, bear hairs and are frequently amelanotic or only slightly pigmented. Because a junctional component is absent, malignant transformation almost never occurs. Microscopy shows infiltration of the dermis by nevus cells arranged in nests. A cell-free collagenous grenz zone (*grenz*, German for border) separates the nevus cells in the dermis from the epidermis. The nevus cells in intradermal nevi typically show polarity, that is, the cellular morphology changes with location. Large type A nevus cells are found in the upper dermis. Type B cells found in the mid-dermis are smaller and often lymphocytoid (they superficially resemble lymphocytes). Type C cells in the lower dermis have little or no melanin and tend to appear fibroblastic with spindled nuclei. In elderly individuals the deeper cells may have a distinctly neural appearance. Benign nevi can infiltrate the deeper structures in the lid and occasionally contain multinucleated giant cells. If one observes mitotic figures, atypical cells with prominent nucleoli, or an intense infiltrate of inflammatory cells in a nevus, or finds "junctional activity" or epithelial involvement in an older patient, the diagnosis may be malignant melanoma.

Compound nevi usually are slightly elevated, papillomatous, and pigmented. The term compound indicates that nevus cells occur both at the junction and in the dermis. Other forms of nevi occasionally are encountered. Blue nevi are composed of heavily pigmented spindled or dendritic melanocytes located in the deeper tissues. The gray blue skin pigmentation in the nevus of Ota (congenital oculodermal melanocytosis) is caused by an extensive blue nevus. Cellular blue nevi can undergo malignant transformation into melanoma (Fig. 12–53).

Malignant melanomas of eyelid skin (Fig. 12–54) are relatively rare tumors that comprise fewer that 1% of eyelid malignancies. The prognosis of skin melanoma depends on the type of tumor and its thickness and depth of invasion. Lentigo maligna melanoma has the best prognosis. It develops in elderly individuals who have lentigo maligna or Hutchinson's malignant freckle. Patients with nodular melanoma tend to do poorly, whereas the prognosis of superficial spreading melanoma is of intermediate severity.

### Adnexal Tumors

A variety of eyelid neoplasms are derived from adnexal structures such as sweat glands and hair follicles. Most are rare. Syringomas are relatively common benign tumors of eccrine sweat glands that occur as multiple flesh-colored nodules on the faces of young women. Histopathology discloses small cysts or comma or tadpole-shaped ductules lined by a dual layer of eccrine ductal epithelium embedded in a dense fibrous stroma (Fig. 12–55). Primary malignant sweat gland tumors also occur on the eyelid. Primary mucus-secreting adenocarcinoma of sweat gland origin, which is probably the fifth most common primary malignant eyelid tumor, has a relatively high incidence (38%) of distant metastasis (Fig. 12–56). Some eccrine adenocarcinomas are comprised of signet ring cells. A malignant variant of syringoma also occurs that infiltrates the lid and orbit deeply, causing stromal desmoplasia analogous to that seen in scirrhous breast carcinoma; it can present with enophthalmos. Apocrine tumors include syringocystadenoma papilliferum (Fig. 12–57) and adenomas and adenocarcinomas of the glands of Moll.

Tumors of hair follicle origin include trichofolliculomas, trichoadenomas, trichoepitheliomas, trichilemmomas, and pilomatrixomas. Most of these "tricky" tumors are rare and are a diagnostic challenge to dermatopathologists. Pilomatrixoma, which often presents as a reddish nodule on the upper lid or brow of young patients, is relatively common (Fig. 12–58). Its eponymic designation (the calcifying epithelioma of Malherbe) and its histopathologic features are memorable. Pilomatrixoma contains sheets of bland, uniform, basophilic cells (hair matrix cells) that readily undergo necrosis, forming eosinophilic shadow cells with ghostly nuclei (Fig. 12–59). Dystrophic calcification characteristically develops in the necrotic areas, and a prominent foreign body giant cell response to the sheets of dead cells typically is observed.

## OTHER LESIONS

Xanthelasmas are soft, flat or slightly elevated, yellowish plaques that typically occur near the inner canthi (Fig. 12–60). They usually are removed to improve cosmesis. Xanthelasmas are predominantly dermal lesions. Histopathologic examination reveals sheets of foamy, lipid-laden histiocytes that tend to aggregate around vessels in the dermis (Fig. 12–61). The epidermis is normal. Although xanthelasmas occasionally signify hyperlipidemia, two-thirds of patients have normal lipids. An indurated xanthelasma-like lesion may occur in association with bilateral orbital infiltration, retroperitoneal fibrosis, and characteristic bone lesions in Erdheim-Chester disease, a rare and potentially fatal systemic disorder.

Multiple waxy nodules located along the eyelid margins that contain acellular eosinophilic hyaline material of unknown composition are found in autosomal recessively inherited lipoid proteinosis, or Urbach-Wiethe disease. Patients who have primary systemic amyloidosis may develop multiple confluent waxy purpuric papules on the eyelid skin that hemorrhage spontaneously or after minor trauma. The AL amyloid deposits are comprised of immunoglobulin light chains. Slightly elevated or umbilicated papules, which may be partially depigmented in Blacks, are an eyelid manifestation of sarcoidosis. Histopathology shows noncaseating granulomas. Multiple eyelid nodules and severe mutilating arthritis occur in patients with multicentric reticulohistiocytosis.

## EYELID MARKERS FOR SYSTEMIC MALIGNANCY

Rare eyelid tumors may serve as clinical markers for internal malignancy in patients with several hereditary syndromes. Multiple trichoepitheliomas (Brooke's tumor) can be inherited as an autosomal dominant trait. Trichilemmomas of the eyelid have been reported in Cowden's multiple hamartoma-neoplasia syndrome, which predisposes to the development of breast cancer in one-third of affected women. Sebaceous adenomas, other sebaceous neoplasms, and keratoacanthomas are found in Muir-Torre syndrome. Patients are at risk for visceral tumors, especially colonic carcinoma. Myxomas of the eyelid (Fig. 12–62) and spotty lentiginous pigmentation of the lids and conjunctiva, which often involves the caruncle and semilunar fold, are ocular markers for cardiac myxomas, endocrine abnormalities, and rare testicular tumors in autosomal dominantly inherited Carney syndrome. Atypical xanthelasma-like lesions that contain xanthoma cells, Touton giant cells, and foci of necrosis are found in patients with necrobiotic xanthogranuloma who may have systemic monoclonal gammopathies and plasma cell dyscrasias.

Other rare malignant eyelid tumors include metastases from distant primary cancers and the trabecular carcinoma or Merkel cell tumor (Fig. 12–63). A cutaneous APUDoma, the Merkel cell tumor typically presents as a violaceous, or reddish blue, nodule. The tumor is a neuroendocrine neoplasm of the skin that has a carcinoid-like histology. Electron microscopy shows dense-core neurosecretory granules, and immunohistochemistry typically shows the dual expression of the epithelial marker cytokeratin and neural markers such as neuron specific enolase. The fatality rate is 20%. Merkel cell tumor should be locally resected with frozen section control of surgical margins.

## LACRIMAL DRAINAGE SYSTEM

Tears are drained into the nose through the nasolacrimal drainage system, which is located nasally and is comprised of the puncta, canaliculi, lacrimal sac, and nasolacrimal duct. The puncta are the openings of the canaliculi. They are located in upper and lower eyelids near the inner canthus. The canaliculi are small tubules lined with epithelium that run from the puncta to the lacrimal sac. The lacrimal sac is located in the lacrimal fossa in the anteromedial wall of the orbit. A downward extension of the lacrimal sac called the nasolacrimal duct enters the nasal cavity on the lateral wall of the inferior nasal meatus. The nasolacrimal duct is enclosed in a bony canal about 12 mm long.

Congenital obstruction of the naso lacrimal duct is a relatively common cause of tearing (epiphora) in infants. It usually is caused by incomplete canalization of the duct near its lower end. Chronic dacryocystitis is the most common cause of nasolacrimal duct obstruction or stenosis in adults. Surgical specimens obtained at dacryocystectomy typically disclose an infiltrate of lymphocytes and plasma cells in the wall of the lacrimal sac. Concretions or casts occasionally are found within the lumina of the canaliculi or sac. They include masses of the gram-positive filamentous fungus *Actinomyces* (Fig. 12–64) and dacryoliths comprised of laminated inspissated protein that may contain fungal elements. Chronic nasolacrimal duct obstruction can predispose to acute bacterial infection of the lacrimal sac (acute dacryocystitis).

Neoplasms of the lacrimal sac are a rare cause of nasolacrimal duct obstruction and recurrent dacryocystitis. In addition to tearing, patients present with a mass in the inner canthal region, which is situated below the medial canthal tendon. Hemorrhage (bloody discharge or epistaxis) and pain are suggestive of a malignant neoplasm.

Most lacrimal sac tumors are papillomatous neoplasms that arise from the epithelial lining of the sac (Figs. 12–65, 12–66). They include exophytic and inverted papillomas comprised of squamous cells, transitional cells, or a mixture of the two. The papillomas may be benign, show focal atypia, or progress to invasive carcinoma. Invasive carcinoma typically arises from papillomas that have an inverted growth pattern. Fewer than one-third of lacrimal gland tumors are nonepithelial. Lymphomas, malignant melanomas, fibrous histiocytomas, hemangiopericytomas, neurilemomas, and angiosarcomas occasionally occur in this site.

## References

### General References

Eagle RC Jr: Specimen handling in the ophthalmic pathology laboratory. Ophthalmol Clin North Am 8:1–15, 1995.

Font RL: Eyelids and lacrimal drainage system. In Spencer W (ed) Ophthalmic Pathology: An Atlas and Textbook. 4th ed. Vol 2. Philadelphia: Saunders, 1996:2218–2437.

Lever WF, Schaumburg-Lever G: Histopathology of the Skin. 7th ed. Philadelphia: Lippincott, 1990.

### Developmental Lesions

Boyd PA, Keeling JW, Lindenbaum RH: Fraser syndrome (cryptophthalmos-syndactyly syndrome): a review of eleven cases with postmortem findings. Am J Med Genet 31:159–168, 1988.

Culbertson WW, Ostler HB: The floppy eyelid syndrome. Am J Ophthalmol 92:568–575, 1981.

Ellis FJ, Eagle RC Jr, Shields JA: Phakomatous choristoma (Zimmerman's tumor): immunohistochemical confirmation of lens-specific proteins. Ophthalmology 100: 955–960, 1993.

Kidwell ED, Tenzel RR: Repair of congenital colobomas of the lids. Arch Ophthalmol 97:1931–1932, 1979.

Mansour AM, Wang F, Henkind P, Goldberg R, Shprintzen R: Ocular findings in the facioauriculovertebral sequence (Goldenhar-Gorlin syndrome). Am J Ophthalmol 100: 555–559, 1985.

Pe'er J, BenEzra D, Sela M, Hemo I: Cryptophthalmos syndrome: clinical and histopathological findings. Ophthalmic Paediatr Genet 8:177–182, 1987.

Schauer GM, Dunn LK, Godmilow L, Eagle RC Jr, Knisely AS: Prenatal diagnosis of Fraser syndrome at 18.5 weeks gestation, with autopsy findings at 19 weeks. Am J Med Genet 37:583–591, 1990.

Schwartz LK, Gelender H, Forster RK: Chronic conjunctivitis associated with "floppy eyelids." Arch Ophthalmol 101:1884–1888, 1983.

Stefanyszyn MA, Hidayat AA, Flanagan JC: The histopathology of involutional ectropion. Ophthalmology 92:120–127, 1985.

Waardenburg P: A new syndrome combining developmental anomalies of the eyelids, eyebrows and nose root with pigmentary defects of the iris and headhair with congenital deafness. Am J Hum Genet 3:195, 1951.

Whitaker LA, Katowitz JA, Jacobs WE: Ocular adnexal problems in craniofacial deformities. J Maxillofac Surg 7: 55–60, 1979.

### Benign Lesions

Boniuk M, Zimmerman LE: Eyelid tumors with reference to lesions confused with squamous cell carcinoma. II. Inverted follicular keratosis. Arch Ophthalmol 69:698–707, 1963.

Kwitko ML, Boniuk M, Zimmerman LE: Eyelid tumors with reference to lesions confused with squamous cell carcinoma. I. Incidence and errors in diagnosis. Arch Ophthalmol 69:693–697, 1963.

Leahey AB, Shane JJ, Listhaus A, Trachtman M: Molluscum contagiosum eyelid lesions as the initial manifestation of acquired immunodeficiency syndrome. Am J Ophthalmol 124:240–241, 1997.

Robinson MR, Udell IJ, Garber PF, Perry HD, Streeten BW: Molluscum contagiosum of the eyelids in patients with acquired immune deficiency syndrome. Ophthalmology 99: 1745–1747, 1992.

Sassani JW, Yanoff M: Inverted follicular keratosis. Am J Ophthalmol 87:810–813, 1979.

Shields JA, Eagle RC Jr, Shields CL, et al: Apocrine hidrocystoma of the eyelid. Arch Ophthalmol 111:866–867, 1993.

**Keratoacanthoma**

Boniuk M, Zimmerman LE: Eyelid tumors with reference to lesions confused with squamous cell carcinoma. III. Keratoacanthoma. Arch Ophthalmol 77:29–40, 1967.

Grossniklaus HE, Wojno TH, Yanoff M, Font RL: Invasive keratoacanthoma of the eyelid and ocular adnexa. Ophthalmology 103:937–941, 1996.

Hodak E, Jones RE, Ackerman AB: Solitary keratoacanthoma is a squamous-cell carcinoma: three examples with metastases. Am J Dermatopathol 15:332–342, 1993.

**Basal Cell Carcinoma**

Doxanas MT, Green WR, Iliff CE: Factors in the successful surgical management of basal cell carcinoma of the eyelid. Am J Ophthalmol 91:726–736, 1981.

Einaugler RB, Henkind P: Basal cell carcinoma of the eyelid: apparent incomplete removal. Am J Ophthalmol 67: 413–417, 1969.

Margo CE, Waltz K: Basal cell carcinoma of the eyelid and periocular skin. Surv Ophthalmol 38:169–192, 1993.

**Squamous Cell Carcinoma and Predisposing Lesions**

Gaasterland DE, Rodrigues MM, Moshell AN: Ocular involvement in xeroderma pigmentosa. Ophthalmology 89: 980–986, 1982.

Lund HZ: How often does squamous cell carcinoma of the eyelid metastasize. Arch Dermatol 92:635–637, 1965.

Marks R, Foley P, Goodman G, et al. Spontaneous remission of solar keratoses: the case for conservative management. Br J Dermatol 115:649–655, 1986.

Morgan RJ: Metastases from squamous cell epitheliomas of the skin. In Epstein E (ed) Controversies in Dermatology. Philadelphia: Saunders, 1884:134.

Scott KR, Kronish JW: Premalignant lesions and squamous cell carcinoma. In Albert DM, Jakobiec FA (eds) Principles and Practice of Ophthalmology: Clinical Practice. Vol 3. Philadelphia: Saunders, 1994:1733–1744.

**Sebaceous Carcinoma**

Doxanas MT, Green WR: Sebaceous gland carcinoma: review of 40 cases. Arch Ophthalmol 102:245–249, 1984.

Hidayat AA, Font RL: Sebaceous carcinoma of the eyelids and caruncle of eyelid and eyebrow: a clinicopathologic study of 31 cases. Arch Ophthalmol 98:844–847, 1980.

Jakobiec FA: Sebaceous tumors of the ocular adnexa. In Albert DM, Jakobiec FA (eds) Principles and Practice of Ophthalmology: Clinical Practice. Vol 3. Philadelphia: Saunders, 1994:1745–1770.

Jakobiec FA, Zimmerman LE, La Piana F, et al: Unusual eyelid tumors with sebaceous differentiation in the Muir-Torre syndrome: rapid clinical regrowth and frank squamous transformation after biopsy. Ophthalmology 95: 1543–1548, 1988.

Margo CE, Grossniklaus HE: Intraepithelial sebaceous neoplasia without underlying invasive carcinoma. Surv Ophthalmol 39:293–301, 1995.

Rao NA, Hidayat AA, McLean IW, Zimmerman LE: Sebaceous gland carcinoma of the ocular adnexa: a clinicopathologic study of 104 cases with five year follow-up data. Hum Pathol 13:113–122, 1982.

Wolfe JT III, Yeatts RP, Wick MR, et al: Sebaceous carcinoma of the eyelid: errors in clinical and pathological diagnosis. Am J Surg Pathol 8:597–606, 1984.

**Melanocytic Lesions**

Margo C: Pigmented lesions of the eyelid. In Albert DM, Jakobiec FA (eds) Principles and Practice of Ophthalmology: Clinical Practice. Vol 3. Philadelphia: Saunders, 1994:1797–1812.

Naidoff MA, Bernardino VB Jr, Clark WH: Melanocytic lesions of the eyelid skin. Am J Ophthalmol 82:371–382, 1976.

**Adnexal Tumors**

Aurora AL, Luxenberg MN: Case report of adenocarcinoma of the glands of Moll. Am J Ophthalmol 70:984–990, 1970.

Lahav M, Albert DM, Bahr R, Craft J: Eyelid tumors of sweat gland origin. Graefes Arch Clin Ophthalmol 216: 301–311, 1981.

Shields JA, Shields CL, Eagle RC Jr, Mulvey L: Pilomatrixoma of the eyelid. J Pediatr Ophthalmol Strabismus 32:260–261, 1995.

Tong JT, Flanagan JC, Eagle RC Jr, Mazzoli RA: Benign mixed tumor arising from an accessory lacrimal gland of Wolfring. Ophthal Plast Reconstr Surg 11:136–138, 1995.

Wright JD, Font RL: Mucinous sweat gland carcinoma of the eyelid: a clinicopathologic study of 21 cases with histochemical and electron microscopic observations. Cancer 44:1757–1768, 1979.

**Eyelid Markers for Systemic Disease**

Bardenstein DS, McLean IW, Nerney J, Boatwright RS: Cowden's disease. Ophthalmology 95:1038–1041, 1988.

Jonsson A, Sigfusson N: Significance of xanthelasma palpebrum in the normal population. Lancet 1:372, 1976.

Kennedy RH, Flanagan JC, Eagle RC Jr, Carney JA: The Carney complex with ocular signs suggestive of cardiac myxoma. Am J Ophthalmol 111:699–702, 1991.

Mansour AH, Hidayat AA: Metastatic eyelid disease. Ophthalmology 94:667–670, 1987.

Robertson DM, Winkelmann RK: Ophthalmic features of necrobiotic xanthogranuloma with paraproteinemia. Am J Ophthalmol 97:173–183, 1984.

**Merkel Cell Carcinoma**

Cummings HL, Green WR: Merkel cell carcinoma of the eyelid: a report of two new cases and a review of the literature. Md Med J 41:149–153, 1992.

Kivela T, Tarkkanen A: The Merkel cell and associated neoplasms in the eyelids and periocular region. Surv Ophthalmol 35:171–187, 1990.

Rubsamen PE, Tanenbaum M, Grove AS, Gould E: Merkel cell carcinoma of the eyelid and periocular tissues. Am J Ophthalmol 113:674–680, 1992.

**Miscellaneous Lesions**

Alper MG, Zimmerman LE, LaPiana FG: Orbital manifestations of Erdheim-Chester disease. Trans Am Ophthalmol Soc 81:64–85, 1983.

Eagle RC Jr, Penne RA, Hneleski IS Jr: Eyelid involvement in multicentric reticulohistiocytosis. Ophthalmology 102: 426–430, 1995.

Feiler-Ofry V, Lewy A, Regenbogen L, Hanau D, Katznelson MB, Godel V: Lipoid proteinosis (Urbach-Wiethe syndrome). Br J Ophthalmol 63:694–698, 1979.

Girard C, Johnson WC, Graham JH: Cutaneous angiosarcomas. Cancer 26:868–883, 1970.

Rosenthal G, Lifshitz T, Monos T, Kachco L, Argov S: Carbon dioxide laser treatment for lipoid proteinosis (Urbach-Wiethe syndrome) involving the eyelids [letter]. Br J Ophthalmol 81:253, 1997.

**Lacrimal Sac**

Pe'er JJ, Stefanyszyn M, Hidayat AA: Nonepithelial tumors of the lacrimal sac. Am J Ophthalmol 118:650–658, 1994.

Ryan SJ, Font RL: Primary epithelial neoplasms of the lacrimal sac. Am J Ophthalmol 76:73–88, 1973.

Stefanyszyn MA, Hidayat AA, Pe'er JJ, Flanagan JC: Lacrimal sac tumors. Ophthalmic Plast Reconstr Surg 10: 169–184, 1994.

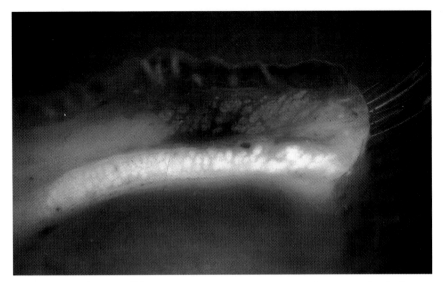

FIGURE 12–1 • **Upper eyelid.** The upper eyelid is roughly rectangular compared to the lower lid which is much shorter and triangular. The anterior surface of the lid is covered by skin. A row of cilia (eyelashes) arises near the lid margin (at right) and curves away from the globe. The white foci seen below are the lobules of the meibomian gland in the tarsal plate, the eyelid's fibrous skeleton. The palpebral conjunctiva is tightly adherent to the back surface of the tarsal plate.

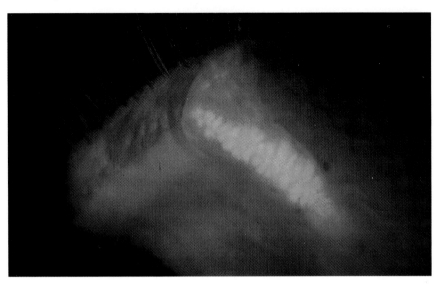

FIGURE 12–2 • **Lower eyelid.** The lower eyelid is roughly triangular and has a much shorter tarsal plate and fewer meibomian glands.

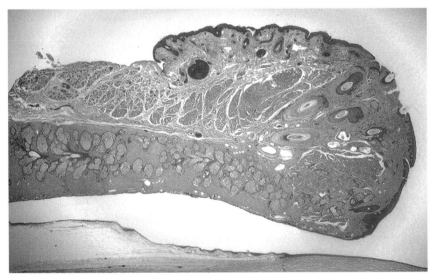

FIGURE 12–3 • **Upper eyelid.** The anterior surface of the eyelid is covered by a delicate layer of skin. The posterior surface is covered by the palpebral conjunctiva, which is firmly adherent to the tarsal plate. The tarsal plate contains large sebaceous glands called the meibomian glands. Eosinophilic bundles of orbicularis muscle are seen in cross section in the connective tissue anterior to the tarsus. Part of the skin is missing at left. Hematoxylin-eosin, ×5.

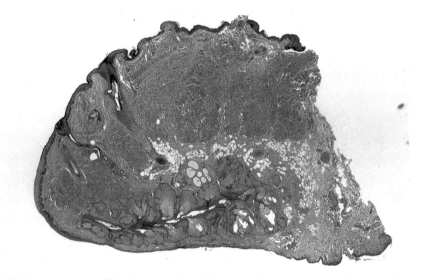

FIGURE 12–4 • **Lower eyelid.** The tarsal plate of the lower lid is much shorter. The lower lid is roughly triangular. Hematoxylin-eosin, ×10.

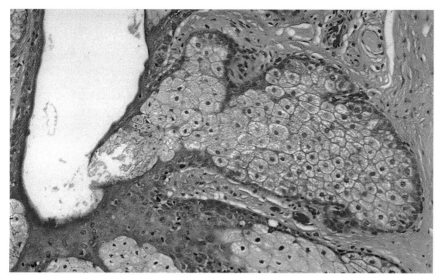

FIGURE 12–5 • **Meibomian gland lobule, eyelid.** Each meibomian gland is composed of multiple sebaceous gland lobules arranged along a central duct, which is oriented perpendicular to the lid margin. Sebaceous glands are holocrine glands; lipidized cells shed into the duct comprise the secretory product. Cellular division occurs in the basal cell layer in the periphery of the lobules. The nuclei become increasingly pyknotic as the cells mature and become lipidized. A flap-like valve of ductal epithelium covers the opening of this lobule. Hematoxylin-eosin, ×50.

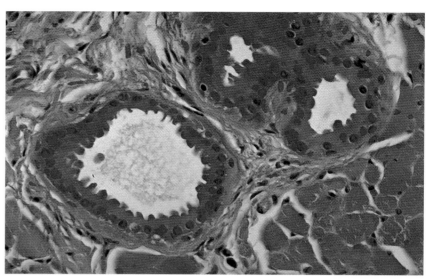

FIGURE 12–6 • **Glands of Moll.** The dilated lumina of these apocrine sweat glands are lined by tall eosinophilic cells capped with the apical snouts that characterize apocrine decapitation secretion. Hematoxylin-eosin, ×100.

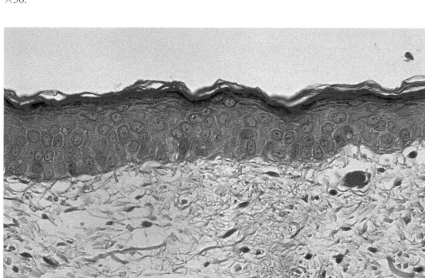

FIGURE 12–7 • **Eyelid skin.** The skin of the eyelid is extremely delicate and lacks rete pegs. The layers of the epidermis include the basal cell layer, the malpighian or prickle cell layer, the granular cell layer, and the superficial keratin layer. Hematoxylin-eosin, ×100.

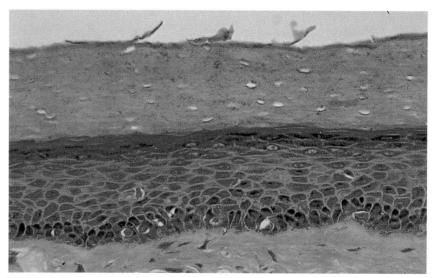

FIGURE 12–8 • **Hyperkeratosis.** The superficial layer of eosinophilic keratin is markedly thickened. The dead cells comprising the mass of keratin lack nuclei. A granular cell layer is present underneath the keratin. The epidermis in this specimen is mildly thickened. Hematoxylin-eosin, ×50.

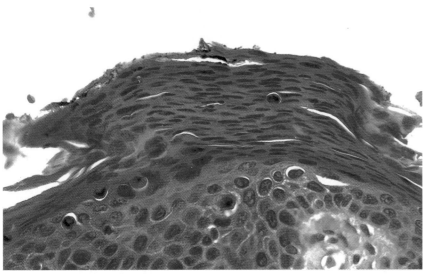

FIGURE 12–9 • **Parakeratosis, actinic keratosis.** The keratin layer retains flattened nuclei, and no granular cell layer is present. Parakeratosis is typically found in actinic keratosis. In this example the epidermis is composed of mildly atypical squamous cells. Hematoxylin-eosin, × 100.

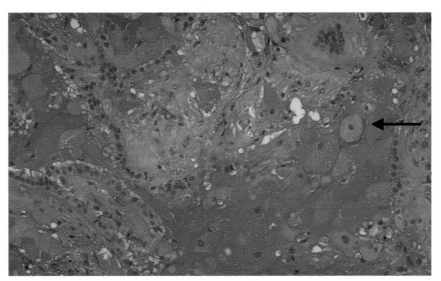

FIGURE 12–10 • **Zimmerman's tumor (phakomatous choristoma).** Phakomatous choristoma is a rare congenital tumor of lenticular anlage that always occurs in the lower medial eyelid or anterior orbit. The tumor is composed of neoplastic lens epithelial cells and segments of thick basement membrane that mimics lens capsule. Swollen cells with eosinophilic cytoplasm that resemble the bladder or Wedl cells of posterior subcapsular cataract are present (arrow). Hematoxylin-eosin, ×50.

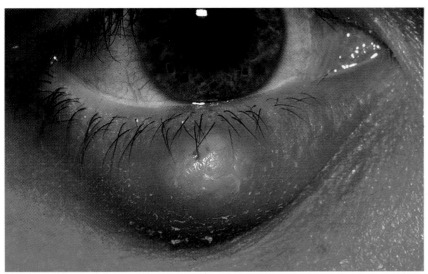

FIGURE 12–11 • **Eyelid abscess.** This localized lid infection is more conspicuous than most hordeolums.

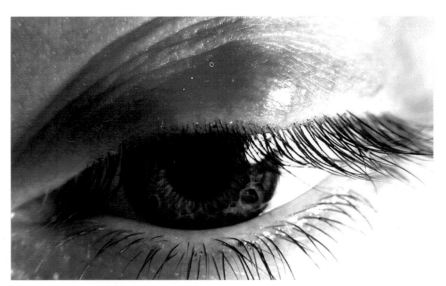

FIGURE 12–12 • **Chalazion.** The focal area of nodular thickening in the upper eyelid represents a chronic granulomatous inflammatory response to irritating lipid material that has escaped from its normal compartment in the lid. Chalazia usually are only mildly tender and inflamed. Recurrent or atypical "chalazia" should be examined pathologically to exclude simulating lesions such as sebaceous carcinoma.

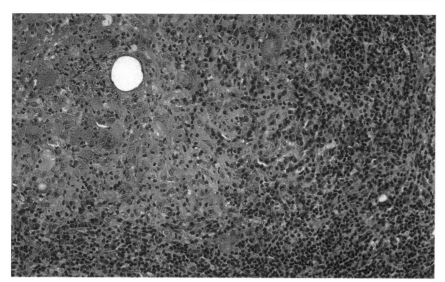

FIGURE 12–13 • **Chalazion.** Pink epithelioid histiocytes and giant cells indicative of chronic granulomatous inflammation surround an empty lipid vacuole. The lipid was dissolved by fat solvents during processing. Empty lipid vacuoles are required for the diagnosis of lipogranulomatous inflammation. The inflammatory infiltrate also contains many plasma cells and lymphocytes. Hematoxylin-eosin, ×100.

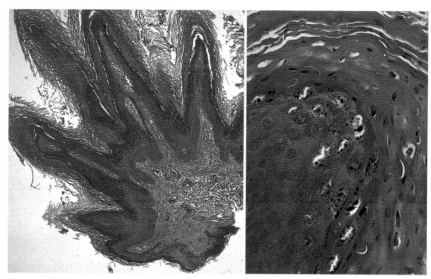

FIGURE 12–14 • **Verruca vulgaris.** Viral papilloma is comprised of spire-shaped fronds of hyperkeratotic epidermis. Parakeratosis and vacuolated cells containing viral inclusions are seen on the crest of the frond (*right*). Hematoxylin-eosin. Left ×25; right ×250.

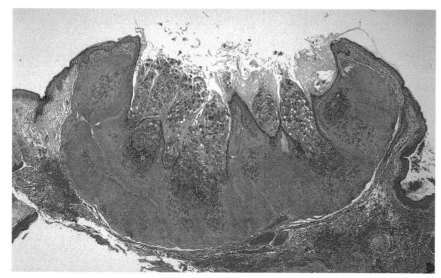

FIGURE 12–15 • **Molluscum contagiosum.** This viral tumor has a typical crateriform configuration. Inclusions of pox virus shed by the infected acanthotic epithelium fill the crater. Hematoxylin-eosin, ×10.

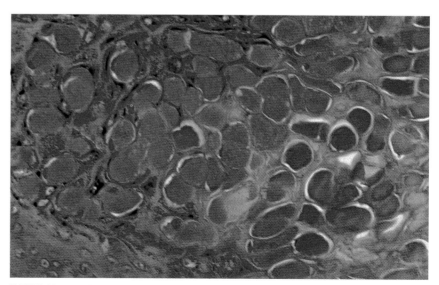

FIGURE 12–16 • **Molluscum contagiosum, Henderson-Patterson corpuscles.** The pox virus infection causes lobular acanthosis of the epidermis. The thickened epidermis contains large, oval intracytoplasmic viral inclusions called Henderson-Patterson corpuscles. The inclusions become increasingly basophilic as they mature. Hematoxylin-eosin, ×100.

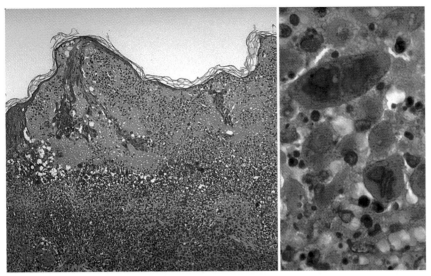

FIGURE 12–17 • **Herpes simplex infection of the skin.** Serous fluid and inflammatory cells fill a herpetic vesicle that has formed within the acantholytic epidermis. The underlying dermis is intensely inflamed. *Inset:* Multinucleated giant cells with Cowdry type A intranuclear inclusions are seen. Hematoxylin-eosin. Main figure ×25; inset ×250.

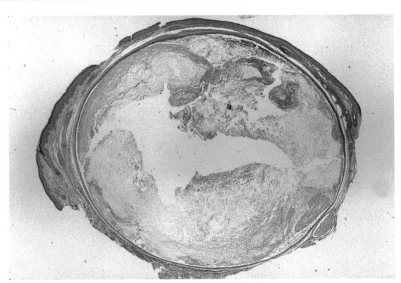

FIGURE 12–18 • **Epidermal inclusion cyst.** Epidermal inclusion cysts typically are round or oval and unilocular. The lumen of the cyst contains laminated eosinophilic keratin, which had a cheesy appearance grossly. The cyst is lined by keratinized squamous epithelium that resembles skin but lacks epidermal appendages. Hematoxylin-eosin, ×5.

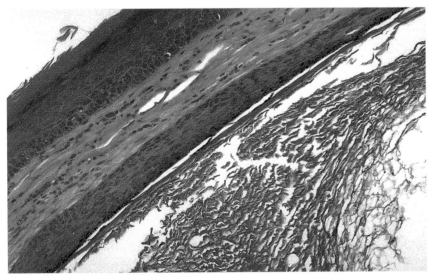

FIGURE 12–19 • **Epidermal inclusion cyst.** The surface of the skin is seen at top left. The cyst is lined by keratinized stratified squamous epithelium resembling epidermis. Laminated keratin fills the lumen. Hematoxylin-eosin, ×50.

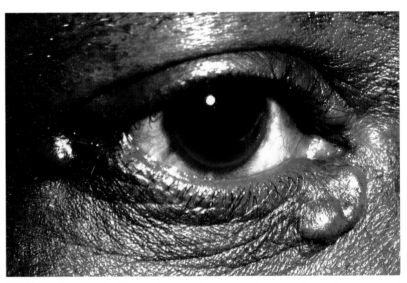

FIGURE 12–20 • **Eccrine hidrocystomas.** Cysts caused by the blockage of eccrine sweat glands often involve the canthal skin. Multiple cysts occur in some patients. They are filled with watery fluid. Eccrine hidrocystomas also are called sweat ductal or sudoriferous cysts.

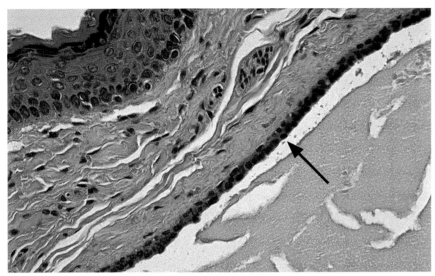

FIGURE 12–21 • **Eccrine hidrocystoma.** The eccrine hidrocystoma (below) is lined by a dual layer of epithelial cells resembling the epithelium of an eccrine sweat gland duct. The lumen is filled with eosinophilic granular debris consistent with serous fluid. The lumen is often branching and multilocular. Hematoxylin-eosin, ×100.

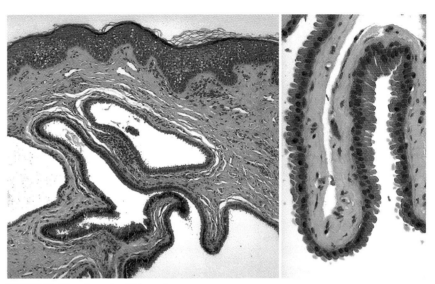

FIGURE 12–22 • **Apocrine hidrocystoma.** Branching lumen of multilocular Moll gland cyst appears empty. The cells comprising the epithelial lining (*right*) are tall and show apical snouts of decapitation secretion indicative of apocrine differentiation. Hematoxylin-eosin. Main figure ×25; inset ×100.

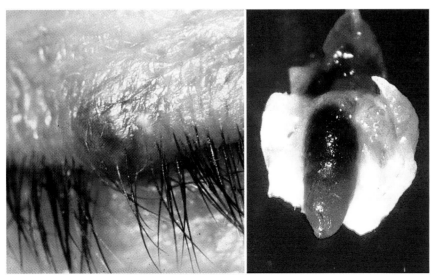

FIGURE 12–23 • **Apocrine hidrocystoma.** Bluish lesion near the lid margin was thought to be a pigmented melanocytic nevus preoperatively. Photograph of another case shows brownish fluid filling the lumen of the cyst.

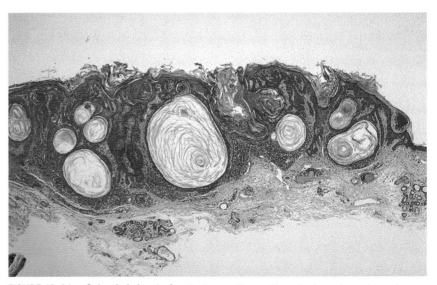

FIGURE 12–24 • **Seborrheic keratosis.** Benign sessile papilloma is situated anterior to the plane of the surrounding skin. The lesion contains many characteristic pseudohorn cysts. Hematoxylin-eosin, ×10.

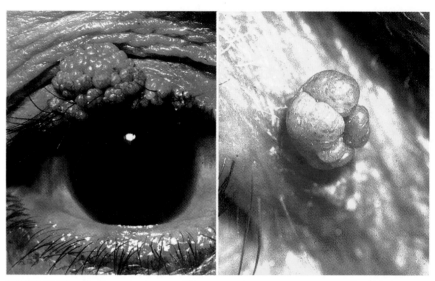

FIGURE 12–25 • **Basal cell carcinoma.** Invasive malignant tumor is localized deep to the plane of the surrounding skin. Surface ulceration is present. Hematoxylin-eosin, ×10.

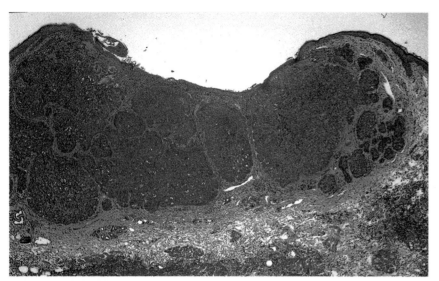

FIGURE 12–26 • **Benign squamous papillomas.** Squamous papillomas are common benign epidermal tumors of the eyelid. They are branching, tree-shaped lesions composed of multiple fronds of benign epidermis.

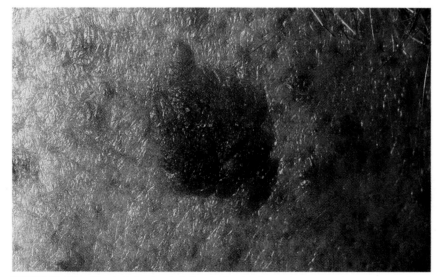

FIGURE 12–27 • **Pigmented seborrheic keratosis.** Sessile papillomatous lesion is situated anterior to the plane of the surrounding skin. Scaly surface reflects hyperkeratosis.

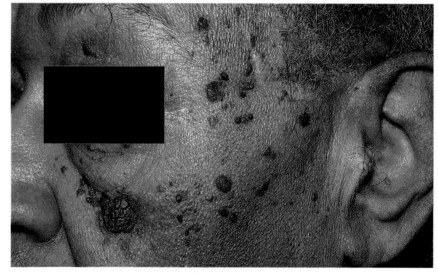

FIGURE 12–28 • **Dermatosis papulosa nigra.** Multiple seborrheic keratoses are seen on the face of this elderly African-American woman.

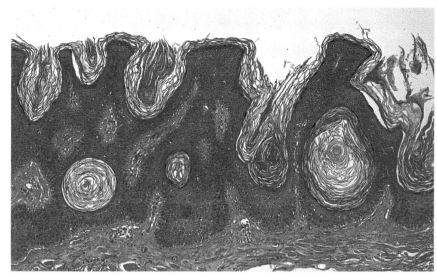

FIGURE 12–29 • **Seborrheic keratosis.** Thick layer of hyperkeratosis covers a sessile papilloma. Characteristic pseudohorn cysts filled with keratin are present. Hematoxylin-eosin, ×25.

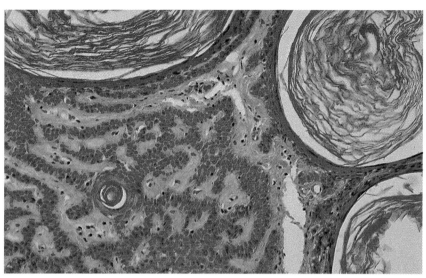

FIGURE 12–30 • **Seborrheic keratosis, adenoid type.** The dermis contains interweaving bands of benign epithelial cells. Several keratin-filled pseudohorn cysts are present. Hematoxylin-eosin, ×50.

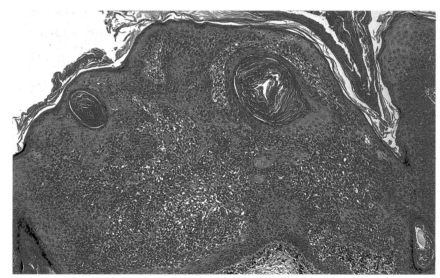

FIGURE 12–31 • **Inverted follicular keratosis.** IFK is thought to be an irritated variant of seborrheic keratosis. Acantholysis and circular foci of squamous cells (squamous eddies) are characteristic histologic features. Hematoxylin-eosin, ×25.

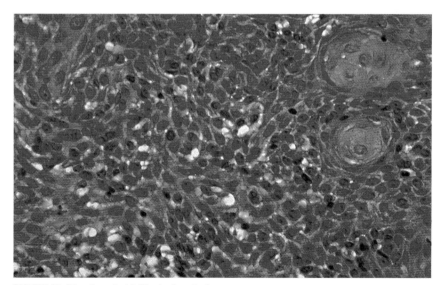

FIGURE 12–32 • **Inverted follicular keratosis.** Several oval foci of squamous differentiation called squamous eddies are seen at right. The smaller basaloid cells show mild acantholysis. Hematoxylin-eosin, ×100.

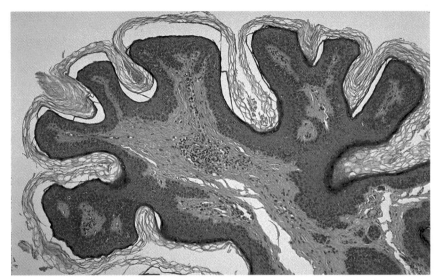

FIGURE 12–33 • **Squamous papilloma.** Multiple fronds or finger-like projections of epidermis comprise the benign epidermal tumor. The epidermal fronds contain a central core of fibrovascular tissue. Hyperkeratosis is present on the surface of this lesion. Hematoxylin-eosin, ×25.

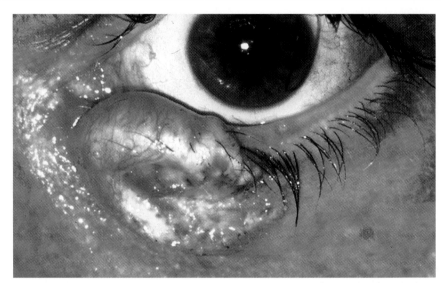

FIGURE 12–34 • **Keratoacanthoma.** Keratin fills irregular crater in a large biopsy-confirmed keratoacanthoma of the lower eyelid. The tumor developed rapidly. Some authorities now believe that keratoacanthoma is a "deficient squamous cell carcinoma" that tends to involute spontaneously.

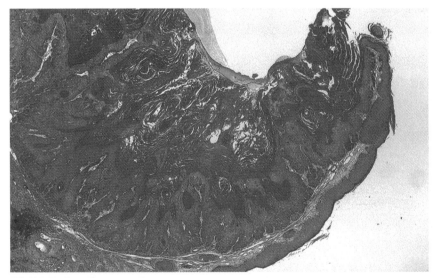

FIGURE 12–35 • **Keratoacanthoma.** A mass of keratin fills the crater-shaped tumor, which is composed of squamous cells with eosinophilic cytoplasm. A lateral buttress of normal skin is seen at right. The base of the lesion has a smooth, "pushing" margin. Hematoxylin-eosin, ×5.

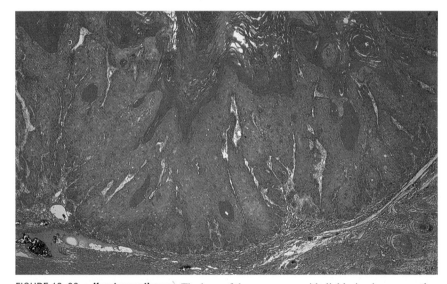

FIGURE 12–36 • **Keratoacanthoma.** The base of the squamous epithelial lesion has a smooth "pushing" margin. A large mass of keratin is seen above. The general configuration of the lesion is important for the histopathologic diagnosis. It usually is impossible to distinguish keratoacanthoma from squamous cell carcinoma in a small incisional biopsy. Hematoxylin-eosin, ×10.

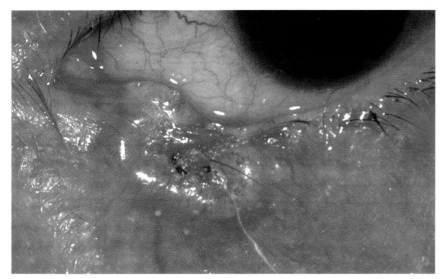

FIGURE 12–37 • **Basal cell carcinoma.** Noduloulcerative basal cell carcinoma of the lower lid has pearly, elevated margins.

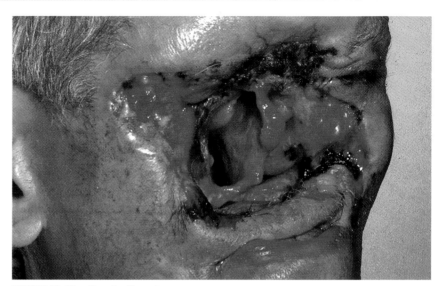

FIGURE 12–38 • **Basal cell carcinoma.** Neglected morpheaform basal cell carcinoma has produced ghastly facial disfigurement.

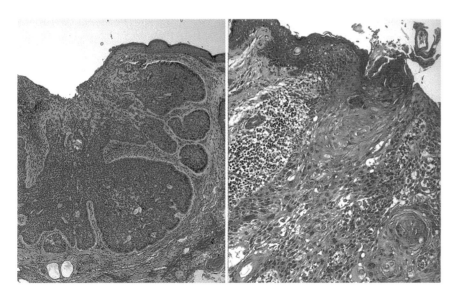

FIGURE 12–39 • **Invasive basal cell and squamous cell carcinomas.** The invasive basal cell carcinoma (*left*) appears basophilic because tumor cells have scant cytoplasm. Invasive squamous cell carcinoma (*right*) is comprised of cells with eosinophilic cytoplasm. Hematoxylin-eosin. Left ×25, right ×50.

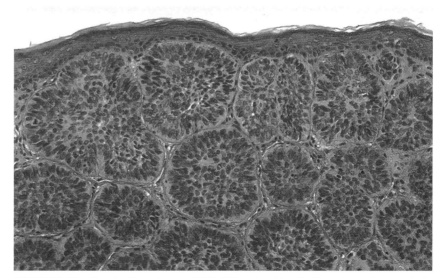

FIGURE 12–40 • **Basal cell carcinoma.** Well-differentiated basal cell carcinoma is comprised of nests of basaloid cells that show peripheral palisading of nuclei. No connection with epidermis is evident in this field. Hematoxylin-eosin, ×100.

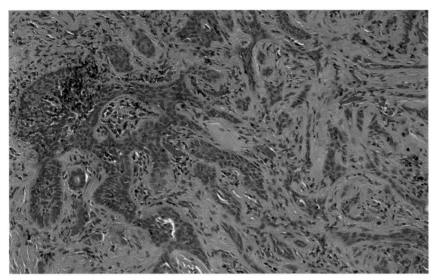

FIGURE 12–41 • **Morpheaform basal cell carcinoma.** Morpheaform basal cell carcinoma is a poorly differentiated variant of basal cell carcinoma that is composed of slender infiltrating tendrils of tumor cells similar to those found in scirrhous breast carcinoma. The margins of morpheaform basal cell carcinoma are often indistinct clinically, and the tumor tends to infiltrate deeply. Hematoxylin-eosin, ×25.

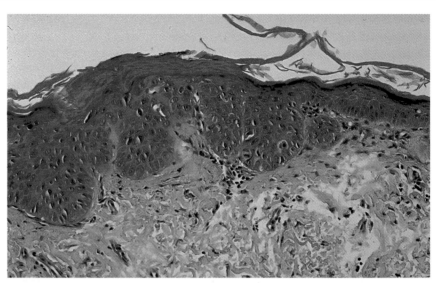

FIGURE 12–42 • **Actinic keratosis.** A surface plaque of parakeratosis covers a thickened segment of epidermis that is replaced by atypical squamous cells. Irregular buds of atypical keratinocytes extend into the papillary dermis at the base of some lesions. The dermis shows actinic elastosis. Normal epidermis is seen at right. Hematoxylin-eosin, ×100.

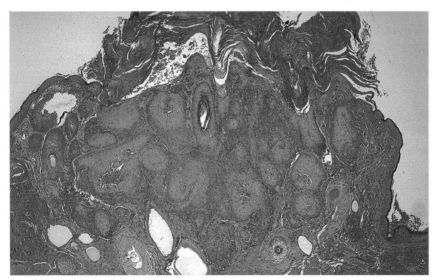

FIGURE 12–43 • **Squamous cell carcinoma.** Eosinophilic nests of squamous cell carcinoma infiltrate the eyelid margin. A thick layer of surface keratinization is present. Hematoxylin-eosin, ×10.

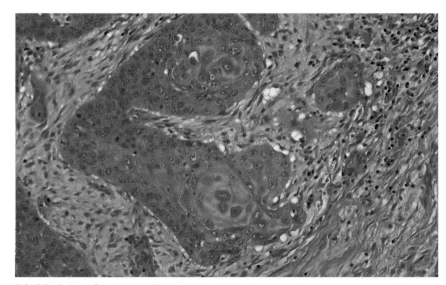

FIGURE 12–44 • **Squamous cell carcinoma.** Infiltrating nests of tumor are composed of neoplastic squamous cells with abundant eosinophilic cytoplasm. Hematoxylin-eosin, ×100.

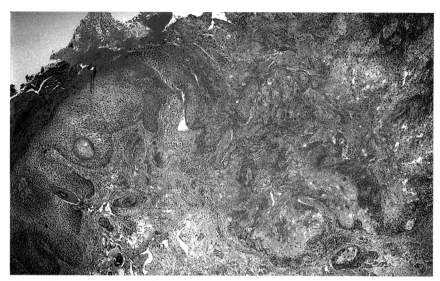

FIGURE 12–45 • **Squamous cell carcinoma arising from actinic keratosis.** Atypical squamous cells remain confined by the basement membrane of the markedly acanthotic epithelium at left. Eosinophilic squamous cell carcinoma invades the dermis at right. The tumor has incited a chronic inflammatory response. Hematoxylin-eosin, ×10.

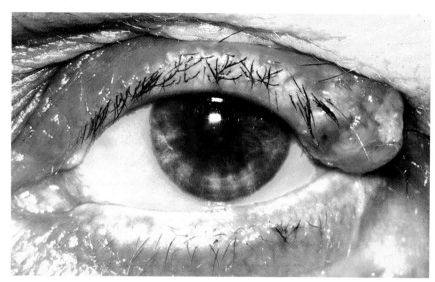

FIGURE 12–46 • **Sebaceous carcinoma.** Upper eyelid tumor is yellow, indicating the presence of lipid.

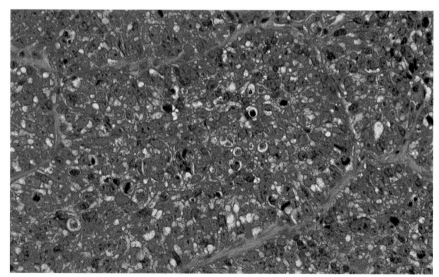

FIGURE 12–47 • **Sebaceous carcinoma.** Tumor is composed of lobules of cells with foamy vacuolated cytoplasm. Numerous mitoses are present. Peripheral palisading is not seen. Hematoxylin-eosin, ×100.

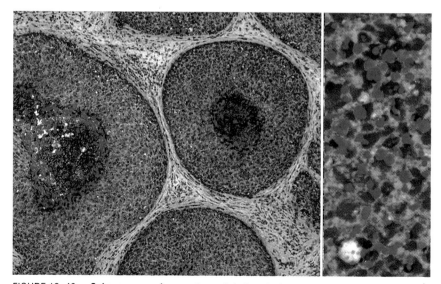

FIGURE 12–48 • **Sebaceous carcinoma.** Large lobules of sebaceous carcinoma show central necrosis (comedocarcinoma pattern) mimicking holocrine secretion. Oil red O stain performed on frozen sectioned material confirms the presence of lipid in cytoplasmic vacuoles. Oil red O. Main figure ×50, inset ×250.

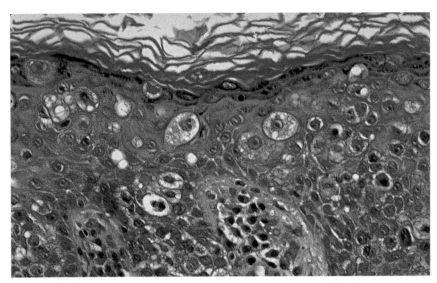

FIGURE 12–49 • **Sebaceous gland carcinoma, pagetoid invasion of eyelid skin.** Individual tumor cells with vacuolated cytoplasm from an underlying sebaceous carcinoma infiltrate the epidermis in a fashion analogous to Paget's disease of the breast. Hematoxylin-eosin, ×100.

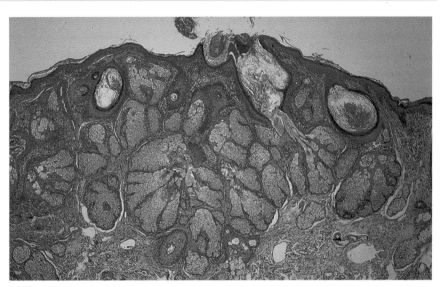

FIGURE 12–50 • **Senile sebaceous gland hyperplasia.** Lobules of mature benign hyperplastic sebaceous glands form a nodule in the dermis. They show typical arrangement around the central duct. The nodule was misdiagnosed as basal cell carcinoma preoperatively. Hematoxylin-eosin, ×10.

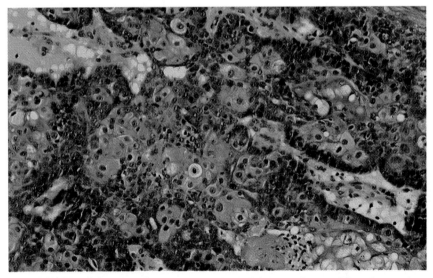

FIGURE 12–51 • **Sebaceous adenoma.** Incompletely lipidized cells comprising a low-grade sebaceous neoplasm form disorderly lobules. Differential diagnosis included sebaceous adenoma or low-grade sebaceous carcinoma. Sebaceous adenomas serve as a clinical marker for systemic malignancy in patients with the Muir-Torre syndrome. Hematoxylin-eosin, ×100.

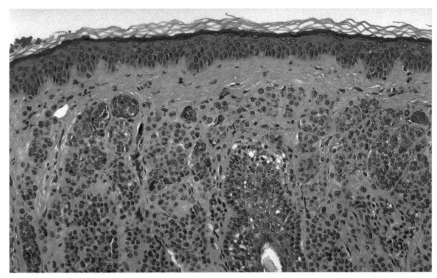

FIGURE 12–52 • **Intradermal nevus.** Nests of benign nevus cells infiltrate the dermis. An acellular "grenz" zone separates the nevus cells from the epidermis. No junctional activity persists. Some of the cells are lightly pigmented. Hematoxylin-eosin, ×25.

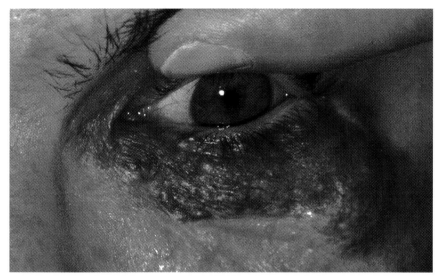

FIGURE 12–53 • **Cellular blue nevus.** Bluish brown discoloration of the lids reflects infiltration of the dermis and orbital tissues by a cellular blue nevus. Patient developed orbital malignant melanoma.

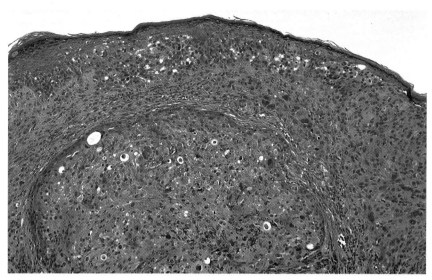

FIGURE 12–54 • **Malignant melanoma, eyelid.** Lobules of frankly malignant melanocytes including epithelioid cells invade the dermis. The basal half of the overlying epidermis is replaced by atypical melanocytic hyperplasia. Hematoxylin-eosin, ×50.

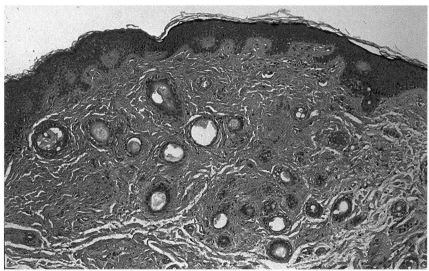

FIGURE 12–55 • **Syringoma.** Syringomas are benign sweat gland tumors. Oval and comma- or tadpole-shaped epithelial ductules are found amidst dense fibrous stroma. The ducts mimic the straight dermal duct of eccrine sweat glands. Syringomas often occur as multiple elevated papules on the facial skin of young women. Hematoxylin-eosin, ×50.

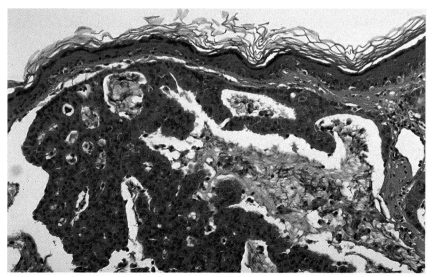

FIGURE 12–56 • **Primary mucus-secreting sweat gland carcinoma.** Pools of mucus surround cords of malignant sweat gland epithelium. Primary sweat gland carcinomas can metastasize but fortunately are rare. A metastasis to the lid from a distant primary carcinoma must be excluded clinically. Hematoxylin-eosin, ×50.

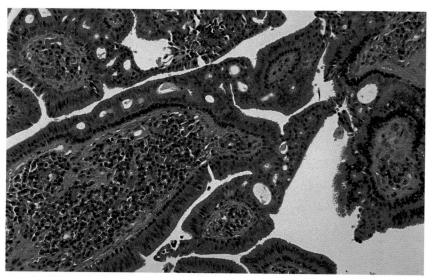

FIGURE 12–57 • **Syringocystadenoma papilliferum.** A papillary proliferation of benign apocrine sweat glandular epithelium lines and partially fills cystic spaces in the dermis. Plasma cells infiltrate the stroma. The overlying epidermis was acanthotic. Hematoxylin-eosin, ×50.

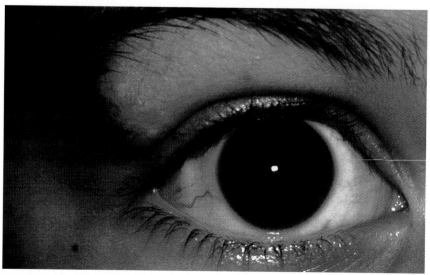

FIGURE 12–58 • **Pilomatrixoma.** Tumor underneath the brow in a child appears clinically as a slightly erythematous subepidermal nodule.

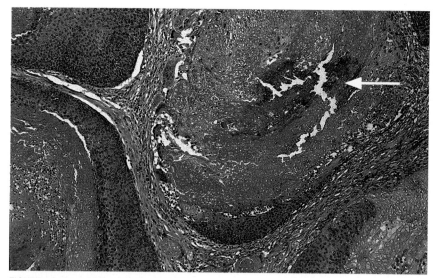

FIGURE 12–59 • **Pilomatrixoma (calcifying epithelioma of Malherbe).** Tumor is comprised of viable hair matrix cells, which are basophilic, and sheets of nonviable eosinophilic shadow cells. Arrow denotes a focus of dystrophic calcification in a necrotic area. Hematoxylin-eosin, ×50.

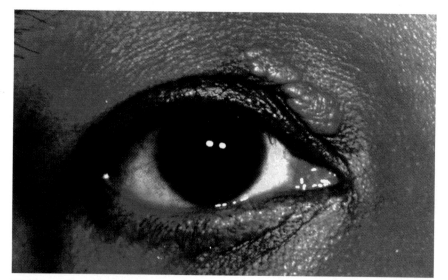

FIGURE 12–60 • **Xanthelasma.** An elevated yellowish plaque involves the inner canthal skin of the upper lid.

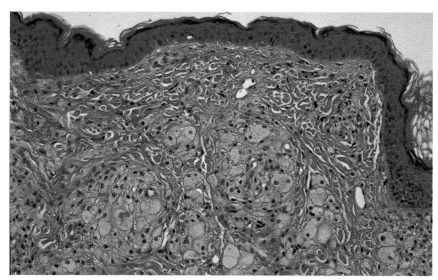

FIGURE 12–61 • **Xanthelasma.** The dermis contains an infiltrate of xanthoma cells (lipid-laden histiocytes). The epidermis is normal. Hematoxylin-eosin, ×50.

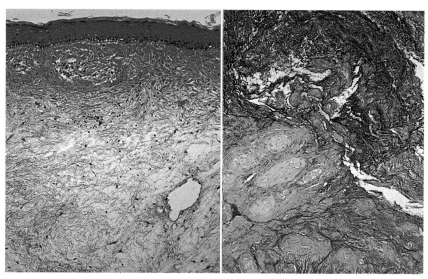

FIGURE 12–62 • **Eyelid myxoma, Carney syndrome.** Lucent pools of relatively acellular mucin are present deep in the dermis. The alcian blue stain (*inset*) confirms the presence of acid mucopolysaccharide. The patient had Carney syndrome, an autosomal dominantly inherited syndrome that includes multiple myxomas, spotty mucocutaneous pigmentation, and endocrine abnormalities. Left: hematoxylin-eosin, ×50; right: alcian blue, ×100.

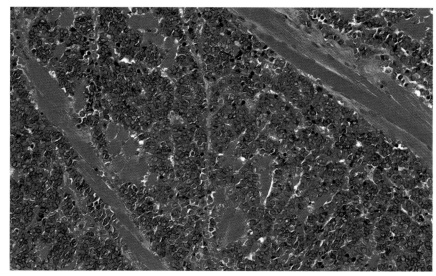

FIGURE 12–63 • **Merkel cell tumor.** Primary neuroendocrine tumor of the eyelid skin infiltrates the orbicularis muscle. The tumor was immunoreactive for keratin, neuron specific enolase, and chromogranin. Hematoxylin-eosin, ×100.

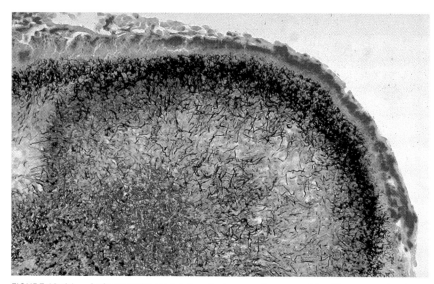

FIGURE 12–64 • **Actinomycotic lacrimal cast.** A mass of gram-positive filamentous fungi removed from a canaliculus has a laminated appearance. Gram stain, ×100.

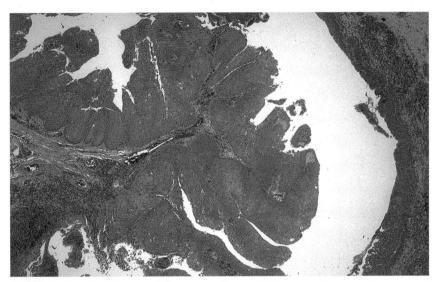

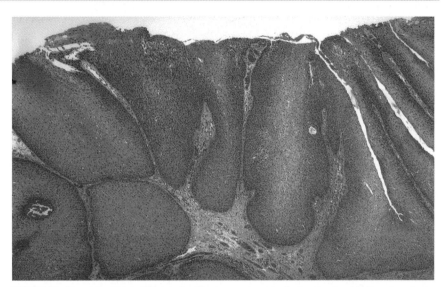

FIGURE 12–65 • **Papilloma, lacrimal sac.** Papillary epithelial tumor fills most of the lumen of the lacrimal sac. Hematoxylin-eosin, ×5.

FIGURE 12–66 • **Inverted papilloma, lacrimal sac.** Acanthotic fronds of epithelium invade the stroma. Most lacrimal gland carcinomas arise from inverted papillomas. Hematoxylin-eosin, ×100.

# CHAPTER 13

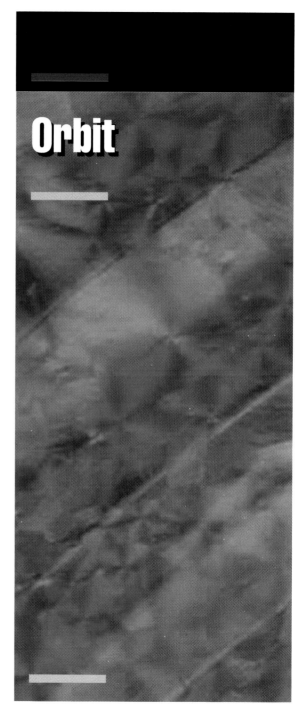

# Orbit

The eye is contained in a protective pear-shaped cavity in the skull called the orbit, which contains about 30 ml of highly specialized tissue (Fig. 13–1). Other orbital contents are the optic nerve, which is a specialized tract of the central nervous system (CNS); smooth and striated muscle; vessels; nerves; fatty and fibrous connective tissue; and the lacrimal gland, a minor salivary gland. The orbit communicates with the intracranial cavity through several fissures and foramina, and several of its bony walls contain paranasal sinuses. The eye and the remainder of the orbital contents, which are delimited anteriorly by a septum of fibrous tissue, are protected by the eyelids, retractable flaps of skin equipped with highly specialized epidermal appendages. The epithelial-lined components of the nasolacrimal drainage system are located in the inferonasal part of the orbit.

Orbital disease is relatively uncommon but diverse in nature. Inflammatory diseases, such as infectious cellulitis and the immunologic disorders thyroid ophthalmopathy and idiopathic orbital inflammation, or "pseudotumor," are encountered most often in general clinical practice. However, the soft tissues of the orbit occasionally give rise to a relatively broad spectrum of primary neoplasms, and the orbit can be involved secondarily by systemic lymphoma, metastases from distant primary cancers, or tumors that arise in neighboring tissues such as conjunctiva, eyelid, paranasal sinuses, or even the intracranial cavity.

The essential clinical manifestation of orbital disease is exophthalmos, or ocular proptosis (see Figs. 13–5, 13–31, below). The eye usually is pushed forward because the orbit is a semiconfined space bounded by bony walls, and most orbital diseases are space-occupying. The proptotic eye may be pushed directly forward (axial proptosis) or in other directions (i.e., down and in) that are determined by and serve to indicate the location of the orbital lesion. For example, tumors of the lacrimal gland, which is located in the superotemporal orbit, typically push the eye inferomedially as well as forward, and mucoceles of the ethmoid sinus in the medial orbital wall cause lateral displacement. Retraction of the eye or enophthalmos occurs occasionally. Causes of enophthalmos include traumatic blow-out fractures of the orbital floor and sclerosing tumors such as metastatic scirrhous breast carcinoma. Other symptoms and signs of orbital disease include pain, loss of vision, and ocular motility disturbances, which may or may not be conspicuous depending on the underlying cause; some orbital tumors (i.e., lymphomas) tend to be well tolerated. Others (i.e., metastatic carcinoma) are more likely to be symptomatic.

## ORBITAL INFLAMMATORY DISEASE

Most orbital disease encountered by the ophthalmologist in general practice is inflammatory in nature. The most common inflammatory diseases of the orbit include infectious orbital cellulitides, noninfectious idiopathic orbital inflammation (inflammatory orbital pseudotumor), and Graves' disease, or thyroid orbitopathy.

Orbital cellulitis usually is caused by the extension of a primary sinus infection into adjacent soft tissues of the orbit (Fig. 13–2). Abscesses can form underneath the periosteum (subperiosteal abscess) or in the orbital soft tissues. Patients with orbital cellulitis have signs of acute inflammation, including erythema, pain and proptosis. Although most orbital cellulitis is caused by bacteria, fungi such as *Aspergillus* or *Mucor*

247

occasionally invade the orbit from primary foci in the sinuses. *Haemophilus influenzae* is an important cause of orbital cellulitis in children. Rarely, a clinical picture resembling orbital cellulitis is caused by an extensively necrotic intraocular retinoblastoma or melanoma. Orbital involvement has been reported in allergic fungal sinusitis (Fig. 13–3).

Mucormycosis (zygomycosis) is a potentially lethal opportunistic infection by saprophytic fungi that usually occurs in acidotic persons, such as poorly controlled diabetics. The fungus is vasotropic and invades orbital vessels, causing thrombosis and necrosis (Fig. 13–4). Histopathology shows both acute and chronic granulomatous inflammation. The hyphae are large and nonseptate and are easily identified in standard hematoxylin-eosin (H&E)-stained sections. Lives occasionally can be saved if an expedient diagnosis is made and antifungal therapy is instituted.

Graves' disease, or thyroid ophthalmopathy, is the most common cause of unilateral or bilateral exophthalmos (Fig. 13–5). Affected patients have an underlying immunologic disorder that is complex and still poorly understood; it affects the thyroid gland and orbital structures, especially the extraocular muscles. The exophthalmos is caused by enlargement of the extraocular muscles (Fig. 13–6). The enlarged muscles contain foci of chronic nongranulomatous inflammation and show endomysial fibrosis and increased quantities of glycosaminoglycans (Fig. 13–7). The tendon of the extraocular muscle and the orbital fat characteristically are noninflamed, a feature that serves to differentiate thyroid ophthalmopathy from idiopathic orbital inflammation (pseudotumor). Visual loss due to compressive optic neuropathy occurs in some patients when the swollen muscle bellies press on the optic nerve in the crowded orbital apex (Fig. 13–8). Corneal complications caused by exposure can also cause visual loss. Graves' ophthalmopathy can occur in patients whose thyroid function test results are high, low, or even normal. Most cases are readily diagnosed by the demonstration of enlarged extraocular muscles on computed tomography (CT) or magnetic resonance imaging (MRI) scans. Few cases are biopsied.

Idiopathic orbital inflammation, or pseudotumor, is relatively common. Although orbital pseudotumor undoubtedly is an immunologic disorder, the details of its immunopathology and the identity of the antigens responsible for inciting the inflammation are unclear. Idiopathic orbital inflammatory pseudotumor is a diagnosis of exclusion, from both clinical and histopathologic standpoints. The presence of fungi, bacteria, and acid-fast organisms, foreign substances, and other specific inflammatory diseases such as Wegener's granulomatosis or sarcoidosis must be excluded with special stains or appropriate tests.

Idiopathic orbital inflammation can affect both adults and children, who may have unilateral or bilateral disease. Although occasional cases are relatively asymptomatic and indolent in their course, idiopathic orbital inflammation classically presents explosively with the acute onset of pain, ocular proptosis, muscle paresis, and sometimes visual loss. The inflammation may be localized to single orbital structures, such as the extraocular muscles (orbital myositis), the lacrimal gland (chronic dacryoadenitis), or the sclera or episclera (scleritis or episcleritis). A diagnostic trial of systemic corticosteroids may be administered to patients suspected of having idiopathic orbital inflammation because the disorder is exquisitely sensitive to steroids.

Biopsy is often performed on patients with orbital inflammatory pseudotumor. Microscopy typically discloses a polymorphous infiltrate of inflammatory cells that may contain lymphocytes, plasma cells, eosinophils, macrophages, and occasionally epithelioid histiocytes (Fig. 13–9). Although vessels ringed or cuffed by chronic inflammation can be seen, it reflects diapedesis of lymphocytes, not true vasculitis. Lymphoid follicles and germinal centers occur in some cases, and fibrosis is often extensive. If the lacrimal gland is involved, its acini are destroyed by the inflammatory process and fibrosis replaces the parenchyma. Fibrosis is particularly marked in the sclerosing type of pseudotumor and is responsible for the typically eosinophilic appearance of specimens under low-magnification light microscopy (Fig. 13–10). This eosinophilia usually distinguishes "pseudotumor" from lymphoid tumors, which are comprised of sheets of basophilic cells. Reactive follicular lymphoid hyperplasia is considered to be an orbital lymphoid tumor by ophthalmic pathologists; it is not called an inflammatory pseudotumor.

If true vasculitis, granulomatous inflammation, and focal necrosis are observed, the patient may have Wegener's granulomatosis. About one-third of patients with Wegener's granulomatosis have ophthalmic manifestations during the course of their disease, and they may present with ocular findings such as orbital infiltration or peripheral corneal ulceration. Clinical suspicion is important because the classic histopathologic features of Wegener's granulomatosis are found in few orbital biopsy specimens (Fig. 13–11). Most patients have concurrent sinus disease. The cytoplasmic anti-neutrophilic cytoplasmic antibody (c-ANCA) test is a helpful diagnostic adjunct but may be negative in the early stages of the disease.

Lacrimal gland biopsy typically discloses discrete noncaseating granulomas composed of epithelioid histiocytes and giant cells in sarcoidosis, which is another diagnosis of exclusion (see Fig. 2–16). Lacrimal gland biopsy occasionally is performed to confirm the diagnosis of sarcoidosis histopathologically.

## ORBITAL TUMORS

A wide variety of benign and malignant primary neoplasms are spawned by the tissues of the orbit. Most of these tumors are relatively rare. Secondary involvement of the orbit by blood-borne metastases, systemic lymphoproliferative disorders, or direct invasion from contiguous structures also occurs. Children and adults are affected by different spectra of orbital tumors.

Primary orbital tumors that are encountered fairly often in adults include cavernous hemangioma, schwannoma, fibrous histiocytoma, hemangiopericytoma, epithelial tumors of the lacrimal gland, and lymphoid tumors. Orbital lymphoid tumors are relatively common. They comprise a spectrum that includes polyclonal reactive lymphoid hyperplasias, cytologically indeterminate atypical lymphoid hyperplasias, and malignant lymphomas comprised of cytologically atypical cells (Figs. 13–12, 13–13, 13–14). Orbital lymphoma is usually a disorder of older patients that is diagnosed on average at age 60 years. The onset of orbital lymphoma is usually insidious. Orbital lymphoid tumors typically present with painless, well tolerated proptosis because the tumor has no fibrous stroma, is soft and pliable, and molds to the globe and other orbital structures. Some patients present with a conjunctival mass or a patch of salmon-colored tissue on the epibulbar surface. The lymphoid infiltrate is often delimited sharply by tissue planes. The latter are evident on imaging studies as linear margins. Lymphomas diffusely infiltrate and thicken the lacrimal gland, which drapes around the globe assuming an appearance that Jakobiec has facetiously termed a "pregnant pancake." The latter contrasts with epithelial neoplasms of the lacrimal gland, which typically are rounded. About 90% of orbital lymphomas involve the superior part of the orbit behind the orbital septum. More than 40% involve the lacrimal gland, usually its palpebral lobe. Bone destruction is rare except in patients with multiple myeloma. When extraocular muscles are involved, usually a single muscle is affected. Motility remains normal because the lymphoma does not stimulate fibrosis.

Macroscopically, lymphoid tumors are soft and friable and tan or salmon-colored (Fig. 13–15). The characteristic salmon hue reflects the presence of many fine capillaries. Ocular lymphomas are extra nodal by definition because the orbit lacks lymphatics and lymph nodes. About two-thirds of ocular adnexal lymphoid tumors are malignant lymphomas comprised of a monoclonal proliferation of B lymphocytes. Most of the lymphomas are low grade lesions composed of well-differentiated lymphocytes (Fig. 13–13). Many are classified as lymphomas of mucosa-associated lymphoid tissue (MALT lymphomas). The remaining orbital lymphoid lesions are polyclonal lymphoid hyperplasias. Knowles and Jakobiec found that approximately one-third of patients who have orbital lymphoid tumors already have, have a history of, or will develop extraocular lymphoma. These authors believe also that classifying ocular lymphoid lesions as benign or malignant histopathologically or as monoclonal or polyclonal immunophenotypically is not a useful predictor of eventual outcome including the occurrence of extraocular lymphoma. In their series, 29% of patients with polyclonal ocular lymphoid proliferations had a history of lymphoma, were found to have concurrent extraocular lymphoma on systemic evaluation, or subsequently developed systemic lymphoma.

Lymphoid tumors of the orbit and ocular adnexa are treated by external beam radiotherapy with appropriate eye shielding if there is no evidence of systemic disease. Chemotherapy should be used if extraocular systemic lymphoma is present; it may be supplemented with adjuvant radiotherapy if ocular regression is subtotal.

Cavernous hemangioma is probably the most common primary orbital neoplasm. This benign vascular tumor typically occurs in middle-aged women. Cavernous hemangiomas cause low-grade proptosis and usually are well tolerated, sparing vision and ocular motility. These benign vascular tumors are well circumscribed, encapsulated lesions that appear dusky-red or purplish blue grossly (Fig. 13–16). They are composed of large, round or oval vascular spaces lined by endothelium separated by thick septa of fibrous tissue that may contain smooth muscle (Figs. 13–17, 13–18). Cavernous hemangiomas show little contrast enhancement on imaging studies because their circulation is relatively stagnant (Fig. 13–19). This feature helps to distinguish them from the much rarer encapsulated vascular tumor hemangiopericytoma, which enhances vividly.

Hemangiopericytoma often has large branching sinusoidal vessels with a "staghorn" configuration that suggests the diagnosis under low magnification (Fig. 13–20). The neoplastic pericytes are enveloped by basement membrane material, which can be demonstrated with the reticulin stain. About 15% of patients with hemangiopericytomas develop distant metastases. Unfortunately, the histologic appearance of the tumor does not always predict metastatic potential; metastatic disease occasionally develops in patients with benign-appearing tumors.

Other vascular lesions that affect the orbit include orbital varices and arteriovenous malformations. Patients with orbital varices often show variable proptosis that depends on the head's position and is increased by the Valsalva maneuver. Histopathology shows a markedly dilated vein that may contain a thrombus (Fig. 13–21). Intravascular papillary endothelial hyperplasia may develop in the thrombosed varix.

Schwannoma or neurilemoma is another well circumscribed orbital tumor. Schwannomas are fairly common neurogenic tumors of adults; they are comprised of a neoplastic proliferation of Schwann cells, the perineural cells that form the myelin sheaths around axons in peripheral nerves. Hence schwannomas usually are associated with a peripheral nerve and may be painful. Microscopy shows an encapsulated spindle cell neoplasm composed of cells with eosinophilic cytoplasm that have indistinct cellular borders and bland elongated oval nuclei. The nuclei are arranged in bands (nuclear palisading) or form structures called Verocay bodies in tumors with the solid histologic Antoni A pattern (Fig. 13–22). The

Antoni B pattern is marked by a loose myxomatous background. Isolated neurofibromas cause diffuse enlargement of the affected nerve and contain axons. They are pseudoencapsulated. Occasionally, schwannomas and neurofibromas are grouped together under the designation peripheral nerve sheath tumor. Schwannomas and isolated neurofibromas are more prevalent in patients who have neurofibromatosis. Malignant peripheral nerve sheath tumors are encountered rarely.

The fibrous histiocytoma is the most common mesenchymal tumor of the orbit in adults. Typically well circumscribed but unencapsulated, fibrous histiocytoma is comprised of spindle cells arranged in a characteristic whirling, pinwheel, or storiform pattern (Fig. 13–23). Benign, locally aggressive, and rare malignant fibrous histiocytomas are recognized. Although benign and locally aggressive fibrous histiocytomas cannot metastasize, they should be totally excised to prevent recurrence. Described in the orbit, solitary fibrous tumor is a spindle cell tumor that shares many features with fibrous histiocytoma (Fig. 13–24). The cells in solitary fibrous tumor are immunoreactive for CD-34 and are arranged in a "patternless pattern."

A variety of rare mesenchymal tumors of fibrous, fibroosseous, smooth muscle, adipose tissue, or cartilaginous derivation occur in the orbit. Other rare primary orbital tumors include endodermal sinus tumor, alveolar soft part sarcoma, granular cell tumor, paraganglioma, primary orbital carcinoid, primary orbital melanoma, retinal anlage tumor, neuroepithelioma, ectomesenchymal tumor, malignant rhabdoid tumor, and primitive neuroectodermal tumor.

Common fibroosseous lesions of the orbital bones include fibrous dysplasia, juvenile psammomatoid ossifying fibroma, and the ivory osteoma. Ivory osteoma is the most common bony lesion in adults. Fibrous dysplasia generally occurs during the first two decades of life, and may spread across suture lines to involve multiple orbital bones. The affected bones have a "ground glass" appearance in CT bone windows (Fig. 13–25). Fibrous dysplasia is composed of irregular trabeculae of immature woven bone surrounded by fibrous stroma (Figs. 13–26, 13–27). The bony trabeculae are not rimmed by osteoblasts and are often shaped like Chinese characters.

Juvenile ossifying fibroma is a more aggressive, expansile lesion that is usually restricted to a single bone. Radiographically it has a sclerotic margin and a less radiodense center. The cellular fibrous stroma of the psammomatoid variant of juvenile ossifying fibroma contains bony spicules that can be confused with psammoma bodies and lead to the misdiagnosis of meningioma (Fig. 13–28).

The orbital bones occasionally are affected by a perplexing group of rare osseous lesions that contain giant cells, including aneurysmal bone cyst, giant cell reparative granuloma, giant cell tumor, the brown tumor of hyperparathyroidism, and eosinophilic granuloma (see below). Osteogenic sarcoma and other soft tissue sarcomas can arise after radiotherapy for retinoblastoma.

## LACRIMAL GLAND

The lacrimal gland is a minor salivary gland that is located in a bony fossa behind the superotemporal orbital rim (Figs. 13–29, 13–30). Lacrimal gland tumors constitute only 10–15% of orbital lesions. Most lacrimal gland lesions encountered in nonreferral clinical practice are inflammatory or lymphoid tumors, which are at least five times more prevalent than primary epithelial tumors. Epithelial neoplasms of the lacrimal gland are rare, but they are important because about half are highly malignant tumors that are potentially lethal.

Granulomatous dacryoadenitis can cause bilateral lacrimal gland enlargement and a characteristic S-shaped lid fissure in patients with sarcoidosis. Keratoconjunctivitis sicca develops in patients with Sjögren syndrome when intense lymphocytic infiltration replaces the parenchyma of the lacrimal gland. Damaged ducts and epimyoepithelial islands persist in the resultant benign lymphoepithelial lesion, and patients are at risk for lymphoma. Cystic dilation of lacrimal gland ducts (dacryops) may simulate a primary lacrimal gland tumor. Concretions, or stones (dacryolithiasis), occasionally form in the ducts of the lacrimal gland.

## EPITHELIAL TUMORS OF THE LACRIMAL GLAND

Compared to other salivary glands, the lacrimal gland gives rise to a relatively limited spectrum of primary epithelial neoplasms. About one-half of epithelial tumors of the lacrimal gland are pleomorphic adenomas or benign mixed tumors, and half are malignant. Lacrimal gland malignancies include adenoid cystic carcinomas, malignant mixed tumors derived from pleomorphic adenomas, and adenocarcinomas that have arisen *de novo*. Mucoepidermoid carcinoma is rare in the lacrimal gland and acinic cell, and Warthin's tumors are almost nonexistent. The lacrimal gland gives rise to a greater proportion of malignant tumors than the parotid gland.

Epithelial tumors of the lacrimal gland typically arise in relatively young individuals whose average age at diagnosis is about 40 years. Several signs and symptoms are important for the clinical evaluation of patients with lacrimal gland tumors: the duration of symptoms, the presence of pain, and the status of the orbital bones on imaging studies. A tumor is probably malignant if it is has been present for less than 6 months, the patient complains of pain, and there is radiographic evidence of bony erosion. Benign pleomorphic adenomas produce a regular, well corticated fossa in the bone, not bone erosion.

Pleomorphic adenoma or benign mixed tumor has a slight male predominance. The patient typically presents with painless proptosis that has been present for a year or more (Fig. 13–31). The eye is displaced inferonasally. Imaging studies disclose a rounded or oval mass that usually involves the gland's orbital lobe. As noted above, the pressure of the slowly enlarging lesion does not destroy bone; rather, it accentuates the lacrimal fossa (Fig. 13–32). Macroscopically, the tumor is well circumscribed and pseudoencapsulated, and its surface is marked by convex bosselations (Fig. 13–33). Sectioning may disclose mucinous or myxomatous areas and hemorrhage. The term *"mixed tumor"* reflects the biphasic mixture of epithelial and mesenchymal elements seen histopathologically (Figs. 13–34, 13–35). The epithelial component includes ducts composed of an inner layer of cuboidal or columnar cells and an outer layer of flattened or spindled myoepithelial cells. The myoepithelial cells typically spindle-off into the stroma, where they may maintain a spindled configuration or undergo metaplasia, forming the mesenchymal part of the tumor that includes myxoid tissue, cartilage, or rarely fat or bone. Electron microscopic studies suggest that pleomorphic adenomas probably are derived from the duct cells of the lacrimal gland.

If pleomorphic adenoma of the lacrimal gland is suspected clinically, the tumor should be totally excised within an intact capsule. Benign mixed tumors should never be biopsied. An orbital recurrence develops in about one-third of patients after incisional biopsy is performed. Recurrent benign mixed tumor can infiltrate orbital soft tissues and even bone and brain, and the recurrences also are prone to malignant degeneration. The rates of malignant degeneration in recurrent benign mixed tumor are 10% and 20% at 20 and 30 years, respectively.

Adenoid cystic carcinoma (Fig. 13–36, 13–37, 13–38, 13–39) is the second most common epithelial neoplasm of the lacrimal gland, constituting 25–30%

of cases. About 60% of cases occur in women. Although the average age at presentation is 40 years, adenoid cystic carcinoma has a biphasic age distribution, and tumors occasionally develop in children. Patients with adenoid cystic carcinoma typically have had symptoms for a relatively short time. The tumor has a propensity for perineural invasion (Fig. 13–36) and can present with pain or numbness, blepharoptosis, and ocular motility deficits. Unfortunately, it may have already extended out of the orbit via nerves before becoming symptomatic.

Adenoid cystic carcinoma tends to be rounded or globular in imaging studies, like pleomorphic adenoma; but the margin of the tumor is often irregular or serrated and it may extend into the medial or posterior orbit (Fig. 13–37). Bone destruction is seen in 80% of cases. Five histologic patterns of adenoid cystic carcinoma are recognized: the cribriform ("Swiss cheese") pattern, the basaloid (solid) pattern, a sclerosing pattern, a tubular pattern with true duct formation, and a comedocarcinoma pattern marked by tumor lobules with central necrosis. A thick basement membrane surrounds the epithelial elements in the cylindromatous variant. The cribriform pattern is characterized by smoothly rounded biomorphic sheets of deceptively bland appearing basaloid cells that contain round pools of mucin that mimic glands (Fig. 13–38). The term adenoid means "gland-like."

The prognosis of adenoid cystic carcinoma of the lacrimal gland is dismal; only 20% of patients survive 10 years. Many fatal tumors invade the middle cranial fossa through the superior orbital fissure. Late pulmonary metastases also occur. Survival correlates with tumor histology; the poorly differentiated basaloid pattern is particularly ominous (Fig. 13–39). If foci of basaloid tumor are found, the 5-year survival is 21% and the median survival 3 years. If no basaloid tumor is found, the 5-year survival increases to 71% and the median survival to 8 years.

The management of adenoid cystic carcinoma of the

lacrimal gland is controversial. An incisional biopsy is performed if the diagnosis is suspected on clinical grounds. Orbital exenteration is performed after the diagnosis is confirmed by a review of permanent sections. The decision to perform a mutilating operation such as orbital exenteration should never be based on frozen section diagnosis. Some authorities recommend *en bloc* resection of the tumor and contiguous bone or radical orbitectomy including the roof and lateral walls of the orbit.

Malignant mixed tumor (pleomorphic adenocarcinoma) usually results from the malignant transformation of benign mixed tumor (Fig. 13–40). Patients with malignant mixed tumors generally are older than patients who have benign mixed tumors. In most cases, the tumor contains a clone of poorly differentiated adenocarcinoma that may show squamous, acinar, or sebaceous differentiation. Patients usually succumb within 3 years with lung and lymphatic node metastases. The prognosis of adenocarcinoma *de novo* is equally poor. Most of these poorly differentiated tumors occur in older men.

Mucoepidermoid carcinoma of the lacrimal gland has a better prognosis than other epithelial malignancies but is rare. Histopathologically, the tumor contains paving stone-like squamous elements and mucus-secreting goblet cells (Fig. 13–41). Treatment includes exenteration or wide local excision.

## SECONDARY ORBITAL TUMORS

Secondary orbital neoplasms in adults include metastases from distant primary tumors and tumors that have invaded the orbit from contiguous structures. Breast carcinoma metastasizes to the orbit most frequently, constituting 42% of 195 orbital metastases in a combined series (Fig. 13–42). Other common sources of orbital metastases are lung (12.8%), prostate (6.7%), and gastrointestinal (4.1%) carcinomas. The primary tumor was unknown in 11.3% of cases.

Tumors that directly invade the orbit include basal cell, squamous cell, and sebaceous gland carcinomas and malignant melanomas of the eyelid, and squamous cell and mucoepidermoid carcinomas and malignant melanomas of the conjunctiva. Secondary orbital tumors also result from the extraocular extension of intraocular tumors, most notably retinoblastoma and uveal melanoma. In underdeveloped countries, retinoblastoma frequently presents as an orbital tumor that requires exenteration (see Fig. 11–4). Sinus carcinomas and lacrimal sac tumors can also invade the orbit. Benign cystic lesions lined by respiratory epithelium called mucoceles occasionally erode through orbital bones and impinge on the orbital contents (Fig. 13–43). Most occur in patients who have chronic sinusitis. Secondary orbital invasion by intracranial meningioma is more common than primary optic nerve meningioma.

## PEDIATRIC ORBITAL TUMORS

Congenital teratomas of the orbit may present at birth with hideously deforming proptosis (Fig. 13–44). The dermoid cyst or cystic dermoid is the most common orbital lesion found in infants and children. Caused by entrapment of surface ectoderm in bony sutures during development, these choristomatous lesions typically are located in the superotemporal quadrant. Cystic dermoids resemble epidermal inclusion cysts histopathologically, but the keratinized stratified squamous epithelial lining also has epidermal appendages such as pilosebaceous units and sweat glands (Fig. 13–45). Hairs are often found mixed with cheesy, keratinous material filling the lumen (Fig. 13–46). Polarization microscopy helps highlight the hair shafts during examination. The epithelial lining of a dermoid cyst may be partially replaced by a layer of foreign body giant cells. A rare variant of dermoid cyst, termed a "conjunctivoid," occasionally is found in the nasal orbit. These unusual dermoids are lined by nonkeratinized epithelium with goblet cells that resembles conjunctiva, but they have epidermal appendages.

Capillary hemangiomas (hemangioma of infancy) and lymphangiomas are the most common vascular tumors of the orbit in children. Involvement of eyelid skin by a capillary hemangioma is readily apparent as a bright red strawberry nevus. Infantile hemangiomas confined to the orbit are more subtle and may present with proptosis and bluish discoloration of the skin. Poorly circumscribed and unencapsulated, these benign vascular tumors are composed of lobules of capillary-caliber vessels or sheets of capillary endothelial cells (Fig. 13–47). The hemangiomas in young infants tend to be quite cellular; capillary lumens appear and enlarge as the lesions mature. Although infantile hemangiomas eventually involute spontaneously, they may be a major cosmetic blemish and often produce potentially reversible visual loss (amblyopia) by causing corneal astigmatism or by occluding the pupil. Nonsurgical therapy includes intralesional injection of steroids and interferon alpha-2a.

Lymphangiomas are poorly circumscribed choristomatous lesions composed of large endothelial-lined channels filled with lymph or serosanguineous fluid (Fig. 13–48). Focal lymphoid infiltrates in the contiguous stroma, which may contain germinal centers, serve to differentiate lymphangioma from cavernous hemangioma, particularly in cases where there has been secondary hemorrhage into the lymphatic vessels. Acute enlargement of lymphangioma is often caused by intralesional hemorrhage, which can produce a blood-filled "chocolate cyst" (Fig. 13–49). Lymphangiomas also may enlarge during upper respiratory infections, presumably because their lymphoid component undergoes hyperplasia. Lymphangiomas are usually quite infiltrative in their growth pattern, and they do not undergo spontaneous involution. Surgical removal may be difficult.

Childhood neural tumors include plexiform neurofibroma found in von Recklinghausen's neurofibromatosis type I and juvenile pilocytic astrocytoma (optic nerve gliomas), which also complicates neurofibromatosis. Plexiform neurofibroma feels like a "bag of worms" when palpated because the malformation is composed of an interweaving plexus of nerves that are markedly enlarged by a proliferation of Schwann cells and mucoid material (see Fig. 1–14). The upper eyelid fissure often has an S configuration on the side of the plexiform neurofibroma.

Rhabdomyosarcoma is the most common malignant orbital tumor of childhood. The tumor presents on average at age 7 and is more common in boys. The possibility of rhabdomyosarcoma should be considered in any child with orbital disease. Orbital rhabdomyosarcoma often grows rapidly and can cause fulminant proptosis. Occasionally, progression is so rapid the tumor is confused with inflammatory disease. Orbital rhabdomyosarcoma affects the superior orbit most commonly and may appear deceptively well circumscribed on imaging studies. About 60% of cases erode through the ethmoidal lamina papyracea in the medial orbital wall. Infrequently, rhabdomyosarcoma arises in the paranasal sinuses and invades the orbit secondarily. Macroscopically, fresh tumor usually is yellow or flesh-colored and may be focally hemorrhagic.

Histologically, rhabdomyosarcoma is nonencapsulated, and its growth pattern is usually infiltrative, although "pushing" margins occasionally are encountered. Several histologic variants of orbital rhabdomyosarcoma are recognized. Most orbital tumors are embryonal rhabdomyosarcomas, which are poorly differentiated neoplasms comprised of spindle and strap cells arranged haphazardly in a loose, myxomatous stroma (Fig. 13–50). Cross striations (Fig. 13–51) are found in fewer than 60% of cases; but rhabdomyoblasts, which appear as globoid cells with abundant eosinophilic cytoplasm, may be present. Immunohistochemistry is used to confirm the diagnosis in most cases (see below). In some instances, special studies including immunohistochemistry or electron microscopy fail to reveal evidence of striated muscle differentiation. Such tumors are called embryonal sarcomas. Botryoid rhabdomyosarcoma is a variant of embryonal rhabdomyosarcoma that is associated with a mucous membrane such as the conjunctiva. Botryoid rhabdomyosarcomas have a multinodular grape-like appearance clinically. Alveolar rhabdomyosarcoma is less common, tends to arise in the inferior orbit, has a characteristic chromosomal translocation [t(2;13)], and tends to have a poorer prognosis. The tumor cells in alveolar rhabdomyosarcoma are enclosed by fibrous tissue septa that resemble alveoli in the lungs (Fig. 13–52). The large polygonal tumor cells have abundant eosinophilic cytoplasm. Pleomorphic or differentiated rhabdomyosarcomas are rare in the orbit and occur in adults.

Orbital rhabdomyosarcomas probably arise from pluripotential mesenchymal cells and are not derived from the dedifferentiation of an extraocular muscle. The diagnosis can be rapidly confirmed by immunohistochemistry, which shows the presence of muscle markers such as muscle specific actin or desmin (Fig. 13–53). Diagnostic transmission electron microscopy can also disclose sarcomeric units and 150 Å myosin filaments. After orbital rhabdomyosarcoma is diagnosed by expedient biopsy, the tumor usually is treated with a combination of radiation and adjuvant chemotherapy. Orbital exenteration is rarely necessary. The survival rate is relatively good (80%) if the tumor has not invaded the paranasal sinuses.

Lymphomas are rare during childhood. If an apparent "lymphoma" is encountered in the orbit of a child, an infiltrate of leukemic cells called a granulocytic or myeloid sarcoma must be excluded. The Leder esterase stain is commonly used to confirm granulocytic differentiation (Fig. 13–54). In the past, granulocytic sarcomas were called chloromas, reflecting a greenish hue caused by myeloperoxidase in some tumors. Infiltration of the orbital tissues by leukemic cells may antedate peripheral leukemia or even bone marrow involvement by several months.

Sinus histiocytosis with massive lymphadenopathy (Rosai-Dorfman disease) can involve the orbit. The histiocytes are S-100 protein-positive and show emperipolesis.

Orbital involvement can occur in Langerhans' cell histiocytosis (histiocytosis X), especially the eosinophilic granuloma variant, which typically causes a cystic or erosive lesion in the superotemporal orbital bone. Biopsy shows a mixture of histiocytes with folded nuclei, eosinophils, and small round osteoclast-like giant cells (Fig. 13–55). The histiocytes stain positively for S-100 protein, and electron microscopy shows racket-shaped Birbeck granules in their cytoplasm.

Most orbital metastases in children stem from neuroblastoma or Ewing's sarcoma. Metastatic orbital neuroblastoma occurs in the late stages of the disease in children known to have the tumor. Metastases from neuroblastoma are often hemorrhagic and cause periocular ecchymoses, an appearance termed "raccoon eyes."

# References

## General References

Henderson JW, in collaboration with Campbell RJ, Farrow GM, Garrity JA: Orbital Tumors. 3rd ed. New York: Raven Press, 1994.

Jakobiec FA, Bilyk JR, Font RL: Orbit. In Spencer W (ed) Ophthalmic Pathology: An Atlas and Textbook. 4th ed. Vol 2. Philadelphia: Saunders, 1996:2438–2933.

Rootman J: Diseases of the Orbit. Philadelphia: Lippincott, 1988.

Shields JA: Diagnosis and Management of Orbital Tumors. Philadelphia: Saunders, 1989.

## Orbital Cellulitis

Hornblass A, Herschorn BJ, Stern K, Grimes C: Orbital abscess. Surv Ophthalmol 29:169–179, 1984.

Macy HI, Mandelbaum SH, Minckler DA: Orbital cellulitis. Ophthalmology 87:1309–1314, 1980.

Shields JA, Shields CL, Suvarnamani C, et al: Retinoblastoma manifesting as orbital cellulitis. Am J Ophthalmol 112:442–449, 1991.

Watters EC, Wallar PH, Hiles DA, Michaels RH: Acute orbital cellulitis. Arch Ophthalmol 94:785–788, 1976.

Weiss A, Friendly D, Eglin K, et al: Bacterial periorbital and orbital cellulitis in childhood. Ophthalmology 90:195–203, 1983.

## Fungal Infection

Chang WJ, Shields CL, Shields JA, et al: Bilateral orbital involvement with massive allergic fungal sinusitis [letter]. Arch Ophthalmol 114:767–768, 1996.

DeJuan E, Green WR, Iliff NT: Allergic periorbital mucopyocele in children. Am J Ophthalmol 96:299–303, 1983.

Ferry AP, Abedi S: Diagnosis and management of rhino-orbitocerebral mucormycosis (phycomycosis). Ophthalmology 90:1096–1104, 1983.

Green WR, Font RL, Zimmerman LE: Aspergillosis of the orbit: report of ten cases and review of the literature. Arch Ophthalmol 82:302–312, 1969.

Houle T, Ellis P: Aspergillosis of the orbit with immunosuppressive therapy. Surv Ophthalmol 20:35–41, 1975.

Klapper SR, Lee AG, Patrinely JR, et al: Orbital involvement in allergic fungal sinusitis. Ophthalmology 104:2094–2100, 1997.

Yohai RA, Bullock JD, Aziz AA, Markert RJ: Survival factors in rhino-orbital-cerebral mucormycosis [review]. Surv Ophthalmol 39:3–22, 1994.

## Thyroid Ophthalmology

Char DH: The ophthalmopathy of Graves' disease. Med Clin North Am 70:97–119, 1991.

Heufelder AE: Involvement of the orbital fibroblast and TSH receptor in the pathogenesis of Graves' ophthalmopathy. Thyroid 5:331–340, 1995.

Hufnagel TJ, Hickey WF, Cobbs WH, et al: Immunohistochemical and ultrastructural studies on the exenterated orbital tissues of a patient with Graves' disease. Ophthalmology 91:1411–1419, 1984.

Netland PA, Dallow RL: Thyroid ophthalmology. In Albert DM, Jakobiec FA (eds) Principles and Practice of Ophthalmology: Clinical Practice. Vol 5. Philadelphia: Saunders, 1994:2937–2955.

Van der Gaag R, Vernimmen R, Fiebelkorn N, et al: Graves' ophthalmopathy: what is the evidence for extraocular muscle specific autoantibodies. Int Ophthalmol 14:25–30, 1990.

Wall JR, Bernard N, Boucher A, et al: Pathogenesis of thyroid-associated ophthalmopathy: an autoimmune disorder of the eye muscle associated with Graves' hyperthyroidism and Hashimoto's thyroiditis. Clin Immunol Immunopathol 68:1–8, 1993.

Werner WC. Modification of the classification of the eye changes of Graves' disease. Am J Ophthalmol 83: 725–727, 1977.

## Idiopathic Orbital Inflammation (Pseudotumor)

Abramovitz JN, Kasdon DL, Satala F, et al: Sclerosing orbital pseudotumor. Neurosurgery 12:463–468, 1983.

Chavis RM, Garner A, Wright JE: Inflammatory orbital pseudotumor: a clinicopathologic study. Arch Ophthalmol 96:1817–1822, 1978.

Hara Y, Ohnishi Y: Orbital inflammatory pseudotumor: clinicopathologic study of 22 cases. Jpn J Ophthalmol 27:80–89, 1983.

Kennerdell JS, Dresner SC: The nonspecific orbital inflammatory syndromes. Surv Ophthalmol 29:93–103, 1984.

Mombaerts I, Goldschmeding R, Schlingemann RO, Koornneef L: What is orbital pseudotumor? Surv Ophthalmol 41:66–78, 1996.

Mottow-Lippa L, Jakobiec FA: Idiopathic inflammatory orbital pseudotumor in childhood. Arch Ophthalmol 96:1410–1417, 1978.

Rootman J, McCarthy M, White V, Harris G, Kennerdell J. Idiopathic sclerosing inflammation of the orbit: a distinct clinicopathologic entity. Ophthalmology 101:570–584, 1994.

## Wegener's Granulomatosis

Bullen CL, Liesegang TJ, McDonald TJ: Ocular complications of Wegener's granulomatosis. Ophthalmology 90:279–290, 1983.

Kalina PH, Lie JT, Campbell RJ, Garrity JA: Diagnostic value and limitations of orbital biopsy in Wegener's granulomatosis. Ophthalmology 99:120–124, 1994.

Koyama T, Matsuo N, Watanabe Y, et al: Wegener's granulomatosis with destructive ocular manifestations. Am J Ophthalmol 98:736–740, 1984.

Perry SR, Rootman J, White VA: The clinical and pathologic constellation of Wegener granulomatosis of the orbit. Ophthalmology 104:683–694, 1997.

Trocme SD, Bartley GB, Campbell RJ, et al. Eosinophil and neutrophil degranulation in ophthalmic lesions of Wegener's granulomatosis. Arch Ophthalmol 109:1585–1589, 1991.

## Lymphoid Tumors

Adkins JW, Shields JA, Shields CL, Eagle RC Jr, Flanagan JC, Campanella PC: Plasmacytoma of the eye and orbit. Int Ophthalmol 20:339–343, 1996.

Eichler MD, Fraunfelder FT: Lymphoid tumors (inflammatory pseudotumor, malignant lymphoma, neoplastic angioendotheliomatosis, pseudolymphoma, pseudotumor, reactive lymphoid hyperplasia). In Fraunfelder FT, Roy FH (eds) Current Ocular Therapy 4, Philadelphia: Saunders, 1995:342–346.

Hidayat AA, Cameron JD, Font RL, et al: Angiolymphoid hyperplasia with eosinophilia (Kimura's disease) of the orbit and ocular adnexa. Am J Ophthalmol 96:176–189, 1983.

Knowles DM, Jakobiec FA, McNally L, Burke JS: Lymphoid hyperplasia and malignant lymphoma occurring in the ocular adnexa (orbit, conjunctiva, and eyelids): a prospective multiparametric analysis of 108 cases during 1977 to 1987. Hum Pathol 21:959–973, 1990.

Margo CE: Orbital and ocular adnexal lymphoma: evolving concepts. Ophthalmol Clin North Am 8:167–177, 1995.

Medeiros LJ, Harris NL: Immunohistologic analysis of small lymphocytic infiltrates of the orbit and conjunctiva. Hum Pathol 21:1126–1131, 1990.

White WL, Ferry JA, Harris NL, Grove AS Jr: Ocular adnexal lymphoma: a clinicopathologic study with identification of lymphomas of mucosa-associated lymphoid tissue type. Ophthalmology 102:1994–2006, 1995.

## Vascular Tumors

Croxatto JO, Font RL: Hemangiopericytoma of the orbit: a clinicopathologic study of 30 cases. Hum Pathol 13:210–218, 1982.

Harris GJ, Jakobiec FA: Cavernous hemangioma of the orbit: an analysis of 66 cases. J Neurosurg 51:219–228, 1979.

Henderson JW, Farrow GM: Primary orbital hemangiopericytoma: an aggressive and potentially malignant neoplasm. Arch Ophthalmol 96:666–673, 1978.

Iwamoto T, Jakobiec FA: Ultrastructural comparison of capillary and cavernous hemangiomas of the orbit. Arch Ophthalmol 97:1144–1153, 1979.

Ruchman MC, Flanagan J: Cavernous hemangiomas of the orbit. Ophthalmology 90:1328–1336, 1983.

## Neural Tumors

Blodi FC: Amputation neuroma in the orbit. Am J Ophthalmol 32:929–932, 1949.

Coleman DJ, Jack RL, Franzen LA: Neurogenic tumors of the orbit. Arch Ophthalmol 88:380–384, 1972.

Krohel GB, Rosenberg MD, Wright JE Jr, Smith RS: Localized orbital neurofibromas. Am J Ophthalmol 100:458–464, 1985.

Rootman J, Goldberg C, Robertson W: Primary orbital schwannomas. Br J Ophthalmol 66:194–204, 1982.

## Mesenchymal Tumors

Bartley GB, Yeatts RP, Garrity JA, et al: Spindle cell lipoma of the orbit. Am J Ophthalmol 100:605–609, 1985.

Dorfman DM, To K, Dickersin GR, et al: Solitary fibrous tumor of the orbit. Am J Surg Pathol 18:281–287, 1994.

Folberg R, Cleasby G, Flanagan JA, et al: Orbital leiomyosarcoma after radiation therapy for bilateral retinoblastoma. Arch Ophthalmol 101:1562–1565, 1983.

Font RL, Hidayat AA: Fibrous histiocytoma of the orbit: a clinicopathologic study of 150 cases. Hum Pathol 13:199–209, 1982.

Font RL, Jurco S III, Brechner RJ: Postradiation leiomyosarcoma of the orbit complicating bilateral retinoblastoma. Arch Ophthalmol 101:1557–1561, 1983.

Guccion J, Font RL, Enzinger FM, et al: Extraskeletal mesenchymal chondrosarcoma. Arch Pathol 95:336–340, 1973.

Hidayat AA, Font RL: Juvenile fibromatosis of the periorbital region and eyelid: a clinicopathologic study of six cases. Arch Ophthalmol 98:280–285, 1980.

Holland MG, Allen JH, Ichinose H: Chondrosarcoma of the orbit. Trans Am Acad Ophthalmol Otolaryngol 65:898–905, 1961.

Jakobiec FA, Rini F, Char D, et al: Primary liposarcoma of the orbit: problems in the diagnosis and management of five cases. Ophthalmology 96:180–191, 1989.

Sanborn GE, Valenzuela RE, Green WR: Leiomyoma of the orbit. Am J Ophthalmol 87:371–375, 1979.

Weiner JM, Hidayat AA: Juvenile fibrosarcoma of the orbit and eyelid. Arch Ophthalmol 101:253–259, 1983.

## Rare Orbital Tumors

Font RL, Jurco S III, Zimmerman LE: Alveolar soft-part sarcoma of the orbit. Hum Pathol 13:569–579, 1982.

Goldstein BG, Font RL, Alper MG: Granular cell tumor of the orbit: a case report including electron microscopic observation. Ann Ophthalmol 14:231–238, 1982.

Gunduz K, Shields JA, Eagle RC Jr, Shields CL, De Potter P, Klombers L: Malignant rhabdoid tumor of the orbit. Arch Ophthalmol 116:243–246, 1998.

Jakobiec FA, Ellsworth R, Tannenbaum M: Primary orbital melanoma. Am J Ophthalmol 78:24–39, 1974.

Lamping KA, Albert DM, Lack E, et al: Melanotic neuroectodermal tumor of infancy (retinal anlage tumor). Ophthalmology 92:143–147, 1985.

Margo CE, Folberg R, Zimmerman LE, Sesterhenn IA: Endodermal sinus tumor (yolk sac tumor) of the orbit. Ophthalmology 90:1426–1432, 1983.

Rootman J, DamJi KF, Dimmick JE. Malignant rhabdoid tumor of the orbit. Ophthalmology 96:1650–1604, 1989.

Tellada M, Specht CS, McLean IW, Grossniklaus HE, Zimmerman LE: Primary orbital melanomas. Ophthalmology 103:929–932, 1996.

Zimmerman LE, Stangl R, Riddle PJ: Primary carcinoid tumor of the orbit. Arch Ophthalmol 101:1395–1398, 1983.

**Osseous and Fibroosseous Lesions**

Blodi FC: Pathology of orbital bones. Am J Ophthalmol 81: 1–26, 1976.

Fu YS, Perzin KH: Non-epithelial tumors of the nasal cavity, paranasal sinuses, and nasopharynx: a clinicopathological study. II. Osseous and fibro-osseous lesions, including osteoma, fibrous dysplasia, ossifying fibroma, osteoblastoma, giant cell tumor and osteosarcoma. Cancer 33: 1289–1305, 1974.

Hoopes PC, Anderson RL, Blodi FC: Giant cell (reparative) granuloma of the orbit. Ophthalmology 88:1361–1366, 1981.

Klepach GL, Ho REM, Kelly JK: Aneurysmal bone cyst of the orbit. J Clin Neuro Ophthalmol 4:49–52, 1984.

Margo CE, Ragsdale B, Purman K, et al: Psammomatoid (juvenile) ossifying fibroma of the orbit. Ophthalmology 92: 150–159, 1985.

Moore AT, Buncic R: Fibrous dysplasia of the orbit in childhood: clinical features and management. Ophthalmology 92:12–20, 1985.

Naiman J, Green WR, D'Heurle D, et al: Brown tumor of the orbit associated with primary hyperparathyroidism. Am J Ophthalmol 90:565–571, 1980.

Spraul CW, Wojno TH, Grossniklaus HE, Lang GK: Reparative giant cell granuloma with orbital involvement. Klin Monatsbl Augenheilkd 211:133–134, 1997.

**Lacrimal Gland Tumors**

Biggs SL, Font RL: Oncocytic lesions of the lacrimal gland. Arch Ophthalmol 95:474–478, 1977.

Bonavolonta G, Tranfa F, Staibano S, Di Matteo G, Orabona P, De Rosa G: Warthin tumor of the lacrimal gland. Am J Ophthalmol 124:857–858, 1997.

Brownstein S, Belin MW, Krohel GB, et al: Orbital dacryops. Ophthalmology 91:1424–1428, 1984.

Cunningham RD: Lacrimal gland tumors. In Fraunfelder FT, Roy FH (eds) Current Ocular Therapy 4. Philadelphia: Saunders, 1995:693–695.

Font RL, Gamel JW: Adenoid cystic carcinoma of the lacrimal gland: a clinicopathological study of 79 cases. In Nicholson DH (ed) Ocular Pathology Update. New York: Masson, 1980:277–283.

Font RL, Gamel JW: Epithelial tumors of the lacrimal gland: an analysis of 256 cases. In Jakobiec FA (ed) Ocular and Adnexal Tumors. Birmingham, AL: Aesculapius, 1978: 787–805.

Font RL, Yanoff M, Zimmerman LE: Benign lymphoepithelial lesion of the lacrimal gland and its relationship to Sjogren's syndrome. Am J Clin Pathol 48:365–376, 1967.

Gamel JW, Font RL: Adenoid cystic carcinoma of the lacrimal gland: the clinical significance of a basaloid histologic pattern. Hum Pathol 13:219–225, 1982.

Grossniklaus HE, Wojno TH, Wilson MW, Someren AO: Myoepithelioma of the lacrimal gland. Arch Ophthalmol 115:1588–1590, 1997.

Iwamota T, Jakobiec FA: A comparative ultrastructural study of the normal lacrimal gland and its epithelial tumors. Hum Pathol 13:236–262, 1982.

Lee DA, Campbell RJ, Waller RR, Ilstrup DM: A clinicopathologic study of primary adenoid cystic carcinoma of the lacrimal gland. Ophthalmology 92:128–134, 1985.

Malhotra GS, Paul SD, Batra DV: Mucoepidermoid carcinoma of the lacrimal gland. Ophthalmologica 153: 184–190, 1967.

Perzin K, Jakobiec FA, LiVolsi V, DesJardins L: Malignant mixed tumors of the lacrimal gland. Cancer 45:2593–606, 1980.

Rose GE, Wright JE: Pleomorphic adenoma of the lacrimal gland. Br J Ophthalmol 76:395–400, 1992.

Rosenbaum PS, Mahadevia PS, Goodman LA, Kress Y: Acinic cell carcinoma of the lacrimal gland. Arch Ophthalmol 113:781–785, 1995.

Shields CL, Shields JA, Eagle RC, Rathmell JP: Clinicopathologic review of 142 cases of lacrimal gland lesions. Ophthalmology 96:431–435, 1989.

Shields JA, Shields CL, Eagle RC Jr, Adkins J, De Potter P: Adenoid cystic carcinoma developing in the nasal orbit. Am J Ophthalmol 123:398–399, 1997.

Tellado MV, McLean IW, Specht CS, Varga J: Adenoid cystic carcinomas of the lacrimal gland in childhood and adolescence. Ophthalmology 104:1622–1625, 1997.

Wagoner MD, Chuo N, Gonder JR: Mucoepidermoid carcinoma of the lacrimal gland. Ann Ophthalmol 14:383–386, 1982.

Wright JE, Rose GE, Garner A: Primary malignant neoplasms of the lacrimal gland. Br J Ophthalmol 76: 401–407, 1992.

**Orbital Metastasis**

Cline RA, Rootman J: Enophthalmos: a clinical review. Ophthalmology 91:229–237, 1984.

Font RL, Ferry AP: Carcinoma metastatic to the eye and orbit. III. A clinicopathologic study of 28 cases metastatic to the orbit. Cancer 38:1326–1335, 1976.

Goldberg RA, Rootman J, Cline RA: Tumors metastatic to the orbit: a changing picture. Surv Ophthalmol 35:1–24, 1990.

Shields CL, Shields JA, Peggs M: Tumors metastatic to the orbit. Ophthalmic Plast Reconstructr Surg 4:73–80, 1988.

Volpe NJ, Albert DM: Metastatic and secondary orbital tumors. *In* Albert DM, Jakobiec FA (eds) Philadelphia: Saunders, 1994:2027–2050.

**Mucocele**

Alberti PWRM, Marshall HF, Black HIM: Frontoethmoidal mucocoele as a cause of unilateral proptosis. Br J Ophthalmol 52:833–838, 1968.

Avery G, Tang RA, Close LG: Ophthalmic manifestations of mucoceles. Ann Ophthalmol 15:734–737, 1983.

Iliff CE: Mucoceles in the orbit. Arch Ophthalmol 89: 392–395, 1973.

**Dermoid Cysts**

Emerick GT, Shields CL, Shields JA, Eagle RC Jr, De Potter P, Markowitz GI: Chewing-induced visual impairment from a dumbbell dermoid cyst. Ophthal Plast Reconstr Surg 13:57–61, 1997.

Jakobiec FA, Bonanno PA: Conjunctival adnexal cysts and dermoids. Arch Ophthalmol 96:1040–1049, 1978.

Shields JA, Kaden IH, Eagle RC Jr, Shields CL: Orbital dermoid cysts: clinicopathologic correlations, classification and management: the 1997 Josephine E. Schueler lecture. Ophthal Plast Reconstr Surg 13:265–276, 1997.

**Pediatric Orbital Tumors**

Ellis FJ, Eagle RC Jr, Shields JA: Phakomatous choristoma (Zimmerman's tumor): immunohistochemical confirmation of lens-specific proteins. Ophthalmology 100: 955–960, 1993.

Ferry AP, Font AP: The phakomatoses. Int Ophthalmol Clin 12:1–50, 1972.

Haik BG, Karcioglu ZA, Gordon RA, Pechous BP: Capillary hemangioma (infantile periocular hemangioma). Surv Ophthalmol 38:399–426, 1994.

Illif WJ, Green WR: Orbital lymphangiomas. Ophthalmology 86:914–929, 1979.

Illif WJ, Green WR: Orbital tumors in children. In Jakobiec FA (ed) Ocular and Adnexal Tumors. Birmingham, AL: Aesculapius, 1978:669–684.

Kivela T, Tarkkanen A: Orbital germ cell tumors revisted: a clinicopathological approach to classification. Surv Ophthalmol 38:541–554, 1994.

Kobrin JL, Blodi FC, Weingeist TA: Ocular and orbital manifestations of neurofibromatosis. Surv Ophthalmol 24:45–51, 1979.

Shields JA, Bakewell B, Augsburger JJ, et al: Space-occupying orbital masses in children: a review of 250 consecutive biopsies. Ophthalmology 93:379–384, 1986.

Woog JJ, Albert DM, Solt LC, et al: Neurofibromatosis of the eyeball and orbit. Int Ophthalmol Clin 22:157–187, 1982.

**Rhabdomyosarcoma**

Abramson DH, Ellsworth RM, Tretter P, et al: The treatment of orbital rhabdomyosarcoma with irradiation and chemotherapy. Ophthalmology 86:1330–1335, 1979.

Ashton N: Embryonal sarcoma and embryonal rhabdomyosarcoma of the orbit. J Clin Pathol 18:699–714, 1965.

Crist W, Gehan EA, Ragab AH, et al: The Intergroup Rhabdomyosarcoma Study III. J Clin Oncol 23:610–630, 1995.

Jakobiec FA, Font RL: Ocular and orbital tumors. In Johanessen JV (ed) The Nervous System, Sensory Organs and Respiratory Tract. Electron Microscopy in Human Diseases. Vol VI. New York: McGraw-Hill, 1979:346–368.

Knowles DM II, Jakobiec FA, Potter G, Jones IS: Ophthalmic striated muscle neoplasms. Surv Ophthalmol 21:219–261, 1976.

Newton WA, Soule EH, Hamoudi AB, et al: Histopathology of childhood sarcomas, intergroup rhabdomyosarcoma studies I and II: clinicopathologic correlation. J Clin Oncol 6:67–75, 1988.

Porterfield JF, Zimmerman LE: Rhabdomyosarcoma of the orbit: a clinicopathologic study of 55 cases. Virchows Arch [A] 335:329–344, 1962.

**Leukemic and Histiocytic Disorders**

Davis JL, Parke DW II, Font RL: Granulocytic sarcoma of the orbit: a clinicopathologic study. Ophthalmology 92:1758–1762, 1985.

Feldman RB, Moore DM, Hood CI, et al: Solitary eosinophilic granuloma of the lateral orbital wall. Am J Ophthalmol 100:318–323, 1985.

Foucar E, Rosai J, Dorfman RF: The ophthalmologic manifestations of sinus histiocytosis with massive lymphadenopathy. Am J Ophthalmol 87:354–367, 1979.

Friendly DS, Font RL, Rao NA: Orbital involvement in "sinus" histiocytosis: a report of four cases. Arch Ophthalmol 95:2006–2011, 1977.

Kincaid MC, Green WR: Ocular and orbital involvement in leukemia. Surv Ophthalmol 27:211–232, 1983.

Kramer TR, Noecker RJ, Miller JM, Clark LC: Langerhans cell histiocytosis with orbital involvement. Am J Ophthalmol 124:814–824, 1997.

Willman CL, Busque L, Griffith BB, et al: Langerhans'-cell histiocytosis (histiocytosis X)—a clonal proliferative disease. N Engl J Med 331:191–193, 1994.

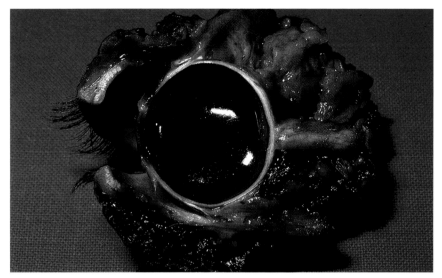

FIGURE 13–1 • **Orbital contents.** The orbital contents include the eye, optic nerve, smooth and striated muscle, vessels, nerves, fatty and fibrous connective tissue, and the lacrimal gland. They are delimited anteriorly by a fibrous tissue septum and protected by the eyelids.

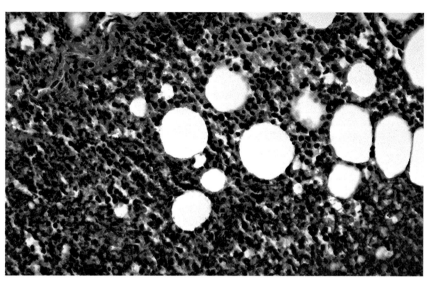

FIGURE 13–2 • **Orbital abscess.** An abscess is a focal collection of polymorphonuclear leukocytes. The polys infiltrating the orbital fat are in various stages of degeneration. Basophilia reflects necrosis. Hematoxylin-eosin, ×100.

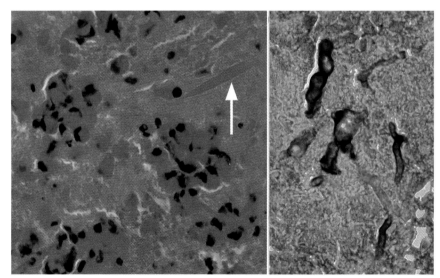

FIGURE 13–3 • **Allergic fungal sinusitis.** Allergic mucin contains clumps of eosinophils and Charcot-Leyden crystals (arrow). *Inset:* Noninvasive hyphae stained with GMS fungal stain. Main figure: hematoxylin-eosin, ×250; inset: Gomori methenamine silver, ×250.

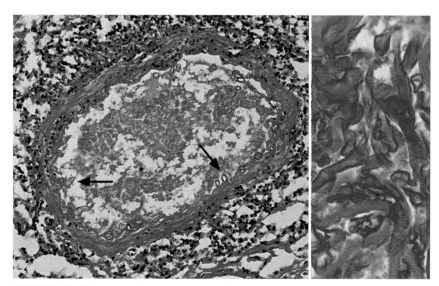

FIGURE 13–4 • **Mucormycosis.** Arrows denote fungal hyphae infiltrating wall of thrombosed vessel. Large branching nonseptate hyphae (*inset*) are readily seen in routine H&E-stained sections. Hematoxylin-eosin. Main figure ×50, inset ×250.

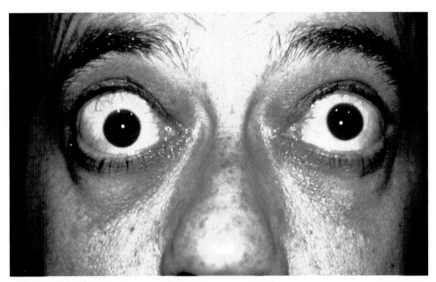

FIGURE 13–5 • **Thyroid ophthalmopathy (Graves' disease).** The patient has bilateral exophthalmos and a characteristic stare. Vertical extraocular muscle imbalance (right hypotropia) reflects fibrosis of the right inferior oblique muscle.

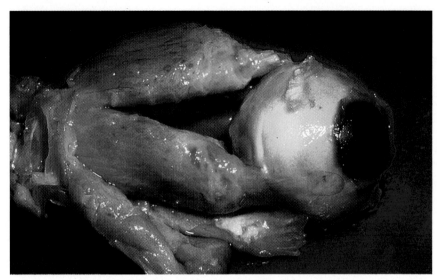

FIGURE 13–6 • **Thyroid ophthalmopathy (Graves' disease).** Postmortem exenteration specimen shows massive enlargement of the extraocular muscles. (Photograph by the author. From Hufnagel TJ, Hickey WF, Cobbs WH, et al: Immunohistochemical and ultrastructural studies on the exenterated tissues of a patient with Graves' disease. *Ophthalmology* 91:1411, 1984. Courtesy of *Ophthalmology*)

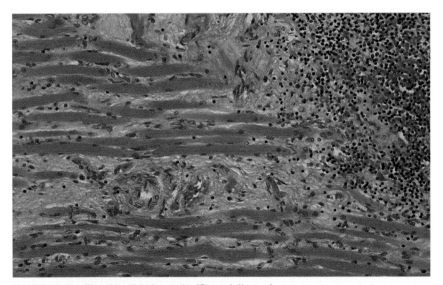

FIGURE 13–7 • **Thyroid ophthalmopathy (Graves' disease).** Extraocular muscle from case seen grossly in Figure 13–5 contains patchy foci of chronic inflammatory cells comprised largely of lymphocytes. The myofibers are separated by fibrosis. The inflammation in Graves' disease characteristically spares the tendons of the extraocular muscles and the orbital fat, features that serve to distinguish the disorder histopathologically from idiopathic orbital inflammatory pseudotumor. Hematoxylin-eosin, ×50.

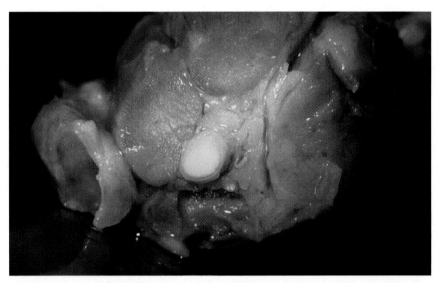

FIGURE 13–8 • **Thyroid ophthalmopathy (Graves' disease).** Optic nerve in the orbital apex of a postmortem specimen is crowded by massively enlarged extraocular muscles. The patient had thyroid optic neuropathy. (Photograph by the author. From Hufnagel, Hickey, Cobbs, et al.: Immunohistochemical and ultrastructural studies on the exenterated tissues of a patient with Graves' disease. *Ophthalmology* 91:1411, 1984. Courtesy of *Ophthalmology*)

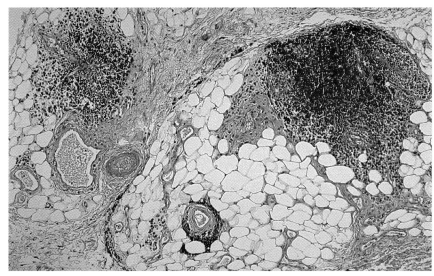

FIGURE 13–9 • **Idiopathic orbital inflammation, orbital fat (idiopathic inflammatory pseudotumor).** The orbital fat contains patchy foci of chronic inflammatory cells. The polymorphous inflammatory infiltrate was comprised largely of lymphocytes and plasma cells. The cuff of cells surrounding the vessel below does not represent true vasculitis. Hematoxylin-eosin, ×25.

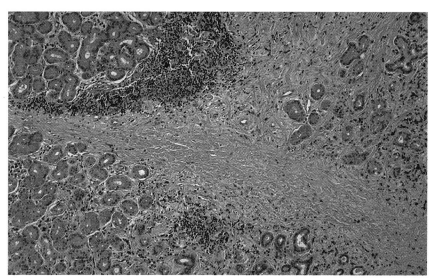

FIGURE 13–10 • **Idiopathic orbital inflammation with fibrosis, lacrimal gland (sclerosing idiopathic inflammatory pseudotumor).** A few residual ductules persist in the eosinophilic, chronically inflamed scar tissue that has replaced the lacrimal gland. Patchy foci of chronic inflammatory cells are present. Higher magnification disclosed a polymorphous inflammatory infiltrate composed largely of lymphocytes and plasma cells.

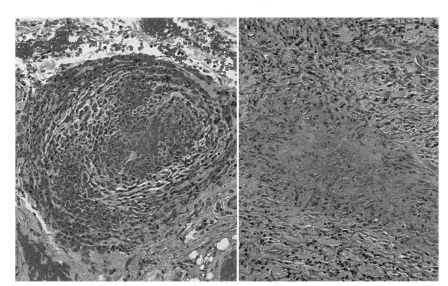

FIGURE 13–11 • **Wegener's granulomatosis.** Granulomatous vasculitis involves an orbital vessel (*left*). Chronic infiltrate contains foci of necrosis (*right*). Both figures: hematoxylin-eosin, ×50.

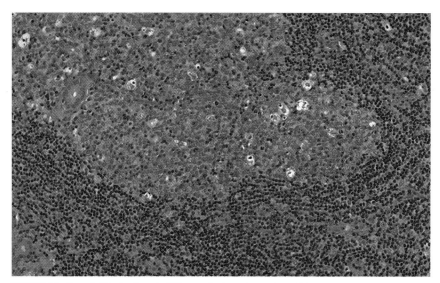

FIGURE 13–12 • **Follicular lymphoid hyperplasia.** The eosinophilic focus above is a germinal center. The clear cells in the germinal center are tingible body macrophages that are antigen presenting cells. Mitoses normally are found in germinal centers. Small well-differentiated lymphocytes surround the germinal center. B lymphocytes predominate in the germinal center and adjacent mantle zone. Hematoxylin-eosin, ×50.

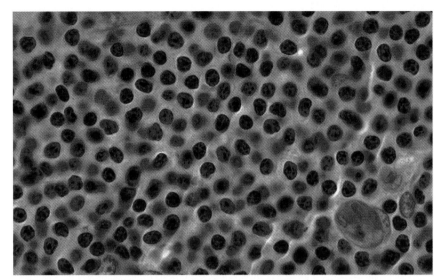

FIGURE 13–13 • **Diffuse non-Hodgkin's lymphoma, well-differentiated lymphocytic type, orbit.** Infiltrate is comprised of monotonous monomorphic sheet of small well-differentiated lymphocytes. Immunophenotypic studies disclosed a monoclonal population of B lymphocytes. Hematoxylin-eosin, ×250.

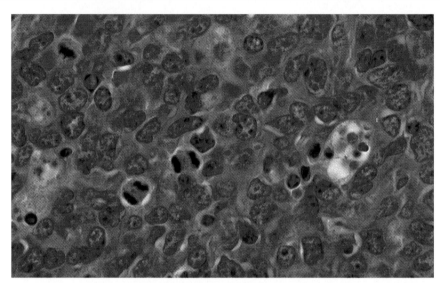

FIGURE 13–14 • **Poorly differentiated malignant lymphoma, orbit.** This obviously malignant tumor is comprised of large, atypical lymphocytes with markedly pleomorphic nuclei. Many cells have nucleoli. Focal necrosis and mitotic activity are present. Hematoxylin-eosin, ×250.

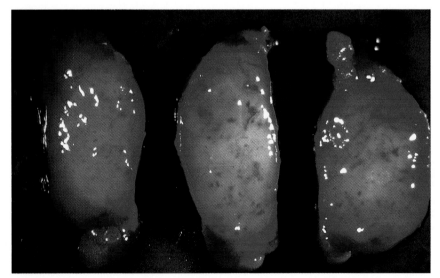

FIGURE 13–15 • **Orbital lymphoma.** Cut surface of a soft orbital tumor has a uniform salmon-yellow color.

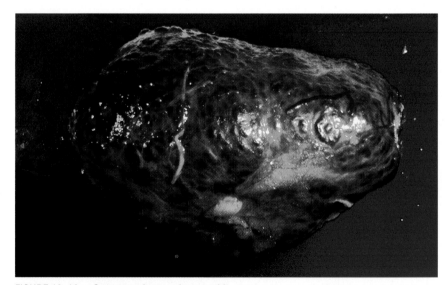

FIGURE 13–16 • **Cavernous hemangioma, orbit.** The well circumscribed encapsulated tumor has a pebbly surface. After fixation cavernous hemangiomas grossly appear deep-blue or purple.

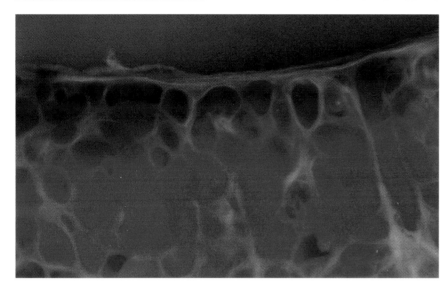

FIGURE 13–17 • **Cavernous hemangioma, orbit.** The benign encapsulated tumor is composed of large blood-filled vascular channels separated by fibrous septa.

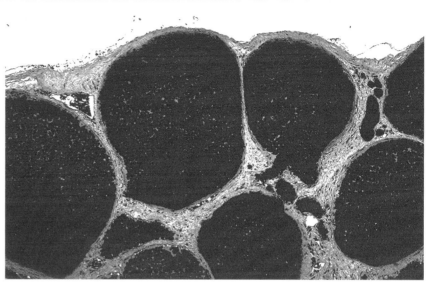

FIGURE 13–18 • **Cavernous hemangioma, orbit.** The large vascular channels comprising the benign vascular tumor are lined by a single layer of endothelial cells. The fibrous septa separating the vessels may contain smooth muscle. Hematoxylin-eosin, × 25.

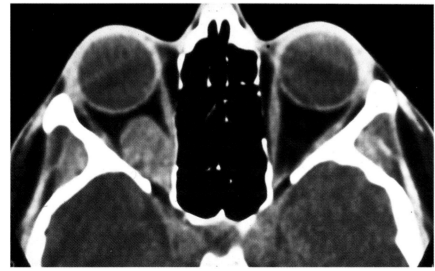

FIGURE 13–19 • **Orbital cavernous hemangioma, CT scan.** The CT scan shows a well circumscribed oval mass within the muscle cone. The differential diagnosis of a well circumscribed orbital tumor also includes schwannoma, hemangiopericytoma, and fibrous histiocytoma.

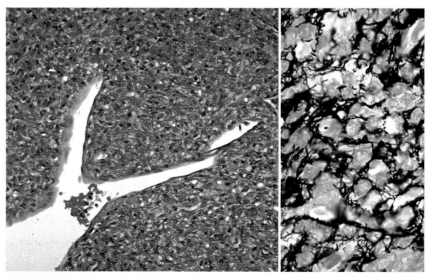

FIGURE 13–20 • **Hemangiopericytoma.** Highly cellular tumor contains a branching staghorn sinusoidal vessel. Reticulin stain (*inset*) highlights the basement membrane encompassing neoplastic pericytes. Main figure: hematoxylin-eosin, ×50; inset: Wilder's reticulin, ×250.

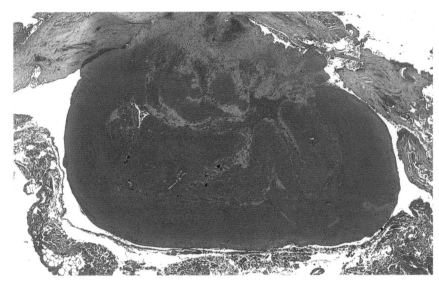

FIGURE 13–21 • **Thrombosed varix, orbit.** A varix is a dilated or ectatic vein. An organized thrombus adheres to the wall of this orbital varix. Hematoxylin-eosin, ×5.

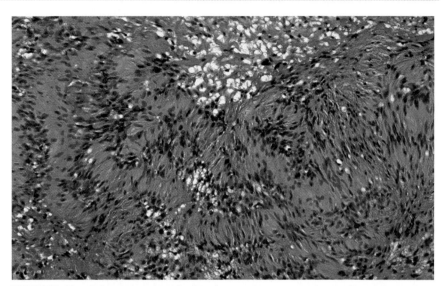

FIGURE 13–22 • **Schwannoma (neurilemoma).** Antoni A portion of a benign peripheral nerve sheath tumor is comprised of highly regimented fascicles of bland spindle cells that show nuclear palisading and enclose tangles of fibrillary processes called Verocay bodies. A small focus of looser myxoid tumor (Antoni B pattern) is seen above. Schwannomas are well circumscribed, encapsulated tumors that are associated with a peripheral nerve. Hematoxylin-eosin, ×100.

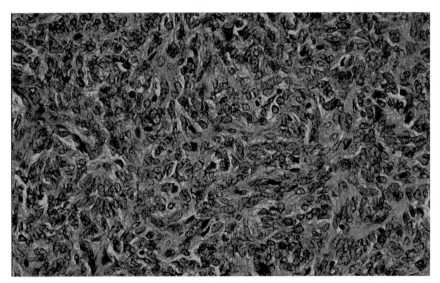

FIGURE 13–23 • **Fibrous histiocytoma.** The spindle cells in a benign fibrous histiocytoma typically are arranged in a whirling storiform, or pinwheel, pattern. The tumor contains a mixture of fibroblastic and histiocytic-like cells. Although they are unencapsulated, benign fibrous histiocytomas usually are well circumscribed. Hematoxylin-eosin, ×100.

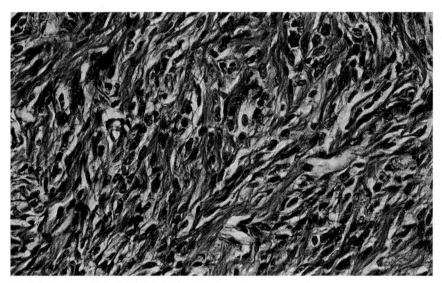

FIGURE 13–24 • **Solitary fibrous tumor.** Spindle cells are arranged in a "patternless pattern." Tumor was immunoreactive for CD-34. (Case presented by Dr. Frederick Jakobiec, 1994 meeting of Verhoeff Society, Rochester, MN)

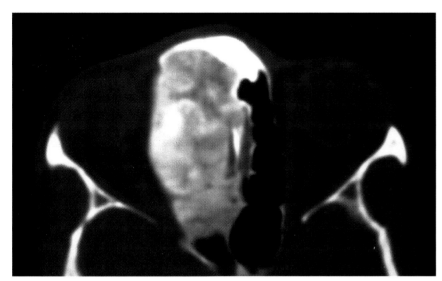

FIGURE 13–25 • **Fibrous dysplasia.** Lesion of nasal bones has "ground glass" appearance on the CT scan. Fibrous dysplasia may spread across suture lines to involve multiple orbital bones.

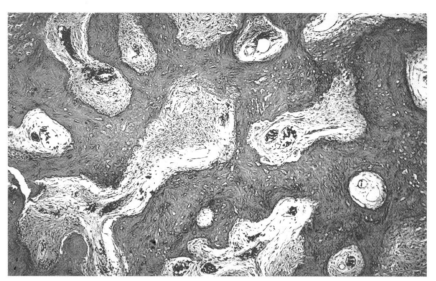

FIGURE 13–26 • **Fibrous dysplasia.** Fibrous stroma contains irregular trabeculae of immature woven bone that are not rimmed by osteoclasts. Fibrous dysplasia represents an arrest in the maturation of bone. Hematoxylin-eosin, ×25.

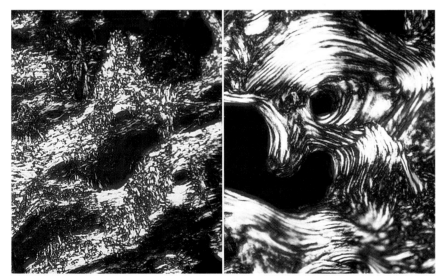

FIGURE 13–27 • **Fibrous dysplasia.** Polarization microscopy of fibrous dysplasia (*left*) discloses an irregular interweaving pattern of collagenous matrix that resembles the fibers in woven cloth. In contrast, collagen fibers in mature lamellar bone (*right*) are arranged in a highly regular parallel lamellae. Both figures: hematoxylin-eosin with crossed polarizers, ×50.

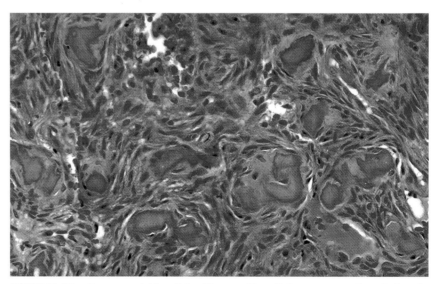

FIGURE 13–28 • **Psammomatoid ossifying fibroma.** The cellular stroma contains spindle cells and small spicules of bone called ossicles that can be confused with the psammoma bodies of a meningioma. This benign lesion found in young individuals has an expansile growth pattern and behaves more aggressively than fibrous dysplasia. It usually does not cross suture lines and is restricted to a single orbital bone. Hematoxylin-eosin, ×100.

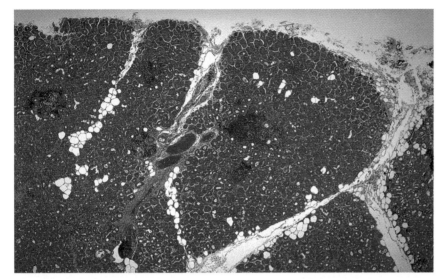

FIGURE 13–29 • **Lacrimal gland.** Fibrofatty stroma separates multiple lobules composed of glandular acini. Patchy foci of chronic inflammation are present. Hematoxylin-eosin, ×10.

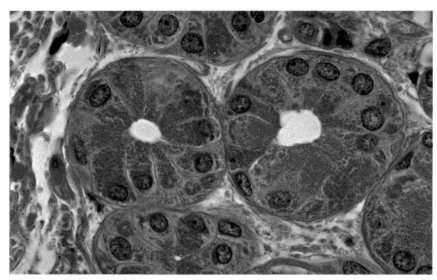

FIGURE 13–30 • **Lacrimal gland, acini.** An inner layer of tall columnar secretory cells and a relatively inconspicuous discontinuous outer layer of contractile myoepithelial cells comprise the acini of the lacrimal gland. Large, intensely eosinophilic secretory granules called zymogen granules are found in the apical cytoplasm of the secretory cells. Hematoxylin-eosin, ×250.

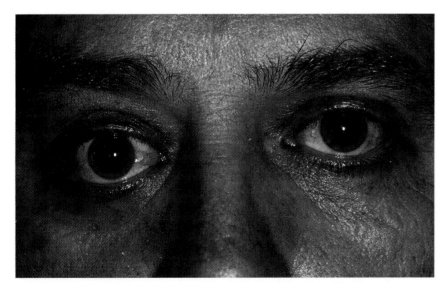

FIGURE 13–31 • **Ocular proptosis, pleomorphic adenoma of the lacrimal gland.** The right eye is pushed forward and inferonasally by a tumor in the superotemporal lacrimal fossa. The patient had slowly developed painless proptosis over several years.

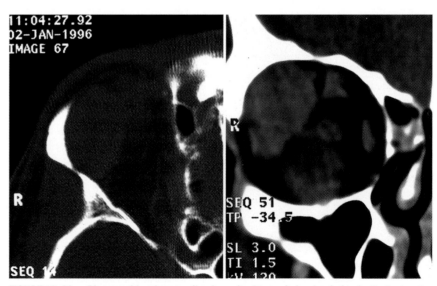

FIGURE 13–32 • **Pleomorphic adenoma (benign mixed tumor), lacrimal gland.** Sagittal and coronal CT scans of the right orbit disclose a well circumscribed tumor that has produced accentuation of the lacrimal fossa.

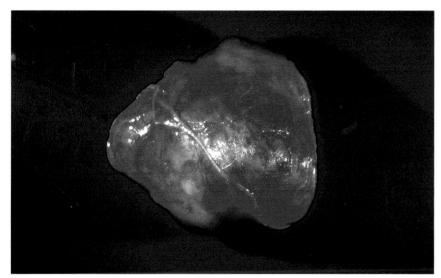

FIGURE 13–33 • **Pleomorphic adenoma (benign mixed tumor), lacrimal gland.** Convex bosselations are present on the surface of a well circumscribed, pseudoencapsulated tumor.

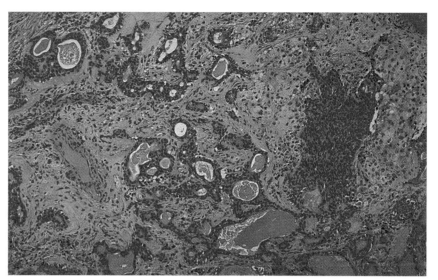

FIGURE 13–34 • **Pleomorphic adenoma (benign mixed tumor), lacrimal gland.** The tumor is comprised of neoplastic ductules of epithelial cells set in a fibromyxoid stroma. The term "mixed tumor" refers to this mixture of epithelial and mesenchymal elements. Hematoxylin-eosin, ×25.

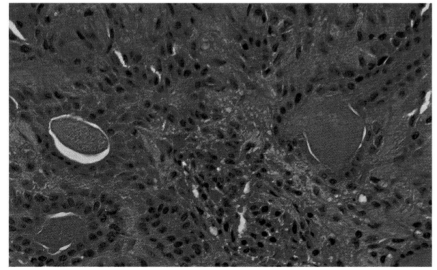

FIGURE 13–35 • **Pleomorphic adenoma (benign mixed tumor), lacrimal gland.** The epithelial ductules are composed of two layers of cells. Myoepithelial cells from the outer layer spindle-off into the surrounding stroma, where they may undergo metaplasia into myxoid tissue, cartilage, or rarely bone. Hematoxylin-eosin, ×100.

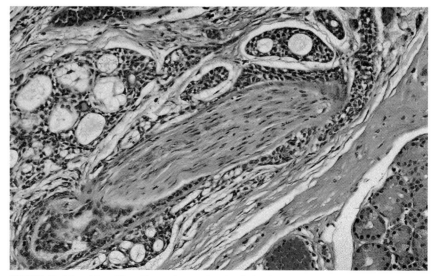

FIGURE 13–36 • **Adenoid cystic carcinoma, lacrimal gland, perineural invasion.** Infiltrative adenoid cystic carcinoma surrounds a large orbital nerve. This highly malignant tumor has a propensity for neural and perineural invasion. Patients may present with pain. Hematoxylin-eosin, ×50.

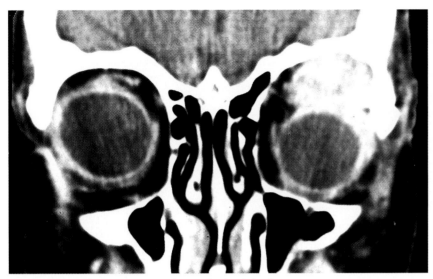

FIGURE 13–37 • **Adenoid cystic carcinoma, lacrimal gland.** The tumor has irregular margins and has produced a scalloped fossa in orbital bone. The tumor developed rapidly and was painful.

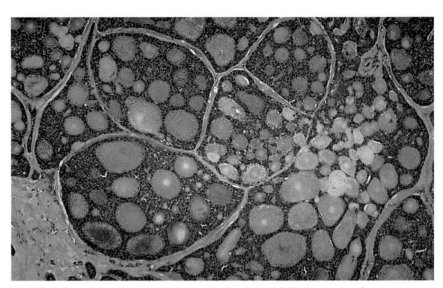

FIGURE 13–38 • **Adenoid cystic carcinoma, lacrimal gland (cribriform pattern).** Multiple pools of mucin impart a "Swiss cheese" appearance to the basophilic lobules of cells comprising the cribriform pattern of adenoid cystic carcinoma. The tumor cells are relatively uniform and have a deceptively bland appearance. Adenoid cystic carcinoma has a dismal prognosis. Hematoxylin-eosin, ×25.

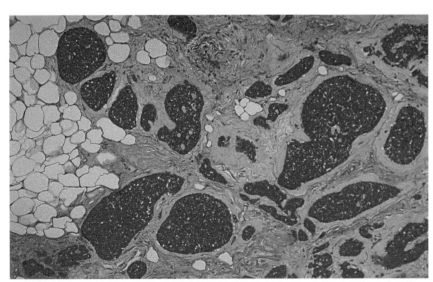

FIGURE 13–39 • **Adenoid cystic carcinoma, lacrimal gland (basaloid pattern).** Poorly differentiated tumor is comprised of solid lobules of deeply basophilic cells with scanty cytoplasm. The absence of peripheral palisading serves to differentiate basaloid adenoid cystic carcinoma from invasive basal cell carcinoma. Tumors with a basaloid component have a poorer prognosis. Hematoxylin-eosin, ×25.

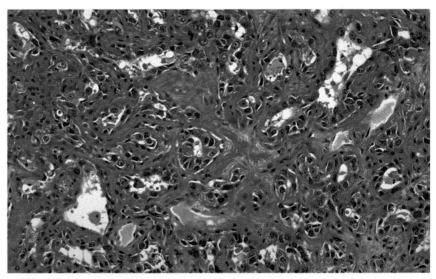

FIGURE 13–40 • **Malignant mixed tumor, lacrimal gland.** The epithelial tubules comprising this field are composed of frankly malignant cells. Most malignant mixed tumors result from the malignant degeneration of a benign mixed tumor. Hematoxylin-eosin, ×50.

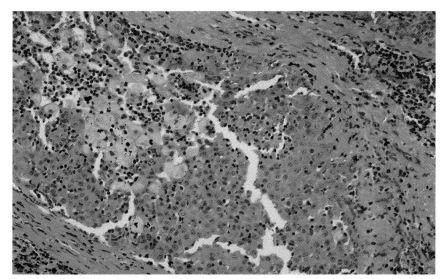

FIGURE 13–41 • **Mucoepidermoid carcinoma, lacrimal gland.** Tumor is comprised of sheets of eosinophilic squamous cells with a "paving stone" arrangement and mucus-producing goblet cells. Mucoepidermoid carcinoma is a rare lacrimal gland tumor that behaves less aggressively than other lacrimal gland malignancies. Hematoxylin-eosin, ×50.

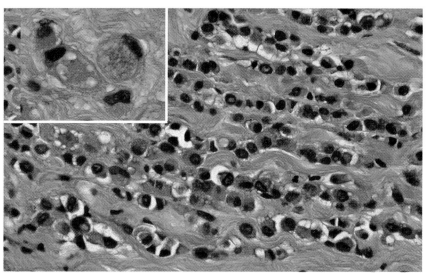

FIGURE 13–42 • **Metastatic breast carcinoma, orbit.** The carcinoma cells are arranged in a linear "Indian file" fashion. *Inset:* Signet ring cells with prominent cytoplasmic vacuoles of mucin. Both figures: hematoxylin-eosin. Main figure ×100, inset ×250.

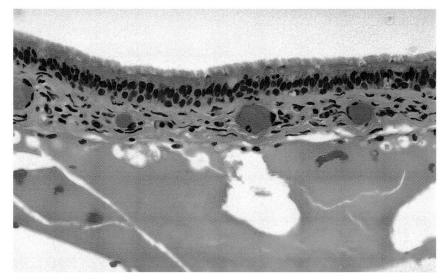

FIGURE 13–43 • **Mucocele.** The mucocele is lined by ciliated respiratory epithelium. Hematoxylin-eosin, ×100.

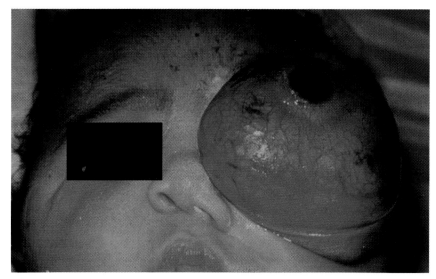

FIGURE 13–44 • **Congenital orbital teratoma.** Congenital orbital tumor produces hideous proptosis. (Case presented by Dr. Harry Brown, 1993 meeting of the Verhoeff Society, Coral Gables, FL)

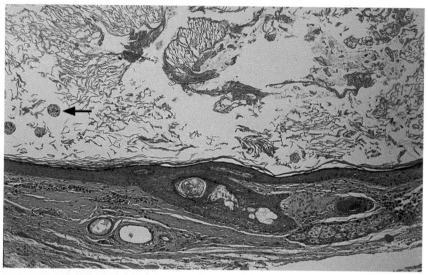

FIGURE 13–45 • **Dermoid cyst.** The cyst is filled with keratin debris and is lined by keratinized stratified squamous epithelium with epidermal appendages that resembles skin. A few hair shafts are mixed with the keratin (arrow). Hematoxylin-eosin, × 50.

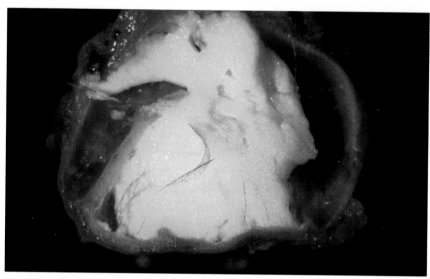

FIGURE 13–46 • **Dermoid cyst.** Sectioned cyst contains cheesy keratin debris and hair shafts.

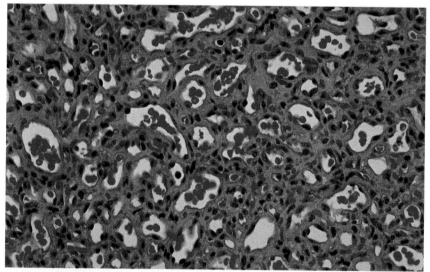

FIGURE 13–47 • **Capillary hemangioma.** This mature capillary hemangioma is composed of a plexus of capillary caliber vessels. Early lesions often are composed predominantly of a solid sheet of endo'helial cells. Vascular lumina develop and become progressively ectatic as the lesion matures. Hematoxylin-eosin, ×100.

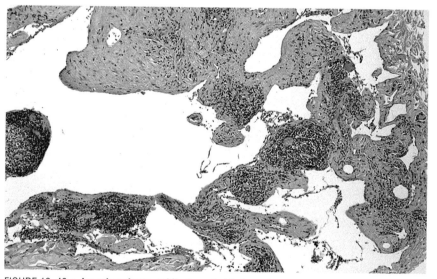

FIGURE 13–48 • **Lymphangioma, orbit.** Lymphoid channels comprising lymphangioma vary markedly in size and shape. They appear empty or contain serous fluid if intralesional hemorrhage has not occurred. Lymphoid foci in intervascular septa help differentiate a lymphangioma with secondary hemorrhage from a cavernous hemangioma. Lymphangiomas typically are unencapsulated and have an infiltrative growth pattern. Hematoxylin-eosin, ×10.

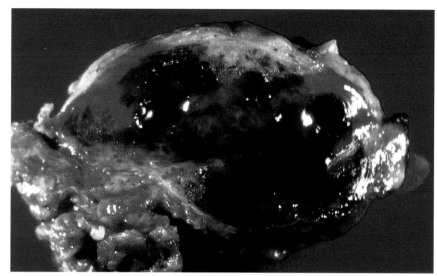

FIGURE 13–49 • **Lymphangioma with secondary hemorrhage.** Blood-filled chocolate cysts caused by secondary hemorrhage into a lymphangioma are evident in this gross specimen. Many lymphangiomas contain blood. Lymphangiomas typically are unencapsulated and exhibit an infiltrative growth pattern.

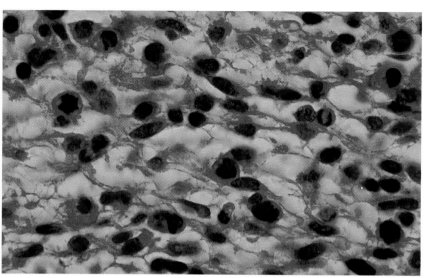

FIGURE 13–50 • **Embryonal rhabdomyosarcoma, orbit.** Syncytium of spindled mesenchymal cells in a loose myxoid stroma constitutes poorly differentiated embryonal tumor. Most orbital rhabdomyosarcomas are classified as embryonal. Hematoxylin-eosin, ×250.

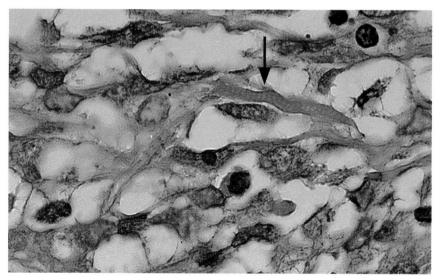

FIGURE 13–51 • **Orbital rhabdomyosarcoma with cross striations.** Arrow points to an eosinophilic strap cell with cross striations. Many embryonal rhabdomyosarcomas lack cross striations. Hematoxylin-eosin, ×250.

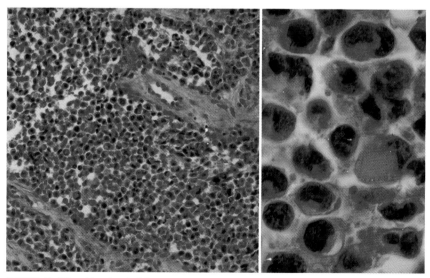

FIGURE 13–52 • **Alveolar rhabdomyosarcoma.** Round, poorly cohesive tumor cells are compartmentalized by fibrous septa that resemble pulmonary alveoli. *Inset:* Large polygonal tumor cells. Several cells have abundant eosinophilic cytoplasm. Hematoxylin-eosin. Main figure ×50; inset ×250.

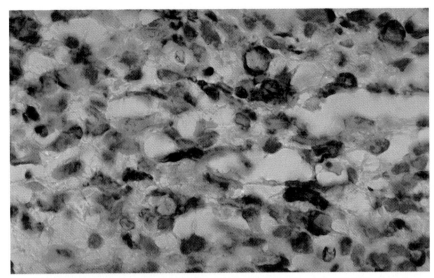

FIGURE 13–53 • **Rhabdomyosarcoma, immunohistochemical diagnosis.** Cells in an embryonal tumor show positive immunoreactivity for muscle marker desmin. Muscle specific actin was also positive. Peroxidase-Antiperoxidase (PAP), ×250.

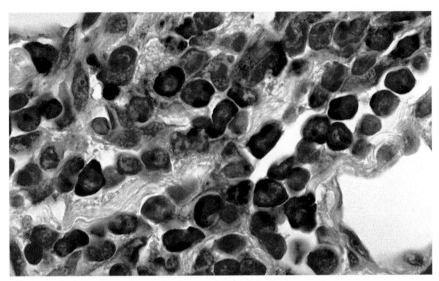

FIGURE 13–54 • **Granulocytic sarcoma.** Positive (red) Leder naphthol AS-D chloroacetate esterase stain confirms the presence of granulocytic differentiation. Granulocytic or myeloid sarcoma must be excluded when an apparent "lymphoma" is encountered in the orbit of a child. Leder stain, ×250.

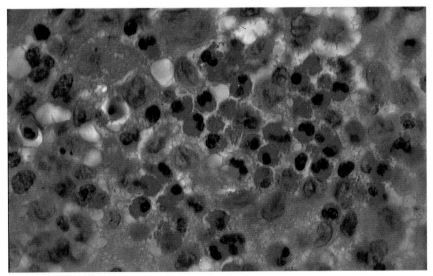

FIGURE 13–55 • **Eosinophilic granuloma, orbit.** Infiltrate is composed of eosinophils, large mononuclear histiocytes with folded nuclei, and small round osteoclast-like giant cells. The eosinophilic granuloma is a localized form of Langerhans' cell histiocytosis that characteristically forms a lytic lesion in the superotemporal orbital bone. The cells stain positively for S-100 protein, and electron microscopy discloses racket-shaped Birbeck granules. Hematoxylin-eosin, ×250.

# CHAPTER 14

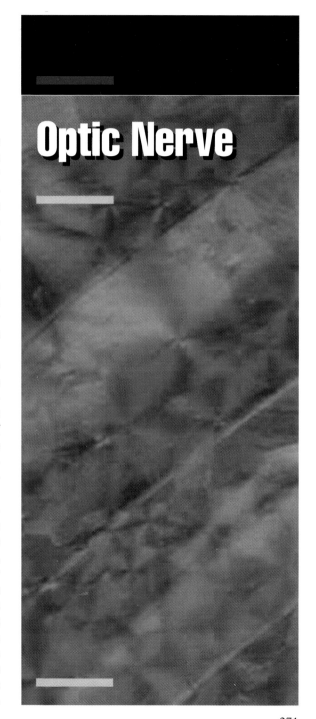

# Optic Nerve

The optic nerve is a tract of the central nervous system (CNS) that connects the eye and the brain. The nerve has intraorbital, intracanalicular, and intracranial portions; and it is about 50 mm in total length. It is comprised of the axons of the retinal ganglion cells, interstitial cells (including oligodendrocytes, astrocytes, and microglia), and fibrovascular septa of the pia mater. The retinal nerve fibers exit the eye through the lamina cribrosa in the posterior sclera and extend to the optic chiasm; they then reach the lateral geniculate body via the optic tracts (Figs. 14–1, 14–2). Behind the lamina cribrosa, the axons are myelinated (Fig. 14–2). Here the nerve measures about 3 mm in diameter. In contrast, the diameter of the optic disk is only 1.5 mm.

Dense collagenous dura, the spidery trabeculated arachnoid, and the vascularized pia mater comprise the meninges of the optic nerve (Fig. 14–3). The optic nerve is encompassed by firmly adherent pia mater, and its substance is compartmentalized by septa of pial connective tissue (Fig. 14–4).

Developmental anomalies of the optic nerve include optic nerve aplasia and hypoplasia, optic pits, optic nerve colobomas, and the morning glory syndrome. Bilateral hypoplasia is often associated with congenital syndromes such as de Morsier's syndrome of septooptic dysplasia, which includes bilateral hypoplastic nerves, absent septum pellucidum, and hemiplegia; and Aicardi's syndrome which affects only females and includes peripapillary chorioretinal lacunae, ectopic retinal pigment epithelium (RPE), agenesis of the corpus callosum, infantile spasms, and mental retardation.

Colobomas of the optic nerve (Figs. 14–5, 14–6) are caused by incomplete closure of the posterior portion of the fetal fissure. Eyes with extensive optic nerve colobomas may be microophthalmic and have a cystic outpouching of the posterior sclera (microphthalmos with cyst) (see Fig. 1–5). The cyst typically is lined by dysplastic neuroectodermal tissue, which communicates with the retina via the coloboma. Optic nerve colobomas occasionally are associated with choristomatous malformations that contain smooth muscle and heterotopic fat.

Optic pits are small crater-like holes that usually occur unilaterally at the temporal margin of the optic disk. Pathogenesis probably is related to anomalous closure of the fetal fissure. Optic pits are frequently complicated by serous detachment of the macula. The subretinal fluid likely is derived from the vitreous.

The morning glory syndrome is an optic nerve anomaly characterized by a funnel-shaped optic nerve head, which appears to contain a central dot of connective tissue believed to be residual Bergmeister's papilla. The retinal vessels emerge from the margin of the disk, which is surrounded by an elevated annulus of disturbed chorioretinal pigment. Bilateral cases occasionally have been associated with midline neurologic and craniofacial anomalies.

Optic disk drusen are globular aggregates of concentrically laminated, calcified material located deep in the substance of the optic nerve head anterior to the lamina cribrosa within the scleral ring (Figs. 14–7, 14–8). Optic disk drusen appear ophthalmoscopically as tan, yellow, or straw-colored glistening or refractile spherical structures. They typically are found in a small, crowded optic disk that has a small or absent cup. Optic disk drusen are unrelated to drusen of the RPE or the heavily calcified epipapillary astrocytomas called giant drusen of the optic disk that occur in some patients with tuberous sclerosis. Optic disk drusen are important clinically because they may be misdiagnosed as papilledema and prompt an unnecessary neurologic evaluation. The pathogenesis of optic disk drusen may be related to blockage of axoplasmic flow in ganglion cell axons within a narrow, crowded scleral canal. Calcified mitochondria dispersed from prelaminar corpora amylacea may provide a nidus for further calcium deposition. Optic disk drusen occur sporadically or may be inherited as an irregular autosomal dominant trait. Disk drusen also occur in association with retinitis pigmentosa and pseudoxanthoma elasticum.

Although optic disk edema (papilledema) classically is associated with elevated intracranial pressure and space-occupying intracranial lesions, swollen optic disks also occur in eyes with acute glaucoma, ocular hypotony, central retinal vein occlusion, juxtapapillary tumors, and severe hypertensive retinopathy (Figs. 14–9, 14–10, 14–11). Optic disk edema does not result from an accumulation of fluid in the extracellular spaces of the disk. Rather, the increase in the volume of the nerve head reflects the intracytoplasmic swelling and thickening of ganglion cell axons caused by blockage of axoplasmic flow in the distorted lamina cribrosa. The pores of the lamina cribrosa are distorted by a pressure gradient between the intraocular pressure and pressure in the retrolaminar optic nerve. A pressure gradient can form if the intracranial pressure is elevated (classic papilledema), the intraocular pressure is low (hypotony), or the intraocular pressure is acutely elevated (acute glaucoma).

Histopathologically, the nerve head is swollen, and the physiologic cup is narrowed (Figs. 14–10, 14–11). The increase in the volume of nerve head tissue displaces the photoreceptors laterally from the margin of the disk. This displacement and an accompanying shallow peripapillary collection of serous subretinal fluid are responsible for enlargement of the blind spot on visual field testing. Folds are also found in the outer retinal layers. Extensive gliosis and axonal loss occur in chronic papilledema.

Optic nerve atrophy is characterized pathologically by shrinkage of the parenchyma of the optic nerve caused by loss of ganglion cell axons (Figs. 14–12, 14–13). The subarachnoid space around the shrunken nerve becomes widened, and the dura may appear redundant and folded. Light microscopy discloses loss of axons and thickening of the pia mater and pial septa. Gliosis may or may not become prominent depending on the cause of the atrophy.

By convention, the terms "primary" or "descending" optic atrophy are applied to atrophy of the nerve caused by lesions in the CNS or orbit. Primary optic atrophy generally is not associated with an ophthalmoscopically visible glial or mesenchymal reaction. Causes of primary optic atrophy include optic nerve trauma, compression by neoplasms or enlarged extraocular muscles in thyroid ophthalmopathy, neurosyphilis, demyelinating diseases including multiple sclerosis, heritable leukodystrophies, and toxic and nutritional optic neuropathies.

Inflammatory, neoplastic, or vascular lesions located in the retina or the vicinity of the optic disk cause secondary or ascending optic atrophy, which is often marked by pronounced alterations in the glial and mesenchymal tissues of the nerve head. Common retinal causes of optic atrophy are chorioretinitis, retinitis pigmentosa, and trauma.

Leber's hereditary optic neuropathy is caused by several point mutations in the subunit 4 gene of mitochondrial DNA encoding NADH dehydrogenase. Mitochondrial DNA is maternally inherited. Leber's hereditary optic atrophy usually presents with subacute progressive bilateral central visual loss in men between age 18 and 30 years. Some patients have disk swelling and telangiectatic peripapillary vessels.

Although retinal ganglion cells and axons are lost in both primary and glaucomatous optic atrophy, cupping of the disk generally occurs in glaucomatous optic atrophy and is not prominent in primary optic atrophy. Schnabel's cavernous optic atrophy is a relatively rare

type of optic atrophy generally found in eyes that have experienced an acute rise in intraocular pressure (Figs. 14–14, 14–15). Light microscopy reveals large spaces in the retrolaminar part of the nerve that are filled with hyaluronic acid. The vitreous humor is thought to be the source of the mucoid material. No gliosis or histiocytic reaction typically is seen. Ischemia is thought to be the cause of rare cases of Schnabel's cavernous degeneration that have occurred in eyes with normal intraocular pressure.

The term optic neuritis refers to involvement of any part of the optic nerve by an inflammatory disease process. The process is called retrobulbar neuritis clinically when the inflammation involves the retrobulbar part of the optic nerve and ophthalmoscopy initially reveals no abnormalities. Multiple sclerosis is a relatively common cause of retrobulbar neuritis. The term papillitis is used when the optic disk is affected, and the process is called neuroretinitis if the peripapillary retina is involved by edema, hemorrhage, and inflammation. Optic neuritis is classified topographically as perineuritis, periaxial neuritis, axial neuritis, and transverse neuritis. It can be caused by bacterial, mycobacterial, viral, mycotic, and parasitic infection as well as by granulomatous disorders such as sarcoidosis and Wegener's granulomatosis (Fig. 14–16). Large granulomas occur on the surface of the optic disk in some patients with sarcoidosis.

Most primary tumors of the optic nerve are optic nerve gliomas and meningiomas. Although melanocytoma (magnocellular nevus) can occur anywhere in the uveal tract, it typically affects the optic nerve head (see Fig. 10–12). Large epipapillary astrocytomas occur in some patients with tuberous sclerosis, and the optic nerve head can be affected by hemangioblastoma in von Hippel-Lindau disease. Rare medulloepitheliomas of the optic nerve have been reported. Combined hamartoma of the RPE and retina (Fig. 14–17) often affects the optic disk and may be associated with neurofibromatosis type 2.

Optic nerve glioma (pilocytic astrocytoma) usually presents between age 2 and 6 years with unilateral visual loss and axial proptosis. Ophthalmoscopy may disclose optic atrophy or papilledema. Strabismus, an afferent pupillary defect and enlargement of the ipsilateral optic canal may be present. There is a strong association with neurofibromatosis type I (10–50%). Optic nerve gliomas cause a fusiform swelling of the optic nerve (Fig. 14–18). The tumor does not invade the orbital tissues because it typically remains confined by the intact dura (Fig. 14–19). Optic nerve gliomas in children are grade I astrocytomas composed of spindly cells that have long, delicate, hair-like processes (Figs. 14–20, 14–21). The term *"pilocytic"* astrocytoma reflects that feature. Eosinophilic clumps of fibrils called Rosenthal fibers are a prominent finding in some tumors. Optic nerve gliomas associated with neurofibromatosis often break through the pia and proliferate in the subarachnoid space within the intact dura (arachnoidal gliomatosis). In such cases the central remnant of the optic nerve may be evident on imaging studies. Arachnoidal gliomatosis may be confused with meningioma in a superficial biopsy. At the present time most optic nerve gliomas are followed conservatively. Surgical excision, usually sparing the eye, may be indicated for high degrees of cosmetically unacceptable proptosis or when the tumor threatens to extend intracranially and involve the chiasm. High grade malignant gliomas of chiasm or optic nerve occur rarely in adults and have a dismal prognosis (Fig. 14–22).

Primary meningiomas of the optic nerve can occur in adults or children, and they may behave aggressively in children. Clinically, optic nerve meningiomas compress the optic nerve, causing optic atrophy and visual loss (Figs. 14–23, 14–24). Ophthalmoscopy may reveal opticociliary (retinochoroidal) venous shunt vessels on the optic disk. Primary orbital meningiomas arise from the meninges of the optic nerve or rarely from ectopic rests of arachnoidal tissue. Primary intracranial meningiomas also invade the orbit secondarily. Most primary meningiomas of the orbit are either meningothelial or transitional (Figs. 14–25). Unlike optic nerve gliomas, optic nerve meningiomas frequently erode through the meninges and invade the soft tissue of the orbit.

# References

### Developmental Lesions

Brockhurst RJ: Optic pits and posterior retinal detachment. Trans Am Ophthalmol Soc 73:264–291, 1975.

Brown GC, Shields JA, Patty BE, Goldberg RE: Congenital pits of the optic nerve head. I. Experimental studies in collie dogs. Arch Ophthalmol 97:1341–1344, 1979.

Eustis HS, Sanders MR, Zimmerman T: Morning glory syndrome in children: association with endocrine and central nervous system anomalies. Arch Ophthalmol 112:204–207, 1994.

Font RL, Zimmerman LE: Intrascleral smooth muscle in coloboma of the optic disc: electron microscopic verification. Am J Ophthalmol 72:452–457, 1971.

Gass JDM: Serous detachment of the macula secondary to congenital pit of the optic nerve head. Am J Ophthalmol 67:821–841, 1969.

Hoyt CS, Billson FA, Ouvrier R, Wise G: Ocular features of Aicardi's syndrome. Arch Ophthalmol 96:291–295, 1978.

Jensen PE, Kalina RE: Congenital anomalies of the optic disk. Am J Ophthalmol 82:27–31, 1976.

Kindler P: Morning glory syndrome: unusual congenital optic disk anomaly. Am J Ophthalmol 69:376–384, 1970.

Lieb W, Rochels R, Gronemeyer U: Microphthalmos with colobomatous orbital cyst: clinical, histological, immunohistological, and electronmicroscopic findings. Br J Ophthalmol 74:59–62, 1990.

Mafee MF, Jampol LM, Langer BG, Tso M: Computed tomography of optic nerve colobomas, morning glory anomaly, and colobomatous cyst. Radiol Clin North Am 25:693–699, 1987.

Pagon RA: Ocular coloboma. Surv Ophthalmol 25:223–236, 1981.

Pollock S: The morning glory disc anomaly: contractile movement, classification, and embryogenesis. Doc Ophthalmol 65:439–460, 1987.

Slamovits TL, Kimball GP, Friberg TR, Curtin HD: Bilateral optic disc colobomas with orbital cysts and hypoplastic optic nerves and chiasm. J Clin Neuroophthalmol 9:172–177, 1989.

Waring GO III, Roth AM, Rodrigues MM: Clinicopathologic correlation of microphthalmos with cyst. Am J Ophthalmol 82:714–721, 1976.

Weiss A, Martinez C, Greenwald M: Microphthalmos with cyst: clinical presentations and computed tomographic findings. J Pediatr Ophthalmol Strabismus 22:6–12, 1985.

Wiggins RE, von Noorden GK, Boniuk M: Optic nerve coloboma with cyst: a case report and review. J Pediatr Ophthalmol Strabismus 28:274–277, 1991.

Zeki SM, Dutton GN: Optic nerve hypoplasia in children: mini review. Br J Ophthalmol 74:300–304, 1990.

### Optic Disk Drusen

Spencer WH: Drusen of the optic nerve: XXXIV Edward Jackson memorial lecture. Am J Ophthalmol 85:1–12, 1978.

Tso MOM: Pathology and pathogenesis of drusen of the optic nerve head. Ophthalmology 188:1066–1080, 1980.

### Optic Disk Edema

Galbraith JEK, Sullivan JH: Decompression of the perioptic meninges for relief of papilledema. Am J Ophthalmol 76:687–692, 1973.

Tso MOM, Fine BS: Electron microscopic study of papilledema in man. Am J Ophthalmol 82:424–434, 1976.

Tso MOM, Hayreh SS: Optic disc edema in raised intracranial pressure. III. A pathologic study of experimental papilledema. Arch Ophthalmol 95:1458–1462, 1977.

### Optic Atrophy

Andersen DR: Ascending and descending optic atrophy produced experimentally in squirrel monkeys. Am J Ophthalmol 76:693–711, 1973.

Brown MD, Voljavec AS, Lott MT, MacDonald I, Wallace DC: Leber's hereditary optic neuropathy: a model for mitochondrial neurodegenerative diseases. FASEB J 6:2791–2799, 1992.

Howell N: Leber hereditary optic neuropathy: how do mitochondrial DNA mutations cause degeneration of the optic nerve? J Bioenerg Biomembr 29:165–173, 1997.

Kerrison JB, Newman NJ: Clinical spectrum of Leber's hereditary optic neuropathy. Clin Neurosci 4:295–301, 1997.

Morris MA: Mitochondrial mutations in neuro-ophthalmological diseases: a review. J Clin Neuroophthalmol 10:159–166, 1990.

Phillips CI, Gosden CM: Leber's hereditary optic neuropathy and Kearns-Sayre syndrome: mitochondrial DNA mutations. Surv Ophthalmol 35:463–472, 1991.

Riordan-Eva P, Wood NW: Mitochondrial disorders in neuro-ophthalmology. Curr Opin Neurol 9:1–4, 1996.

**Glaucomatous Optic Atrophy**

Gong H, Ye W, Freddo TF, Hernandez MR: Hyaluronic acid in the normal and glaucomatous optic nerve. Exp Eye Res 64:587–595, 1997.

Kalvin NH, Hamasaki DI, Gass JDM: Experimental glaucoma in monkeys. I. Relationship between intraocular pressure and cupping of the optic disc and cavernous atrophy of the optic nerve. Arch Ophthalmol 76:82–93, 1966.

Shields CL, Eagle RC Jr: Pseudo-Schnabel's cavernous degeneration of the optic nerve secondary to intraocular silicone oil. Arch Ophthalmol 107:714–717, 1989.

Zimmerman LE, deVenecia G, Hamasaki DI: Pathology of the optic nerve in experimental acute glaucoma. Invest Ophthalmol 6:109–125, 1967.

**Optic Neuritis**

Laties AM, Scheie HG: Sarcoid granuloma of the optic disk: evolution of multiple small tumors. Trans Am Ophthalmol Soc 689:219–233, 1970.

Miller NR: The optic nerve. Curr Opin Neurol 9:5–15, 1996.

Newman NJ: Neuro-ophthalmology: the afferent visual system. Curr Opin Neurol 6:738–746, 1993.

Newman NJ: Optic neuropathy. Neurology 46:315–322, 1996.

Warner J, Lessell S: Neuro-ophthalmology of multiple sclerosis. Clin Neurosci 2:180–188, 1994.

**Optic Nerve Gliomas**

Borit A, Richardson EP Jr: The biological and clinical behavior of pilocytic astrocytomas of the optic pathways. Brain 105:161–187, 1982.

Dutton JJ. Gliomas of the anterior visual pathway. Surv Ophthalmol 38:427–452, 1994.

Lewis RA, Gerson LP, Axelson KA, et al: Von Recklinghausen's neurofibromatosis. II. Incidence of optic gliomata. Ophthalmology 91:929–935, 1984.

Miller NR, Illif WJ, Green WR: Evaluation and management of gliomas of the anterior visual pathways. Brain 97:743–754, 1974.

Rush JA, Younge BR, Campbell RJ, MacCarthy CS: Optic glioma: long-term follow-up of 85 histopathologically verified cases. Ophthalmology 89:1213–1219, 1982.

Spoor TC, Kennerdell JS, Martinez AJ, et al: Malignant gliomas of the optic nerve pathways. Am J Ophthalmol 89:284–292, 1980.

Stern J, Jakobiec FA, Housepian E: The architecture of optic nerve gliomas with and without neurofibromatosis. Arch Ophthalmol 98:505–511, 1980.

**Optic Nerve Meningiomas**

Dutton JJ: Optic nerve gliomas and meningiomas. Neurol Clin 9:163–177, 1991.

Dutton JJ: Optic nerve sheath meningiomas. Surv Ophthalmol 37:167–183, 1992.

Karp LA, Zimmerman LE, Borit A, Spencer W: Primary intraorbital meningiomas. Arch Ophthalmol 91:24–28, 1974.

Marquardt MD, Zimmerman LE: Histopathology of meningiomas and gliomas of the optic nerve. Hum Pathol 13:226–235, 1982.

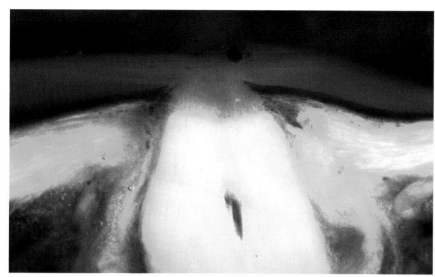

FIGURE 14–1 • **Longitudinal section of optic nerve showing termination of myelination at lamina cribrosa.** Creamy yellow myelin normally terminates abruptly at the posterior margin of the lamina cribrosa. The myelinated part of the nerve is about 3 mm in diameter.

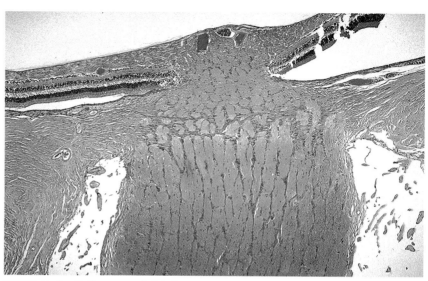

FIGURE 14–2 • **Optic nerve and disk, longitudinal section.** The myelinated part of the optic nerve behind the lamina cribrosa is approximately twice the diameter of the optic disk. Hematoxylin-eosin, ×10.

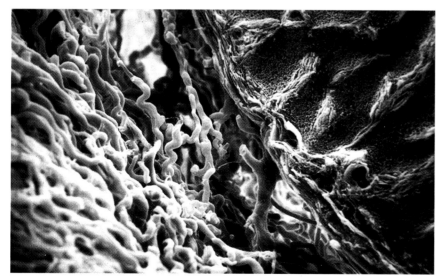

FIGURE 14–3 • **Optic nerve meninges.** The cleft separating the optic nerve at right and the dura at left is the subarachnoid space, which is bridged by spidery arachnoidal processes. Pia mater covers the external surface of the optic nerve. Septa of the pia extend into the substance of the nerve, compartmentalizing its axons. Scanning electron micrograph.

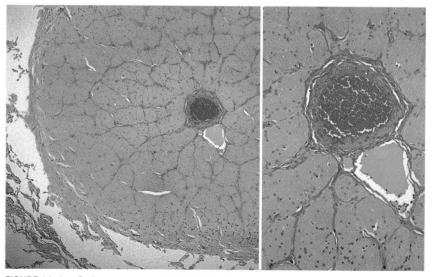

FIGURE 14–4 • **Optic nerve, transverse section.** The parenchyma of the nerve is compartmentalized by delicate pial septa. The central retinal artery and vein share a common adventitial sheath. Hematoxylin-eosin. Left ×25; right ×50.

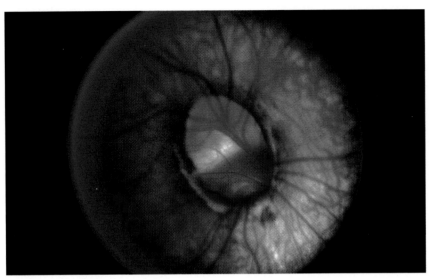

FIGURE 14–5 • **Optic nerve coloboma.** Optic nerve colobomas are caused by incomplete closure of the fetal fissure.

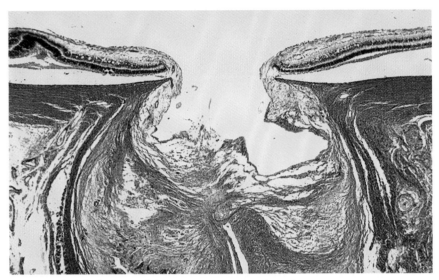

FIGURE 14–6 • **Optic nerve coloboma.** Hematoxylin-eosin, ×5.

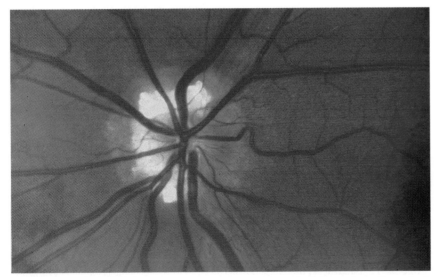

FIGURE 14–7 • **Optic disk drusen.** Anterior substance of the optic disk contains yellow spherical refractile bodies. Optic disk drusen may be misdiagnosed clinically as papilledema.

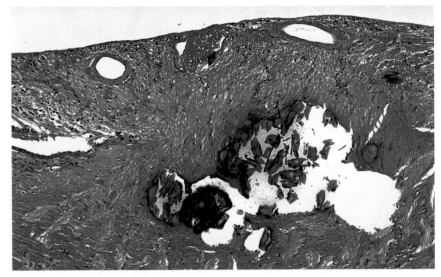

FIGURE 14–8 • **Optic disk drusen.** A conglomeration of calcareous deposits is present in the optic nerve anterior to the lamina cribrosa. The drusen have fractured during sectioning. They were unsuspected, and the specimen was not decalcified. Hematoxylin-eosin, ×25.

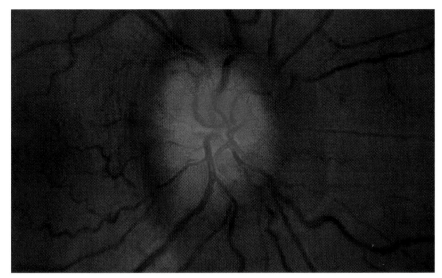

FIGURE 14–9 • **Optic disk edema.** The optic nerve is swollen and injected, and it has blurred margins. Concentric folds are seen in the adjacent retina.

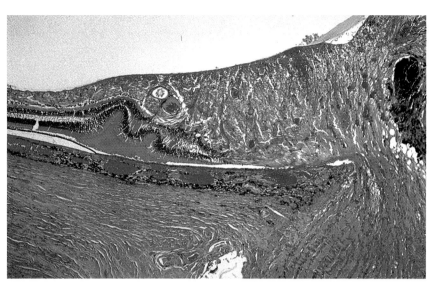

FIGURE 14–10 • **Optic disk edema, secondary to juxtapapillary melanoma.** The optic nerve head is compressed by an infiltrating juxtapapillary tumor, causing blockage of axoplasmic flow. The photoreceptors of the swollen optic nerve are displaced laterally and the peripapillary retina is detached by serous fluid. Folds are noted in the outer retina. Hematoxylin-eosin, ×25.

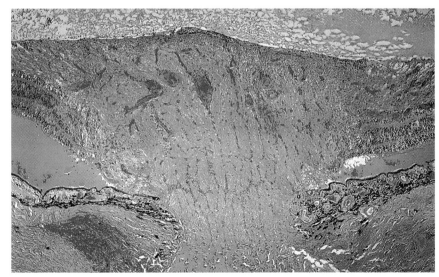

FIGURE 14–11 • **Optic disk edema, hypotony.** The optic disk is massively swollen. The photoreceptors are displaced laterally, and a shallow exudative retinal detachment is present. Severe hypotony caused by uveitis was the cause of the disk edema. Hematoxylin-eosin, ×25.

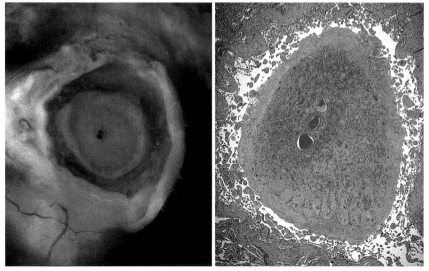

FIGURE 14–12 • **Optic atrophy.** The optic nerve is atrophic, and the subarachnoid space is widened. The severity of the optic atrophy makes the meninges appear redundant. Photomicrograph (*right*) shows marked thickening of pia and pial septa and atrophy of axons. Hematoxylin-eosin, ×10.

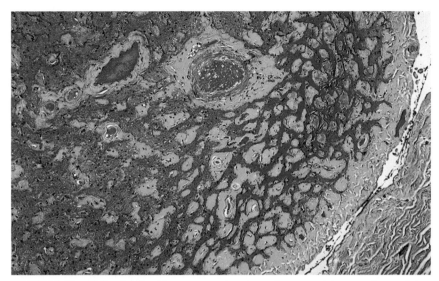

FIGURE 14–13 • **Optic atrophy.** Transverse section shows that most of the parenchyma of the severely atrophic optic nerve has been replaced by blue-staining collagenous connective tissue. The pia and pial septa are markedly widened. Masson trichrome, ×25.

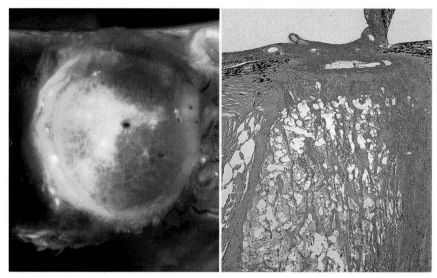

FIGURE 14–14 • **Schnabel's cavernous optic atrophy.** Diameter of transversely sectioned optic nerve is markedly widened. Small cystoid spaces replace myelinated parenchyma. Photomicrograph of longitudinally sectioned nerve (*right*) shows many pools of clear watery mucoid material behind the lamina cribrosa. Hematoxylin-eosin, ×10.

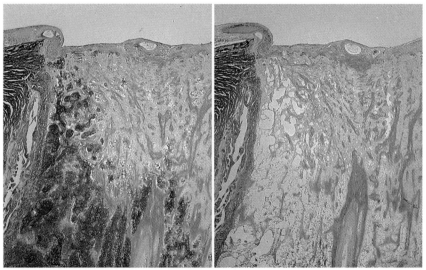

FIGURE 14–15 • **Schnabel's cavernous optic atrophy.** Clear spaces in retrolaminar optic nerve stain intensely for acid mucopolysaccharide (*left*). Positive staining is abolished by pretreatment with hyaluronidase, indicating that the substance is hyaluronic acid (*right*). Both figures: Hale's colloidal iron for AMP, ×10; *right:* after hyaluronidase digestion.

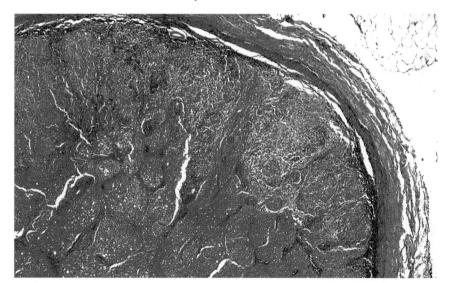

FIGURE 14–16 • **Sarcoid optic neuropathy.** The parenchyma of the nerve contains a prominent focus of chronic granulomatous inflammation comprised of pale-staining epithelioid histiocytes and lymphocytes. The inflammation is concentrated in the periphery of the nerve. Hematoxylin-eosin, ×25.

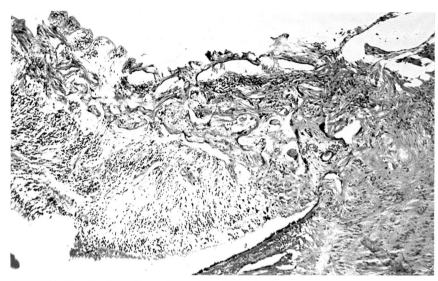

FIGURE 14–17 • **Combined hamartoma of the RPE and retina.** Strands of hyperplastic RPE infiltrate the thickened and disorganized peripapillary retina. A fibroglial membrane adheres to the inner surface of the retina. Hematoxylin-eosin, ×50.

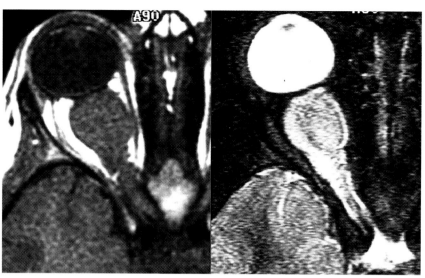

FIGURE 14–18 • **Optic nerve glioma.** Magnetic resonance scans show fusiform swelling of the optic nerve. Left: T1-weighted image; right: T2-weighted image.

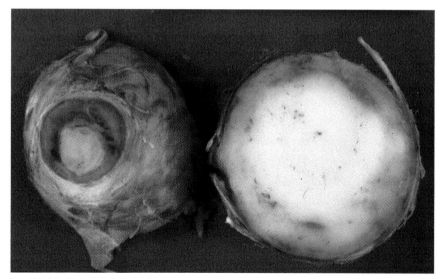

FIGURE 14–19 • **Optic nerve glioma.** Meninges of a markedly swollen nerve are intact. (Courtesy of Dr. Jerry Shields, Wills Eye Hospital).

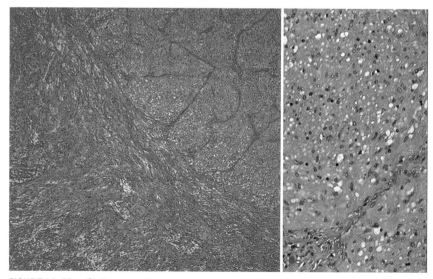

FIGURE 14–20 • **Optic nerve glioma.** Extensive arachnoidal gliomatosis is evident in peripheral part of tumor (at left). Proliferation of bland astrocytes is evident in intertrabecular space at right. Hematoxylin-eosin. Left ×10; right ×50.

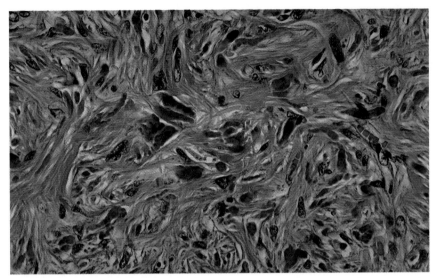

FIGURE 14–21 • **Optic nerve glioma.** Cells comprising a low-grade pilocytic astrocytoma of the optic nerve have slender cellular processes. Tumor contains many PAS-positive Rosenthal fibers. Periodic acid-Schiff, ×100.

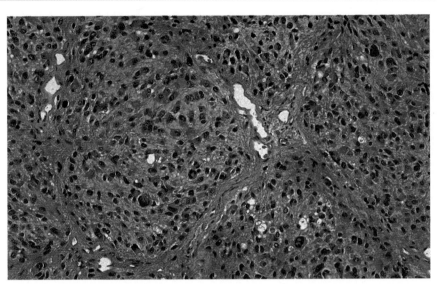

FIGURE 14–22 • **Malignant glioma, optic nerve.** Hypercellular tumor is composed of highly atypical glial cells with hyperchromatic pleomorphic nuclei. Hematoxylin-eosin, ×100.

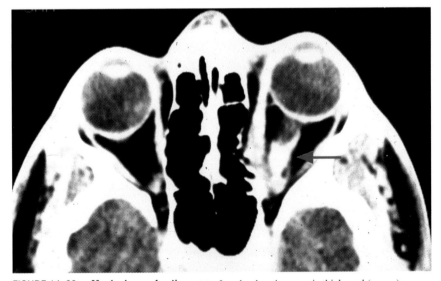

FIGURE 14–23 • **Meningioma of optic nerve.** Involved optic nerve is thickened (arrow).

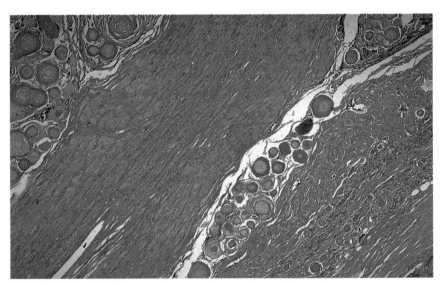

FIGURE 14–24 • **Optic nerve meningioma with psammoma bodies.** Many large psammoma bodies are present in the part of the tumor compressing the optic nerve. The patient had neurofibromatosis. Hematoxylin-eosin, ×10.

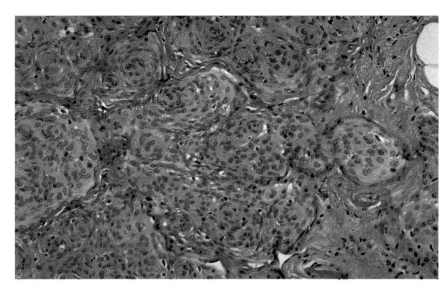

FIGURE 14–25 • **Meningothelial meningioma, optic nerve.** Whorls of bland meningothelial cells comprise this tumor. Psammoma bodies are not present. Most meningiomas cannot metastasize but are locally infiltrative. Orbital meningiomas arise primarily from the optic nerve sheath or invade the orbit secondarily from the intracranial meninges. Rare ectopic meningiomas derived from extradural meningothelial rests have been reported. Hematoxylin-eosin, ×100.

# CHAPTER 15

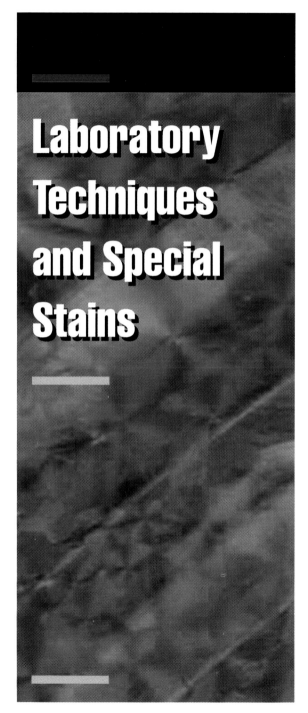

# Laboratory Techniques and Special Stains

This chapter discusses the basic principles of practical ocular histopathology and summarizes techniques used in the handling, gross dissection, and submission of enucleated eyes and other ocular specimens for routine histopathologic examination. Special histochemical and immunohistochemical stains also are discussed.

## FIXATION

Routinely, unopened enucleated eyes are fixed for at least 24 hours by total immersion in a relatively large volume (50–100 ml) of 10% neutral buffered formalin. The large volume of fixative is necessary because the solution must penetrate the sclera. Bouin's solution (bright yellow) should not be used because it hardens the sclera, making eyes difficult to section. Newer alcohol-based fixatives are also unsatisfactory because they precipitate protein in the vitreous and interfere with gross examination. Enucleated eyeballs should be briefly rinsed in running tap water to remove excess fixative prior to handling.

## SPECIMEN ORIENTATION

Determination of laterality (right or left eye) is a prerequisite for proper specimen orientation. The laterality of an eye is determined by identifying key anatomic landmarks. They include the long posterior ciliary vessels, which appear as blue lines on the posterior sclera on either side of the optic nerve in the horizontal plane; the cornea, whose horizontal diameter is usually 1 mm longer than its vertical diameter; and the insertions of the superior and inferior oblique muscles. The inferior

oblique muscle lacks a tendon; its fibers insert directly into the sclera in the inferotemporal quadrant. The nasal end of the muscular inferior oblique insertion lies close to the fovea. The shiny tendinous insertion of the superior oblique muscle is located superiorly and temporally and is an excellent landmark for the superior pole of the eye. After the horizontal meridian and the superior pole have been located, the nasal and temporal sides of the eye are readily identified. It is important to remember that both oblique muscles insert on the temporal side of the eye and their fibers run nasally. The temporal arc of the posterior sclera is 30 degrees longer than the nasal arc because the optic nerve enters the eye 15 degrees nasal to the posterior pole.

## MEASUREMENT

The oriented eye is measured using calipers or a millimeter ruler. Standard measurements include the anteroposterior, horizontal, and vertical diameters of the eye, the length of the optic nerve segment attached, the horizontal and vertical diameters of the cornea, and the size of the pupil (Fig. 15–1). Important pathologic features such as wounds, lacerations, and tumors should also be measured. Most normal human eyes are slightly less than 1 inch in diameter (24 mm), and the normal cornea is approximately 1 cm in diameter (11 × 10 mm).

It is easier to section an eye if the optic nerve is removed first. The nerve is sectioned 1–mm posterior to the sclera to avoid "button-holing" a deeply cupped nerve head. A transverse section of the optic nerve is always submitted if the nerve has not been cut flush with the globe. The surgical margin is marked with India ink or indelible colored pencil before the nerve is removed. The optic nerve segment is always removed before the globe is opened to preclude potential contamination of the surgical margin with intraocular tumor. This point is especially important if the eye contains retinoblastoma, which tends to invade the optic nerve. Surgeons occasionally submit the optic nerve in a separate container. In such specimens, blood-staining and crushing serve to identify the true surgical margin.

## INSPECTION AND DESCRIPTION

The general consistency and character of the eye are noted. Descriptive terms commonly used are normal, soft, collapsed, ruptured, lacerated, hard, and phthisical, among others. Before it is opened, the external surface of the eye is carefully and systematically examined with the dissecting microscope, starting anteriorly. The cornea is usually slightly hazy in fixed or postmortem specimens. The presence of corneal opacities, scars, vascularization, ulcers, band keratopathy, wounds, and incisions are described and measured when appropriate. The shape and size of the pupil, the color of the iris, and the presence and location of iridectomies and surgical iris colobomas are recorded. If the cornea is hazy, iris defects may be disclosed by transillumination.

The rest of the globe is carefully inspected looking for signs of surgical or nonsurgical trauma or extraocular tumor extension. The presence, type, location, and size of wounds, scars, vitrectomy ports, sutures, and prosthetic devices such as retinal implants, explants, and encircling bands and tube shunts should be precisely noted. The use of "clock hours" (e.g., "between 1 and 3 o'clock") is helpful when describing wounds and other important lesions. Drawing a diagram of the findings on the pathology protocol facilitates description and permits reconstruction of the gross description if the dictation is lost.

## TRANSILLUMINATION

Eyes are transilluminated before they are opened to disclose occult pathology that may not be evident on external examination. Transillumination is performed by holding the eye directly in front of a bright light in a darkened chamber. Transillumination is especially helpful during the orientation of eyes that contain intraocular tumors, particularly uveal malignant melanomas (Fig. 15–2). Pigmented melanomas usually cast a dark shadow on the sclera. When clinical data are absent, transillumination may disclose signs of previous surgery (e.g., an iridectomy) that are an indication for vertical sectioning. Eyes that are filled with blood or contain dense gelatinous exudate often transmit light poorly. Staphylomas and cyclodestructive procedures cause increased light transmission.

## DISSECTION

Microscopic sections are cut from a paraffin block that contains a short, cylindrical segment of the ocular tissue called the pupil-optic nerve, or P-O segment. The P-O segment includes most of the cornea, iris, and pupil anteriorly and the optic nerve posteriorly.

When tissue is submitted for histopathologic examination, care must be taken to ensure that the microscopic sections include important lesions such as tumors, lacerations, or incisions. The presence and location of the ocular pathology determines how the eye is opened. It is routine practice to open eyes horizontally if they do not contain wounds or other focal lesions. Horizontal P-O sections include the macula as well as the pupil and optic nerve.

Most eyes that have had prior surgery are opened vertically to include superior limbal surgical wounds in the microscopic sections. This category includes most eyes that have had cataract surgery or filtering

procedures for glaucoma. If an eye with a small superior cataract incision is opened horizontally, the microscopic sections do not include the wound and the pathologist cannot document its presence.

Traumatic lacerations and intraocular tumors can occur anywhere. Such eyes are opened along the meridian that includes the main part of the lesion. The localization of intraocular tumors by transillumination greatly aids sectioning.

## SECTIONING TECHNIQUE

We currently section eyes using one-half of a standard double-edged razor blade that has been snapped in half within its protective wrapper (Fig. 15–3). The two ends of the blade are held between the apposed surfaces of the thumb and forefinger, and a gentle sawing and pushing motion is used. During the initial cut the eye is steadied with the nondominant hand and held cornea side down on the cutting block. Guidelines drawn on the eye with colored pencil facilitate sectioning and ensure that the eye maintains proper orientation. The first cut is begun just external to the dural sheath of the optic nerve and should enter the periphery of the anterior chamber anteriorly. The two dome-shaped caps of tissue that are removed are called calottes (French for visorless cap). The initial calotte includes about one-fifth to one-fourth of the peripheral anterior chamber. The central P-O segment should be about 8–10 mm thick. The globe is placed cut surface down on the cutting board during removal of the second calotte. Eye protection (glasses, goggles, or face shield) is worn during the initial cut to protect against splashes of fixative, which can occur if the intraocular pressure is high.

Any material that flows from the eye during sectioning (blood, crystals, pigment-tinged fluid, silicone oil) is described. Gritty, hard, or even impenetrable intraocular material may be encountered. When this happens, possibilities include intraocular bone, a calcified cataractous lens, or the optic of a prosthetic intraocular lens. Intraocular bone is a common finding in phthisical eyes. Eyes that contain bone must be decalcified before they are submitted. In some instances decalcification is prerequisite for sectioning.

Every specimen is examined carefully and systematically with the dissecting microscope, and macrophotography is performed if indicated. Disturbing light reflexes are minimized by immersing the specimen in 60% "grossing" alcohol during gross examination and macrophotography. The calottes are retained in alcohol as "wet tissue" and may be retrieved if additional sections or studies are necessary.

## ROUTINE HISTOPATHOLOGY: DEHYDRATION, EMBEDDING, AND MICROTOMY

The P-O segment is embedded in a block of paraffin wax to facilitate cutting the microscopic sections. Because water and wax are not miscible, the aqueous fixative and water in the tissue must be removed before the specimen can be embedded, a process called dehydration. Tissue is dehydrated by passing it through increasing concentrations of ethanol until absolute ethanol is reached. The dehydrated tissue is then transferred to xylene, which is miscible with both absolute alcohol and paraffin, and then infiltrated with molten paraffin under vacuum. After infiltration, the specimen is placed in a plastic mold filled with molten paraffin. The paraffin is cooled and hardens into a block, which fits into the chuck of a rotary microtome. The support provided by the surrounding paraffin matrix allows the tissue to be sectioned thinly (6–8 $\mu$m). The thin slices of paraffin and tissue are then floated onto the surface of a heated waterbath, which causes the paraffin to expand. The tissue sections are then

mounted on glass slides, which are heated in an oven to promote tissue adherence.

## STAINING

Most human tissues are relatively transparent unless they contain endogenous pigment (Fig. 15–4). To facilitate examination, microscope slides are stained with dyes such as hematoxylin and eosin that color certain tissue components. Because aqueous solutions of these stains usually are used, the tissue sections must be deparaffinized and rehydrated before they can be stained. This is done by immersing the slides in successive baths of xylene, absolute alcohol, and then decreasing concentrations of alcohol and water. After staining, the tissue subsequently is dehydrated and coverslipped.

In most laboratories, routine histopathologic sections are stained with hematoxylin and eosin (H&E) (Fig. 15–5). Hematoxylin is a basic dye that binds to acidic materials including the DNA in the nuclei of cells (Fig. 15–6). Eosin (tetrabromofluorescein) is acidic and stains basic substances such as proteins pink (Fig. 15–7).

The H&E staining provides helpful diagnostic color cues. Lesions comprised of cells with scanty cytoplasm tend to look blue or basophilic during microscopy. Examples of basophilic lesions include inflammatory infiltrates, lymphoid tumors, retinoblastoma, and basal cell carcinoma. Necrosis, calcification, and DNA deposition in eyes with retinoblastoma also appear blue. In contrast, cells that have abundant cytoplasm (e.g., squamous cells or epithelioid histiocytes) appear pink. Squamous cell carcinomas usually are eosinophilic. Normal ocular structures comprised largely of connective tissue such as the cornea, sclera, and lens appear pink in H&E sections. Protein-rich subretinal fluid, amyloid, and exfoliation material are also eosinophilic.

The periodic acid-Schiff (PAS) stain is a routine stain in most ophthalmic pathology laboratories because it vividly highlights the thick basement membranes of the eye (lens capsule and Descemet's membrane). PAS stains materials that contain unsubstituted vicinal glycol groups (CHOH–CHOH). The vicinal glycol groups are oxidized to dialdehydes (CHO–CHO) by periodic acid, and the Schiff reagent (leucofuchsin) reacts with the dialdehydes, forming complexes that range in color from red to magenta. In addition to basement membranes and aggregates of basement membrane material such as guttae and cuticular drusen, PAS stains glycogen, some mucins (e.g., conjunctival goblet cells), and many but not all fungal hyphae.

## SPECIAL HISTOCHEMICAL STAINS

A variety of special histochemical stains occasionally are ordered in the ophthalmic pathology laboratory to demonstrate the presence of microorganisms and highlight special structures and materials in histologic sections. Special stains for microorganisms are ordered most often. They include modifications of the Gram stain for bacteria called the Brown and Hopps and the Brown and Brenn stains (Fig. 15–8), the Gomori methenamine silver (GMS) stain for fungi (Fig. 15–9), and several acid fast stains for mycobacteria (Fig. 15–10). The Dieterle and Warthin-Starry silver impregnation techniques for spirochetes, *Bartonella*, and *Legionella* occasionally are ordered (see Fig. 4–15). Fungi and yeast forms are impregnated with silver and appear black against a green counterstain in the GMS stain. The Ziehl-Neelson and Fite-Firaco acid fast stains are used to demonstrate the acid fast organisms that cause tuberculosis, leprosy, and nocardiosis. The organisms appear red ("red snappers") against a blue background.

Several histochemical stains are used to demonstrate the presence of metals in tissue. They include the

Perls' Prussian blue reaction for iron and the Von Kossa and alizarin red stains for calcium. The iron stain is used to demonstrate the deposition of iron in ocular epithelial structures in hemosiderosis and siderosis (see Fig. 3–20) and in corneal iron lines (see Fig. 5–36). The iron deposits are blue. The Von Kossa stain for calcium stains the anionic material that binds with calcium (see Fig. 6–5). This silver stain stains calcium deposits black. The alizarin red stain forms complexes with calcium, which appear red against a green counterstain. The ruthenium red stain and rhodanine stains for copper are relatively nonspecific and are used infrequently.

The Masson trichrome stain stains collagen blue and cells red; it is used to demonstrate the presence of fibrosis (see Figs. 8–23, 14–13). Masson trichrome is the histochemical stain of choice for granular corneal dystrophy (see Fig. 5–47). Stains for acid mucopolysaccharides (AMP) include alcian blue, Hale's colloid iron for AMP, and mucicarmine. The first two stain mucin blue because the histochemical reaction is based partially on the iron stain. AMP stains are used to demonstrate mucin production in tumors and for the assessment of corneal dystrophies. They are the stains of choice for macular corneal dystrophy (see Fig. 5–52). The Verhoeff-van Gieson stain for elastic tissue demonstrates the internal elastic lamina in arteries (e.g., temporal artery biopsies) and the excessive production of elastic components (elastotic degeneration) in pterygium and pinguecula (see Figs. 4–23, 5–29). In the latter, the elastotic degeneration stains black, and the reaction is not quenched by pretreatment with elastase. The reticulin stain is used for the assessment of certain neoplasms such as hemangiopericytoma and lymphomas (Fig. 13–20).

Although amyloid can be stained with the metachromatic stain crystal violet and the fluorescent stain thioflavine T, the congo red stain is generally used in clinical practice. The amyloid deposits stain light or-

ange and show apple green birefrigence during polarization microscopy (see Fig. 4–24). Congo red is the stain of choice for lattice corneal dystrophy (see Figs. 5–49, 9–14).

Other histochemical stains that occasionally are ordered include the Fontana-Masson stain for melanin, the luxol fast blue stain for myelin, the Bodian stain for axons, and the oil red O (ORO) stain for lipid (see Fig. 12–48). ORO must be used on frozen-sectioned tissue because fat dissolves during normal tissue processing.

## OTHER OCULAR SPECIMENS

Other tissue specimens processed by ophthalmic pathology laboratories are eyelid, conjunctival, and orbital biopsies, corneal buttons obtained at penetrating keratoplasty, ocular evisceration and orbital exenteration specimens, and intraocular biopsies including intraocular tumors that have been locally resected.

Unoriented biopsies of soft tissue with no obvious epithelial lining are measured and described. The description should include the color and consistency of the tissue and any distinguishing characteristics. Large specimens should be sectioned before submitting them.

Unoriented skin lesions and other specimens with an epithelium must be embedded on the side so the resultant sections include a cross section of the epithelium. Benign skin lesions (papillomas, cysts) usually are excised with a surrounding ellipse of skin. Large ellipses should be bisected and the two new cut surfaces marked with blue pencil as a guide for embedding. If a specimen has been oriented by the surgeon (using sutures or diagrams), the margins should be examined, which usually is done by submitting a number of designated tissue segments in separate cassettes.

Full-thickness eyelid resection usually is performed to remove malignant tumors such as basal cell or seba-

ceous carcinomas. Separate nasal and temporal margins are submitted to determine if the tumor has been totally excised (Fig. 15–11). The true surgical margin is marked with ink or colored pencil before the specimen is dissected. The central part of the resection (main specimen) is sectioned perpendicular to the lid margin in a bread-loaf fashion and totally submitted. The nasal and temporal margins of an eyelid resection are readily determined if the laterality (OD vs. OS) and location (upper or lower lid) of the specimen are known. The upper eyelid can be distinguished by the length of the tarsal plate and its roughly rectangular configuration. The lower lid is approximately triangular.

Many malignant tumors of the eyelid are excised with frozen section control of surgical margins. After the frozen sections are prepared, the marginal tissue samples are fixed in formaldehyde and submitted for permanent control sections. It is unnecessary to reexamine the margins of the main fixed tissue specimen because the true surgical margins have already been examined in frozen sections.

Corneal buttons obtained at penetrating keratoplasty usually are bisected before submission. The halves are wrapped in tissue to avoid specimen loss.

Conjunctival biopsies tend to roll or ball-up in fixative, making assessment of margins nearly impossible. Conjunctival biopsies should be gently spread stromal-side down on heavy paper or cardboard tags before they are immersed in fixative (Fig. 15–12). If this is done, the specimen is fixed as a flat sheet, which is much easier to manipulate and section. Thin slices of cucumber are also effective mounts for conjunctival specimens.

Ocular evisceration involves excision of the cornea and a rim of surrounding sclera and removal of the intraocular contents including uvea, retina, and vitreous. The scleral shell is left behind in the orbit. Although evisceration does not totally prevent the development of sympathetic uveitis, some oculoplastic surgeons prefer to eviscerate eyes because postoperative ocular motility is superior. The large corneoscleral button and the intraocular contents are bisected and entirely submitted.

Orbital exenteration involves removal of the eye and all of the orbital contents. Orbital exenteration usually is performed when the orbit contains an unresectable primary tumor or has been invaded by an eyelid or conjunctival malignancy. Exenteration specimens are large and multiple surgical margins must be submitted. Orientation must be maintained during dissection. Before dissection, the surgical margin (external aspect of the specimen) is marked by coating the specimen with India ink. Immersing the ink-coated specimen in Bouin's fixative binds the ink to the tissue.

Temporal artery biopsy is performed to rule out giant cell arteritis (see Fig. 8–18). To avoid skip lesions, an adequate biopsy should be at least 2 cm long. After fixation, the artery is divided into a series of transverse segments, which are embedded cut-surface down. It is much easier to interpret transverse sections. Arteries that are positive for giant cell arteritis may appear thickened and opacified on gross examination.

## FROZEN SECTION DIAGNOSIS

Frozen sections are prepared from fresh, unfixed tissue that is flash frozen in liquid nitrogen or refrigerated isopentane. The frozen tissue is sectioned with a refrigerated microtome called a cryostat and is stained with a rapid H&E technique. Sections usually are ready for interpretation within 10 minutes or less.

The most common indication for frozen section diagnosis in ophthalmic pathology is the intraoperative examination of surgical margins during excision of malignant eyelid tumors. In orbital surgery, frozen sections are used to determine if the tissue obtained is representative or adequate for diagnosis. The decision to exenterate an orbit should always be based on examination of the permanent sections.

Rapid diagnosis is the main advantage of frozen section diagnosis, but speed has its price. The technical quality of frozen sections is invariably inferior to that of routine sections prepared from paraffin-embedded tissue. The quality of frozen sections usually is sufficient to determine if a basal cell carcinoma or some other common eyelid tumor has been totally excised. In many instances, the final diagnosis of orbital lesions must be deferred to permanent sections. One should remember that frozen section diagnosis consumes valuable tissue that might be better utilized if it were fixed in formaldehyde and processed routinely for light microscopy.

## LYMPHOID TUMORS

Many ocular adnexal lymphoid tumors are low-grade malignant lymphomas. Immunophenotypic analysis frequently is necessary to determine if the cells comprising the infiltrate are monoclonal and therefore neoplastic or are polyclonal and reactive. Only a limited number of immunohistochemical stains for lymphoid markers can be performed on formaldehyde-fixed, paraffin embedded tissue (Fig. 15–13). They include the L26 stain for B cells and the UCHL stain for T lymphocytes. Stains for immunoglobulin light chains, necessary to determine if an infiltrate is monoclonal, usually are unsatisfactory. "Immuno" is optimally performed on fresh, unfixed tissue, using either frozen sections or flow cytometry. Both techniques require fresh, unfixed tissue, which should be expeditiously forwarded to the laboratory in a closed moist chamber to prevent drying. Many pathologists also prefer to fix part of a lymphoid tumor in a special mercury-containing fixative called B-5, which must be prepared fresh as required.

## SPECIAL TECHNIQUES

Immunohistochemistry is a relatively new powerful technique that uses antibodies to detect the presence of specific antigens in tissue. It is helpful from the diagnostic standpoint because the expression of certain antigens is limited to specific cell types. For example, a pathologist can be reasonably confident that a poorly differentiated orbital tumor is a metastatic carcinoma if its cells react with antibodies against epithelial cell markers such as cytokeratin and, in turn, are not immunoreactive with antibodies against antigens expressed by leukocytes or melanoma cells.

A wide variety of monoclonal antibodies directed against fairly specific cellular antigens (or epitopes) are commercially available for use in clinical diagnostic immunohistochemistry. Most of these antibodies work well in sections prepared from routinely processed paraffin-embedded tissue. Antibodies frequently used in ophthalmic pathology are discussed below.

Tissue sections for "immuno" are cut, placed on polylysine-coated "+" slides, which promote tissue adherence and are deparaffinized and hydrated. A battery of primary antibodies directed against a series of potential antigens are then applied and allowed to react with the tissue (Fig. 15–14). The choice of antibodies depends on the histopathologic differential diagnosis.

A second antibody of a different class (made in another species), directed against the first class of antibody, is then applied (Fig. 15–15). Binding of the second antibody occurs if the primary antibody has reacted with its complementary antigen. Although techniques and reagents vary, the second, or occasionally the third, antibody is labeled with an enzyme (usually peroxidase) that reacts with a substrate called a chromogen to produce a colored reaction product (Fig. 15–16). Usually brown, the reaction product is deposited in the tissue and serves as a permanent marker for the presence of the antigen. Appropriate negative and positive controls are mandatory to ensure that results are accurate and meaningful.

An important group of monoclonal antibodies are directed against cytoskeletal components called intermediate filaments, which are fibrous polypeptide molecules found in most eukaryotic cells. They are called intermediate filaments because their diameter (8–10 nm) is intermediate between that of actin microfilaments (4 nm) and microtubules. The intermediate filaments found in different classes of cells vary in their chemical composition and immunoreactivity. They are useful markers in diagnostic immunohistochemistry because they tend to be specific to cell type, and the relative specificity is retained after neoplastic transformation. Five distinct classes of intermediate filaments are recognized: (1) cytokeratins, which are found in epithelial cells and carcinomas; (2) vimentin in mesenchymal cells and sarcomas; (3) desmin in striated and smooth muscle cells (in association with vimentin); (4) glial filament protein, also called glial fibrillary acidic protein (GFAP) in glial cells and gliomas; and (5) neurofilaments in neurons and paraganglia cells.

Antibodies directed against leukocyte common antigen (LCA), melanoma specific antigen (HMB-45), S-100 protein, Leu-7, epithelial membrane antigen (EMA), factor VIII, and *Ulex* lectin are often used. LCA (CD45), which is expressed by most inflammatory and lymphoid cells, is used to determine whether a tumor is lymphocytic in nature. HMB45 is an excellent marker for malignant melanoma cells, but, its name notwithstanding, it is not totally specific. HMB45 is particularly helpful in the evaluation of amelanotic tumors that might be melanomas. S-100

protein is an important marker for neural lesions such as orbital schwannomas and neurofibromas, and it stains many melanomas. Leu-7, which binds to myelin proteins and to natural killer lymphocytes, is another excellent marker for neural tumors. EMA is derived from human milk globule membranes, which are found on the surfaces of many epithelial cells. When used in conjunction with antibodies against cytokeratins (the intermediate filaments found in the cytoplasm of epithelial cells), positive immunoreactivity for EMA can confirm that a tumor is a carcinoma. Anti-EMA antibodies stain the periphery of cells because the antigen is located within the cell membrane. Factor VIII, CD34, and the *Ulex* lectin are markers for vascular endothelial cells. *Ulex* lectin is a plant protein that binds nonimmunologically to the H substance of the ABO system.

A wide variety of antibodies that react against antigens on different types of lymphocytes are used in the evaluation of lymphoid infiltrates and neoplasms. Many of these antibodies/antigens have an alphanumeric designation that includes the prefix CD which stands for "cluster of differentiation." Immunohistochemistry is used to determine whether the lymphoid infiltrate is comprised largely of B lymphocytes (most ocular lymphomas contain more than 60% B cells) or T lymphocytes (reactive inflammatory infiltrates are comprised largely of T cells). Antibodies directed against immunoglobulin light chains (kappa or lambda) are used to determine if the infiltrate is monoclonal and therefore probably a neoplasm. If a lymphoid infiltrate is composed mainly of T cells that express both kappa and lambda light chains, the infiltrate is polyclonal, probably is reactive, and is not a malignant lymphoma. Although optimal results are still obtained if "immuno" is performed on fresh tissue (frozen sections or flow cytometry), several antibodies are available that can differentiate between B and T lymphocytes in paraffin embedded tissues.

Practical immunohistochemical analysis employs a battery of antibodies directed against potential tissue markers. Diagnosis is determined by the tumor's pattern of positive and negative immunoreactivity to the panel of antibodies. For example, both malignant melanoma and schwannoma usually express S-100 protein, but the melanoma should also be immunoreactive for HMB-45 and nonreactive for Leu-7. In contrast, the schwannoma should be Leu-7 positive and HMB-45 negative. Likewise, a spindle cell carcinoma should express cytokeratin but should be negative for other spindle cell tumor markers such as vimentin, desmin, HMB-45, Leu-7, S-100, and smooth muscle actin. Similarly, rhabdomyosarcoma and leiomyosarcoma both express the mesenchymal markers vimentin and the muscle marker desmin, the intermediate filament found in smooth and striated muscle. The leiomyosarcoma is distinguished by its positive staining for smooth muscle actin, which is expressed only in the smooth muscle tumor.

In ophthalmic pathology, immunohistochemistry is often used in the workup of a poorly differentiated neoplasm that might be metastatic carcinoma, metastatic melanoma, or a poorly differentiated lymphoma. Most orbital tumors in elderly patients are either lymphomas or metastatic carcinomas. In this clinical scenario, the antibody panel should include epithelial markers cytokeratin and EMA as well as LCA and HMB-45 to rule out lymphoma and melanoma, respectively.

If a tumor proves to be a cytokeratin-positive metastatic carcinoma and the patient is not known to have cancer, additional stains occasionally can help identify the primary tumor. Specific markers that can identify primary tumors include a marker for breast and other apocrine tumors called gross cystic disease protein; chromogranin, which is found in the granules of neuroendocrine carcinomas; thyroglobulin; prostate specific antigen; and carcinoembryonic antigen, a marker for gastrointestinal tumors. The character of the cytokeratin expressed by the cells also may be suggestive; for example, squamous cell carcinoma generally expresses high-molecular-weight basic cytokeratins.

Immunohistochemistry is used infrequently for diagnosing of intraocular tumors because it usually is possible to distinguish between primary uveal melanoma and metastatic carcinoma, which constitute most of the lesions, in routine sections. "Immuno" is used more often for assessing fine-needle aspiration biopsies, which often yield relatively few cells. "Immuno" occasionally is required to distinguish between malignant melanoma and leiomyoma and schwannoma of the uvea.

## OTHER DIAGNOSTIC TOOLS

*Transmission (TEM)* and *scanning (SEM) electron microscopy* serve as adjuncts to routine histology in diagnostic pathology laboratories, and are tools in ocular research. TEM is still used selectively for the diagnosis of tumors and unusual lesions, but it has been supplanted to some extent by immunohistochemistry, which is less expensive, faster, and less labor-intensive. SEM shows the three dimensional shape of objects at high magnification and resolution, and it can reveal patterns of disease that are not immediately obvious in sectioned material (see Fig. 8–37). A scanning electron microscope equipped with an x-ray analysis attachment can rapidly determine the elemental composition of materials such as foreign bodies.

*Flow cytometry* is primarily used in ophthalmic pathology for immunophenotypic analysis of adnexal lymphoid lesions. A suspension of unfixed cells is prepared and is reacted with antibodies directed against selected antigenic markers. Suspended in fluid, the cells flow rapidly through a thin tube past detectors that are able to detect and accurately quantify them. Flow cytometric analysis of lymphoid tumors requires fresh, unfixed tissue. Flow cytometry also can be used to measure the DNA content of tumor cells and assess the ploidy of neoplasms. It has not proved especially beneficial for evaluating ocular tumors.

*In situ hybridization* occasionally is used to detect the presence of organisms such as viruses in tissue sections. The technique employs nucleic acid probes whose sequences are complementary to the DNA of the organisms that are being sought. *In situ* hybridization is used to detect the presence of human papilloma virus in conjunctival tumors.

The *polymerase chain reaction* (PCR) is used to detect the presence of organisms by amplifying species-specific parts of their genetic material. The technique uses two single-stranded DNA primers that are complementary to segments of the target organism's DNA. DNA synthesis is catalyzed by a heat resistant form of DNA polymerase obtained from *Thermus aquaticus*, a bacterium isolated from a hot spring in Yellowstone National Park. Repeated cycles of thermal denaturation, annealing, and synthesis amplifies the sought-after segment of DNA a millionfold, producing quantities that are large enough to detect. Southern blot analysis is used to identify the DNA.

## OPHTHALMOLOGISTS AND THE PATHOLOGY LABORATORY

Effective and accurate communication is the most important element in the relationship between the practicing ophthalmologist and the pathology laboratory. Pathologists are consultants who require accurate clinical data to provide their clinical colleagues with optimum service. Few physicians would refer a patient to a consultant without a clinical summary or letter of introduction, yet specimens constantly arrive in pathology laboratories with few or no clinical data.

Ophthalmologists usually communicate with the pathology laboratory in writing, using the pathology slip or transmittal form. Information on the slip should include the age, sex, and race (if pertinent) of the patient, the laterality and location of the lesion, the operation performed, the clinical impression (preoperative diagnosis), the postoperative diagnosis if different, and any other appropriate clinical information. If the specimen is a globe, the visual acuity and intraocular pressure also should be listed. Many surgeons do not realize that satisfactory completion of pathology slips is a requirement of hospital and laboratory accrediting organizations such as the Joint Commission on Accreditation of Health Care Organizations (JCAHO) and the College of American Pathologists.

The patient's age and sex should always be listed. Age is an important factor in the interpretation of melanocytic lesions of the conjunctiva. Junctional nevi of the conjunctiva do occur rarely in children, but a "junctional nevus" in a middle-aged or elderly patient is almost always primary acquired melanosis, a precursor of conjunctival malignant melanoma. The sex of the patient is important when assessing metastatic disease. Breast carcinoma is the most common source of ocular metastases in women but is rare in men. The patient's race should be noted if it is pertinent and important from a clinical standpoint. For example, certain tumors such as uveal melanoma occur infrequently in patients of African ancestry, whereas sarcoidosis is common.

"Lesion" is not a particularly helpful or informative preoperative diagnosis. Always list the diagnosis if you are fairly certain what the "lesion" is, or at least indicate important entities that you would like to rule out. Your clinical impression is important because it may influence how your specimen is processed. For example, if the pathologist knows that you are concerned about sebaceous carcinoma, she or he usually reserves some "wet tissue" for possible fat stains, which may be necessary to confirm the diagnosis in poorly differentiated cases. Fat stains cannot be done if the entire specimen has been embedded in paraffin because the fat is dissolved by the solvents used for processing. Although routine tissue processing precludes staining for fat, fixation does not. Fresh, unfixed tissue is easier to cut, but frozen sections still can be prepared from formalin-fixed tissue.

Direct personal communication with the pathologist is advised if the case is unusual or important, you are concerned about the diagnosis, or you have questions about proper specimen handling. Call the pathologist if you have questions or concerns. Personal contact is the fastest, most efficient (and most confidential) means of conveying important clinical data. Furthermore, it decreases the likelihood that the specimen will be mishandled and may give the pathologist additional insight that can contribute to an accurate diagnosis. The pathologist is the best guide to laboratory services and may be able to suggest additional tests, techniques, or methods of tissue processing that can facilitate diagnosis. She or he can also inform you about special fixation or processing requirements (e.g., fresh tissue for flow cytometric analysis of lymphoid tumors).

Personal communication is always best if you think the specimen may need special stains or special procedures such as electron microscopy. Requesting that a certain stain be applied without discussing the case beforehand is tantamount to the pathologist instructing the surgeon what operation to perform and what instruments to use. The pathologist usually knows what stains and procedures are indicated (assuming that he or she is aware of the problem and has been supplied with adequate clinical data). You should also speak to the pathologist directly if you need photographs for presentation or publication. Photography is not done routinely, and its cost is not reimbursed. You are asking the pathologist to expend his or her time and resources to do you a favor.

If possible, you should personally hand-deliver important specimens to the laboratory. This ensures that the specimen arrives expeditiously and is not misplaced in the operating room or lost in transit. It also evidences your interest and concern.

Batching and submitting multiple specimens excised from different locations in a single container is dangerous. It occasionally is done by ophthalmologists who believe that they are excising multiple benign cysts or papillomas. If one of the lesions proves to be an unexpected malignancy (e.g., an incompletely excised basal cell carcinoma), its location is then unknown.

All ophthalmologists are encouraged to visit the pathology laboratory and microscopically review their cases with the pathologist. Always review the histopathology with the pathologist if your clinical impression and the pathologic diagnosis are discordant; it is well to question diagnoses also that are unexpected or make no sense. If you remain unsatisfied, request that the case be sent in consultation to an experienced ophthalmic pathologist. Finally, always forward rare or unusual ocular lesions to ophthalmic pathology laboratories that can appreciate their significance and that have the experience and expertise to process and evaluate them.

# References

Eagle RC Jr: Immunohistochemical diagnosis of intraocular lesions. Int Ophthalmol Clin 33:211–221, 1993.

Eagle RC Jr: Immunohistochemistry in ophthalmic pathology. In Laibson PR (ed) The Year Book of Ophthalmology, 1990. St. Louis: Mosby-Year Book, 1990:133–136.

Eagle RC Jr: Photographic tips for the ophthalmic pathology laboratory. In Wilson R (ed) The Year Book of Ophthalmology, 1997. St. Louis: Mosby, 1997:341–354.

Eagle RC Jr: Specimen handling in the ophthalmic pathology laboratory. Ophthalmol Clin North Am 8:1–15, 1995.

Karcioglu ZA (ed): Laboratory Diagnosis in Ophthalmology. New York: Macmillan, 1987.

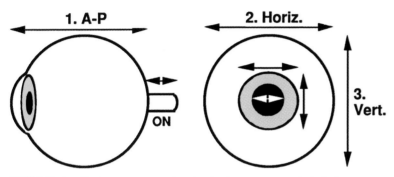

FIGURE 15–1 • **Ocular measurements.** Standard measurements include the anteroposterior, horizontal, and vertical diameters of the eye, the length of the optic nerve segment, the horizontal and vertical diameters of the cornea, and the size of the pupil.

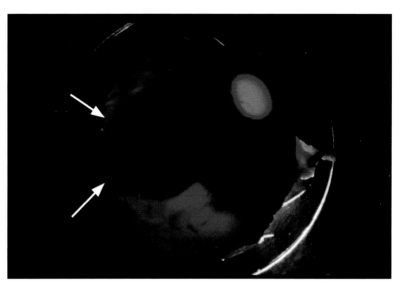

FIGURE 15–2 • **Transillumination.** Transillumination of eye containing a ciliochoroidal melanoma. Arrows point to a round shadow cast by the choroidal part of this pigmented tumor. The pupil glows brightly.

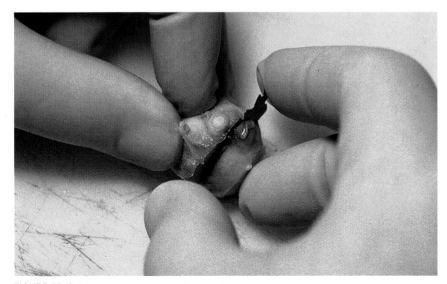

FIGURE 15–3 • Sectioning technique for the globe.

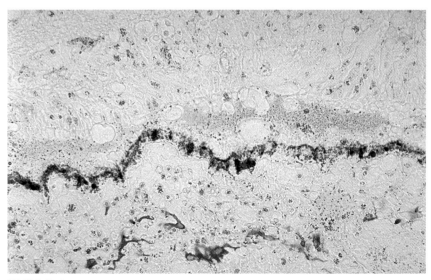

FIGURE 15–4 • Unstained section. Presence of endogenous pigment allows identification of RPE and choroidal melanocytes. Unstained section, ×100.

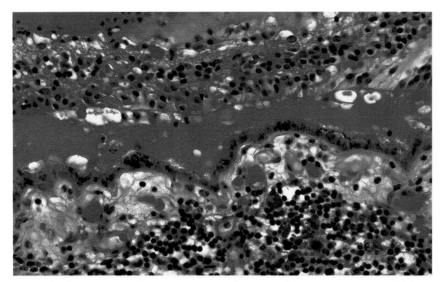

FIGURE 15–5 • H&E-stained section (same area as in Figure 15–4). A shallow retinal detachment and chronic nongranulomatous choroiditis are present. Hematoxylin- eosin, ×100.

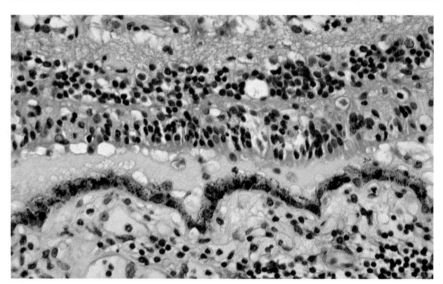

FIGURE 15–6 • Hematoxylin-stained section (same area as in Figure 15–4). Basic dye stains DNA in cellular nuclei, highlighting the retinal layers and choroidal inflammation. Hematoxylin, ×100.

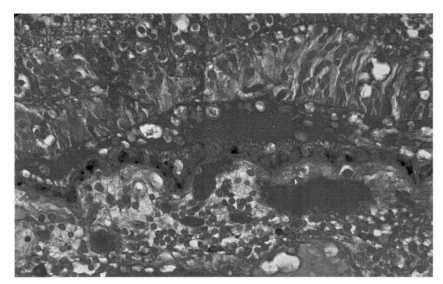

FIGURE 15–7 • Eosin-stained section (same area as in Figure 15–4). Acidic dye stains cytoplasm, erythrocytes in choroidal vessels, and protein. Eosin, ×100.

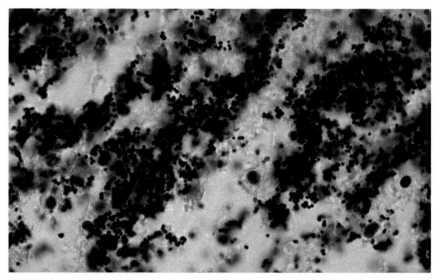

FIGURE 15–8 • Tissue Gram stain discloses myriad gram-positive cocci in exudate from eye with endophthalmitis. Brown and Hopps, ×250.

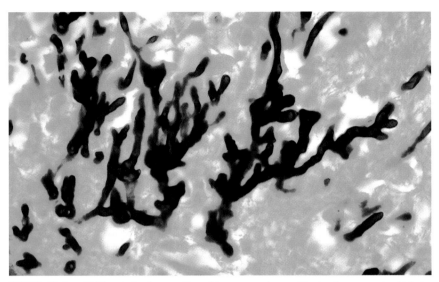

FIGURE 15–9 • GMS stain for fungus. Branching septate *Aspergillus* hyphae are stained black by silver impregnation. Gomori methenamine silver, ×250.

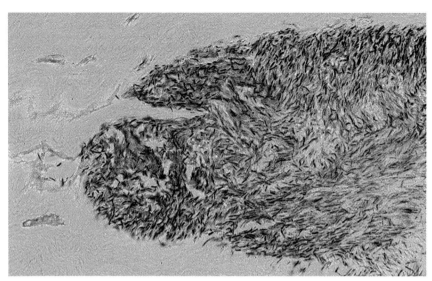

FIGURE 15–10 • Acid fast stain discloses a large colony of atypical mycobacteria in the stroma of an infected cornea. Ziehl-Neelson, ×250.

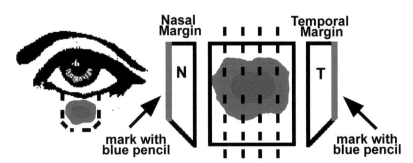

FIGURE 15–11 • Sectioning technique for full-thickness eyelid resection of a malignant tumor.

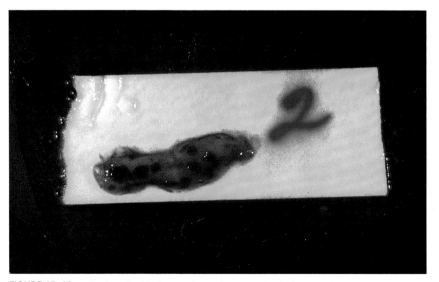

FIGURE 15–12 • Conjunctival lesions such as this nevus should be spread on cardboard prior to fixation to minimize distortion.

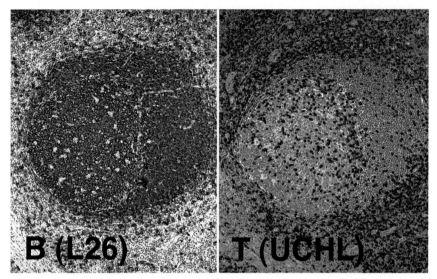

FIGURE 15–13 • Immunohistochemical stains for lymphocytes. L26 stain for B cells (*left*) and UCHL stain for T cells (*right*) work well on routine paraffin sections. B cells are localized to the follicular center and mantle zone in the tonsil. T cells predominate in interfollicular zones. Both figures: Peroxidase-Antiperoxidase (PAP), ×50.

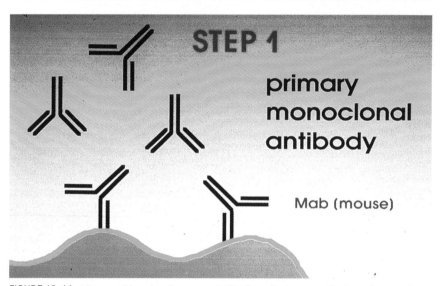

FIGURE 15–14 • Immunohistochemistry, step 1. Binding of primary antibody to tissue antigen.

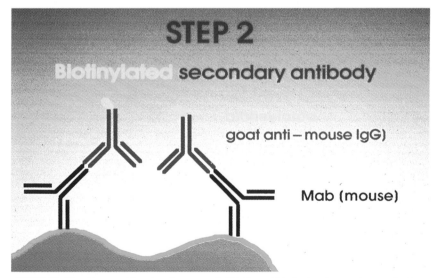

FIGURE 15–15 • Immunohistochemistry, step 2. Binding of biotinylated secondary antibody to primary antibody.

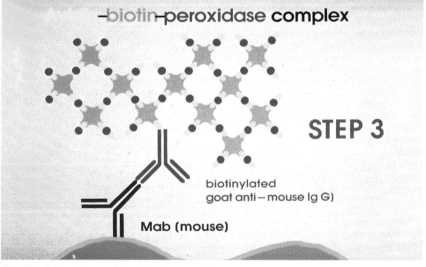

FIGURE 15–16 • Immunohistochemistry, step 3. Avidin–biotin–peroxidase complex and chromogen form a colored reaction product that permanently marks the site of antigen.

# INDEX

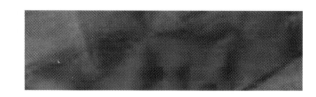

Note: Page numbers in *italics* indicate figures.

ISBN 0-7216-7809-2